Bryan McAskill's Book of Natural Remedies

Volume 1:
Simple, Approved
Self-Care Solutions
for Common
Health Conditions

BRYAN MCASKILL

ISBN: 979-8-218-46123-2

Forward:

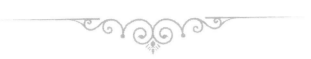

This book was almost entitled, "Bryan McAskill's LOST Book of Remedies" because…..I literally lost it. First, I misplaced my flash drive I had this book saved on. Then, I was editing and deleting some sections and accidentally clicked "select all" and hit the backspace button and automatically hit save as I do after writing and had to just sit there and think of what to do next. Fortunately, I had the majority of this book besides a few sections I worked on that week saved to another flash drive. And then, my phone broke that I had many notes saved on with remedies for various conditions. So, I took a break and focused on other things

This was all during a time where several of my peers and loved ones, we lost their presence in their physical form due to health issues, addictions, personal choices, or accidents. I spent much of my time in reflection to help process everything going on at this time. I was working on the development of a community garden and farm where I live which helped to re-connected and united all of us in the area. But I was very unmotivated in my personal pursuits. I allowed myself to detach from the responsibilities and obligations I placed upon myself such as writing and working on this book. This was challenging as I was growing many of the plants I would recommend for various conditions; but was not writing about them. Through much support and guidance, I was motivated enough to get back on track and continue working on this book. I am glad to add this text to the world as it is my belief that having a few steps to begin with on your own, we can speed up and further clarify the healing process of various conditions and get closer to reaching optimal health and longevity in the number of years that we live, and the quality of those years while we are here in this form.

I've remained sober while surrounded by drugs, alcohol, abuse, chemicals, and influence, while remaining focused living amongst the most distracting times in world history. My recommendations in this book support ways to keep this constant in your life as well to help promote both quality, and quantity in life. Quality in regard to standard of living without hindrances, illness, or disease, and quantity in the number of years in your lifespan.

As this book was being written and now being published, I am studying to receive a Ph.D. in Holistic Medicine and Healing Nutrition. Hopefully by Volume 2, I can achieve this prestigious honor. I hope to continue to add more to my *Book of Natural Remedies* series over the course of my lifespan in order to add more helpful information and resources until they become common knowledge, and we can identify warning signs and symptoms much earlier so these diseases and conditions that plaque our societies can be eradicated and become more foreign than common.

What I have learned is to let your own personal health and wellness journey speak for itself and serve as an example for what is most helpful and beneficial. No one likes being told what to do or that they are wrong about something. It is my hope that many can use this text to serve as a written document outlining some of the unknown barriers that continue to plague our health and be able to set a new starting point on how we can approach healing from specific conditions as needed.

Preface:

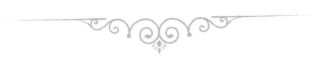

When we look at health, we often highlight the main features within an item or meal and then overlook everything else. We list out nutrients and minerals such as, "B-vitamins", calcium, magnesium, hydrogen, etc., while ignoring things such as how much saturated fat, or sodium is in an item. On a deeper level, we may consume something high in calcium, but the body cannot properly absorb minerals such as calcium without an adequate amount of magnesium so, if we are not getting enough of both of these minerals, we will not actually hold onto the amounts we believe we are consuming, and unknowingly become deficient in several categories. We must consume in abundance what we need, but not always in quantity. The phrase "less is more" accurately describes the process of gathering and absorbing nutrients and minerals. The items that are abundant in nutrients and minerals come from nature; not from an artificial substance, chemical, manufacturing warehouse, or from pharmaceuticals. Fresh fruit, vegetables, grains, nuts, seeds, and herbs contain what we need without containing many ingredients that essentially cancel out our absorption of many nutrients and minerals and reduce the quantity of what we consume.

I've always tried to share anything I've come across that can be helpful. If it's been helpful for me, then it can be helpful to others is a mindset I maintained through much of this process. However, it was not until the application of helping others, did I understand that this is not always the case. For example, eating mostly fruits have helped me achieve health I never could have imagined, but there are specific fruits (citrus) that can trigger severe symptoms for those with conditions such as herpes or gut issues. Doing a routine colon cleanse and consuming natural herbs for testosterone (because I'm a male) has helped me feel as though I've hit a "reset" button on my body and feel restored. A colon cleanse or increase in testosterone for those with cervical or prostate cancer can contribute to this condition spreading. I've had to look myself in the mirror more often during each step, in order to better connect the dots. This has come with much criticism and resistance from my peers and for those who follow me. My intention has never been to mislead anyone, but I admit recommendations I've made in the past have unknowingly made the path to greater health much longer than it could have been for clients I've worked with on their health goals and various conditions. Over time, I've come to see what keeps us all connected rather than what differences we individually subscribe to as the foundation of our healing.

What eventually inspired me to begin documenting information again was that it occurred to me that the only time people meet with a medical doctor regularly, is when there is a disease present. More often than not, people will receive an "antidote" in the form of a prescription and go back home. These antidotes are often what become the mask of a disease. We take in small amounts of things that do not absorb well into our bodies, and when it becomes too much, stress and tension within the body builds, and sets the foundation for sickness and disease. Avoiding unnecessary trips and scheduling to meet with a doctor can save a lot of unnecessary stress and concern, and also lessen the dependance upon those in the medical field. When dealing with many health conditions, we're recommended to meet with a physician; not a nutritionist, dietician, or a member of the holistic community. This is a major flaw in the medical system in regard to effectively treating conditions and health issues.

Another reason I was inspired to continue writing this book was, seeing all of the updates in technology. When I was a young child, I remember seeing huge computers taller than I am today and using a lot of hardware in order to properly utilize these machines. Today, we have apps on our personal phones that contain all of the software they had in hundreds of the machines I saw when I was younger. For us to make these strides in technology while everything has appeared to remain unchanged, I naturally began looking more into what else has relatively remained unchanged over the past few centuries, the human body.

We have learned more about how the human body functions through technological research and scientific research. Much of this is through trial and error in the form of studies and experiments using lab rats and other participants. Enough research has been completed where we can generally grasp how each organ and system in the body functions. It has debatable on what helps the most, but what has remained clear is what items harm the body the most. Without going into detail here, anything that does not provide many nutrients and minerals will inevitably harm the body. What also has remained consistent is that medical doctors do not seek to enforce strict protocols or educate around items the most detrimental to our health to help avoid these things. As more items are introduced that cause harm, standard protocols within the medical science field should change just like any other system. But they have not. They still uphold the same standard documented by practitioners thousands of years ago.

These systems being firm on their stance, should note consistent progress then, right? But here we are today, with disease being more common than anything else, and death due to preventable ailments being at an all-time high. It is safe to say that the medical industry is working with outdated technology, both, its hardware in the form of machinery they use, and its software with the tools they remain open to utilizing. Preventative treatment has become almost non-existent today outside of holistic practitioners.

How the medical system/industry operates today will only result in one of two scenarios:

1. The medical industry acknowledges that there are no medicine(s) that can properly make up for any nutritional deficiencies that we can achieve through what we consume, or…

2. The inevitable decline of the medical industry as we know it where there will first be a strong fight to remain dependent and reliant upon them for all aspects of our health through the use of forced vaccinations, introduction to newer drugs to mask conditions better, and altering the environment where being sick often is normal. Then they will eventually become reduced to researchers who report data and information compiled by doing research studies, to then be echoed by medical doctors and practitioners to their patients.

Whichever scenario presents itself first, our mission to is prepare proactively and preventatively by consuming that which heals the body, while working to nourish our cells throughout our lifespan.

The final, and most obvious reason I began documenting information in order to create this book, was the fact that I personally have not known anyone who has transitioned from "natural causes" as everyone has passed of some disease or attack. Being able to provide natural remedies to be applied to help reverse conditions and decrease the many preventable causes of death, became the driving force behind documenting and organizing information when working on this book. Our health is in our hands, and we must work to make the necessary changes to promote health and longevity. It is my hope to have those who purchase this book, to apply and share information put together in this text and add onto it to help themselves, their families, loved ones, and complete strangers, while providing the children access to everything written in this book so they grow up with this knowledge.

Healing Protocol(s)

I've had people ask for recommendations regarding with cancer, anemia, arthritis, and many more, who years later, after reversing their conditions naturally (without pharmaceuticals) notify me that they were consuming items detrimental to their health such as, candy, junk items, high-fat, and high-sugar, and items that are well-known carcinogens (cancer-causing) but **were still able to reverse their condition.**

Now, what does this mean?

Can we have "cheat" meals? Can we heal our bodies even if we don't abstain from items, we may have become accustomed to consuming? Does this mean I can reverse my condition without committing to changing my entire lifestyle?

Short Answer: Yes, but…

Longer Answer:

Yes, but… it is not encouraged. Anything we commit to we most likely will not meet its full expectations. Those who get married write vows and may not entirely stick to those throughout the course of their marriage and lifespan. But they use these as guidelines for helping them remain on track and headed in the correct direction. We must treat our diets/lifestyle the same way. Whatever we do the most, in addition to whatever we prioritize as a necessity will have a direct impact on the outcome we desire. Just because we do not stick to something 100% does not mean that all hope is lost. We must remain persistent, with urgency and clarity, while being specific on what we do regarding certain conditions.

A simple way to achieve this is to steer your focus on learning and understanding each of the systems in the body. Don't forget that although the human body is very complicated and complexed, there are only so many organs and system in which the body operates. Study these first, and then search what is impacting your condition the most. Then follow a standard protocol that I recommend in order to contribute to your progress and pursuit of optimum health and longevity. If you wish to learn more about each system in the body as well as herbal applications for each, make sure to purchase a copy of my book entitled, *Healing Herbs For The Human Body Systems: An Introduction to Human Physiology and Herbal Applications.*

Standard Healing Protocol:

My recommendations for will always go as followed when working to heal the body (disease or not) in addition to the guidelines to follow for each condition outlined in this text:

1. Fasting more regularly

2. Clean Lymphatic System (movement)

3. Removing all processed foods. Drastically reduce or remove all items that are difficult to digest while working to heal.

4. Colon cleanse

5. Load up on iron rich items to clean the blood

6. Maintain a cleaner, plant-based/plant-centered lifestyle and use herbs to support treating condition.

It is important to incorporate #1, #3, and #6 into your lifestyle year-round so that you only have a few steps to focus on. Others will need to make additional steps which can prolong the healing process and will take much more work.

#1 - Fasting More Regularly

Fasting is a specific time period where one abstains from consuming. You may avoid consuming certain foods or any food/drink altogether. There are various forms of fasting such as, intermittent fasting (choosing a designated time period where you do not eat, only drink water), liquid fasting (only liquids), dry fasting (not eating or drinking), and many others. Making this step is necessary to allow the body to gear its focus on accurately assessing what its needs are, even for a short time period. The body regulates many systems within when we provide it an opportunity to have an extended period of time to do this. Think of cleaning your home, but having an entire day (uninterrupted) to do this; you will get a lot more completed and get rid of more things that may be taking up space or are unnecessary.

Take it upon yourself to do this more often than not to help guide your healing journey specifically for you. For more in-depth information about fasting, which also includes specific plans to follow, and recipes, I encourage you to purchase my book entitled, *Fasting: A Guide To Health and Wellness.*

#2 – Cleaning Lymphatic System

The lymphatic system is a network of tissues and organs that help rid the body of toxins, waste, and other unwanted materials. The primary function of the lymphatic system is to transport lymph, a fluid containing infection-fighting white blood cells, throughout the body. Our body being mostly fluids, we must work to properly clean this system so that any accumulated waste materials will no longer be a part of it. These waste materials contribute to excess inflammation and instability with the inner workings of the body to continue proper flow. We help push along the waste materials held within the lymphatic system through repetitious movements such as jogging, walking, jump rope, yoga, or rebounding (bouncing in a small trampoline). Movement is medicine.

#3 - Removing All Processed Foods.

Regardless of your opinion of removing these items, they take several hours to digest prior to absorbing any minerals and benefits. The body does not need this extra work. It's important to address this step and be mindful of ways to make this adjustment whether it's a lifelong change or not. Processed and commercialized dairy products contain an excess number of hormones and chemicals which break down the body and processed foods do not provide anything nutritionally necessary in the body that can be absorbed while the body worked to filter the toxins in these items. Processed meats are carcinogens (cancer-causing) and are extremely high in sodium which contributes to many health issues outlined in this text. All junk foods essentially do not provide the body with anything useful after digestion, so it turns into waste. This excess waste simply gets in the way of the natural flow of each system in the body.

#4 - Colon cleanse

Again, reduce the additional work the body has to do. Medical Doctors will often prescribe Magnesium-Citrate to serve as a laxative. The problem with taking a laxative is that it does not properly clean the colon as it just pushes out waste already located within the digestive tract that would be discharged later on. You want to allow the body to properly clean the colon by clearing out waste sitting in the colon and intestines. The average person has about 15-20 pounds of waste sitting in their colon. Many will suggest eating more fiber, but you don't want to ever overcome during this time period. The colon also communicates with different areas of the body and works to gather nutrients we consume. When our colons are stuffed or backed-up, we may consume enough of what we need, but our bodies do not properly absorb it. This is why we must work to do a colon cleanse and then continue to keep it clean just like anything else. There are many suggestions and recommendations to follow in many sections of this text.

#5 - Load up on iron rich items

Iron is the mineral that helps transport nutrients in the body to wherever they need to go or are most needed. Keeping these passageways clear is best for absorbing nutrients, vitamins, and minerals, and helping the body identify what is waste and not needed. We must consume enough iron, but also not consume what robs us of iron which are processed foods and items difficult to digest as we send blood to the colon to help create mucus that pushes waste material through the digestive tract. Even if you consume 100% of everything that the body needs, if you do not consume enough iron regularly, these vitamins, nutrients, and minerals will not get to their destinations, and you will continue to show signs and symptoms of illness.

#6 - Maintain lifestyle and use herbs to treat condition.

This is where we can welcome in an abundance of creativity. Once your lifestyle is more consistent and has a stronger foundation, it can become more flexible (ex. think of a bamboo plant which is typically tall and thin, but its foundation is very strong. It can bend and flex, knowing it will return to center with ease).

This stage will encourage trying new recipes that follow guidelines you're already use to and working with ingredients you have not worked with much before. Different combinations of flavors and new habits begin to form such as your wake-up and sleep routines, and seeking out more opportunities to try new activities that benefit your health such as meditation, yoga, Pilates, hiking, pottery, arts and crafts, or whatever you wish to explore with a clearer view and a healthier, more adaptable and open mindset.

At this each stage in this generic protocol you can apply to each condition outlined in this text, I encourage you to apply the following phrase:

My path may not be predetermined but the objective(s) remain the same.

10 Daily Pronouncements

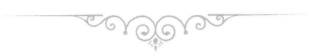

In addition to following standard protocol in the previous section, I would like to encourage you to follow ten daily pronouncements to help keep you on your healing journey. These are to be incorporated however you see fit, not in any order. But, they are to serve not as reminders, but as declarations for doing things intentionally and living mindfully.

(Execute these deliberately with intention daily)

1. Place of Solitude

Mandatory period for peace. Pitstop for the soul. Go to a space where you can mentally and physically calm the body and the mind. Create this space in your home, in your community, or in your mind. Tap in to shed anything not serving you well, promote positive thinking, and use a conduit for mental therapeutics. Meditation, prayer, and visualization are to be used in your place of solitude.

2. Commune With Nature

Time spent observing nature. Going for a walk, sitting home listening to rainstorm, watch animals crawl or fly by (or eat). Observe with intention to connect patterns that serve you well.

3. Ritual of Physicality

Exercise or other controlled, physical movement. Learn to defend oneself. Be peaceful, not harmless.

4. Live Nourishment

Consume only that which nourishes the body in abundance. Natural foods that can be consumed raw or cooked further. Fruits and vegetables are already cooked by the sun.

5. Acknowledge Abundant Knowledge

Lifelong learning is in everything. Seek out gaining knowledge in anything of interest. Keep your mind sharp and your time occupied.

6. Selective Reading(s)

Choose and decide wat you want to learn and gather resources. Help teach others what you have learn without misinforming. Hand select texts you have at your disposal to further understand. Read texts that guide you.

7. Personal Reflection

Only you live your life and hold your thoughts. Create moments where you can reflect upon parts of your personal journey. Before the closing of each day, process and analyze how your day went. Leave behind what's not needed, and retain what will help you tomorrow.

8. Vibrational Absorption

Listen in to the sounds of your environment. Sounds helps us feel what we cannot see. Crucial part to our awareness is sound. Create your own sounds through instrument(s) or listen to music for better balance. Absorb these vibrations to set order within the body and mind.

9. Spoken Word / Mantra

Boost your awareness and concentration. Create your own joyful feelings. Stimulate balance. Self-counsel by quieting the fluctuations of the mind. Chant your mantra to yourself to decrease negative thought and set your intention on instilling peace and tranquility.

10. Simplicity

Avoid complications. Reduce acquiring things you don't need. Keep decisions simple to create fewer steps in your journey; the fewer steps there are, the more effectiveness is welcomed into your lifestyle. Reduce the number of decisions daily to remain calm and promote more stillness. Less stimulation equals more concentration. More room for appreciation while there are fewer distractions. Keeping things simple increases your chances to reveal your personal uniqueness to the world around you and within you.

What Is Dis-ease In Our Bodies?

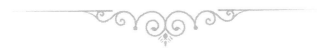

(from Healing Herbs For The Human Body Systems:
An Introduction to Human Physiology and Herbal Applications by Bryan McAskill)

We have been told that disease is the result of germ, virus, or bacteria. However, we have learned this from modern medicine science that has only existed for a few centuries. Disease at its core is a microbe generated from the body when erosion begins. Erosion begins when there is no oxygen and/or when there is mineral depletion. Being deprived of oxygen and minerals will create and promote these conditions. When the body is deprived of nutrients, excess mucus is created to serve as a buffer until the body and the cells get what they need. Foods and materials that are detrimental to our health create additional mucus and promote *cell proliferation* which is when cells become divided to create more cells in an effort to make up for the cells that have died. This often creates a condition referred to as "Abnormal Cell Growth" which is defined as the condition known as *Cancer*, or these cells are turn into tumors.

Along with excess mucus being in the body, this mucus will fill in the gaps that are deprived of oxygen.

If you lock a vegetable in a sealed oxygen-free box for a month it will begin to erode and become filed with maggots and parasites. Now, how did these insects get into this sealed box? Did they sneak in at night when no one was looking? Are they tiny magicians and can snap their fingers and appear in the box? No…. these insects came from WITHIN the vegetable as they deteriorate. Same things can be said for us humans and our bodies.

We have forgotten that our bodies contain all of the elements that we can identify and name within the universe. Therefore, our bodies, can create these very same diseases that we attempt to avoid.

ALL disease has its origin with being deprived of something. How does this happen? Well, how many foods do you eat that do not contain many of the necessary minerals your body needs? Wouldn't this be the start? And what keeps you alive? Isn't it the foods that you consume? So, if you do not consume the nutrients that you need, erosion will begin in the body. This will decrease the electricity at which your body operates which will cause deficiencies. The body will pull Calcium and Magnesium from the bones and create things like arthritis, or your bones will break although you don't notice any symptoms. The body will pull Iron form the blood and you will start to become anemic. The body will continue on this path until it cannot anymore, and disease will prevail.

This is the importance of consuming natural things in tune with the cosmic procession. Our bodies contain all of the elements in the universe, so we have a specific code/frequency at which our bodies operate. Eating low frequency/dead foods that provide little to no nourishment, and items filled with artificial chemicals, these will all contribute to breaking your body apart and your own self-destruction.

Wherever you are in the world, there will be various herbs that are more assessable to you than others. This book is not for the use of taking herbs to independently treat and/ or diagnose specific diseases and illnesses; although you should find yourself using herbs to help support a current condition or symptom(s). Herbs, medications, natural, or alternative treatments will not be effective if your diet is unhealthy. You cannot add something to a toxic environment and create peace; you will need the rest of the environment to conform to the principles established within what nature has provided.

What Does It Mean To be "Healthy"?

We have gotten away from what is natural, and this has in turn, confused, and complicated what it means to be "healthy". Many feel that a "well balanced diet" is best for optimum health and longevity, but what does a well-balanced diet consist of? Does this mean that you can just eat a little bit of everything, regardless of its' nutritional content? Our health is determined by our nutrition.

The Origin of the words we use is called Etymology. The Etymology of the word "Nutrition" stems from the 15th century Latin word "nutritionem" which meant "to nourish, suckle, or feed". The stem "nu-tri" in suffix form translates to "nau-tri" or "(s)nau" which means "to swim". Your nutrition must swim around and through the body without barrier. Consuming foods with chemicals, GMOs, and bacteria (factory made, processed) slows down your body's ability to absorb and identify necessary minerals and nutrients that it needs, which leads to overconsumption, or malnutrition (mineral depletion).

No matter which angles you look at it, all nutrients needed for the body are various compositions of minerals that are required for our bodies. A well-balanced diet, therefore, consists of minerals that we need in the correct proportions that will assimilate within our bodies.

We must accurately address our needs. Just like the body system(s) are not separate from one another, neither are our symptoms or their treatments. There would be no need to incorporate an herb that promotes muscle growth if you have bone and joint pain, since this would only add to your ailments. We need to incorporate herbs that are helpful for our primary ailments, but also those that support a healthier body. If your lifestyle is unhealthy, and you find relief for a primary issue within your respiratory system you have through using herbs, your body will then shift its' attention to a secondary issue within the body somewhere else. This cycle will continue until you eventually start back at your primary issue/ailment or develop a worse issue you could not properly address over time. This is why the lifestyle you live will create these conditions. Although many may be caught off guard or surprised, there are no victims when it comes to the body creating and developing an environment that promotes and attracts a disease or illness.

"The Healing Crisis"

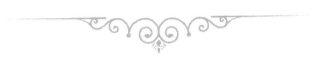

When you set your mind on healing, the body responds. Many will seek advice without first acknowledging that what they are currently doing and what they're consuming is the issue, and only reference individual items others have consumed as a barometer for what "works" or is "helpful". This is how information gets confusing, and we are often left wondering what the best option may be and leaving us overwhelmed at identifying our next step. This is what I refer to as "The Healing Crisis".

When you truly focus on your healing, you will feel difficulties and challenges, but you will know the difference. If you feel uneasy or sick, you will know the difference. If you are cleansing or detoxing, you will know the difference. You will know when something is not right and what your body is working through. Others who have been through this may not disclose to you or anyone else what was most challenging for them and/or if they tried to take any shortcuts or withdrew. Again, you will know the difference the more you work through these internal mental and physical challenges. You will notice things such as why others do not have cravings for certain items, what habits you want to change next, and will look at things more holistically where all things you do contribute to your overall goals and objectives.

Now, working on healing the body from an illness or disease, understand that this is not a game. You'll go through your own healing crisis while others do as they please. It will feel lonely and unfair. But remember that you are doing the work not many choose to do and redirect your journey through the trenches many avoid their entire life. The moment you decide to work on healing, everything you do will go under a microscope for your body and your mind to examine and respond to. This will increase stress and you may feel overwhelmed, but this is what remaining still and being discipline is for. It does not take much effort to find a store and buy something. Stillness and discipline are training yourself for what you do in the moment.

You may have consumed the same items and have maintained the same habits for many years now. The difference now, is setting the intention behind what you consume so that the body can respond differently than what you are used to in order to get everything back aligned. Once you begin, everything will shift, and you will become more like water where you adapt to ongoing changes with urgency and quickness. This is how wisdom enters your soul where your body will tell you what's needed, and you will be able to carry this throughout your journey.

There's no comfort in the growth zone and there's no growth in the comfort zone. These both represent sides of the "Healing Crisis" that makes its way into our lives in various forms so that we can transcend what is needed, at the time it is needed. You are not late, and you are not behind. Once you begin your journey, you're quite literally just beginning. Make sure to enter with enthusiasm and willingness to change so that you can get the most out of your personal pursuit for overall health and well-being.

Acknowledgments

Throughout writing this text I've had many peers and loved ones, as well as peers and loved ones of others who have passed on from health conditions that are outlined in this book. It was challenging writing certain sections of this text as many thoughts and memories of these people would pass by, but this also helped keep me motivated to continue to write knowing something in this book may help someone one day.

It is not my intention to provide a simple list of recommendations and believe it may have saved their lives, but to use this text to help share preventative changes to be aware of and adjustments we can all start with before engaging in full-time treatment of any kind. I did share recipes, remedies, and recommendations with many while writing this book. I did not hold or gatekeep any information I believe would be helpful to those in need in those moments. I am proud to have gathered more evidence of how useful and practical recommendations covered in this text can be after sharing certain sections or recommendations.

I would like to thank all of those who have encouraged me to continue working on this book as well as all of the professors, doctors, researchers, herbalists, scientists, and holistic lifestyle practitioners mentioned in this text who provided additional information to share. I am truly grateful to connect with and collaborate with so many generous individuals in their respective fields.

Herbal Dosages	
Dosage	(Varies from person to person. Best practice is to take lowest dosage and increase to recommended dosage).
Infants (to 3 years)	Consult a professional practitioner and/or Herbalist.
Children (3-10 years)	One-third of an adult dosage. (See adult dosage recommendations)
Children (11-16 years)	Half an adult dosage. (See adult dosage recommendations)
Adults	Tea: 2-3 cups per day (no more than 1tbsp per serving of herbs; dried or fresh) Decoctions: 2-3 cups per day Tinctures: 1 teaspoon 2-3 times per day
Seniors (65+)	Tea: 2-3 cups per day (no more than 1tbsp per serving of herbs; dried or fresh) Decoctions: 1-2 cups per day Tinctures: 1 teaspoon 2-3 times per day
How To Use:	
Fresh Herbs	• Internal and external use • Potency varies according to plant species and parts of plant being used
Freeze-Dried Herbs	• Internal and external use • Last longer than fresh or dried herbs
Prepared Products	• Internal and external use • Use according to label directions
Prepared Teas	• Internal use • Use according to package directions
Dried Herbs	• Internal and external use • Stay fresh for about one year. • Leaves should have some green, scent, and flavor when healthy
Tinctures	• Internal and external use • Plant extract in water, or alcohol solution; to help remain potent for several years. • Follow label instructions on bottle. • Can store for 12 months
Tinctures (Sample Recipe)	• 3oz of dried herb chopped finely, 16oz plant extract (or alcohol) • Combine and place in covered glass bottle. • Store in dark, shaking daily for two weeks minimum. • Strain and store in a dark labeled bottle. • Dosage: 10-30 drops 2-3 times a day (drops depend on what herb is used)

Decoction	• Internal and external use • Barks, Berries, Roots, Rhizomes, and Stems are boiled and steeped in water. • Dosage: 1 cup 3-4 times per day • Storage: 24 hours
Decoction (Sample Recipe)	• 1oz of fine chopped dried herb, 1 pint of spring water • Add Bark, Berries, Roots, and Stems if desired. • Simmer for 20 minutes, cool and then strain
Creams & Ointments	• External use only • Potent; use only as directed
Infusions	• Internal and external use • Leaves, Flowers, and Seeds are boiled and steeped in water. • Dosage: 1 cup 3-4 times per day • Storage: 24 hours
Infusion (Sample Recipe)	• 1oz of dried herb, 1 pint of boiling water • Steep for 10-15 minutes. • Strain
Compress	• External use only • Drench bandage with infusion or tincture, apply to affected area
Powders	• Internal and external use • Mix with sprig water, juice, or smoothie
Gargles/Mouthwash	• Use antiseptic herbs only
Baths	• Aromatic bath: add 1-2 pints of strained herbal infusion or add2 2-3 drops of essential oil to bath. • Hand Bath: place cool infusion in bowl and immerse hand in for 5-10 minutes. (This is particularly good for those with arthritis). • Foot Bath: pour infusion in hot water. Dip feet in for 10 minutes. • Body Wash: dip cloth into cool tepid infusion and bathe areas that is desired.
Plaster	• External use for irritated skin • Similar to a "poultice" (explained in next section) • Herb is placed between two bandages and applied to affected area. • Prevent herb from direct contact with skin
Poultice	• External use; use fresh, dried, or powdered herbs. • Place fresh herb on affected area; secure with bandage • Make infusion from dry herb and drench bandage or dressing. • Place dried herb on bandage and apply to affected area. • Mix paste from powdered herb and cold water. • Spread on bandage and apply to affected area
Essential Oils	• External use only • Concentrated oil is extracted from herbs. • Used for aromatherapy

Combinations To Avoid

There are a variety of suggestions and recommendations made throughout this book. Dietary adjustments regarding specific foods, herbs, and other items that may serve you well for particular conditions, but do not necessarily go well with one another. Please note that this is not a comprehensive list and is meant to be used as a precaution based upon what you may already incorporate into your lifestyle, and what you plan to incorporate as you work towards a healthier lifestyle.

If You Have…	And Take…	Avoid	Because
Allergies	Antihistamines such as: Diphenhydramine (Benadryl), hydroxyzine (Atarax), and astemizole (Hismanal)	Sedative herbs such as: Valerian, valerian root, skullcap, and passionflower.	They may increase the medication's sedative effects and lead to constant drowsiness, headaches, and fatigue.
Angina	Beta-blockers such as: Propranolol (Inderal)	The following herbs: Fumitory and Broom.	They will increase beta-blockers which will slow your heart rate significantly.
Anxiety	Hypnotic and mild sedative drugs such as: Flurazepam (Dalmane), diazepam (Valium), and alprazolam (Xanax). Triazolam (Halcion)	Yohimbe, cowslip, mistletoe, passionflower, skullcap, valerian. Grapefruit juice.	These increase the drug's effects and can become sedative. Boosts the absorption of these drugs into the bloodstream and can lead to overdose.

If You Have...	And Take...	Avoid	Because
Asthma	Theophylline (Theo-Dur) Ephedrine or Pseudo-ephedrine	Charcoal and Gua-rana St. John's Wort Ephedra Tannins found in: Black tea, green tea, and uva-ursi.	Increases drug's effects. Can lower blood levels of the drug. Intensifies the drug's effects. Interfere with the drug's absorption and interferes with blood flow.
Autoimmune condition or an inflammatory disease (tendonitis, allergies, or asthma)	Drugs that suppress the immune system such as: Corticosteroids like prednisone *=(Deltasone) Aspirin	Immune-boosting herbs such as: Astragalus, echinacea, reishi, and maitake. Ginkgo Biloba	They counteract one other's effects. Increases blood-thinning properties of these medications.
Congestive Heart Failure or Atrial Fibrillation	Digitalis medications such as: Xdigitoxin (Crystodigin) or digoxin (Lanoxin). Digoxin (Lanoxin)	Coltsfoot, motherwort, hawthorn, goldenseal, aloe, fumitory, licorice, lungwort, queen-anne's lace St. John's Wort Licorice	These impact the cardiovascular system and can create complications or increase the drug's effects. Lowers blood levels of the drug. Decreases potassium in the body leading to the risk of the drug's toxicity.
Constipation	Laxative drugs such as: Docusate (Colace), and polybophil (FiberCon)	Aloe, plantain, rhubarb, cascara sagrada, senna, and yellow dock.	Also have laxative effects than can lead to a leaky gut.
Cough	Codeine	Tannins such as: Black tea, green tea, red raspberry leaf, and uva-ursi.	These interfere with the drug and counteract one another.

If You Have...	And Take...	Avoid	Because
Depression	SSRI (selective reuptake inhibitor), antidepressants such as fluoxetine (Prozac), sertraline (Zoloft), or paroxetine (Paxil). MAO (monoamine oxidase) inhibitor depressants such as phenelzine (Nardil) or tranylcypromine (Parnate).	Sedative herbs such as: Passionflower, skullcap, and valerian. St. John's Wort Butcher's broom, gingko biloba, capsicum, and ginseng.	These increase the drug's effects. Can cause "serotonin syndrome" where a person is lethargic and confused. Can cause serious reactions.
Headache or Fatigue	Drugs containing caffeine such as: Excedrin No Doz, or Vivarin.	Creatine Asian ginseng, ephedra, guarana, yerba mate, and yohimbe.	Decreases effect of drugs and drugs offset ability to absorb creatine. These will trigger anxiety, insomnia, high blood pressure, and rapid heartbeat.
Heart attack, atrial fabulation, venous thrombosis, pulmonary embolism, or stroke	Anticoagulants such as warfarin (Coumadin)	Angelica, black haw, bromelain, buchu, cat's claw, chamomile, devil's claw, dong quai, feverfew, garlic, ginger, ginkgo biloba, ginseng, horse chestnut, irish moss, kelp, lungwort, papaya leaf, pau d'arco, red clover, and yarrow. St. John's Wort	These increase drug's effects and can lead to additional complication in the circulatory system. Can lower blood levels of the drug.
Heartburn or gastro-esophageal reflux disease (GERD)	The gastrointestinal stimulant known as "cisapride" (Propulsid)	Grapefruit juice Menthol-containing herbs such as peppermint and spearmint.	Can inhibit intestinal enzymes that can irritate the gastrointestinal tract. Can trigger worse symptoms of reflux.

If You Have...	And Take...	Avoid	Because
High Blood Pressure	Diuretics such as: Furosemide (Lasix), and indapamide (Lozol).	Buchu, cornsilk, dandelion, uva ursi, and yarrow. Cowslip, cucumber, dandelion, and horsetail. Cascara sagrada, aloe, black walnut, and senna.	These are also diuretics and can present worsening symptoms. Increase the drug's effects. These promote the depletion of potassium in the body.
High Blood Pressure (from congestive heart failure)	Calcium-blockers such as: Amlodipine (Norvasc), diltiazem (Cardizem), or nifedipine (Procardia) Felodipine (Plendil) ACE (angiotensin converting enzyme) inhibitors such as: Captopril (Capoten) or enalapril (Vasotec)	Grapefruit juice Black cohosh, cat's claw, dandelion, fumitory, goldenseal, irish moss, kelp, queen anne's lace, and yarrow. Arnica, blue cohosh, ephedra, licorice, garlic, and hawthorn. Grapefruit juice Ephedra, licorice, garlic, and hawthorn.	Boosts drug absorption into the bloodstream. These increase the drug's effects. These decrease the drug's effects and can disrupt the blood flow leading to either high blood pressure or low blood pressure. Boosts the absorption of this drug. Disrupts circulatory system.
High Cholesterol	Statins such as: Atorvastatin (Lipitor), simvastatin 9Zocor), or pravastatin 9Pravachol).	Grapefruit juice	Inhibits intestinal enzymes that creates toxicity when taking this drug.
Menopausal Symptoms	Ethinyl estrodiol (Estinyl), conjugated estrogens (Premarin), or estradiol (Estrace). Conjugated estrogens (Premarin).	Grapefruit juice Blue cohosh	Boosts absorption of drug Interferes with drug and increases the drug's effects.
Nicotine Addiction	Any drugs containing nicotine	Blue cohosh, tobacco	Increases drug's effects

If You Have...	And Take...	Avoid	Because
Pain	Aspirin	Angelica, black haw, bromelain, cat's claw, chamomile, fenugreek, feverfew, garlic, gingko, horse chestnut, kelp, lungwort, pau d'arco, red clover, wintergreen, and yarrow	These reduce the clotting tendency of the blood and can cause the blood to thin too much.

List of Drugs Derived from Plants

Common Drugs Derived from Plants		
Drug/Chemical	Action	Plant Source
Acetyldigoxin	Cardiotonic	Digitalis lanata (Grecian foxglove, woolly foxglove)
Adoniside	Cardiotonic	Adonis vernalis (pheasant's eye, red chamomile)
Aescin	Anti-inflammatory	Aesculus hippocastanum (horse chestnut)
Aesculetin	Antidysentery	Frazinus rhychophylla
Agrimophol	Anthelmintic	Agrimonia supatoria
Ajmalicine	Treatment for circulatory disorders	Rauvolfia sepentina
Allantoin	Vulnerary	Several plants
Allyl isothiocyanate	Rubefacient	Brassica nigra (black mustard)
Anabesine	Skeletal muscle relaxant	Anabasis sphylla
Andrographolide	Treatment for bacillary dysentery	Andrographis paniculate
Anisodamine	Anticholinergic	Anisodus tanguticus
Anisodine	Anticholinergic	Anisodus tanguticus
Arecoline	Anthelmintic	Areca catechu (betel nut palm)
Asiaticoside	Vulnerary	Centella asiatica (gotu cola)
Atropine	Anticholinergic	Atropa belladonna (deadly nightshade)

Common Drugs Derived from Plants		
Drug/Chemical	Action	Plant Source
Benzyl benzoate	Scabicide	Several plants
Berberine	Treatment for bacillary dysentery	Berberis vulgaris (common barberry)
Bergenin	Antitussive	Ardisia japonica (marlberry)
Betulinic acid	Anti-cancerous	Betula alba (common birch)
Borneol	Antipyretic, analgesic, anti-inflammatory	Several plants
Bromelain	Anti-inflammatory, proteolytic	Ananas comosus (pineapple)
Caffeine	CNS stimulant	Camellia sinensis (tea, also coffee, cocoa, and other plants)
Camphor	Rubefacient	Cinnamomum camphora (camphor tree)
Camptothecin	Anti-cancerous	Camptotheca acuminata
(+)-Catechin	Hemostatic	Potentilla fragarioides
Chymopapain	Proteolytic, mucolytic	Carica papaya (papaya)
Cissampeline	Skeletal muscle relaxant	Cissampelos pareira (velvet leaf)
Cocaine	Local anesthetic	Erythroxylum coca (coca plant)
Codeine	Analgesic, antitussive	Papaver somniferum (poppy)
Colchiceine amide	Antitumor agent	Colchicum autumnale (autumn crocus)
Colchicine	Antitumor, antigout	Colchicum autumnale (autumn crocus)
Convallotoxin	Cardiotonic	Convallaria majalis (lily-of-the-valley)
Curcumin	Choleretic	Curcuma longa (turmeric)
Cynarine	Choleretic	Cynara scolymus (artichoke)
Danthron	Laxative	Cassia species
Demecolcine	Antitumor agent	Colchicum autumnale (autumn crocus)
Deserpidine	Antihypertensive, tranquilizer	Rauvolfia canescens
Deslanoside	Cardiotonic	Digitalis lanata (Grecian foxglove, woolly foxglove)
L-Dopa	Anti-parkinsonism	Mucuna species (nescafe, cowage, velvetbean)

Common Drugs Derived from Plants		
Drug/Chemical	Action	Plant Source
Digitalin	Cardiotonic	Digitalis purpurea (purple foxglove)
Digitoxin	Cardiotonic	Digitalis purpurea (purple foxglove)
Digoxin	Cardiotonic	Digitalis purpurea (purple or common foxglove)
Emetine	Amebicide, emetic	Cephaelis ipecacuanha
Ephedrine	Sympathomimetic, antihistamine	Ephedra sinica (ephedra, ma huang)
Etoposide	Antitumor agent	Podophyllum peltatum (mayapple)
Galanthamine	Cholinesterase inhibitor	Lycoris squamigera (magic lily, resurrection lily, naked lady)
Gitalin	Cardiotonic	Digitalis purpurea (purple or common foxglove)
Glaucarubin	Amoebicide	Simarouba glauca (paradise tree)
Glaucine	Antitussive	Glaucium flavum (yellow hornpoppy, horned poppy, sea poppy)
Glasiovine	Antidepressant	Octea glaziovii
Glycyrrhizin	Sweetener, treatment for Addison's disease	Glycyrrhiza glabra (licorice)
Gossypol	Male contraceptive	Gossypium species (cotton)
Hemsleyadin	Treatment for bacillary dysentery	Hemsleya amabilis
Hesperidin	Treatment for capillary fragility	Citrus species (e.g., oranges)
Hydrastine	Hemostatic, astringent	Hydrastis canadensis (goldenseal)
Hyoscyamine	Anticholinergic	Hyoscyamus niger (black henbane, stinking nightshade, henpin)
Irinotecan	Anticancer, antitumor agent	Camptotheca acuminata
Kaibic acud	Acaricide	Digenea simplex (wireweed)
Kawain	Tranquilizer	Piper methysticum (kava kava)
Kheltin	Bronchodilator	Ammi visaga

Common Drugs Derived from Plants		
Drug/Chemical	Action	Plant Source
Lanatosides A, B, C	Cardiotonic	Digitalis lanata (Grecian foxglove, woolly foxglove)
Lapachol	Anticancer, antitumor	Tabebuia species (trumpet tree)
a-Lobeline	Smoking deterrent, respiratory stimulant	Lobelia inflata (Indian tobacco)
Menthol	Rubefacient	Mentha species (mint)
Methyl salicylate	Rubefacient	Gaultheria procumbens (wintergreen)
Monocrotaline	Topical antitumor agent	Crotalaria sessiliflora
Morphine	Analgesic	Papaver somniferum (poppy)
Neo-andrographolide	Treatment of dysentery	Andrographis paniculate
Nicotine	Insecticide	Nicotiana tabacum (tobacco)
Nordihydroguaiaretic acid	Antioxidant	Larrea divaricata (creosote bush)
Noscapine	Antitussive	Papaver somniferum (poppy)
Ouabain	Cardiotonic	Strophanthus gratus (ouabain tree)
Pachycarpine	Oxytocic	Sophora pschycarpa
Palmatine	Antipyretic, detoxicant	Coptis japonica (Chinese golden thread, goldthread, Huang-Lia)
Papain	Proteolytic, mucolytic	Carica papaya (papaya)
Papaverine	Smooth muscle relaxant	Papaver somniferum (opium poppy, common poppy)
Phyllodulcin	Sweetener	Hydrangea macrophylla (bigleaf hydrangea, French hydrangea)
Physostigmine	Cholinesterase inhibitor	Physostigma venenosum (Calabar bean)
Picrotoxin	Analeptic	Anamirta cocculus (fish berry)
Pilocarpine	Parasympathomimetic	Pilocarpus jaborandi (jaborandi, Indian hemp)
Pinitol	Expectorant	Several plants (e.g., bougainvillea)
Podophyllotoxin	Antitumor, anticancer agent	Podophyllum peltatum (mayapple)

Common Drugs Derived from Plants		
Drug/Chemical	Action	Plant Source
Protoveratrines A, B	Antihypertensives	Veratrum album (white false hellebore)
Pseudoephredrine	Sympathomimetic	Ephedra sinica (ephedra, ma huang)
nor-pseudoephedrine	Sympathomimetic	Ephedra sinica (ephedra, ma huang)
Quinidine	Antiarrhythmic	Cinchona ledgeriana (quinine tree)
Quinine	Antimalarial, antipyretic	Cinchona ledgeriana (quinine tree)
Quisqualic acid	Anthelmintic	Quisqualis indica (Rangoon creeper, drunken sailor)
Rescinnamine	Antihypertensive, tranquilizer	Rauvolfia serpentina
Reserpine	Antihypertensive, tranquilizer	Rauvolfia serpentina
Rhomitoxin	Antihypertensive, tranquilizer	Rhododendron molle (rhodo-dendron)
Rorifone	Antitussive	Rorippa indica
Rotenone	Piscicide, Insecticide	Lonchocarpus nicou
Rotundine	Analgesic, sedative, tranquil-izer	Stephania sinica
Rutin	Treatment for capillary fragility	Citrus species (e.g., orange, grapefruit)
Salicin	Analgesic	Salix alba (white willow)
Sanguinarine	Dental plaque inhibitor	Sanguinaria canadensis (bloodroot)
Santonin	Acaricide	Artemisia maritma (worm-wood)
Scillaren A	Cardiotonic	Urginea maritima (squill)
Scopolamine	Sedative	Datura species (e.g., Jimson-weed)
Sennosides A, B	Laxative	Cassia species (cinnamon)
Silymarin	Antihepatotoxic	Silybum marianum (milk thistle)
Sparteine	Oxytocic	Cytisus scoparius (scotch broom)
Stevioside	Sweetener	Stevia rebaudiana (stevia)
Strychnine	CNS stimulant	Strychnos nux-vomica (poi-son nut tree)

Common Drugs Derived from Plants		
Drug/Chemical	Action	Plant Source
Taxol	Antitumor agent	Taxus brevifolia (Pacific yew)
Teniposide	Antitumor agent	Podophyllum peltatum (may-apple or mandrake)
Tetrahydrocannabinol (THC)	Antiemetic, decreases ocular tension	Cannabis sativa (marijuana)
Tetrahydropalmatine	Analgesic, sedative, tranquilizer	Corydalis ambigua
Tetrandrine	Antihypertensive	Stephania tetrandra
Theobromine	Diuretic, vasodilator	Theobroma cacao (cocoa)
Theophylline	Diuretic, bronchodilator	Theobroma cacao and others (cocoa, tea)
Thymol	Topical antifungal	Thymus vulgaris (thyme)
Topotecan	Antitumor, anticancer agent	Camptotheca acuminata
Trichosanthin	Abortifacient	Trichosanthes kirilowii (snake gourd)
Tubocurarine	Skeletal muscle relaxant	Chondodendron tomentosum (curare vine)
Valepotriates	Sedative	Valeriana officinalis (valerian)
Vasicine	Cerebral stimulant	Vinca minor (periwinkle)
Vinblastine	Antitumor, Antileukemic agent	Catharanthus roseus (Madagascar periwinkle)
Vincristine	Antitumor, Antileukemic agent	Catharanthus roseus (Madagascar periwinkle)
Yohimbine	Aphrodisiac	Pausinystalia yohimbe (yohimbe)
Yuanhuacine	Abortifacient	Daphne genkwa (lilac)

*** *(From: Taylor, Leslie. Plant-Based Drugs and Medicines. Square One Publishers, 2000, Garden City Park, N.Y.)*

Table of Contents

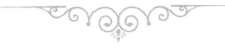

Acne

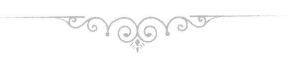

If you were to ask your doctor if poor digestion was the cause for your acne, they would say "No". This is why Dermatologists only provide assistance with covering up the issues, which may help on a small scale by protecting the body from absorbing everything by adding a layer on top of it, but this does not present a direct treatment, and is why Dermatologists won't provide a more direct treatment that can be adopted by all. "Acne has generated an entire industry of high-priced dermatologists and an incredible laundry list of very potent and expensive medications, including topical and oral antibiotics" – Dr. Andre Rubman (N.D., naturopathic physician and founder of the Southbury Clinic for Traditional Medicine in Connecticut (USA).

We are not deficient in any form or medications, lotions, or creams. These items simply work to provide what minerals we may often become deficient in due to diet. Clearing up the diet is essential for providing a cure. This begins in the digestive system.

The Gastrointestinal (GI) Tract is the body's primary organ for elimination. When the GI Tract is loaded with excessive toxins (biochemical toxins generated by saturated fats in animal products, hydrogenated fats generated in processed foods, refined sugars, coffee, and alcoholic beverages), the body looks for an additional location to store these toxins. The additional location that is often chosen (if not the liver, kidneys, or the blood) is within what are known as the "sebaceous glands" which are oil-secreting glands in the skin that generate pimples when they are filled with waste.

When the GI Tract is filled often with anti-inflammatory foods and fatty acids (nuts, seeds, most fruits), the skin can use these to break down waste internally and result in clearer skin. Most topical creams will contain fatty acids, but the issue comes from the many other chemical that are present within these lotions, creams and supplements which can contribute to acne issues long term.

Remedies:

Fatty Acids

Fatty acids (omega-3, omega-6, and omega-9) are a form of *polysaturated fat* which work to help provide the body (particularly the skin) build healthy cell membranes. These help maintain the skin's barrier which assist with maintaining hydration and absorbing nutrients, and results in keeping the skin healthy and appearing younger.

Common Sources of Fatty Acids: Brazil Nuts, Walnuts, Kola Nuts, Avocados, Bananas, Sea Vegetables (Nori, Wakame, Hijiki, Sea Moss, Bladderwrack), Coconut, Coconut Oil, Olive Oil, Grapeseed Oil, Avocado Oil, Mushrooms, Quinoa, Wild Rice.

Antioxidants

Antioxidants can help stop the formation of free radicals. Free radicles are unstable molecules that cause oxidative damage ("internal rust" or "ash") within the cells. When this damage occurs in the skin cells, this can prolong the effects of acne as the skin (and cells) will take longer to heal and can cause lasting damage that causes a person to become more susceptible of having acne due to weaker cells in the area.

Common Sources of Antioxidants: berries, leafy green vegetables, natural spring water, okra, cherries, dates, raisins.

Zinc

The body uses the mineral Zinc to breakdown bacteria in the body and helps strengthen the immune system. When we do not properly breakdown bacteria that is accumulated when acne is present, acne will remain and continue to reappear over time.

Common Sources of Zinc: chickpeas, mushrooms, zucchini, squash, okra, Brazil nuts, and walnuts.

*Zinc: 15 milligrams a day within diet is recommended.

Iron

Note: women are often most susceptible to having acne 2-3 days before their periods. Being proactive during this time period is essential for best results.

Keeping the blood clean of toxins is necessary for clearer skin. Anything you put onto your skin goes into the bloodstream. Anything you consume that contains toxins, will also enter the bloodstream to be filtered out. Keep the blood's iron content full helps increase the body's alertness for removing toxins.

Common Sources of Iron: quinoa, wild rice (not black rice), chickpeas/garbanzo beans, kale, nuts (particularly walnuts), hemp seeds, dates, dried apricots, watercress

Iron Rich Herbs: sarsaparilla, burdock (and root), guaco, chainey root, monkey ladder, chickweed, yellowdock

Tea Tree Oil

Many studies, including a recent one published in the *Australian Journal of Dermatology*, suggest that using tea tree oil on mild or moderate acne can be highly effective. You can mix several drops of tea tree oil into your usual face products or apply a few drops directly to a blemish as a spot treatment. Follow instructions on label for specific dosage.

Cut Out The Processed Sugar and Oils

The sugars and oils in processed foods, "junk items" such as, cakes, cookies, pizza, processed animal meats, and items cooked in grease flood the bloodstream with carcinogens (cancer-causing substances). These oils are removed via our sweat glands, but do not offer the same protection as things like fatty acids, so they begin to corrode and create skin issues. When we do not eat for a bit of time and then fill our stomach with candy, soda, or any processed sugar, your pancreatic enzymes jump in to take care of the increased sugar intake. Then your insulin overshoots and you go into "reactive hypoglycemia" (low blood sugar – even through you just consumed sugar). Your adrenal glands bring adrenaline in to help mobilize the stores of glycogen sugar in your liver to combat the low blood sugar levels. This adrenaline rush stimulates a sudden increase in heart rate (tachycardia).

This is why we want to plan regular meals and avoid consuming any processed sugars. The hypothalamus part of the brain relaxes when it knows what to expect. This process disrupts the blood flow within the body where the body is not able to effectively clean beneath the skin properly to clear out toxins and bacteria. Keep a regular dietary regimen to help the hypothalamus relax and don't send it mixed signals by consuming processed sugars, especially on an empty stomach.

Remove The Dairy

Dairy contains many carcinogens and mucus-forming materials that attempt to make their way out of the body through the skin, creating acne and poor skin health. The majority of the time, dairy is accompanied in items that contain processed sugars or oils. From candy to pizza, these substances are together and remain detrimental to our health. They create hormonal imbalances which sends excess hormones into the bloodstream and accumulates bacteria in the body. These substances must be removed in order to reduce their impact on the body. Dairy presents an additional obstacle due to the fact that dairy makes it more difficult for the body to absorb Iron, especially for women. Women are often encouraged to consume dairy due to hormonal imbalances, or a person may crave these items during menstruation. You want to avoid that which blocks you from absorbing anything that is necessary to the body. Dairy is not helpful.

Look for hidden ingredients in items you consume that may contain dairy in them and find replacements.

Colon Cleanse

Acne is one of the first noticeable signs of constipation. Clean the digestive tract by starting with the colon.

(Follow this regimen for 30 days minimum)

1.   Herbal Colon Cleanse (Cascara sagrada, Rhubarb Root, Prodijiosa, and Black Walnut Hull). Mix about 1 tablespoon of each herb together, boil water and place ½ tablespoon of mixed herbs into 8oz cup of water. Strain our herbs and drink twice a day.

2.   Elderberry, Sea Moss, Bladderwrack, and Ginger Tea at least 3 times a week

3.   Iron-rich Herbs Daily (Sarsaparilla, Guaco, Burdock Root – in capsule or tea form)

4.   Other herb to add to diet: Holy Basil, Quassia, Mullein, and Vervain

Apple, Onion, Colon Cleanse Recipe

1 Apple

1 Large Onion

1 Handful of Pectin (The white part of the citrus. When you peel an orange or lime, that white part you see)

Direction: Blend together with water.

Dosage: Eat about 3 to 4 oz in the morning.

Tamarind Juice ("agua de tamarindo ")

(from 21 Day Liquid Fast, by Bryan McAskill)

• 15 dried tamarind pods

• 2 quarts water, divided

• 1/2 – 3/4 cup date sugar

Step 1: bring half the water to a boil in a large pot over high heat.

Step 2: While you are waiting for the water to boil, prepare the tamarind pods. Remove the brittle outer shell and pull off as many strings as you can. Discard the shell and strings.

Step 3: After the water comes to a rolling boil, remove it from the heat and place the inner portion of the tamarind and the sugar in the water. Let the tamarind soak for about 1 hour and 30 minutes.

Step 4: At this point, the water will have cooled down. Use your fingers to squeeze out the hard tamarind seeds and remove the remaining strings; discard them.

Step 5: Place the liquid and remaining pulp in a blender and process until the pulp is fully blended into the water.

Step 6: Run the liquid through a strainer

Step 7: Pour your delicious agua de tamarindo into a pitcher, add the rest of the water, and refrigerate until cold.

Acupressure

Traditional Chinese Medicine (TCM) sees acne as a problem with "chi" energy (energy that that keeps vital components of the body moving freely. This occurs when the "liver chi" is blocked and out of balance and the lymphatic system needs attention. In other words, when the systems in the body responsible for removing waste are overloaded.

There are 4 specific acupressure points for pre-menstrual acne. Stimulating the points of SP6 and SP9 helps release congestive energy during the menstrual cycle. While simultaneously stimulating points LV3 and LV4 helps to open further release toxicity from the body. Applying pressure to these points helps the body stimulate and open these detoxifying channels within the body. waste can flow more freely and become less clogged while promoting its elimination from the body through dietary adjustments.

If you do not have a professional acupuncturist to go to (many will not agree to focusing exclusively in these areas) here's a routine, you can incorporate into your daily regimen.

At least twice a week, sit upright in a chair and use your thumb to make circular movements in a clockwise direction in and around each of the 4 points for about 1-minute each. Press hard enough to cause slight discomfort, but not enough that you want to stop.

Change Your Makeup:

Us a non-oil-based makeup if you use makeup and are prone to acne. Incorporate more internal health cleansing to help alleviate acne issues at its core.

Read Labels:

Avoid products that go onto the skin that contain the following: lanolin's, isopropyl myristate, sodium lauryl sulfate, laureth-4, C and D dyes. These chemicals irritate the skin and are not absorbed well into the body.

Stop Popping Pimples:

Pimples are formed from inflammation. Squeezing pimples or whiteheads can add to the inflammation. You can break open a wall or skin pour and make it susceptible to outside toxins. Yes, clearing out pus will help a pimple heal quicker, but by not addressing the core reason pimples are formed, you should expect another pimple to show itself shortly after.

Note: you do want to attack blackheads as squeezing them won't create more pimples. The inside of a blackhead (blocked pour) is solid. Removing this allows more skin pours to breathe which can contribute to your overall skin health.

Give Dry Skin Extra Care:

Dry skin is sensitive. Be careful of what you put onto dry skin as well as any pressure you putt onto those areas.

Proper Hydration:

Help your skin by consuming more water-filled items such as: watermelon, cucumber, berries, pears, mango, peaches, and most importantly, natural spring water. Consuming these items will allow the body to hold onto more water as compared to just drinking water.

Exfoliate

Get an exfoliating brush and gently brush areas of the skin to help keep them clean and also to help identify any sensitive areas where pimples or acne may show up.

Herbal Lymphatic System Cleanse Recipe:

The lymphatic system moves waste materials around and out of the body. It is likely that every bit of acne you may have has come directly through the lymphatic system. You will want to help slowly clean out excess waste in this system.

Mix together the following herbs and mix together (about ½ tablespoon of each)

Red Clover, Burdock, Yellow dock, Blessed Thistle, and Licorice Root

Bring 1 quart of water to a boil and add 1 ounce of combined herbs. Turn off heat and steep for 30 minutes. Drink two cups a day daily for 90 days (yes it can take a while to cleanse the lymphatic system).

*You can refrigerate the unused portion for up to a week.

In addition to cleaning the lymphatic system, incorporating herbs that support the liver, nourish the blood, and fight infections of healing acne. are all crucial to eliminating the issue.

Hydrotherapy:

A weekly steam bath for your face can help keep your pours clean.

Simple Hydrotherapy Recipe:

Using a 1 teaspoon-sized tea bag, prepare an 8oz cup of Yarrow (herb) tea. Steep for 30 minutes and add it to a steaming pot of water. Lean over the steaming water for 5-10 minutes, holding a towel over your head to keep the steam on your face and not directly on your hair. You should stand over about 12 inches away from the steaming water, so it does not burn your skin. If your acne is bad, do this routine 2-3 times a week. If not, you can use this routine once a week to keep your skin feeling well.

Skin Care Routines:

From: Fasting: A Guide To Health And Wellness, by Bryan McAskill)

Anti-Acne Face Mask

Ingredients: 1 key lime (juiced), 1 teaspoon of agave nectar, 7-10 fresh basil leaves

Instructions:

- Mash fresh basil leaves. Mix well with key lime juice and agave nectar until smooth.
- Apply this mixture to clean skin. Allow to dry for 30 minutes. Rinse with water and pat dry
- Repeat three times weekly

Smoothing Face Mask

Ingredients: 1 cucumber, seeded, 1 key lime (juiced)

Instructions:

- Peel and chop one cucumber. Put the pieces in a blender and mix until smooth.
- Mix 1 teaspoon of key lime juice with 1 teaspoon of cucumber juice.

- Use a cotton ball to apply to clean skin. Leave on for 20 minutes. Rinse with cool water and pat dry.

- Repeat daily. You can store cucumber juice in the refrigerator for repeated use.

Remove Dark Spots Mask

Ingredients: 1 papaya, ½ teaspoon of key lime juice

Instructions:

- Blend or mash up a soft ripe Papaya into a puree. Make sure there are no lumps. Add ½ teaspoon of key lime juice and mix together.

- Apply the face mask onto your clean face and let it dry for 15-30 minutes.

- Wash away with water. No more than three times a week. re

Natural Face Mask

Ingredients: 1 tablespoon of agave, 1tablespoon of plum tomato

Instructions:

- Blend plum tomato until you get a smooth puree

- Stir in agave

- Apply mixture onto your face and let it sit for about 15 minutes

- Wash off with cold water and pat face dry

- For more firm skin, mix in 1 tablespoon of sea moss power and 1 tablespoon of bladderwrack powder of this mix and leave on your face for 30 minutes before washing off.

Sea Moss Facial Scrub

Ingredients: 2 tablespoons of Sea Moss Gel, spring water, dry brush or exfoliating brush

Instructions:

- Add 2 tablespoons of Sea Moss Gel to a bowl

- Add water slowly to a bowl (about ½ cup). You can add more water if needed, but depends on preference)

- Mix together well

- Apply Gel to face and rub into your skin. You can apply with a dry brush or exfoliating brush if you want a deeper clean.

- Wash off your face with water and pat to dry

Natural Deodorant (Option #1)

Ingredients: 1 key lime (cut in half), 1-2 tablespoons of coconut oil

Instructions:

- Rub key lime on your underarms and pat to remove liquid from running down
- Massage in with a small amount of coconut oil. If you feel a slight burning sensation when you apply key lime, wash off with water and use less next time

Natural Deodorant (Option #2)

Ingredients: ½ cup of Coconut oil, 1 tablespoon of Sea Moss Gel, ½ cup of shea butter, 1 tablespoon of key lime juice

Instructions:

- Mix all ingredients together and store in a glass airtight container overnight
- Mix well together before each use
- Use 1 teaspoon of mixture and massage in and pat to dry

Addictions

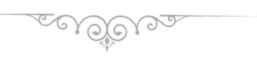

All addictions have a root cause. The root cause, however, does not determine the dependency on things such as alcohol, drugs, gambling, or some other addictive behavior. All addictions have certain items that can be helpful but the main target area for all addictions is the biochemistry of the brain and body. The main culprit that impacts the biochemistry of the brain and body is, **_Sugar_**.

"I believe that people with addictive personalities are sugar-sensitive" says Kathleen DesMaisons. Ph.D., and President and CEO of Radiant Recovery, which is a treatment facility centered around alcoholism, drug addiction, and compulsive behaviors located in Albuquerque, New Mexico, USA.

Too much sugar in any form (from junk foods, refined carbohydrates, and alcohol) directly impacts the biochemistry of the brain and body in two ways.

1. Raises serotonin which is a natural chemical in the brain the controls mood and emotions. When a sudden burst of serotonin is increased, it is short lived. Typically, serotonin is that arousal feeling when doing enjoyable activities such as exercise, stretching, meditation, cooking, etc). when serotonin is boosted from sugary foods, it wears off quickly and often makes people feel worse, where they experience symptoms of depression, anxiety, and low self-esteem; all contributing to the development of addictive behavior.

2. Sugar boosts the pleasure neurotransmitters in the body referred to as "beta-endorphins" which trigger impulsive behavior and cravings for more sugar.

To put it more simply, sugar helps to create the ideal biochemical environment for addiction.

Remedies:

Key Adjustments To Make:

1. Have something in your system first thing in the morning. Key Limes in water or fruit smoothie are ideal as they provide many nutrients while being easy to digest. When you don't consume anything upon awakening, your blood-sugar levels, beta-endorphins, and serotonin levels are not balanced; this is not ideal for those battling addiction.

2. Have a mid-day and evening meal planned ahead time. When you make time for regular meals, you're less prone to snack and indulge into typical sugar cravings. You teach your body to start AND stop which is vital when battling addictions.

3. Move from white foods to brown foods. White foods such as baked goods, cakes, cereals, and common pastas are made from white flours. Incorporating more brown versions of these items such as, Quinoa Rice, Spelt, Rye, and Kamut Breads, Chickpea Pasta, and Amaranth, can help you become healthier while consuming some of your typical meals.

4. Identifying "hidden" sources of sugar is very crucial to establishing a more solid foundation for yourself. These items are often hidden in plain sight (on ingredient labels) by having complicated names. Besides looking for _**sugar**_ on ingredient labels, you will also want to search for these common words:

Barley malt, brown rice syrup, cane juice, fruit juice concentrate, galactose, glucose, high-fructose corn syrup, honey, lactose, corn sweetener, corn syrup, malted barley, malto-dextrin, maltose, mannitol, sorbitol, xylitol, maltitol, microcrystalline cellulose, molasses, polydextrose, dextrin, dextrose, fructose, fructo-oligosaccharides, raisin juice, raisin syrup, sucanat, and sucrose. There are many more, but these are the most common.

Generate An Honest List Pros & Cons For Addiction

(the "Pro" list is if the addiction continued while the "Con" list is in opposition of the addiction).

Pro: Write down what you enjoy. Examples can include, "Helps me unwind after working all day", "Tastes good", or "Makes me feel good".

Con: Then write down the benefits of removing this addiction from your life. Examples can include, "I'll have more time to spend with family", "I'll be healthier", I'd be more productive with my time", or "I would save some money".

Take note of each Pro and Con you can come up with (ask for suggestions if you cannot think of any and write them down) and focus on using the "Con" list as daily reminders to achieve more regularly.

Create Distance

Work to incorporate some steps to create space between yourself and your addiction. If your addiction is food-related, don't write it on your shopping list, or place it behind some healthier options so it's not so easily assessable. If you have a drug addiction, call a friend instead, take a walk, or (with caution) delete you suppliers phone number; "with caution" is due to uncontrollable urges that may lead to other behaviors detrimental to health and well-being. Using drugs is neve recommended, but make sure this step can be achieved without increased harmful behaviors to self or others before considering.

Keep Busy

Keeping busy can promote engagement with mor enjoyable activities which help boost the neurotransmitters in the body and essentially help satisfy that need in a healthier way.

Avoiding Anticipated Behaviors:

AA (Alcoholics Anonymous), NA (Narcotics Anonymous) and other self-help programs work to teach members to avoid people, places, and things that are associated with their addictions.

Support groups provided necessary structure for an addict. Where there is structure, there is support and guidance, which are often what is needed the most when working to overcome any addiction.

Herbal Remedy For Alcoholism
(this is not a "cure" but helps deter and reduce cravings)

(Follow this regimen for 30 days minimum)

- Colon Cleanse (Cascara sagrada, Rhubarb Root, Prodijiosa, and Black Walnut Hull). Mix about 1 tablespoon of each herb together, boil water and place ½ tablespoon of mixed herbs into 8oz cup of water. Strain our herbs and drink twice a day.
- Elderberry, Sea Moss, Bladderwrack, and Ginger Tea at least 3 times a week
- Iron-rich Herbs Daily (Sarsaparilla, Guaco, Burdock Root – in capsule or tea form)
- Other herb to add to diet: Holy Basil, Quassia, Mullein, and Vervain

Iboga

Tabernathe iboga ("ibogaine"), a shrub commonly found in West and Central Africa has been known to be used for treating strong addictions to substances such as, cocaine, nicotine, and alcohol, among others.

Ibogaine has been shown to reduce cocaine and morphine self-administration in laboratory animals, and reduction of alcohol intake by alcohol-preferring rats. This compound essentially works to reduce the rewarding effects of substances such as nicotine in animals.

Ibogaine may work in reversing the effects of opiates on gene expression, with resulting impacts on neuroreceptors, returning them to a pre-addiction condition (Brackenridge, 2010).

Furthermore, addictive loops and pathways in the brain are reversed (He et al., 2005).

This plant can be viewed within a similar realm as psychedelic mushrooms which have begun to reemerge as legitimate, consistent treatment for conditions impacting mental health disorders.

Similar to psychedelic mushrooms, caution is at the forefront given its force with even very small dosages. Side effects can be unknown which can deter many from using this as a treatment as the structure of treatment is difficult to define.

Psychedelics (caution)

There are various forms of psychedelics which range from mushrooms which contain psilocybin which is the compound found in "magic mushrooms", to *mescaline* which is the active compound in the peyote cactus which is known to produce psychedelic effects. There is still much research to be conducted on psychedelics, so you want to do so under guidance of a shaman or experiences healer. There is evidence of psychedelics working to encourage the growth of new connections between neurons in the brain. This ability of the brain to make new connections is called *plasticity*. Brain plasticity involves the ability of the nervous system to change its activity in response to intrinsic or extrinsic stimuli by reorganizing its structure, functions, or connections, which impact how the brain functions and responds during challenges such as mental health. States such as Oregon and Colorado have allowed psychedelics to be use medically under assisted adult use, where other states such as California, Michigan, Minnesota, Washington, and Massachusetts, have several cities where psychedelics are decriminalized under possession.

Allergies

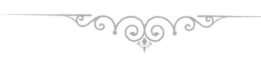

Allergies area result of the body's immune system overreacting to what many consider to be a harmless substance (dust, peanuts, pollen, etc.). 1 in 5 Americans battle with sneezes, coughing, chest tightness, itchy eyes, rashes, and wheezing, which are all contributors to developing regular allergies.

Allergies can come in many forms and can be triggered by almost anything. Allergies are most commonly triggered by allergens which stimulate the immune system which promotes a list of common responses such as sneezing, coughing, or having itchy eyes. These allergens enter through four main areas:

1. Ingestion (eating or drinking something such as peanuts or shellfish),
2. Injection (getting a vaccine such as a penicillin shot),
3. Absorption Through The Skin (poison ivy), or
4. Inhalation (breathing in dust or pollen).

Allergies being triggered by innumerable sources makes it very difficult to know what to avoid until you know what the trigger is. "You'll find a bit of everything in house dust" says Thomas Platts-Mills, M.D. house dust can often set the foundation for allergies and also present regular triggers indoors and outdoors. Rather than try to avoid all triggers to your allergies, there are many reasonable options you can accommodate for prior to any dietary adjustments or restrictions.

Besides dust and pollen-related allergies, there are things like sea-food allergies. For these, it is recommended to go to the source. Identify what you may get from sea animals and sea creatures and get those nutrients and minerals elsewhere (just like we can for land animals). In this section, we will review common triggers for allergies and adjustments to incorporate into your lifestyle to begin alleviating your condition.

Remedies:

Reduce and Breakdown The Excess Mucus

Any item that takes longer than 30-minutes to digest will trigger a response for the body to generate additional mucus to push it along the digestive tract. This is that "full" feeling we get after eating particular items. We want to avoid the commons items that first take long to digest to alleviate the gut, intestines, and digestive tract. These items include meats (land and sea animals), dairy, foods cooked in grease, oily foods, and processed items containing white flour and/or white sugar such as, cakes, chips, cookies, and candy.

After removing these items from your lifestyle, you should notice significant improvement with experiencing relief of your symptoms and overall better health. The next step is to breakdown ("thin out") any additional mucus to reduce symptoms and make it easier to expel this mucus from your body. As you incorporate a plant-based lifestyle, many foods in your diet that already breakdown/thin the excess mucus such as, berries, cucumbers, oranges, watercress, onions, and common herbs such as, ginger, cayenne pepper, eucalyptus, mullein leaf, burdock root, and many more.

As you avoid consuming items that contribute to excess mucus production which are low in fiber, and consume that which thins out the mucus, over time, your body will not feel congested, and the digestive system will experience relief, which will relive you of your symptoms. It does take time, but for more day-to-day adjustments you can make, refer to the rest of the remedies listed in this section.

Air-Out Your Space

Allowing air to flow freely throughout your living or workspace is best for reducing any stagnant bacteria in the air that can trigger your symptoms. Air conditioning is great for keeping a steady flow of air in your area. If you want something less intrusive, a rotating fan will get the job done.

Even in the winter (when it's not snowing or raining) you may let air flow through a few windows or door for few minutes. You do not want your home or workspace to get cold, but you do not want to keep the same air confined within the same space for too long. You also want to remain mindful of any household pets you have if you choose to open a door or window to not let them out.

Air Filter

When you use an air filter you want to keep the door closed so the machine doesn't get overwhelmed with too much air to filter. Take note of what section of the room may need the most work and place your air filter there. it would be helpful to do some cleaning of any dust prior to installing an air filter.

De-humidifier

You want to keep the air moving but you want to avoid having too much humidity as humidity can be a breeding ground for mold. Mold for anyone is highly toxic but can immediately trigger symptoms for those with allergies.

Deep Clean Your Carpets

Many forms of dust and bacteria can hide in carpets and rugs. Having an area rug can be a better option since it can be moved easier and dusted properly, unlike area rugs and carpets that are installed wall to wall. If you have strong allergies, it would be best to hire a professional cleaning to come in at least once a month to properly clean you rugs and carpets. This can seem like nuisance but is worth the investment long-term. Dust mites are also very common to hide in carpets and should be removed at all costs. You may also want to strongly consider removing all carpets and rugs to keep your space clean.

Avoid Smoke

Cigarette smoke is a strong irritant for those with allergies and should be avoided. Not only will everyone breathe easier, but the smoke will also not seep into your rug, carpet, furniture, or air within your living space or office.

Isolate Your Pets

Dander and hair from pets can be almost impossible to track and collect daily as it can flow or be shed anywhere. Creating a designated area for your pet to spend most of their time is ideal as it can help alleviate cleaning up hair and dander throughout your house. Cleaning your pet's area at least once a week should be the standard in your home to regularly remove any debris.

Seal Up Your Beds

Encasing your pillows, mattress, and bedframe in allergen-proof covers is essential to reducing your direct contact with potential allergens. Search for fabrics that are tight knit to help reduce dust mites from settling in as well.

Laundry (Hot Cycle)

All linins should be washed at 130-degrees Fahrenheit to help rid them of dust mites and various waste materials. After your water has turned on for your wash, simply check the temperature with a thermometer.

Create A Sanctuary Space

If you do not have an entire room you can use for this space, work on creating an area that can be dedicated to free space and simplicity. Try to not use your bedroom for this space to maximize the amount of "flow" you have in your home. You want to use your bedroom for rest only. If you are very limited on space, try gathering some storage bins or organizational containers and clearing out a closet space where you can reposition items as needed when spending time in your sanctuary.

Avoid White Flour and White Sugar

"Sugar and white flour weaken the immune system and rob the body of energy" says Dr. Metzger, M.D., Ph.D., medical director of Helena Women's Health in San Francisco, California, and Palo Alto, California. When excess sugars and white flour are consumed, this creates an enormous workload on the digestive system and due to their toxicity, the immune system t-cells respond by treating this as a foreign invader. The body can do without the additional immune response which can be better served focusing on other areas of the body and avoid accumulating waste within the body. These items contribute to gut/intestinal issues which trigger responses from being in contact with allergens. White flour and white (artificial/processed) sugars take longer to digest than most other foods and contain poorly absorbed carbohydrates which can also irritate the gut.

Note:

An image we can keep in mind is a water barrel. When this barrel is full, anything added to it will make it spill over. In the case of allergies, the allergen and whatever triggers symptoms of allergies are what make this barrel spill over. It is recommended to incorporate the following into your dietary regimen to avoid your barrel from spilling over.

1. Fasting. There are many different Fasting methods. Research various methods and choose what is best for you at the moment. Fasting involves scheduling a designated time period where you do not consume solid items. Liquids are recommended such as water and fruit/vegetable smoothies (unless you are doing a water fast or dry fast). Fasting will allow your barrel to decrease what's inside by naturally cleansing out what's not needed and allow your body wo properly work to reduce the body's response to allergies without your barrel overflowing.

2. Sauna/Hot Yoga. Heat helps the body release stored toxins that come from fat cells and go into the blood and travel into the skin cells to then be released. Hot Yoga can create a more physical movement aspect towards removing toxins from the body and help release some toxins that may be "trapped" in various spots in the body. Allowing

the body to move and flow is best practice for reducing many of the symptoms associated with allergies.

3. Nettle (Herb). Rather than list out many herbs that are helpful to reducing each symptom connected to allergies, it is recommended to simply incorporate one herb known as "Nettle" into your daily life to help with this condition. To maximize the effectiveness of this herb, you should begin taking it several prior to the time of year allergies begin to display themselves more regularly in your life. You may use 2 teaspoons of this herb in dried form for tea to drink daily. Capsules: take two 300-milligram capsules up to three times a day. Freeze-dried Nettle is more concentrated and take a few days to "kick in". It would be best to begin Fasting until this herb begins to show its benefits to you for best results.

4. Massages. You can massage the outside circles of your eyes (from the top part of your cheekbones to just under your eyebrows). Work to move in a circular motion (clockwise or counterclockwise) for 3-4 minutes each way. Do this massage sequence 2-3 times a day to help the nose and eyes breath and improve circulation in the areas most affected by allergies.

My Personal Remedy:

- Green juices (green plants: cucumbers, dark leafy greens, green apples, zucchini, etc)
- Kamu kamu powder and Amla berry extract.

*drink green juices 2-3 times a day. After about two weeks, you can graduate (yes, celebrate) to fruit juices with items you do not have a reaction to. Do this several times following it with kamu kamu powder and amla berry extract until you see a difference.

Mix together kamu kamu powder and amla berry extract in equal parts (follow directions on labels). Mix in with warm (or at least room temperature) water and drink two times a day. Water amount can vary so aim for about two 14-16pz glasses of water for this.

Quick Tips:

If you're experiencing signs and symptoms of allergies, but remain uncertain of where it is coming from, check with any of the following tests to help determine where your allergies are being triggered by:

1. ALCAT (antigen leucocyte cellular antibody test) – measures reactions to mold, foods, or chemicals.

2. Bronchial Inhalation Challenge Testing – detects sensitivity to chemicals and environmental factors in the air.

3. Cytotoxic Testing – blood test that is used to detect chemicals and food allergies.

4. EAV (electroacupuncture testing) – uses electroacupuncture techniques to detect a variety of allergies (most common in Europe).

5. Enzyme Potentiated Desensitization – uses enzymes in small amounts to help desensitize a person from their allergies.

6. Kinesiology Testing – test where a Doctor measures your muscle strength holding various items. Weakness indicates you are allergic or sensitive to a substance

7. NAET (Nambudripad's Allergy Elimination Technique) – provides a holistic approach that involves acupuncture, chiropractic care, and physical movements to stop allergens from producing symptoms.

8. Patch Testing – used to diagnose direct contact allergies.

9. Provocative Neutralization Therapy – therapy that works specifically to prevent, block, and neutralize reactions to the identifies trigger/substance.

10. RAST (radioallergosorbent test) – blood test used to detect allergies from common foods, pollen, dust, mold, and dander.

11. Serial Dilution Endpoint Titration Testing – tests for inhalant and food allergies.

Alzheimer's Disease

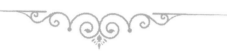

Alzheimer's disease is a condition where the brain begins to deteriorate significantly. Doctors will often offer only two treatment methods for this condition. The first is a prescription of Donepezil ("Aricept") which is given to promote the natural chemical in the brain known as "acetylcholine" which is responsible for memory. The second treatment offered is a regular prescription of synthetic vitamin E pills to help slow down the destruction of brain cells.

The primary issue with both of these treatment methods is that neither address the main cause of Alzheimer's which is, excessive aluminum and heavy metal absorbed within the cells of the brain. Medical Doctor's recommendations only gloss over what can be effective and work to improve memory while slowing down symptoms. What the medical institutions have not put into modern practice is that symptoms such as decreased memory and the deterioration of cells within the brain, are a result of what's being deprived to the body and the many factors that get in the way of maintaining memory and healthy cells such as the foods we eat, and the chemicals that are consumed daily.

For Alzheimer's the following steps need to be addressed:

(Caution: You should use the remedies discussed below as only a part of an individual treatment program from those who have experience treating this condition).

1. Regenerate Brain Cells

    a. Focusing on reducing the consumption of heavy metals. It is strongly recommended to not consume food or beverage from a can as well as medical pharmaceuticals that have a high content of heavy metals. Items in cans are filled with "preservatives" which serve to take the role of embalming the items to extend their lifespan. The heavy metals in cans seep into the foods and drinks and is absorbed by these items (and cannot just be washed off) waiting for you to consume them in which these same heavy metals go into the bloodstream after not being able to absorb within the body and creates heavy metal toxicity.

2. Protect Mental Energy / Cleaning The Colon

    a. The colon is essentially the "2nd brain" within the body which sends along signals back and forth to one another. When one is consuming toxic materials (and eventually craving these materials) the other will believe it's necessary and create a dependence. Cleaning up mucus and heavy metals within the bloodstream, while working to regenerate the cells within the brain will take some time. Cleaning the colon in the meantime is essential for reducing noticeable signs and symptoms of Alzheimer's disease.

3. Removes Toxins From The Blood

    a. The blood goes everywhere within the body. Having chemicals (most notably heavy metals) in the bloodstream sends them directly to the brain. As the brain absorbs the blood it needs to survive, it is laced with chemicals that promote deterioration. Best practice for removing toxins in the body is to stop consuming them. Start with items that come in a can followed by processed items ("junk foods", starches, artificial sugars, and white flours).

        i. The blood needs Iron to thrive. Loading up on Iron from plant sources is most vital as Iron from a plant source easily absorbs into the body of living beings.

        ii. Common Sources of Iron are: Wild Rice (not black rice), Quinoa, Chickpeas (Garbanzo Beans), Kale, Walnuts, Hemp Seeds, Dates, Dried Apricots, and Watercress).

        iii. Common Herb Sources for Iron are: Sarsaparilla, Burdock (and Burdock Root), Guaco, Chainey Root, Monkey Ladder, Chickweed, and Yellowdock.

        iv. Also refer to recipes for cleansing heavy metals provided at the end of this section.

4. Protect The Brain Cells

    a. Omega-3 fatty acids are essential to protecting the brain cells. Consuming these in abundance are a necessary part of the healing process. Common sources are: Walnuts, Brazil Nuts, Avocados, Hemp Seeds, Hemp Milk, Walnut Oil, Olive Oil, and Sea Vegetable such as Nori, Hijiki, Bladderwrack, Kelp, and Dulse.

5. Keep Physically Active

    a. Physical movement helps keep the brain stimulated and set regular tasks and challenges for the brain to complete. Regular exercise helps the brain build new brain cells as well, according to Dharma Singh Khalsa, M.D., President and Medical Director of the Alzheimer's Prevention Foundation in Tucson, Arizona, USA.

6. Boost/Expand Mental Capacity

    a. This step can come in many forms from releasing toxins from the body, to stimulating the brain by doing crossword puzzles or sudoku. The main thing is to challenge the brain without placing a burden on it. When approaching Alzheimer's disease through a nutritional lens, there are two specific herbs (many others as well) that provide necessary needs that are deficient when Alzheimer's is present (blood flow to the brain, and reduction of oxygen due to excess consumption of heavy metals). The two herbs to work into lifestyle are:

        i. Gingko Biloba – helps to increase blood flow to the brain (when toxins are not present in the bloodstream, the brain is able to remain alert and active without hindrance).

        ii. Blue Vervain – increases oxygen delivery to the brain. The body has to be in a stable condition for it to be receptive enough to absorb the increased oxygen intake flowing towards the brain.

**These herbs can be taken in capsule form (two 300mg twice a day) or in tea form (about 2 teaspoons of each twice daily).

Note: Again, these recommendations do not present a "cure" by themselves alone. The healthy lifestyle as a whole is what helps to reverse various conditions. These steps are necessary pieces to incorporate immediately and upon onset of diagnosis.

Removal of Heavy Metals In The Body

This entails an extensive process of elimination as heavy metals can be stored anywhere within the body. There is also no official "end" to track either. The goal when working to regularly cleanse heavy metals from the body is to incorporate what is needed, while also eliminating items that contain heavy metals continuously.

Heavy Metal Remover Smoothie:

2 handfuls of Kale

½ cup of Cilantro

2 Green Apples (sliced)

1 tablespoon of Hemp Seeds

this smoothie should be in the regular dietary regimen for those who have Alzheimer's.

HEAVY METAL DETOX PLAN:

Focused on removing metallic ingestion in excess amounts:

- Aluminum (no canned foods)
- Mercury (no fish or sea animal)
- *Formaldehyde (no junk foods, starches, alcohol, or unnatural juices)
- Eliminate inorganic compounds listed above that are alien to your alkaline body structure. Elements that decrease electrical maintenance & output are necessary when reversing disease and illness.

It is believed that there are natural forms of formaldehyde that develop via interactions with the metabolism process. However, the formaldehyde we see listed as an ingredient (or not listed) is a substance that is mostly a chemical known as "Formalin" which is a solution that works to disinfect household products, soy products, hydrated animal products, and sprayed onto many fruits and vegetables.

FEATURES TO KNOW:

Detoxification requires the adequate use of all organs in your human system. No tissue is more important than any other tissue (organs, glands, nodes, etc.).

Optimization of your Brain and Nervous System will aid the flushing of toxins out of the body. Through your Kidneys, Liver & other detoxifying organs of the body. You will want to make the following items the foundation of your diet to help address areas most in need with this condition:

Sea Vegetables:
Sea moss, Kelp, Dulse, Nori, Bladderwrack, Hijiki

Fruits:
Wild Blue Berries, Apricots, Seeded Grapes, Plums, Cantaloupes, Cherries, Key Limes, Tamarind

Vegetables:
Chaga Mushroom, Avocado, Tomatoes (Cherry/Plum), Cucumber, Nopales (Cactus)

Chlorophyllics:
Calaloo, Dandelion, Lettuces, Turnip Greens, Wild Arugula, Watercress, Nopales (Mexican Cactus)

Seeds:
Hempseeds, Sesame Seed

Nuts:

Brazil Nuts, Walnuts, Cashews

Herbs:

Red Clover, Blue Vervain, Blessed Thistle, Ginger, Bugleweed, Hops, Sage, Valerian, Elderberry, Cayenne Pepper.

Other Key Components:
- Sweating expels pollutants
- Sun (direct contact) as often as possible is strongly encouraged
- Quality sleep aids in mineral structure rejuvenation within the body
- Light to moderate intensity walking, jogging, running for exercise (cardiovascular health)

TOOLS:
- Steamer (no oils)
- Juicer (less fiber) - pro fast mineral reactions aka metabolism

Conclusion:

Stick to the plan listed in this section while implementing many of the tips provided within this section. It may seem like an extensive list and may even seem overwhelming. I do want to encourage you to start by first identifying changes you're comfortable with making and understand that this is not a lifetime change as you take necessary steps towards your healing. As you experience a steady decrease in symptoms, I am confident that you will develop a higher attunement with your body and its' needs and be able to identify the next steps in your journey. You will enter the "healing crisis" arena during your healing. Just work to remain calm and not to worry. All parts of the healing process have their place.

There is still much more research to be conducted for this condition but no matter what may be added, it is most important to remove what is not helpful which this section has begun to cover.

Anal Itching, Fissures, and Discomfort

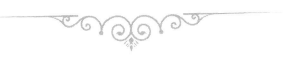

The most common issue in this area of the body are hemorrhoids which are swollen veins which can create immense discomfort. Fissures are breaks in the skin (ulcer) which tear open and make passing a stool very difficult. These issues, if not treated correctly will become chronic issues that remain present for an extended period of time. Most anal fissures and conditions like hemorrhoids heal within a few weeks. Although surgery can often be avoided in most anal discomfort, there are many remedies that can be applied to provide relief.

Remedies:

Fiber and Fluids

Avoid these conditions by loading up on fiber (to digest and break down stools) and fluids (water, tea, smoothies) so the body can make your stools softer and allow them to be released with minimum discomfort. General rule you can follow is to load up on fresh fruits and vegetables, whole grains, and drinking 6-8 glasses of water a day. It is recommended for women to aim towards 21-25 grams of fiber a day, while men aim between 30-38 grams of fiber a day.

Common sources of Fiber: garbanzo beans, lentils, brussels sprouts, sweet potatoes, avocado, pears, sunflower seeds, flax seeds, hazelnuts, apples and berries (high pectin fruits) and onions.

Don't Scratch Or Itch

This may be difficult but resist your urge to scratch or itch this area as you can further tear the skin and make the condition worse. A better option can be to pat the area and gently applying pressure with a cloth to avoid scraping and tearing the skin or creating a rash.

Lose Extra Weight

Extra weight can cause a person to sweat more during basic tasks which can irritate these issues. If anal itching, hemorrhoids, or fissures are a common occurrence for you, shedding any extra weight you normally don't carry around is best to lose. Additional pounds can often be brought on by overeating, lack of exercise, or stress so it is a good idea to weight yourself on a scale somewhat regularly to remain aware of your body weight to notice any imbalances.

Soak In A Hot Tub

This is not always an option but being able to do so will help with relaxing the muscles in the body (particularly around the anal sphincter) which reduce much of the discomfort of any anal issue.

Avoid Spicy or Pickled Foods

Spicy foods make us sweat but also promote bowel movements. You want to have regular bowel movements, just not very often during this time.

Specialized Pillows

A donut-shaped pillow or water-filled pillow can help decrease pain by protecting this area.

Exchange Toilet Tissue With Facial Tissue

Toilet tissue is often rougher than we may imagine when we do not have fissures or discomfort. Facial tissues often contain some form of moisturizer which can provide a softer texture during this time.

Wipe Softly

Make sure to wipe your area of discomfort softly and take your time. One swift or aggressive wipe can prolong your condition for several more weeks. You may run a piece of your toilet or facial tissue under your faucet to soften it as well to avoid further irritating your area.

My Personal Remedy For Itching and Discomfort:

(Mix together the following):

2 teaspoons of Thyme

1 teaspoon of Nettle

1 teaspoon of Dandelion

1 teaspoon of Burdock

Boil 4 cups of water and bring to a boil. Pour water into cup (with herbs) and let steep for 12-15 minutes. Let cool, then strain. Drink twice a day while following other remedies covered in this section. Can apply directly onto skin but will want space to air dry if possible.

Anemia

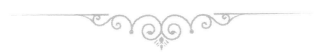

Take a moment to look at your wrist. See your blue veins? That's due to the hemoglobin which is comprised of a protein that contain 4 iron atoms at its core. Iron is only naturally produced in one place (nature). Iron comes from the core of dying stars. Just look at what the core of our planet is made of (iron). We are also dying stars as we come from stardust.

Anytime you look at your veins keep in mind that you are looking at what you are built from, and kept alive by, stardust.

Anemia is not only brought on by iron deficiency as commonly believed. There are several different forms of anemia. This condition can result from other deficiencies as well. Such as, copper, riboflavin ("vitamin B2"), folic acid ("vitamin B9"), cobalamin ("vitamin B12"), and tocopherol ("vitamin E"), all can create forms of anemia as all of these minerals and nutrients require the production of red blood cells which are low when anemia is present. Iron, is simply a mineral that serves as the body's free transportation service, transporting nutrients to where they need to go. Without enough iron, nutrients don't get where they need to go and even if you're consuming what you need, if you do not get enough iron regularly, your deficiencies will remain present.

Common Forms of Anemia:

Iron anemia:

Primary deficiencies: iron and riboflavin ("vitamin B2")

Pernicious anemia:

Primary deficiency: cobalamin ("vitamin B12")

Megaloblastic anemia:

Primary deficiencies: folic acid ("vitamin B9", and cobalamin ("vitamin B12")

Hemolytic anemia:

Primary deficiencies: tocopherol ("vitamin E", copper)

If you're currently on medications your goal should be to consume more natural foods so you will not rely on them to live. Consuming the right kind of iron is a simple, but necessary step to achieve this goal. Iron is a mineral that serves as the body's free transportation service, transporting nutrients to where they need to go. We must consume an adequate amount of nutrients needed to begin with in order for them to be transported to their correct and most needed location(s) in the body.

Medications provide Iron in the form of Iron-oxide which come from heavy metal and ferrous sulfate which is an inorganic chemical that is used to create additional red blood cells. However, without being able to properly absorb essential minerals, the body is creating artificial red blood cells that die out and do not maintain their structure long. This material has to then be filtered out of the body along with the heavy metals in prescription pills, which create chaos in the body starting with the blood and ending with kidney and liver filtration; causing issues that begin to overwork the detoxifying organs in the body.

So, after taking these medications and supplements, the body cannot readily absorb minerals, produce its own healthy red blood cells long term, and ends up creating an additional workload for the liver and kidneys and leads to their destruction.

The body simply needs the right form of Iron (iron-fluorine) which come from plants. These are easily digestible and void of heavy metals (only containing vital trace minerals). They can enter the bloodstream and keep it's need maintained without interference from absorbing unrecognizable substances. Iron is the mineral in our bodies that transport nutrients. Consuming minerals, nutrients, and phytonutrients must remain at the forefront of diet and lifestyle, where Iron serves as the vehicle taking them where they need to go in order to fulfill our cellular needs.

The oxygen-carrying protein (hemoglobin) becomes deficient mostly for women during their menstrual cycles when they lose blood. If you are a woman and lose blood often or experience heavier cycles and you do not work to load up on your natural forms of Iron, your body will experience a plethora of undesirable signs and symptoms of discomfort.

Remedies:

Riboflavin ("vitamin B2")

Riboflavin helps the body use nutrients such as carbohydrates, fats, and proteins for energy, and additionally functions as an antioxidant.

Common sources of riboflavin: tomatoes, avocado, sunflower seeds, dandelion greens, swiss chard, kale, quinoa., and edible sea vegetables (Nori, Wakame, Hijiki, Sea Moss, Bladderwrack).

Folic Acid ("vitamin B9")

This is a synthetic man-made vitamin that is added to fortified foods (foods that have vitamins and minerals added to them). It's comprised of several "B-vitamins" but B9 by itself is put together separately to be added to foods. Items that are naturally nutrient-dense should have the combination of "B-vitamins" needed to produce folic acid (vitamin B9).

Common sources of folic acid: avocado, turnip greens, swiss chard, kale, lettuce, dandelion greens, sunflower seeds, oranges, kiwi, quinoa, and wild rice.

Cobalamin ("vitamin B12")

Is naturally created via bacterial synthesis in the gut. Cobalamin is a bacterium that is part of every growing plant that we consume. However, this is often washed off during processing that it is no longer present on these items, and we do not consume this bacterium. Animals will consume foods while they are still in the ground and absorb a larger quantity of cobalamin that goes into their muscle tissue and can be absorbed by anything that eats them. However, eating an animal is a longer route to getting access to this bacterium, and we are unsure if they even have an adequate amount to be absorbed based upon their diets/lifestyle. We can gain consistent access to this bacterium by simply eating more fresh foods that are not processed, and by growing our own foods. The fewer stops from the farm to your table, the better your chances are of gaining access to absorb this healthy bacterium.

We essentially only need about 1 microgram of B12 a day. When we repeatedly do not meet this need, it can become noticeable, but we don't need nearly as much B12 as we do calcium, magnesium, or any other mineral. Since we have worked to kill off any form of bacteria (harmful or helpful) most people remain deficient. If we consume that which is natural and work on eating locally grown produce and growing our own plants (even something small to put in a window at home) we can consume enough B12 and do away with any B12 deficiency (and many others) so that B12 deficiency is no longer a topic of decision.

You will want to go to local markets and farmer's markets in your area where there is a shorter "farm to table" distance where B12 will remain more present in some capacity. Also growing some of your own plants at home or a t a local garden will be best.

Copper

This mineral works to lower LDL (bad) cholesterol and increase HDL (good) cholesterol, helps balance iron metabolism and absorption, produces red blood cells, supports the immune system, and turns sugar into energy for the cells, among many other tasks. 2 milligrams of copper daily will be a sufficient enough for the body to perform its daily tasks and responsibilities.

Common Sources of Copper: blackberries, blueberries, guava, apricots, bananas, leafy green vegetables, avocado, sunflower seeds, mushrooms, spring onions, and you can drink sparingly from a copper vessel or bottle.

Iron

Iron is a mineral that transports nutrients, minerals, and phytonutrients all throughout the body so they can fulfill their main tasks and responsibilities. The body uses this mineral to create a protein (*hemoglobin*) that's in red blood cells and carries oxygen to the cells in the body, and *myoglobin*, which is a protein that provides oxygen to the muscles. Without iron, nothing we consume really gets where we need them to go and will create deficiencies that will lead to various illnesses. The inability to promote the productions of red blood cells that iron provides for us, will reduce the bones' ability to produce bone marrow which sends off these red blood cells into the bloodstream and into our immune systems.

Natural Sources of Iron: Wild rice, chickpeas/garbanzo beans, dandelion greens, sarsaparilla, burdock, yellow dock, chapparal, and prunes.

Common Herbs High In Iron:

Sarsaparilla, sarsil berry (berry from the plant of the Sarsaparilla), guaco, conconsa, lily of the valley, purslane, kale, dandelion, lam's quarters, burdock, blue vervain, yellow dock, chickweed, anamu.

Items that rob you of iron:

- chocolate
- cow's milk
- coffee (yes, decaffeinated coffee too and those weight loss coffees as well)
- soda
- yeast
- artificial sugars and food dyes
- foods high in oxalic acids ("oxalates") such as, cauliflower, broccoli, spinach, soy, potatoes, dates, raspberries, navy beans, cashews, and baked potatoes with skin (baked potatoes, French fries, etc). Oxalates deplete and interfere with iron absorption.

- losing blood (this can happen during cycles but not replacing and replenishing your iron when this happens is the issue).

If you choose to implement Iron supplements into your lifestyle, understand that Ferrous Sulfate will not properly provide you with what you need. Ferrous Gluconate, Iron Gluconate, and Iron Picolinate digest and absorb much easier into the body as compared to Ferrous Sulfate and should be sought out within the ingredient labels on products. It is strongly recommended to incorporate more natural items such as those listed above, however, everyone can be at different stages in their journey.

Note: women who experience losing blood once a month through menstruation should aim around 15 milligrams per day of Iron, where Men can aim for 10 milligrams per day.

Many medical doctors confuse anemia for many other conditions or mark them off as stress related, nervous tension, or difficulty managing emotions. Rather than wait for your doctor to figure this out, there are two simple methods for testing if you have anemia.

1. Press down for about 2-3 seconds on one of your fingernails. Press right down against the nailbed as the area will turn whiter. Release and note how long it takes for that area to return to its normal state. It should only take a second or two to return to normal. If it takes longer, then you may be anemic or begin moving in that direction if you do not work to reduce this issue.

2. Gently pull down you bottom eyelids and view the color of your blood vessels underneath. If they appear to be pale, then you may be anemic.

Remove Dairy From Your Diet

Dairy presents an additional obstacle due to the fact that dairy makes it more difficult for the body to absorb Iron, especially for women. Women are often encouraged to consume dairy due to hormonal imbalances, or a person may crave these items during menstruation. You want to avoid that which blocks you from absorbing anything that is necessary to the body.

Avoid Alcohol and Artificial Sugars

Alcoholic beverages and artificial sugars often deplete the body of many essential minerals which can make anemia much worse and also trigger symptoms for often.

Caffeine

This is listed above to avoid as it inhibits iron absorption. Coffee, black tea, soda, and chocolate are some of the more common items that contain caffeine that should be avoided.

Aromatherapy

Essential oils can be very helpful to relieving physical discomfort for anemia. If your skin is cold and "clammy" it is advised to put 1-2 drops of Ginger oil on the area. If your skin is drier, you want to want hydrate as much as possible and use a dry brush for the affected area.

Anger

Anger itself is not the problem. Trouble arises when anger becomes uncontrollable. Anger is an emotion that we must release in nondestructive ways. Many get angry and "take it out" on people, things, or even themselves. We must always work to not leave behind or create more waste than what is produced. When a person punches a hole in a wall, not only does the wall need to be fixed, but their hand has to heal from being cut, bruised, or damaged. We can simply opt for other methods and to remedy the situation that do not create destruction. Dealing with anger by causing damage to self or others often leads to more anger a definitely more reminders which can linger on. It is my recommendation to not mask over your anger but get underneath it to understand your true feelings. There may be sorrow, fear, or impatience at its core; anger is simply outside of the core being expressed.

Individual and/or group therapy are great tools for self-reflection and evaluation to detect triggers as well as offering a positive space to receiving encouraging feedback. However, many therapists and psychologists lack training in areas specifically around anger. Outside of credentials, there are three questions I encourage you to ask your therapist or psychologist to identify if they have adequate training for what you may need to effectively work on your anger.

1. What do you believe about anger?
2. Have you been trained to help clients deal with their anger outside of talk therapy?
3. Have you done your own anger work? (follow up question) If so, how?

These questions will tell you if you can rely on your therapist for anger specifically, or if you can simply add on other supports or activities outside of therapy.

If you do not get your anger "out" it will linger inside of you.

"Nobody makes you angry; you decide to use anger as a response."

— BRIAN TRACY —

There's a short story/lesson that often comes to mind when thinking about anger. This lesson displays where anger resides and the need for dealing with anger internally rather than externally. You can view this story/lesson below. It is recommended you read this and take a moment to reflect upon how to apply this to you own life when in various situations.

Empty Boat

A monk decides to meditate alone, away from his monastery. He takes his boat out to the middle of the lake, moors it there, closes his eyes and begins his meditation.

After a few hours of undisturbed silence, he suddenly feels the bump of another boat colliding with his own. With his eyes still closed, he senses his anger rising, and by the time he opens his eyes, he is ready to scream at the boatman who dared disturb his meditation.

But when he opens his eyes, he sees it's an empty boat that had probably got untethered and floated to the middle of the lake.

At that moment, the monk achieves self-realization, and understands that the anger is within him; it merely needs the bump of an external object to provoke it out of him.

From then on, whenever he comes across someone who irritates him or provokes him to anger, he reminds himself, "The other person is merely an empty boat. The anger is within me."

There are bound to be countless empty boats in our daily lives; each trying its best to provoke us. Realize and understand too that the anger is within us. Just as Brian Tracy said that nobody made us angry but that we decided to use anger as a response. We cannot prevent these empty boats from bumping into us and provoking us, but we certainly can choose how we want to response to them.

Remedies:

Twisting A Towel

Grab any towel of medium to long length. Twist it as much as you can while letting out and frustration, grunts, or noises. Much tension when angry is stored in the jaw. It can help to yell or shout while doing this to help release any anger stored in the body. It is also encouraged for you to say out loud "I am angry" during short breaks you take from this activity to help acknowledge the moment as it begins to diminish.

Punch A Pillow

This may seem like a recommendation for a child as it is a common response for young people but, it can be very effective in reducing your anger while not breaking anything. As we grow older, we get bigger and stronger and often associate strength with power, and power with control. So, we tend to destroy objects or move things when angry and justify our position as we achieve "success" in breaking or moving a heavy object. This may appear to temporarily decrease your anger, but more often than not, you just have a sudden burst of testosterone, and your body works to stabilize itself and you're able to calm yourself. Punching a pillow is a form of physical aggression, but nothing is getting harmed, and pillows often do not get destroyed by hitting them; if they do, they are easily replaceable and won't cause damage to your hand or body.

Screaming

If you have a controlled, private setting at your disposal, yelling out loud is an effective way to diminish your anger. Yelling as opposed to formulating insults or threat towards others, is very different. When we yell obscene gestures or insults towards others, we are using our brain power to select words or phrases which only create more complexity to how you express your anger. Just yelling noises out loud allows you to not hold any tension in your jaw, while refocusing on how your body is feeling in the moment. Although it is not recommended, it you must yell curse words, hurtful phrases, or obscenities, do so while you're by yourself. Feel free to lock yourself in your car with the windows rolled all the way up if you need a personal space to yell also.

Break Something!

Yes, this sounds like it is disagreeing with what has been stated so far but, here is a recommendation to break items in a controlled setting that you have to travel to; not items within your home that you are attached to or belong to others. There are places where you can break glass, windows, or other objects to express your anger. Often people who are angry need to hear something outside of themselves making noise, so they know their anger is being expressed and their efforts are leading towards less anger to be expressed in the moment.

If there are not places as described that will provide space to break objects, search through your kitchen and find some plates that would break easily that you can dispose of. You can place a sheet on a wall or place a few on the floor in a room as you clear the area where you can throw your plates to break them. A few strong sheets may be needed anyway to help gather and throw out broken pieces of glass.

Exercise

Focusing on an activity such as exercise can help channel your anger around an activity as you work to express yourself. Gradual, controlled movements are best to help a person express themselves while staying grounded. Aerobic exercises such as walking or jogging, are great due to the consistent repetition and ability to simplify while processing what may have caused or triggered your anger.

Breathing

You will want to breathe in slowly and deeply through the nostrils and release through the mouth. This ways of inhaling and exhaling prevents any air from getting "caught" within this process. It is recommended to make some noise (whatever comes most natural to you) when exhaling through the mouth. Release any locked tension and work to release any anger on the surface as you dig a bit deeper with every breath. Breathing is a very crucial piece to the emotional well-being of a person which can be stabilized through deep breathing exercises.

Valerian, Chamomile, and Passionflower (herbs)

These herbs are known for helping relax the body by promoting calmer feelings and lowering stress. Supporting your mood is a great proactive approach for those working to better cope and/or reduce/avoid their anger and contributing factors. Take 2 teaspoons of any of these herbs to drink in tea form twice a day. It can serve you well to make drinking at least one cup of tea once a day to help set your intention for the day or relax the body before you get moving. Any of these teas mentioned can help induce sleep when consumed at night as well which can help to further relax the body and the mind to help balance your emotions.

Commit To Not Expressing Your Anger Onto Others (it belongs to you)

Our main supports often want to alleviate our symptoms as much as possible, but not too often are they equipped with the tools that are most helpful. We may often be challenged by others, and it can be difficult to accurately identify what to do in the moment when we are asked by someone else. This creates a high risk of acting out our anger elsewhere, making things worse, or potentially ruining a good friendship or relationship. Not that dealing with anger has to always be dealt with in private, but expressing your anger onto others can be unwarranted and also not well received. It is best to have identified outlet for expressing your anger, where you may disclose to a close friend or support ways you can continue to troubleshoot what may be helpful. Having this approach instead changes your dialogue from identifying problems you may not know the answers to, to identifying potential solutions to consider.

Individual or group therapy is strongly encouraged for having an outlet for verbally expressing your anger in a controlled setting with a professional who often has the therapeutic tools that can remain supportive as you work through these challenges.

Cognitive Behavioral Therapy (CBT)

CBT is a therapeutic approach where clients learn to do the following:

- Cope better with difficult life situations
- Positively resolve conflicts in relationships
- Deal with grief more effectively
- Mentally handle emotional stress caused by illness, abuse or physical trauma
- Overcome chronic pain, fatigue and other physical symptoms

The specific steps in Cognitive Behavioral Therapy include:

- Identification of situations or circumstances in your life that lead to trouble
- Awareness of your thoughts and emotions surrounding anger triggers
- Acknowledgement of inaccurate, negative thought patterns
- Relearning of healthier, positive thought patterns

Very few risks are associated with cognitive behavioral therapy, and you will likely explore painful feelings and emotions, but you will do it in a safe, guided manner. Cognitive Behavioral Therapy (CBT) is considered a short-term approach and generally lasts about 10 to 20 sessions depending upon your specific disorder, the severity of your symptoms, the amount of time you've been dealing with anger symptoms, your rate of progress, your current stress levels, and the amount of support you receive from friends and family. Engaging in CBT will help work to take an assessment of the root of your anger to help it dissolve and re-wire your responses to typical triggers, resulting in decreased anger and anger expression.

Angina (Angina Pectoris)

Heart disease is one of the most common health issues in the world. Prior to the very well-known, *heart attack*, conditions like Angina are present. Angina occurs in the body when the heart does not receive enough blood and oxygen. The heart not getting enough blood and oxygen will present an immense amount of pressure from your shoulder and arm to your neck, jaw, and parts of your back. The pain tends to be more persistent in men, while women mostly in the chest and have shortness of breath.

This condition is often triggered by stress, emotional instability, heavy metals being present in the body, alcohol, cigarette smoking, extreme temperatures, and excessive physical exertion due to all of these placing a great demand on the heart's need for oxygen and blood (which is carried by oxygen). When the arteries around the heart are filled with plaque caused by mucus causing foods, this narrows the supply of blood and oxygen that can get to the heart. The level of pain if directly associated with the amount of plaque around the heart.

Medical doctors will work to implement prescriptions such as Nitroglycerin (brand name: Nitro-lingual) to treat this condition. This prescription only places a small band aid on a massive wound. It does not get to the core of the issue which is <u>plaque</u>. Removing foods which are mucus forming while consuming certain foods which promote blood flow are essential towards treating this condition. If you were to have an Angina attack the prescription medication coenzyme Q10 (coQ10) will be distributed to you. This prescription presents the chemical version of the Q10 that's located within every cell in the body that work to remain a power charge for each cell, particularly the heart muscle. Those who take coQ10 drastically reduce their need for Nitroglycerin medication. Now, you do not want to simply swap one medication for another when you can address this condition at its core by cleaning up plaque around the heart within the body, but you do want to receive what is helpful if an attack were to present itself so that you can recover while getting started on healing from this condition. A daily dose of 90 to 180 milligrams of coQ10 is typically recommended.

Remedies:

EDTA (ethylenediaminetetraacetic) Chelation Therapy

Rather than the very risky (and very expensive) coronary bypass surgery, Chelation Therapy provides ethylenediaminetetraacetic acid (a natural amino acid-like molecule in the body) which binds with and works to remove excess heavy metals and break down plaque from the arteries. Unstable oxygen molecules set the foundation for all coronary artery conditions. Heavy metals trigger the symptoms. Removing heavy metals, in turn, removes the triggers of the symptoms and allows a person to work through healing from this condition without interference (as long as they are making necessary dietary adjustments). Chelation treatments are administered two to three times a week and last about 3 hours long. Treatments continue for a total of 25 to 40 treatments. It is crucial to work with a doctor who has experience with Chelation Therapy. The premise of Chelation Therapy is spot on as it targets the bloodstream, however, doctors do this by injection. Following the guidance of a Holistic Herbalism, Healer, or Nutrition Practitioner can provide an alternative to this form of therapy by introducing natural methods to address the internal issues of removing heavy metals via the within the bloodstream, along with dietary recommendations for removing plaque and toxins from the system.

Working with the condition of Angina presents a vicious cycle of ailments. The heart functions off of creating energy from (healthy) fats. But when the heart is deprived of oxygen it cannot carry blood to the designated area. When a stronger blood flow is achieved, the heart will tend to burn sugar (glucose) for energy until it receives a regular supply of oxygen again. When this happens, the body creates lactic acid build up from waste materials due to the heart working overtime, and then presents the same symptoms of Angina.

What needs to take place is for the body to receive what is needed, but also for the body to recognize it is there. When the heart is working excessively, it may not process what's there (yes, even blood or oxygen) and miss out on the opportunity to absorb them and remain deprived.

Tocopherol (Vitamin-E)

What we refer to as Vitamin E (tocopherol) is actually a fat-soluble nutrient that is important to vision, reproduction, and the health of your blood, brain, and skin. This nutrient is found in abundance in bell peppers (particularly red bell peppers), walnuts, leafy green vegetables, mangos, and avocados. Working these into your lifestyle more often will allow the body to properly recognize and absorb key nutrients, especially blood and oxygen. "Vitamin-E" helps to increase the body's receptors and help stop the formation of blood clots.

Warm Showers And Baths

These help to dilate (open) the blood vessels and allow blood to flow easier. Opening up the passageways of blood circulation can help reduce repeated episodes of Angina. You do want to make sure your bathroom has a good exhaust fan or window to circulate the air well. Steam can reduce the amount of oxygen in the room and can make symptoms of Angina worse.

Clean The Colon

Reduce the additional work the body has to do. Doctors will often prescribe Magnesium-Citrate to serve as a laxative. The problem with taking a laxative is that it does not properly clean the colon as it just pushes out waste already located within the digestive tract that would be discharged later on. You want to allow the body to properly clean the colon by clearing out waste sitting in the colon and intestines. The average person has about 15-20 pounds of waste sitting in their colon. Many will suggest eating more fiber, but you don't want to ever overcome during this time period.

Natural Ways To Clean The Colon:

Herbal Tea Recipe (dried herbs)

- 1 tablespoon of Burdock Root
- 1 teaspoon of Rhubarb Root
- 1 teaspoon of Yellowdock

*Drink 1-2 cups of this tea daily for 5 days. Take 2 days off to track progress and repeat for about 1 month. This will not completely clean you colon but will set the foundation for keeping your colon clean as you make necessary dietary adjustments.

Tamarind Juice ("agua de tamarindo ")

(from 21 Day Liquid Fast, by Bryan McAskill)

- 15 dried tamarind pods
- 2 quarts water, divided
- 1/2 – 3/4 cup date sugar

Step 1: bring half the water to a boil in a large pot over high heat.

Step 2: While you are waiting for the water to boil, prepare the tamarind pods. Remove the brittle outer shell and pull off as many strings as you can. Discard the shell and strings.

Step 3: After the water comes to a rolling boil, remove it from the heat and place the inner portion of the tamarind and the sugar in the water. Let the tamarind soak for about 1 hour and 30 minutes.

Step 4: At this point, the water will have cooled down. Use your fingers to squeeze out the hard tamarind seeds and remove the remaining strings; discard them.

Step 5: Place the liquid and remaining pulp in a blender and process until the pulp is fully blended into the water.

Step 6: Run the liquid through a strainer

Step 7: Pour your delicious agua de tamarindo into a pitcher, add the rest of the water, and refrigerate until cold.

Delete The Meat

Pretty much everyone can have their own opinions on this as both side of the argument to consume or not consume meat as supported by science (just depends on which view of science you are viewing from). What must be understood is that all animals flesh takes several hours just to digest. This places an incredible burden on the digestive tract, the organs, and the blood. It is strongly encouraged to search up any benefits you may be getting from meat and look elsewhere for additional options. A well-balanced diet (this is, a diet where you are getting an assortment of essential minerals and hydration) will provide you with this. Consuming fruits daily, hydrating with water, and cooking an assortment of vegetables while also consuming grains and nuts will provide you with what you need.

Doctors will advise you to avoid foods high in cholesterol, but this is the "bad" cholesterol they are referring to, which only comes from animal products; the "good" cholesterol comes from our liver. So, removing meat from your lifestyle (at least during this time when working to heal) will serve you well of completing this step of reducing your cholesterol consumption.

Exercise (later in the day)

As much as we want to encourage daily exercise first thing upon awakening, this is to be approached with caution when dealing with Angina. The "fight or flight" hormones in the body (cortisol and norepinephrine) increase overnight and peak in the daytime. When this occurs, it can lead to the body providing a brief "spark" of energy which can send the heart overboard and worsen symptoms. No sprinting or heavy lifting first thing in the morning. Do these exercises later in the day when hormones decrease.

Eat Lightly

Developing a Fasting regimen may seem too extreme but may be necessary for long-term health. A way to work towards developing a regular Fasting routine is to eat lightly. Do not have large meals or overconsume more than needed. Only eat when appetite is there; do not eat just based on what time of the day it is when you typically eat. Provide the inner workings of your body with a much-needed break and allow any excess waste to move its way out before consuming something.

Avoid Smoke

This should go without saying but smoking will only contribute to many of the symptoms that remain present with Angina. Even second-hand smoke can trigger or worsen symptoms after exposure. If you smoke or are regularly around those who smoke, this would be a good time to make some necessary adjustments with where you spend your time and working to reduce any habit you may have acquired over time in your life.

Provide Some Stillness Into Your Life

Emotional stress is one of the primary triggers for those with Angina. Working in more breathing exercises, meditation, or light yoga, can provide an outlet conducive to relieving things such as tension and anxiety which make the demand for blood and oxygen levels increase and can make Angina worse.

Ankle Sprain

An ankle sprain is when the ligaments and connective tissues are stretched out further than they want to go. To recover, excess inflammation surrounds these areas so that they can reduce their chances of being irritated and can focus on healing.

What we typically do for an ankle sprain (or any type of sprain) and work immediately on reducing the inflammation (swelling) by applying a variety of cold and warm solutions. We place ice packs on it followed by a heat pad or warm towel. This may contribute to reducing the inflammation around the injury, but then the injury itself is exposed and left to heal on its own. We then believe that once we can move around alright with minimal pain due to adjusting to out pain tolerance, that out injury is "healed", and we can go back to our normal routine. This is how injuries linger on. These old remedies only put a band-aid on a more serious injury.

The body naturally produces the inflammation when injured as a response that there is support needed. This inflammation is not essentially the very same substance that is produced from consuming foods that create excess mucus/inflammation. This form of inflammation that surrounds injuries is a type of substance that breaks down into white blood cells that surround the injury. This is why our appetite usually diminishes whenever we have an injury due to white blood cells being responsible for detecting injuries, disease, and harmful bacteria. As the body shifts it focus to these more often, there is less attention given to appetite so the body can work on healing itself.

The main thing we don't want to do is immediately remove the inflammation/white blood cells from an injured area as it is there to help provide protection. You want your injury to have additional layers of protection. Putting ice followed by a warm towel or heated pad on an injury, sends a fabricated response to the body where it believes the injury is healed and sends the white blood cells to other areas in the body. We want to keep some sort of protection around our injury as we work to heal; even once we're active. What happens most often is we put on a brace or some sort of wrap as a support which does not effectively help long term, until someone like an athlete can train to repair in their off-season. We should not have to wait until an off-season or until we make time to train on healing our injuries. We can focus on meeting their needs by slowly alleviating the support that is there over time to help heal.

Remedies:

R.I.C.E. Method

R.I.C.E. stands for, Rest, Ice, Compression, and Elevation. These four steps can be helpful to reducing the main challenges when it comes to a sprained ankle.

1. Rest – this step is simply resting the affected area by limiting its movement from physical activity.

2. Ice – this step involves a plan for how to apply ice effectively. You begin by applying ice to the area for about 15-20 minutes, then allow the skin to warm itself for about 15 minutes, and then you reapply the ice. You do this about every 3-hours while awake. Although we do not want to rely upon ice, applying ice will help signal the body when to stop sending white blood cells to the area. If we immediately do not ice and do not apply any other method, the swelling may be more than what is needed and take longer to heal.

3. Compression – applying some sort of pressure will also stop fluid from making its way to the affected area. Blood flow can function as normal and can help push out any accumulation of waste from the injured area. This step goes along with the previous step as you are applying pressure by wrapping an Ace Bandage or some elastic wrap over the ice, so the entire area is covered. You want to not wrap too tight or too loose to not disrupt blood flow.

4. Elevation – you want to keep the injured area elevated so that the blood flow is not as strong so that waste and/or excess fluids do not make their way into the affected area. For lower body injuries, it is recommended to keep elevation above the height of the hip (ex. sitting down with an ankle injury, foot should be elevated above the area where the hip is). For upper body injures, it is recommended to keep elevation above the heart.

Urine Wrap and Soak

A helpful remedy to help alleviate swelling, but not sending the white blood cells away, is a form of Urine Therapy. Filling up a plastic bag (same bag you would ordinarily use for ice) with your own urine and wrapping it around your ankle will help apply heat and pressure but contain many minerals where the body can detect them and know how many white blood cells are needed. Our urine is intelligent. It contains many vital minerals and parts of our DNA which can communicate more with our injury than a bag of ice or a heated towel can.

After the warmth of the urine wears off, you can choose to soak the affected area in your urine as well. You can start by pouring some onto a small towel and allowing to soak while elevated. You want to place a small collection pan or tray for any liquid that may run off just as you would when soaking a towel with water. As your swelling decreases and you become active again, it is recommended to continue to soak your previously injured area(s) in your urine after training or any strenuous exercise.

Arnica Cream

Make your own Arnica Salve to apply to area. If you know an herbalist, you should be able to find Arnica Salve to purchase to use during this time.

My Personal Arnica Salve Recipe:

1. You need to infuse your carrier oil with Arnica and St. John's Wort herbs. Place your dried herbs in a sterile (boil before using) glass jar. I use 1 cup of Arnica and 2 tablespoons of St. John's Wort.

2. Next, add the carrier oils. I use 1 cup of olive oil and 1 cup of coconut oil.

3. Now you will need to infuse the oil. There are several ways to infuse oils with herbs.

   • Solar Infusion Method: this is considered to be the best method. To solar infuse your oil, simply place your jar of oil and herbs in the sun for at least 4 weeks. Swoosh the jar occasionally. This makes the best oil but clearly takes much time to complete.

   • Slow Cooker Method: to use a slow cooker, place a towel in the bottom of your slow cooker and set you jar of oils and herbs in it. Fill the cooker halfway with water and set to warm or low for 8-10 hours. Gently swoosh the jar occasionally until finished.

   • Double Boiler Method: to use the double boiler method, place your jar of oil and herbs into a pot filled with water. Warm the jar over low heat for at least an hour. Then lower the heat (the longer the time the better). Gently swoosh around the jar every 10 minutes or so.

4. Once your oil is infused with the Arnica and St. John's Wort, it is time to strain the herbs out of the oil. I place a metal strainer with unbleached mullein cloths on top of s glass dish, then pour the oils and herbs onto it.

5. Allow the oils to drain through the herbs and cloths, dripping into the container. Don't be impatient during this step. It will take time.

6. Typically, I end up with about 1 1/2 cups of infused oil.

7. Most will add an essential oil but feel free to skip this step for now. It is now more important to pour the oil into your storage container(s). I use glass jars but some prefer plastic or tin. The oil will be hot, so proceed with caution.

8. Allow the jars to cool. It will form into a nice salve rather quickly.

9. Apply the cooled salve to affected area and rub in gently. Wash off after a few hours to avoid any contamination.

Anxiety

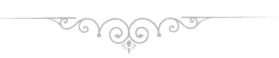

Shortness of breath, worrying, feeling restless, sweating, and difficulty remaining focused are the most common signs of anxiety showing itself. How anxiety is typically treated is by trying to work around these issues. The difficulty that comes with anxiety is that it will be on display in almost any setting at almost any time. This is difficult to plan for, which then makes a person feel more anxious.

The primary treatment provided for Anxiety are medication such as Xanax (alprazolam) and Valium (diazepam); both of which are tranquilizers. They aim to stunt the growth of a person's symptoms. Although this may appear helpful, using tranquilizers are addictive. They can create dependence early on upon use and re-create the same challenges when these medications are not present and available. Your brain and body can develop a strong dependence on tranquilizers within just a few weeks. Relying on tranquilizers interferes with a person being able to engage in activities that are truly helpful.

With Anxiety present for a long time being untreated, we literally train ourselves to worry until it becomes a habit in which we feel vulnerable (worry) if we are not worrying. This vicious cycle plagues many when there are not skills being taught or habits being reformed. Those who have been diagnosed with Anxiety (by displaying symptoms for more than 6 months) tend to be very intuitive, great listeners, and very sympathetic, according to Dr. Drummond, M.D., associate medical director of the Seacoast Mental Health Center in Portsmouth, New Hampshire, USA.

When Anxiety is present, the excessive worrying and restlessness causes the blood to feel restricted (along with breathing) which creates magnesium deficiency and low CO2 (carbon-dioxide) levels. Magnesium is responsible for regulating the nerves in the body (among other responsibilities). Whenever you are low on magnesium, the response your body will give will mimic many of the symptoms attributed to anxiety, as well as trigger symptoms for those already diagnosed with Anxiety.

Anxiety as a whole, mimics stress. What must be understood is that stress expressed as anger creates sale within the body. A nucleus of an atom can only hold 2 electrons in the 1st valance (outer layer) and 8 in the remainder valences. When we get upset or frustrated (heat rises) this causes the sodium (Na) molecule to throw electrons off. This makes it unstable and causes it to create a bond with whatever is compatible with it in its' current state (this is called "Covalent Bonding"). In this case, the sodium (Na) molecule is now compatible with chloride (Cl) because chloride produces "free" electrons to the body which the sodium molecule is looking to replace. Chloride maintains metabolism and energizes the cells.

Now you have Na + Cl which is NaCl, which creates Sodium Chloride aka "salt".

We can eat right but if we're around people who get us upset or situations that make us upset, we'll continue to accumulate salt within the body. These people and situations will create the same thing we're looking to escape from. Salt is a crystal. All crystals serve as conduits for healing (good energy in, bad energy out). Salt however, especially coupled with an unhealthy environment (the body), will cause the body to remain negative and only be capable of projecting negatives words, feelings, or behaviors. In a more positively functioning environment/body, stress turns into motivation and positive movement expression. This is why eating right (in my opinion) helps support further positivity and improvement.

Remedies:

Magnesium

Magnesium deficiency can be directly met through what a person consumes. Low CO_2 levels are a bit more complicated as we have to create an environment that is conducive to breathing, while keeping this area of the body (respiratory system) clear in addition to the blood flow being positive so that it can properly absorb the oxygen being produced by the CO_2 (carbon dioxide) within the body.

Magnesium deficiency often leads to:

- insomnia
- body aches
- leg cramps
- osteoporosis
- migraines

Common Foods and Spices High In Magnesium: Avocado, Chickpeas, Bananas, Pumpkin Seeds, Butternut Squash, Kale, Green Beans, Lettuce, Arugula, Cucumber, Tomatoes, Dates, Figs, Collard Greens, Chives, Walnuts, Kelp, Sesame Seeds, Dandelion Greens, Sunflower Seeds, Quinoa, Millet, Parsley, Tamarind, Basil, Dill, Ginger, Oregano, Thyme

Also any CBD (cannabidiol) products are helpful. CBD Oils are almost pure magnesium.

To test the purity of a CBD Oil, send to a lab for testing or you should feel a steady decline in needing to rely on this substance after your need has been met regularly.

Common Medicinal Herbs good for Magnesium:

Nettle leaf, Horsetail, Red Clover, Sage, Nopal

Breathing Exercises:

(Some of these are adapted from James Nestor's Book *Breathe: A New Science Of A Lost Art*)

30 Nostril Breathes

For this exercise, you will simply take a total of 30 breathes by breathing in and out only using the nostrils 30 times. Focus on increasing how deep your breath gets during this exercise to avoid feeling light-headed or dizzy.

If you do begin feeling light-headed or dizzy at any time, you may stop this exercise and hydrate by drinking water to help recover.

If you need a visual aid, feel free to look at each number as you inhale and exhale until you are completed with this exercise

1 2 3 4 5 6 7 8 9 10 11 12 13 14 15 16 17 18 19 20 21 22 23 24 25 26 27 28 29 30

Pursed Lip Breathing

This simple breathing technique makes you slow down your pace of breathing by having you apply deliberate effort in each breath. You can practice pursed lip breathing at any time.

How To Do This Exercise:

- Relax your neck and shoulders.
- Keeping your mouth closed, inhale slowly through your nose for 2 counts.
- Pucker or purse your lips as though you were going to whistle.
- Exhale slowly by blowing air through your pursed lips for a count of 4.

Alternate Nostril Breathing

Alternate nostril breathing is a yogic breath control practice. In Sanskrit, it is known as *nadi shodhana pranayama*. This translates as "subtle energy clearing breathing technique."

This exercise works to lower stress, symptoms of anxiety, increase CO_2 (Carbon-Dioxide) absorption within the body, and can improve cardiovascular health.

You can practice alternate nostril breathing on your own, but you may want to ask a yoga teacher to show you the practice in person so you can make sure you're doing it correctly.

Focus on keeping your breath slow, smooth, and continuous to help you to remember where you are in the cycle.

How To Do This Exercise:

- Sit in a comfortable position with your legs crossed.

- Place your left hand on your left knee.

- Lift your right hand up toward your nose.

- Exhale completely and then use your right thumb to close your right nostril.

- Inhale through your left nostril and then close the left nostril with your fingers.

- Open the right nostril and exhale through this side.

- Inhale through the right nostril and then close this nostril.

- Open the left nostril and exhale through the left side.

- This is one cycle.

- Continue for up to 5 minutes.

- Always complete the practice by finishing with an exhale on the left side.

Diaphragmatic Breathing (#1)

Belly breathing can help you use your diaphragm properly. Do belly breathing exercises when you are feeling relaxed and rested. Practice diaphragmatic breathing for 5 to 10 minutes 3 to 4 times per day. When you begin you may feel tired, but over time the technique should become easier and should feel more natural.

How To Do This Exercise:

- Lie on your back with your knees slightly bent and your head on a pillow. You may place a pillow under your knees for support.

- Place one hand on your upper chest and one hand below your rib cage, allowing you to feel the movement of your diaphragm.

- Slowly inhale through your nose, feeling your stomach pressing into your hand. Keep your other hand as still as possible.

- Exhale using pursed lips as you tighten your stomach muscles, keeping your upper hand completely still. You can place a book on your abdomen to make the exercise more difficult. Once you learn how to do belly breathing lying down you can increase the difficulty by trying it while sitting in a chair. You can then practice the technique while performing your daily activities.

Diaphragmatic Breathing (#2)

(Adapted from Dr. Elke Zuercher-White, Ph.D., psychologist)

Phase 1:

- Lie on your back on a bed or carpeted floor. Place one or two pillows on your stomach. Watch the tops of the pillows from the corner of your eye. As you breathe in, your diaphragm should expand, raising the pillows upward. and when you breathe out, the pillows should move down again.

Phase 2:

- Lie on your back without the pillows and put one hand over your navel. Look at the ceiling or close your eyes as you take deep, controlled breaths. With your hand, feel your stomach move up and down.

Phase 3:

- Repeat phase 2, but now focus your attention on your diaphragm and feel it move up and down. Essentially "become one" with your breathing.

Phase 4:

- Sit upright on a sofa or couch, leaning back so that you can watch your stomach area. Watch your diaphragm move up as you breathe in and down as you breathe out.

Phase 5:

- Sitting up straight, repeat phase 4 but with better posture as you should begin to get more comfortable. Make sure your upper chest and shoulders are still.

Phase 6:

- While standing upright, repeat phase 5.

Breath Focus Technique

This deep breathing technique uses imagery or focus words and phrases. You can choose a focus word that makes you smile, feel relaxed, or that is simply neutral to think about. Examples include peace, let go, or relax, but it can be any word that suits you to focus on and repeat through your practice. As you build up your breath focus practice you can start with a 10-minute session. Gradually increase the duration until your sessions are at least 20 minutes.

How To Do This Exercise:

- Sit or lie down in a comfortable place. Bring your awareness to your breaths without trying to change how you are breathing. Alternate between normal and deep breaths a few times. Notice any differences between normal breathing and deep breathing. Notice how your abdomen expands with deep inhalations. Note how shallow breathing feels compared to deep breathing. Practice your deep breathing for a few minutes.

- Place one hand below your belly button, keeping your belly relaxed, and notice how it rises with each inhale and falls with each exhale.

- Let out a loud sigh with each exhale.

- Begin the practice of breath focus by combining this deep breathing with imagery and a focus word or phrase that will support relaxation. You can imagine that the air you inhale brings waves of peace and calm throughout your body. Mentally say, "Inhaling peace and calm." Imagine that the air you exhale washes away tension and anxiety. You can say to yourself, "Exhaling tension and anxiety."

4-7-8 Breath

The 4-7-8 breathing technique, also known as "relaxing breath," involves breathing in for 4 seconds, holding the breath for 7 seconds, and exhaling for 8 seconds.

This breathing pattern aims to reduce anxiety or help people get to sleep. The 4-7-8 breathing technique requires a person to focus on taking a long, deep breath in and out. Rhythmic breathing is a core part of many meditation and yoga practices as it promotes relaxation. Dr. Andrew Weil teaches the 4-7-8 breathing technique, which he believes can help with the following:

Reducing Anxiety

Helping a person get to sleep

Managing Cravings

Controlling or reducing anger responses

Dr. Weil is a celebrity doctor and the founder and director of the University of Arizona Center for Integrative Medicine.

How To Do This Exercise:

- Before starting the breathing pattern, adopt a comfortable sitting position.

- To use the 4-7-8 technique, focus on the following breathing pattern: empty the lungs of air

- Breathe in quietly through the nose for 4 seconds
- Hold the breath for a count of 7 seconds
- Exhale forcefully through the mouth, pursing the lips and making a "whoosh" sound, for 8 seconds
- Repeat the cycle up to 4 times

Lion's Breath

Lion's breath is an energizing yoga breathing practice that is said to relieve tension in your chest and face. It is also known in yoga as Lion's Pose or simhasana in Sanskrit.

How To Do This Exercise:

- Come into a comfortable seated position. You can sit back on your heels or cross your legs.
- Press your palms against your knees with your fingers spread wide. Inhale deeply through your nose and open your eyes wide. At the same time, open your mouth wide and stick out your tongue, bringing the tip down toward your chin.
- Contract the muscles at the front of your throat as you exhale out through your mouth by making a long "ha" sound. You can turn your gaze to look at the space between your eyebrows or the tip of your nose.
- Do this breath 2 to 3 times in a row a few times.

Resonant or Coherent Heart Breathing

Resonant breathing, also known as Coherent Breathing, is when you breathe at a rate of about 5 full breaths per minute. You can achieve this rate by inhaling and exhaling for a count of 5. Breathing at this rate maximizes your heart rate variability (HRV), reduces stress, and, according to one 2017 study, can reduce symptoms of depression when combined with Iyengar yoga.

How To Do This Exercise:

- Inhale for a count of 5.
- Exhale for a count of 5.
- Continue this breathing pattern for at least a few minutes.

Additional Remedies To Help Reduce Symptoms:

Take Your Space

Go to (or create) a space designated for you to relax. Include colors and textures that you enjoy the most and leave room for open space so that you can allow air to flow. Place images or pictures that help you feel more positive and optimistic. Add anything that helps promote a calmer mind and a calmer body to reduce anxiety-provoking thoughts or feelings of tension that are not detrimental to your health.

Practice Your Relaxation Techniques

Taking time to practice your relaxation techniques when you're not triggered helps the body build repetition. We often have skills that we know of and reminders to set, but when we don't practice them regularly, it becomes difficult to apply these skills and use them effectively. Then we begin to worry about our ability to work through these challenges and promote the same signs and symptoms of Anxiety that we are trying to avoid.

Meditation

The practice of meditation allows one to clear their mind and relax while controlling their breathing. Some find it helpful to create a "blank slate" and not think of anything, while others simply try to observe their thoughts as they pass by as they work to remain still. Guided meditation can provide additional relief as you can be guided by another person without the pressure of meditating "correctly".

Make Contact With Others

Feeling connected help to reduce Anxiety. Although public places can trigger Anxiety, it can be helpful to go to a restaurant, park, or event to help be around others even if you do not communicate with anyone. Having even small, brief encounters with others can drastically help reduce your symptoms as well.

Become More Realistic (Get The Facts)

We tend to worry when we have to figure something out or remain unsure about something. Start by decreasing your worrying by becoming a bit more logical and search for information you want to know. You do not have to reach any predetermined "finish line" or become an expert. Just try to dismantle some of what you may be wondering about. A practice to remain optimistic is with any question you have that you can provide clarity to, you can view this as being 1% closer to becoming less worried.

Reduce The Stimulation

Cut out any noises you can, turn off the phone and/or TV, and move further away from any outside noises. All noises around us get our attention on some level. Reducing or eliminating many of these noises allows us to focus on other things much easier and feel calmer as we are less stimulated.

Write Things Down

When you write things down, you don't have to think about them as much. Journaling or just writing down can help you begin to dissolve those racing thoughts that have been on your mind all day.

Create Plan To Go To Sleep

We must give ourselves time to relax. We do not just stop everything all at once. Creating a plan can help your body settle in and prepare for extended rest. Put aside any tasks you have to complete and clear out time to "add less stress" to your day. We often achieve more success when we plan for something. Planning a bedtime routine for yourself (and your family) can be essential with reducing your anxiety and feeling rested to start your next day.

Fast From Television

Besides being visually stimulated later at night which can make it difficult to sleep, new shows that are available can take up much of your personal time. The daily News stations can present an obstacle as they can add to your list of worries and concerns. Whether it's news about the traffic, weather, violence, or health emergency. Do away with this and prepare your daily routine ahead of time and plan to make any necessary adjustments as needed.

Find Something To Laugh At

Laughter can help defuse any danger or excessive worrying. If you can find a way to laugh an anything that may be causing you distress, this can be helpful to claim some power of what may have you worried or concerned. Try to think ahead and ask yourself if you will laugh at this situation in the future.

Cut Out The Caffeine

"Nothing is worse for anxiety than caffeine" says Bernard Vittone, M.D., psychiatrist and founder of the National Center for the Treatment of Phobias, Anxiety, and Depression in Washington, D.C., USA. Coffee, soda, chocolates, and medication such as Excedrin are all caffeine stimulants which impact the neurotransmitters in the brain. If you thought anxiety was tough to manage before, adding caffeine stimulants is the equivalent to adding a tornado to a snowstorm you are trying to escape from. Do what you can to remove this additional barrier. Work in replacements such as herbal tea instead of coffee in the morning (mix roasted Dandelion Root with Black Walnut Hull and Blessed Thistle for a natural stimulant with a similar taste). Swap out your sodas for fruit smoothies to give you a natural energy boost with no crashing. And work in more fruits to snack on instead of chocolate, especially in the evening.

If you consume a lot of coffee and don't believe it is impacting your anxiety, try this:

- Abstain from consuming coffee (and hopefully other caffeine products) for 5-7 days. Then proceed to drink 2-3 cups in one sitting and observe how you're feeling. You will notice tightening of muscles, restlessness and become more worried.

Avoid Alcohol

Alcohol is a stimulant. Upon initial ingestion you feel relaxed, but then you can become more worries and restless.

Individual and/or Group Therapy

Therapy is a safe space to process your thoughts objectively. Being able to collaborate with a professional on self-reflection, identifying and practicing useful skills, while working to alleviate signs and symptoms is a crucial piece towards overcoming your Anxiety. Simply talking with friends and family is not the same as engaging in therapy. Therapists will present resources, an unbiased opinion, and challenge you to review what is helpful and what is not. Therapists will not just tell you what you want to hear, but understand their role in providing help and guidance. The tools a Therapist can provide will help you narrow down your focus and have a designated time and place for when you will work on dissolving signs and symptoms of Anxiety. Having a predetermined time and space to work on your skills will help reduce many symptoms by itself as you can plan ahead and prepare yourself before each session.

How To Choose A Therapist When You Have Anxiety

Ask Yourself The Following:

• Do I feel safe and at ease upon meeting this person?

• Do they have a sense of humor?

• Are they treating me with respect and dignity?

• Are they willing to explain their strategies, goals, and treatment with me?

• Are they non defensive and kind?

• Can they understand my background and cultural heritage? If so, how?

• Am I treated like an equal?

- Do I feel safe disclosing my innermost feeling and thoughts to this person?
- Am I able to receive homework in between sessions to continue to work on my treatment goals and objectives?

Clean The Liver

The liver sends out the good cholesterol our body needs. When the body is overworked, the liver becomes backed up and cannot send out toxins. Most toxins are filled with chemicals which end up in the bloodstream and can immediately trigger symptoms and impact neurotransmitters in the brain (i.e. "send mixed signals). The liver is one of the primary detoxifying organs in the body. Keeping this organ clean will help to remove many of the chemicals and excess waste we do not need in our body.

Tips on how to clean the liver:

Herbal Teas:

1. The herb called Palo Azul is very helpful for cleaning the liver and breaking down toxins.

   (How To Prepare: take 1 large piece or 2-3 medium sized pieces of this herb and place them in a boiling pot of water for approx. 60 minutes. Strain out the herbs and drink 1 cup a day for about 24-30 days).

2. As mentioned above as a coffee replacement, mixing Roasted Dandelion Root, Black Walnut Hull, and Blessed Thistle, can serve as a natural detoxifier which can help provide some relief for the liver.

   (How To Prepare: take 1-2 cups of each herb and mix well together in a bowl or container. Boil water while placing about 1 tablespoon of mixture into a cup and pour boiling water into cup. Let sit for about 10 minutes and then strain out the herbs. You can drink hot or let cool off and add ice for an "Iced coffee". Store herbs in a zip lock bag or container and you can let your drink sit in the fridge overnight as well.

3. Liver Detox Tea
   - Ingredients: Burdock Root, Sarsaparilla, and Yellow Dock. About 750mg/each (about ¼ teaspoon each herb in powder form per 8oz water). Dosage changes for dried herb to about twice this amount at least.
   - Burdock Root helps promote urinary tract health and healthy liver function. Promotes clear, healthy skin.
   - Sarsaparilla contains biochemicals called saponins that may promote clear, healthy skin.
   - Yellow Dock is classified as a bitter herb that helps promote digestion. High in iron.

Remove Artificial Foods

Processed foods, carbonated drinks, candies, and so forth, weight down the Liver and provide an additional workload to its schedule. When the Liver is overworked, it can neglect to detoxify any or all these substances which is mostly the case when these are consumed regularly.

Valerian Root (herb)

This herb can be used for best results. Taking 150-300 milligrams of this herb can help the nerves relax in the body, promote stillness, help you fall asleep faster and improve sleep quality.

Common Herbal Teas

Try making some tea to relax. Not only does the warmth of the tea help relax the blood vessels, but there are also many herbs that provide a calming effect on your nerves, thoughts, uneasiness, and your body as a whole to help reduce symptoms of anxiety. Herbs to incorporate can include: lavender, valerian, chamomile, hops, lemon balm, and passionflower. Make sure to get these herbs in their natural state or dried form for best results. Avoid commercialized brand-name products as there are often many chemicals included.

To Make Tea:

- Take 1-2 teaspoons of any herb mentioned above and place into cup.
- Boil a few cups of water.
- Pour boiling water into cup of herbs and let steep for about 10-15-minutes.
- Strain herbs and enjoy.
- Aim to drink some tea at least once a day but you can drink any of the herbs listed in this section twice a day.

Psychedelics (caution)

There are various forms of psychedelics which range from mushrooms which contain psilocybin which is the compound found in "magic mushrooms", to *mescaline* which is the active compound in the peyote cactus which is known to produce psychedelic effects. There is still much research to be conducted on psychedelics, so you want to do so under guidance of a shaman or experiences healer. There is evidence of psychedelics working to encourage the growth of new connections between neurons in the brain. This ability of the brain to make new connections is called *plasticity*. Brain plasticity involves the ability of the nervous system to change its activity in response to intrinsic or extrinsic stimuli by reorganizing its structure, functions, or connections, which impact how the brain functions and responds during challenges such as mental health. States such as Oregon and Colorado have allowed psychedelics to be use medically under assisted adult use, where other states such as California, Michigan, Minnesota, Washington, and Massachusetts, have several cities where psychedelics are decriminalized under possession.

Arrythmia

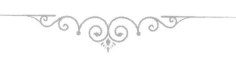

When the heart skips a beat (irregular heartbeat) due to stress, this can create the condition known as "Arrythmia". Medical doctors will attempt to prescribe drugs that will work to calm the heart (beta-blocker) or a calcium channel blocker to attempt to regulate your body's heartbeat. "I believe the allopathic, medicine-based approach to curing benign arrythmia is often ineffective" says Seth Baum, M.D., an integrative cardiologist and founder of the Baum Center for Integrative Heart Care in Boca, Raton, Florida, USA.

Remedies:

Yoga

Stress being the main culprit in the development of Arrythmia, it only makes sense to do stress-reducing activities such as Yoga. Although a full Yoga routine of class can seem demanding, starting off with basic poses can be helpful. A pose such as the "Dead Pose" is simple enough to do daily. To do this pose all you have to do is lie on your back on any comfortable but flat surface. Place your arms by your sides, palms facing up, and breathe easily while keeping your focus on your breath. Whenever you begin thinking about something else, bring your mind back to your breath. Try this for about five minutes a day and/or whenever you start to feel stress linger on.

Apply Pressure to Your Adrenal Glands (Qigong)

Whenever you stimulate the adrenal glands in the body (which are responsible for regulating blood pressure as well as the body's response to stress) it will create awareness for the body to adequately address its needs involving blood pressure, stress, metabolism, and the immune system among other things. Whenever you are stressed, the adrenal glands pump out hormones they irritate and overstimulate the heart muscle where it begins to race, flutter, or skip a beat.

Start by making a closed fist with both hands and place them behind your back (knuckles facing your lower back). Your hands should be pressing against your lower back (right near your kidneys) just above your waist, but below the ribs. Slowly rub your hands against this area up and down until the area is warmer. Do this for about 2-3 minutes each time at least twice a day.

Quiet Down

Yelling and raising your voice can trigger stress and also work up the heart. You want to remain calm while working away from this condition. Spending time in silence but also remaining silent will be very beneficial for you. Take up a hobby such as reading to help keep you occupied without using your voice.

Magnesium

One primary needs the body calls for when Arrythmia is present is, Magnesium. Too little magnesium in the body does not allow the system to charge the muscles and nerves for optimum performance. Having enough magnesium in the body can help these areas remain charged and can directly calm the heart.

Common Foods and Spices High In Magnesium: Avocado, Chickpeas, Bananas, Pumpkin Seeds, Butternut Squash, Kale, Green Beans, Lettuce, Arugula, Cucumber, Tomatoes, Dates, Figs, Collard Greens, Chives, Walnuts, Kelp, Sesame Seeds, Dandelion Greens, Sunflower Seeds, Quinoa, Millet, Parsley, Tamarind, Basil, Dill, Ginger, Oregano, Thyme

Also, any CBD (cannabidiol) products are helpful. CBD Oils are almost pure magnesium.

To test the purity of a CBD Oil, send to a lab for testing or you should feel a steady decline in needing to rely on this substance after your need has been met regularly.

Common Medicinal Herbs good for Magnesium:

Nettle leaf, Horsetail, Red Clover, Sage, Nopal

Common Herbs To Help Combat Arrythmia:

Hawthorn (particularly its berries) help treat heart issues and blood vessels. Conditions such as Congestive Heart Failure (CHF), low and high blood pressure, high cholesterol. And atherosclerosis ("hardening of the arteries") can benefit from consuming this herb.

Suggested Dosage:

Brewed Tea (Leaves)

Three times daily after meals; 1 teaspoon of leaves and flowers/ 8 oz boiling water

- **Dried powder:** 300-1000 mg orally three times daily
- **Liquid extract:** 0.5-1 ml orally three times daily
- **Tincture:** 1-2 ml orally three times daily
- **Solid extract:** 1/4-1/2 teaspoon orally once/day
- **Syrup:** 1 teaspoon orally two to three times daily

Leaf/Flower

- **Extract:** 160-900 mg/d orally div two to three times daily
- **Powder:** 200-500 mg orally three times daily
- **Tincture:** 20 drops orally two to three times daily

Passionflower

There are about 500 known species of Passionflower. This extended family of plants are known as *Passiflora Incarnata*. This plant goes by many common names such as "Purple Passionflower" or "Marypop". This plant works to boost the level of Gamma-aminobutyric (GABA) in the brain which helps to decrease brin activity that promote relaxation and quality sleep.

Arthritis

The origin of "arthritis" is:
"Arthron" – joint "Itis" – inflammation

When the cartilage (cushion between the bones) begins to break down and inflammation is abundant in the body, the set the foundation for the condition known as, "Arthritis". There are more than 100 forms of this condition. When you break down and diminish its structure, symptoms begin to dissolve. The most common form of this condition are: 1. Osteoarthritis (when the cartilage in the joints begin to break down), and 2. Rheumatoid Arthritis (when the immune system misidentifies a part of the body as a foreign invader and attacks it).

The most common medications that are prescribed are: Aspirin, Ibuprofen, Indomethacin, and Aleve. These may alleviate symptoms in the moment, but in the long run, thy make the condition worse. Any relief will feel great, and the body will be receptive to it. The issue with short term relief is that the majority of the symptoms remain beneath the surface (untouched) and will settle deeper into the body until a drastic measure is needed such as surgery, or a complete overhaul of diet and lifestyle within a short period of time which can be extremely challenging for most. Extended reliance on medication that appear to provide short term relief creates other issues such as clogging up the digestive tract which can cause internal bleeding when trying to digest.

The cold temperatures freeze inflammation that's already present in the body and make moving around difficult, especially during the colder months. Inflammation around the bone joints and ligaments remain lubricated as long as there is regular movement. But once you are not active (typically at nighttime after daily tasks are complete) inflammation begins to get stagnant and hardens, which severely limits mobility. Simply not eating foods that cause inflammation can greatly reduce symptoms and difficulties of this condition.

Remedies:

Fasting

All forms of Fasting can help reduce inflammation within the body. besides expelling things like mucus, Fasting helps promote the elimination/detoxifying organs in the body to remove excess waste and contribute to the body locating and removing inflammation in the body and help alleviate many of the symptoms of Arthritis. You can learn much more about Fasting in my book entitled, *Fasting: A Guide To Health And Wellness*, which comes with descriptions of different forms of Fasting, recipes, and plans to stick to.

Cayenne Pepper On Everything!

Cayenne Pepper is a great expectorant. Going by my definition, when consuming an expectorant, you can EXPECT waste and mucus to be removed from the body. Going by the technical definition, you will simply be removing phlegm through the air passageways. Adding Cayenne Pepper to meals or sprinkling Cayenne Pepper Powder onto dishes filled with sauteed vegetables or grains such as Cayenne, or adding to fruits such as Mango are simple ways to work this into your diet to help remove any excess inflammation.

Common Foods and Herbs Most Helpful For Arthritis:

Sea Moss

Besides being abundant in many of the minerals we need to fulfill out cellular needs, Sea Moss is particularly high in potassium-chloride which help to break down inflammation.

White Willow Bark

A natural chemical known as "Salicin" serves as an anti-inflammatory which reduces pain within the nerves in the body and do away with much of the lingering pains from Arthritis.

Melons

Melons provide an abundance of hydration and anti-inflammatory properties that will help flood the body with what it needs to help remove the stiffness within the joints. It is recommended to partake in a 3-5 day Fast consisting of only melons. More advanced methods can involve going an entire month or several weeks only consuming melons and a select number of other fruits which will decrease inflammation in the body while providing direct relief to the bones and joints.

Berries

Specifically, blackberries, blueberries, and raspberries are all anti-inflammatory items that help break down inflammation which being very easy to digest.

Nopal and Prickly Pears

Besides reducing inflammation, the items decrease blood sugar and lower cholesterol; both of which contribute to hardening inflammation.

Kelp

This sea vegetable works to reduce inflammation at the cellular level. For this reason, it can help reduce any dire need for prescription "painkillers". If you are currently on any painkiller medications, Kelp can help reduce your symptoms and help to get you off these medications and can be taken daily.

Ginger

Helps reduce various pains and inflammation. Working in herbs such as Ginger (which can be taken in capsule form as well) help set daily reminders of your goal to reduce your symptoms while not adding anything that will contribute to or worsen your symptoms. One of Ginger's ingredients (gingerol) helps promote anti-inflammatory propertied you need to break down inflammation within the body.

Guggul ("Guggulu")

The herb is very powerful and healing for those with arthritis. Best to purchase a tincture of this herb where you can take ¼ teaspoon with 1/2 teaspoon of water about 30 minutes before every meal to provide relief. You do not want to rely on several meals a day while working to heal, but this mixture can be taken 3 times a day at the most. After about 1 month you should experience significant improvements. This herb works its way all the way to the bone while working to reduce stiffness and swelling.

Oils To Incorporate (or avoid)

The reason oils are very helpful are that they often contain the fatty acids that we are deficient in when experiencing symptoms of Arthritis or any joint or bone pains. Four specific fatty acids are to be focused on when a person has Arthritis. They are:

1. Alpha-linolenic Acid (LNA) Acid

2. Eicosatetraenoic Acid (EPA)

3. Docosahexaenoic Acid (DHA)

4. Gamma-linolenic Acid (GLA)

These four fatty acids not only help reduce inflammation, but they also help repair a weakened immune system that has been battling a disease and toxic environment for an extended period of time.

Maha Narayan Oil

The oil can be difficult to find in its purest form but has helped many (from personal experience). I have witnessed many with Arthritis apply this oil to their skin and experience immediate relief. Some have had arthritis for decades while others were recently diagnosed and had similar reports. This oil can be applied similar to a massage oil to your most sensitive areas as it works to provide relief around the joints of your bones.

Walnut Oil

Can be added lightly to vegetables and cooked meals. Provides fatty acids, healthy fats such as Omega-3 and offer powerful antioxidant properties. Helps improve memory and concentration as well.

Coconut Oil

This oil can be applied directly to the skin but also added to juices and smoothies. This oil provides a simple addition to your diet that is easy to work in you daily regimen.

Grapeseed and Avocado Oil (for cooking)

These oils are best for cooking as they are high in fatty acids and also digest easily without interruption. These oils do not often stick like most other oils and can be added to salads.

Canola Oil, Soy, and Vegetable Oils

These toxic substances provide zero nutritional benefits. Canola oil, soy, or "vegetable" oils do not digest well. These substances remain intact and create a very difficult task for the body to digest and search for any nutrients to hold into. Due to these substances remaining almost intact when digesting, they contribute to clogging up the intestinal walls and make digesting anything more difficult afterwards.

Breathing Techniques

("Hara Breathing")

Place your hand (palm facing down) right below your navel. Inhale slowly while expending your belly into your hand. Set your intention and practice visualizing your body adapting around your condition to make the condition less powerful. Practice this breathing exercise for a few minutes every day for best results of relaxing the body and soothing your joint and bone pain.

Acupressure

Exercise #1: Spine

The spine is the primary crossroad of all the meridians (pathways of energy in the body). when you increase the flow/energy within the spine, ease of pain can travel throughout the body.

Start by rolling a towel into a tube shape (preferably the length of your spine) and lay down on your bed, wooden board, or comfortable surface while the towel is underneath the right side of your spine. As you lay there, take slow, controlled breaths, and press down on a specific point on your hand ("S13") located right underneath the knuckle on your smallest finger. From this point, press upwards at a slight angle toward your ring (4th) finger. Press firm enough and repeat until you experience relief. Start with your right hand and then repeat with your left hand.

Note: Only lay down with towel under your back if you can lay down comfortably. If not, remove towel.

Exercise #2: Spine and Hips

Start by sitting upright in a chair. Then, let your head drop forward and bend until your shoulders meet with your knees or thighs. If you can only bend slightly forward do not go past discomfort. Also, if you feel dizzy, stop this exercise, hydrate and go back to sitting upright until your dizziness goes away. Breath deep into your navel while down (similar to the Hara Breathing mentioned earlier in this text) and work to release tension in the body in the spine and hips. Continue this exercise and work to stretch deeper until you can place your arms inside of your thighs and touch your ankles.

While down touching your ankles, take your thumb (or any finger that can reach) and press on point "K16") which is located about an inch below the peak of the anklebone on the inside part of each foot. Press down steadily for 4-5 breaths or as long as you feel comfortable. Then proceed to press down on the same location but pressure point located on the outside of the foot (point "BL62").

If you can, try reaching down and applying pressure to all four pressuring e points at the same time while also massaging around each area to provide relief.

Exercise #3: Fingers, Wrists, and Arms

Pressure point "TW5" can provide much relief to the areas surrounding the hands and arms. This pressure point is on the outside of the upper arm, about two inches from the wrist, and right in the middle of your arm between the two bones. Press firmly on this spot for about one to minutes.

Exercise #4: Feet and Toes

For relief in the feet and toes, you want to locate pressure point "GB41"). This is located between the fourth and fifth toe (your big toe is your first toe). Beginning at the web between these toes, press firmly between the toes directly on the bone towards the ankle. Press for about 1-2 minutes each side, one foot at a time, and repeat as needed until you notice relief.

Exercise #5: Large Joints In The Body

The large joints in the body are typically, the shoulders, knees, elbows, and hips; essentially any joint connecting two main bones/areas of the body are considered "large joints". There are two main points to focus on for large joints which are, "TW5" and "GB41". You should already know where TW5 is as listed earlier in this text. GB41 is located towards the top part of the bone in your 4th toe (away from the toe). If you cannot reach GB41, you may use a soft tool or cane-like object to press down on this area. You do want to be careful to not press down much harder on any point more than the others; they are all equally necessary and damage to these areas can worsen your symptoms.

Exercise #6: Lay Down

A lot of the aches and pains we have is just tension or areas of the body that have remained stagnant for lack of relaxation and/or movement. Start by lying flat on your back (preferably on a flat surface) and bend your knees so that your feet are flat on the surface about 12 inches from the rest of your body. elevate your head slightly off of the surface with a pillow or small stack of books and rest your hands on your stomach alongside your ribs while your elbows remain at your side.

Remain in this position until you feel your shoulders, neck, lower back, and various parts of your back relax. Allow these areas to become softer and softer for about 12-15 minutes. Do this daily as a part of your morning or evening routine to help alleviate any tightness or pressure in these areas.

Asthma

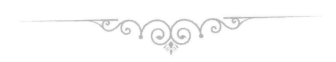

If you look for a medical cure for Asthma, you'll come across symptoms and side effects that are worse than the condition itself. Medical treatment often involves some sort of surgery or prescription medication which comes with additional issues even if the primary issue is resolved. Medical doctors will treat the symptoms as opposed to the cause of asthma. The cause of Asthma is excessive mucus buildup (inflammation) that has made its way into the respiratory system (particularly the throat and nasal passages). Simply reducing (hopefully eliminating) foods that create inflammation will rid your body of asthma.

Remedies:

Reduce or Remove The Meat

Animal flesh (both land and sea animals) creates Uric Acid in the body. Not only does this take hours to digest and breakdown due to not having fiber, but it also builds upon the inflammation and mucus that is already in the body. When the body is met (internally) with a large buildup of substances, it works to break it down but also pushes it into other areas in the body to assist with breaking it down as the body works to address the other needs within the body. This compounds the problem initially as each system in the body is being exposed to this unnecessary substance. Removing Uric Acid, even for a predetermined time period, will work to eliminate symptoms as well as triggers of Asthma. You'll want to incorporate more plants while not overeating to reduce symptoms across the board.

...And The Dairy

Dairy products at their core are what's known as "lactic acid". Lactic Acid is a colorless, syrupy organic acid formed in sour milk and produced in the muscle tissues during strenuous exercise. Whenever there is an absence of oxygen, lactic acid builds up in the body. This is why whenever we exercise and feel "sore" it is lactic acid that has built up. This is also why it is important to not load up on unhealthy foods immediately after working out to reduce the amount of mucus present in the body so the body can focus on repairing muscle tissues. Consuming lactic acid (dairy) creates additional strain on the muscular system and when exercising, the body will rely more upon the respiratory system (heavily breathing), and this is why many experience asthma symptoms and asthma attacks whenever they are physically active. Removing this substance from you diet and lifestyle is essential to not only reducing symptoms of Asthma but being able to breathe easier and retain the body's oxygen levels.

...Also White Flour and White Sugar

Starches (potatoes, GMO products, breads, common rice, products containing white flour and white sugar) breakdown into a substance known as "Carbonic Acid". This substance is a dissolvable substance when in water that is comprised of elements that are in oxygen, hydrogen, and carbon. Being comprised of these minerals, the body wants to hold onto it. The issue with this is that when it enters the body from an unnatural source such as the items listed above, this substance breaks down in the body (which is mostly comprised of water) and enters the blood stream where it is then sent (in trace amounts) to various areas of the body. This substance can directly impact brain and nerve function where the body is not able to immediately recognize potential triggers and often will lead to some sort of attack (asthma attack, heart attack, stroke, etc). This substance essentially clogs the body, particularly the passageways that connect all of the systems within the body. This same substance is only released from the body in a gaseous state (goes from a solid food, to breaking down into a liquid, to being released as a gas). Gasses are released from the body through the respiratory system. Having additional work to do, the respiratory system (in addition to breathing) also must release this gas; now you have air going in and out at the same time. This will immediately trigger and create symptoms of Asthma.

Simply removing the substances mentioned above will be enough to drastically reduce and hopefully remove this condition from your body. if you have enough preparedness and discipline to remove these items, you do not need to continue reading this excerpt and can proceed to the next condition.

Asthma is not just a childhood issue. Children are just triggered more due to being more active. Asthma accounts for about 500,000 hospital visits a year across all ages.

My Personal Remedy For Asthma (and Pneumonia):

Step 1: Commit to remove all dairy for 14 days straight. (will help much more if all meats are removed as well).

Step 2: Drink Mullein Leaf, Guaco, Red Willow Bark, Elderberry, and Dandelion Root.

**Add some Linden Flower herb to your tea if u want to get fancy lol

Dosage for each herb:

2 to 4 years = 2 teaspoons (once/day)

4 to 7 years = 1 tablespoon (once/day)

7 to 11 years = 2 tablespoons (once/day)

12+ = 2 tablespoons (can drink more regularly per day; or more than 8oz cup).

Additional Remedies:

Get A Peak-Flow Meter

This is a device available at most drugstores that measures the speed at which air leaves your lungs. It can not only shed light on how severe your symptoms may be but can detect an oncoming attack you are not away of and should prepare for. A reading between 80-100 indicates that your breathing is healthy. The lower the score, the more risk you are to experience severe symptoms and triggers. It is recommended to keep a journal where you track your levels during the day as well as activities you are doing so you can increase your awareness around when you are most susceptible to triggers and when you are not.

Allergies and Plant Pollen

Allergies are the most common trigger of Asthma so it would benefit you to know what items to avoid during this time. Plant Pollen often is the main allergy that remains present, particularly during the warmer months. It is recommended to stay indoors between 5am and 10am whenever possible on dry, hot, and windy days when pollen counts are the highest. Try to keep your windows closed as often as possible during the day and use a fan to help circulate the air (for now). These are small adjustments to make that are not meant to be a life sentence, but simply, adjustments to make while working to heal your condition.

Turn On Your Bathroom Fan

Mold can accumulate wherever moisture is present. Although we want to avoid mold at all times, even small amounts can trigger symptoms while hiding out in spaces you cannot see. Make sure to use a fan in the bathroom and even crack a window to avoid moisture from building up. Also make time to wipe your floor tiles as well to help remove any additional moisture that you may ignore.

Open Windows When Cooking

Keeping the air clean can reduce toxins being released into the air which can impair passageways to breathing. Turning on your exhaust when cooking can also help.

Wash Your Pets

Dander is a leading cause and trigger for Asthma. Many families go without having a pet due to someone in the home being allergic to a specific animal. However, this does not tell the whole story as we cannot be allergic to an animal; we become triggered by the pet dander left by them when they shed. Cleaning your pet (not just washing them) by scrubbing them and removing excess dander will help significantly with keeping your air and your pet clean.

Dust Control

Dust can accumulate almost anywhere. From picture frames to ceiling fans, to rugs and floors. You want to as often as possible clean these areas of dust, so they don't accumulate and put additional toxins into the air.

Keep A Pest-free Home

Rodents, roaches and small bugs can trigger symptoms as they leave debris in various areas and die off which contributes to debris in most common areas of the household. One of the simplest ways to control bugs (particularly roaches) is to sprinkle boric acid in areas where they are most likely to be (drainpipes, kitchen and bathroom baseboards). Do this and you can reduce a need for an exterminator who may be able to get rid of the bugs, but the chemicals they will spray into the air can present triggers and worsen the quality of air in your home which you want to avoid.

Maintain A Smoke-Free Home

Cigarette smoke is extremely irritating for those with Asthma. Other forms of smoke such as Marijuana and even candles can irritate the air. We do not want to just settle for whatever is "less harmful" but remain helpful. If you or someone "has" to smoke, make sure there is plenty of ventilation or simply go outside so the air does not get trapped in the home.

Remain Physically Active

Putting science aside, maintaining an active lifestyle will do much more for relieving your symptoms than a sedentary lifestyle would do for you. Exercising in warmer areas can be more helpful than colder air which can irritate symptoms. Swimming is a great exercise for those with Asthma as moist air will help soothe the airways in the body and reduce potential attacks while engaging in strenuous exercise.

Breathing Exercises

We tend to breathe a certain way which naturally adjusts to the condition. Its intention is to do its job without being an interference. Although this can appear helpful, it further promotes more of the same type of breathing. Breathing exercises can help to retrain the muscles in the repository system and work to treat this condition at its core.

Stress Control

Practicing Yoga, Meditation, and Mindfulness will help to reduce the stressors in the body. when the body experiences stress, many of the muscles will tighten up which can trigger symptoms. These exercises also help to open the airways in the body as well.

Wash Your Hands

Asthma often leads to developing more colds during the colder months. These colds will present with having more "sniffles" and running noses. During the day we touch many things such as paper, doorknobs, money, other people's hands –not keeping them clean can contribute to these same issues.

Flush Your Sinuses

There are many store-bought products and devices available to help flush the sinuses. Sinus infections will make symptoms worse over time. try to look at flushing your sinuses as "mucous drainage" because that's what you are doing. A simple remedy goes as followed:

Mix ½ teaspoon of fine-grained sea salt in 1 cup of warm water. Pour solution into your cupped palm and inhale it through one nostril while holding your other nostril closed (temporarily). You want to repeatedly blow out of the nostril you just inhaled through to help discharge any mucous that is trapped. Then repeat with your other nostril. Do this as often as possible, not just when you get a cold or feel sick to remain proactive with this condition.

Load Up On Flavonoids

Flavonoids are items that look like tiny crystals located in foods that fight inflammation. Common foods such as onions, apples, berries, and prickly pears, flavonoids give these items their color. Flavonoids not only strengthen the capillary walls which can make breathing easier, they are antioxidants, so they also work to protect the airways from pollution.

Magnesium

Magnesium is a mineral that works to decrease muscle tension and airway spasms. Having enough magnesium in your reserves by consuming enough of it regularly can help to reduce symptoms as well as the severity of attacks if you experience one.

Common Sources Of Magnesium: Avocados, Bananas, Chickpeas, Tamarind, Basil, Dill, Ginger, Oregano, Thyme, Butternut Squash, Brazil Nuts, Okra, Leafy Green Vegetables, Nopal, CBD (cannabidiol) products are helpful.

Omega-3 Fatty Acids

When an Asthma attack occurs, the lungs become inflamed and makes it harder to breathe. Omega-3 Fatty Acids help breakdown inflammation in the lungs. Sea herbs and vegetables such as Wakame, Nori, Bladderwrack, Hijiki, Kelp and Dulse can provide you with a necessary amount of Omega-3. Cooking with avocado oil and grapeseed oil can help increase (and maintain) your daily consumption of Omega-3.

Common Fatty Acid Sources: (Brazil Nuts, Walnuts, Kola Nuts, Avocados, Bananas, Sea Vegetables (Nori, Wakame, Hijiki, Sea Moss, Bladderwrack), Coconut, Coconut Oil, Olive Oil, Grapeseed Oil, Avocado Oil, Mushrooms, Quinoa, Wild Rice.

Licorice Root (Herb)

This herb contains many anti-inflammatory properties particularly for the lungs. For best results, get this herb in a tincture form, add 20-40 drops into a cup of hot water and let cool until water is room temperature. Drink slowly and do this about three times a day.

Nettle (Herb)

This herb helps to clear the sinuses because it contains a form of histamine that helps control allergic reactions and breathing. A histamine is a natural compound released by cell in the body to help relieve the muscles and tension in the body as it works to break down inflammation.

Cayenne Pepper

Helps to thin out mucous in the body for it to be expelled from the body. Adding Cayenne pepper to meal will help reduce the amount of inflammation in the body. You may notice having a runny nose or light coughing when consuming cayenne pepper, but this is a good thing. When you initiate mucous being expelled from the body you do not have to worry as it is expected.

Potassium

This essential mineral helps the muscles and nerve relax which can help reduce the severity of an Asthma attack and help reduce overall symptoms.

Common Potassium Sources: squash, zucchini, bananas, avocado, dried apricots, and herbs such as, guaco (also high in iron), conconsa (has the highest concentration of potassium phosphate), lily of the valley (rich in iron fluorine and Potassium phosphate).

Athlete's Foot

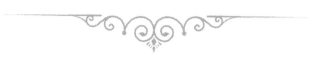

You do not have to be an athlete to have Athlete's Foot. This condition is a simple fungal infection. What prolongs this condition is the fact that we are typically on our feet throughout the day. Athlete's Foot is a fungal infection that breeds best under warm, moist conditions (which are most present with Athletes; hence the name "Athlete's Foot").

Remedies:

Change Your Shoes and Socks

If you encounter Athlete's Foot, you should avoid wearing the same pair of shoes two days in a row, and if you sweat during the day, it would be in your best interest to change socks during the day to avoid any contact with moisture.

Leave Uncovered And Constant Rest

Leaving your foot uncovered anytime possible will help to avoid any blisters from coming up. Providing constant rest will always be best for help limit activity and allowing the foot to heal.

Sea Salt Solution

Make sure to soak your foot in salt water to help reduce the swelling and excess perspiration. Take about 2 teaspoons of sea salt per pint of warm water. Soak your foot in this for about 5-10 minutes at a time and then let dry before repeating until you notice differences.

Rub In Baking Soda

Add room temperature water to 1 tablespoon of baking soda and rub together. This will create a paste. Rub this paste onto affected area and settle for a moment. Then rinse off and dry thoroughly. Repeat daily and as needed.

Scrub Off Dead Skin

As your condition begins to heal, you can easily become reinfected as the fungus attaches to dead skin cells. You will want to scrub (softly) off the dead skin cells surrounding the affected area. Pay extra attention to the spaces in between your toes as these can offer breeding grounds for these kinds of conditions during the day and even while you sleep.

Take Care Of Your Toenails

Keeping your toenails clean are necessary for this condition to heal. You want to get a toothpick and scrape just underneath you nails to remove any debris or waste. It is recommended to use a small nail file during this time to help avoid clipping then unevenly or leaving cracks/niches for the fungus to collect in and reinfect the area.

Proper Footwear

You'll want to avoid plastic materials as they can provide a wet spot of moisture for the fungus to collect and grow. Footwear that allows air to flow in are best although you will want to regularly remove them during the day if you are active during the day.

Dry And Clean

Make sure to clean the insides of your shoes and footwear to avoid moisture from collecting. Add powder if desired and regularly wipe clean until dry so moisture does not settle in.

Cover Your Feet In Public Settings

Most of the time, athlete's foot is acquired from doing simple things like walking barefoot in a gym, locker room, or shower at the gym after a workout. Put on a sock or some material on your feet at all times. Ideally you will want to have on your shoes, but make sure they are close by or at least have them close enough that you do not have to walk far or across any space where moisture collects.

Avoid Refined Sugars

Refined sugars most often found in "junk foods" and candies are to be avoided in general, but especially during this time if you have this condition. These foods create fungus but also allow current fungi to remain in the body and flourish.

Astragalus (Herb)

This herb helps boost the immune system tremendously. Astragalus helps to repair many issues involving the skin and fungal infections in the body; making it the ideal herb to use during this time. about 1-2 teaspoons of this herb (in dried form) is best for tea up to twice a day. This herb is commonly sold in capsule form. Depending on the size of the capsules you should consume around 2800mg a day. Most capsules are 700mg so about 4 capsule a day would be best. It is recommended to take 2 (700mg) capsules in the daytime, 1 capsule mid-day, and 1 with dinner.

A fungal infection that takes a long time to overcome can be attributed to not following protocol for healing, or that your immune system is not strong enough to work on this condition that impacts only one, relatively small area on the body which should ever take long when the immune system is strong.

My Personal Herbal Compound Remedy:

Ingredients:

2 teaspoons of Benzoin Tincture (benzoin is the gum resin/sap from the trunk of trees in the Styrax family)

5 drops of Lavender Essential Oil

5 drops of Thyme Essential Oil

- Mix well together and massage affected area and then apply to the rest of your entire foot.

- Let your feet dry for about 5 minutes before walking around again.

- This mixture is watery, so it is recommended to blow dry or pat to dry with a cloth or small towel.

*Note: for best results, use this remedy at night so that you can limit your activity afterwards and let this mixture absorb into the body and work to relieve this condition while you sleep.

Attention Deficit Hyperactivity Disorder (ADHD)

We often associate ADHD with children who have difficulty paying attention and sitting still (although these are difficult for anyone to do). The issue to come up over time is that children are taught ways to manage their symptoms without working towards eliminating their symptoms. They grow up to become adults who learn more complexed ways to maneuver around these very same symptoms, although they may look different for an adult at work than they do for a child in a school or after school program.

Common symptoms of ADHD include: easily distracted, forgetful, disorganized, restlessness, and/or impulsivity.

What is important to note are the many items that are consumed that increase and promote these most common symptoms. In addition to the many distractions that can contribute symptoms, we must shift our focus on where the distractibility, forgetfulness, disorganization, restlessness, and impulsiveness are coming from, the body. And what maintains the body? What we put inside of it when we consume. We must work to limit how these responses are triggered and acquired by not contributing them. It is essential to creating a living vessel (body and mind) that is not conducive to such behaviors and impulses.

Note: this does not immediately stop all medications as the impact can vary greatly and you would not want to compound other challenges to work through. You do want to focus on diet/lifestyle by removing chemicals as you work to wean yourself (or others) off of common medications. Dosage decrease can be closely monitored initially, followed by a more permanent lowered dosage, and continued on until medications are no longer needed.

Here are the most common medications distributed to those who are diagnosed with ADHD:

ADHD (Attention-deficit Hyperactivity Disorder)	
CHEMICAL NAME	BRAND NAME(s)
Stimulant Meds	
Amphetamines	Adderall, Dexedrine, Dextrostat, Vyvanse
Methylphenidates	Ritalin, Concerta, Metadate, Focalin, Quillivant, Daytrana (patch)
Non-Stimulant ADHD Meds	
Atomoxetine	Strattera
Clonidine	Catapres, Kapvay
Guanfacine	Tenex, Intuniv

Medications are introduced with the intention of interrupting the signals in the brain to help halt or reduce certain impulses, which inevitable lead to changes in behavior. Medications are used to interfere with the way neurons in the brain (responsible for impulses) send, receive, and process signals. The issue with this is, that as long as you use medications and grow older, these impulses are not the same, and medication dosages or other challenges are often increased. In addition, if medications are not consumed, the body has to adjust without the ability to receive and redirect the signals in the brain.

Remedies:

No More Dyes!

We must work to not complicate this ever-changing process by consuming unnatural chemicals which distort the signals that are getting the brain such as the chemicals in many processed foods and drinks. Consuming these items only adds *interest* the present symptoms involving attention.

Red 40	Linked to hyperactivity, aggression, allergies, and learning disorders. One of the most common toxins linked to cancer. This dye comes from coal tars.	Drinks, candy, medications
Yellow 5	Linked to hyperactivity, low sperm count, and cancer.	Gelatin, candy, cereals, junk foods, chips
Yellow 10	Linked to infertility, attention difficulties, mood disturbances	Allowed in cosmetics

Blue 1	Linked to hyperactivity, brain and bladder tumors, and chromosome damage	Ice cream, yogurt, candy, drinks
Blue 2	(Same as Blue 1)	Soft drinks, cereals, candy

These are not the only chemicals to avoid but are the most present that contribute directly to attention difficulties.

These same chemicals are most present in processed foods that are laced with a variety of sugars. A study conducted by the University of South Carolina concluded that the more sugar hyperactive children consumed, the more destructive and restless they became. Another study conducted at Yale University indicates that high-sugar diets may increase inattention in some kids with ADHD.

These sugars are not always simply listed as "sugar" on the list of ingredients. There are many names that are used in place of sugar to help hide what is used in certain products. Names such as, *corn sweetener, ethyl maltol, corn syrup, dextrose, fructose, fruit juice concentrates, glucose, high-fructose corn syrup, invert sugar, lactose, maltose, malt syrup, raw sugar, sucrose, sugar syrup, Florida crystals, cane sugar, crystalline fructose, evaporated cane juice, corn syrup solids, malt syrup, barley malt, rice syrup, caramel, panocha, muscovado, molasses, treacle, and carob syrup*, among others. We want to do away with consuming these sugars to not trigger and promote certain symptoms.

A more recent study has ADHD linked to Iron deficiency. A 2014 study published in the Annals of Medical & Health Sciences Research found that Iron deficiency was increasingly associated with Attention Deficit Hyperactivity Disorder (ADHD). The blood is Iron and goes everywhere in the body. The blood travels throughout the body continuously. Iron is the electrical charge the body uses to function. When there is an Iron deficiency, the blood cannot flood the spaces it travels to at full strength. Areas such as the brain, will experience a slower (or lower) blood flow which impairs the brain's ability to build solid synapses (neurons communicating to one another) and dendrites within the brain (left-right brain communication) which become impaired, which in turn is displayed as distractibility, forgetfulness, disorganization, restlessness, and impulsiveness, which are all present within the condition of ADHD.

As we work to help aide the brain, our other brain (the gut) deserves equal attention. The gut is responsible for sending signal throughout the body, particularly to the brain in your head. These two brains communicate to one another to assist one another in identifying each of their needs. Our gut can and should be cleaned of whatever is not needed through diet. There are many ways to do this, but understand that doing so, is one step closer towards the goal of re-wiring the brain in a way that it can remain alert and respond effectively to outside stimuli that can promote the many symptoms of ADHD. As a new foundation is created at which one operates, symptoms become less extreme, and over time, become less present until they can dissolve.

Cleaning The Colon

For Adults:

(for children, cut dosages in half to 1/3 the amount listed)

Colon Cleanse Tea: 1 teaspoon of Cascara Sagrada, ½ teaspoons of Black Walnut, and 1 teaspoon of Rhubarb Root for about 10-12oz of tea. This tea is very bitter. But you want this tea to be bitter so that it can break down what is not needed in the body. If this tea is too difficult for you to adjust to, you can always search for these herbs or colon cleanses available in capsule form. You will want to try this tea prior to fasting to identify which option will be best for you during your liquid fast. Cleaning the Colon is vital for survival. The Colon is a part of the gut which is essentially our 2nd brain. It holds onto leftover waste and materials that create inflammation in the body and directly trigger many symptoms of disease. Without a clean colon, the body cannot function well as a whole.

Duration: 5-6 consecutive days at a time. Do for 5 days then take at least 2 days off.

Ingredients:

Cascara Sagrada (1 teaspoon)

Black Walnut hull (1/2 teaspoon)

Rhubarb Root (1 teaspoon)

Prodijiosa (1 teaspoon) – if applicable/available to you.

Water 8oz (boiling)

*You can do any combination of these herbs or take individually for this cleanse. You do not need every ingredient, but this cleanse works best when including all herbs mentioned above.

This cleanse is probably the most important to our health. The colon is essentially our second brain and is a part of the large intestine which works to remove waste from the body. The colon is responsible for holding a temporary storage of feces, but also reabsorbing water and minerals necessary to our health.

Cleaning The Blood

Blood Cleanser Tea: 2-3 pieces of Sarsaparilla (dried herb), 1 tablespoon of Burdock, and 1-2 pieces of Guaco (dried herb).

This tea supplies the body with an adequate amount of Iron which helps to filter out toxins that are in the blood. When the blood is deficient in Iron, this allows for toxins that are consumed to be spilled over into the bloodstream when the liver and kidneys are not able to filter waste materials out of the system. This tea you can drink at any time, but it is best to consume at the halfway point or closer to the end of this 5-Day Liquid Fast to allow your body to adjust to consuming liquids so it can prepare for absorbing necessary nutrients it needs to enhance the removal of toxins from the body. Consuming this tea towards the end of this fast example, will help you feel more energized during a time that you would begin to feel more fatigued. There is no place in the body where blood does not flow. It is vital to keep the blood clean. When the blood is clean, the body can function better and be able to detect any potential issues that may be present much faster. If there is a condition that may be an underlying issue for your body, detecting it quicker by keeping the blood clean allow you to address these concerns much earlier.

Common Foods High In Iron: Quinoa, Wild Rice (not black rice), Chickpeas, Kale, Nuts (particularly Walnuts), Hemp Seeds, Dates (and Date Sugar), Dried Apricots, Watercress, Raisins, Dandelion Greens

Common Herbs High in Iron: sarsaparilla, burdock (and root), guaco, chainey root, monkey ladder, chickweed, yellow dock

Fasting is a great time to work in many of these herbs as well as directly experience the many benefits these herbs provide the body.

Tamarind Juice (also to clean colon):

*   15 dried tamarind pods
*   2 quarts water, divided
*   1/2 – 3/4 cup date sugar

Step 1: bring half the water to a boil in a large pot over high heat.

Step 2: While you are waiting for the water to boil, prepare the tamarind pods. Remove the brittle outer shell and pull off as many strings as you can. Discard the shell and strings.

Step 3: After the water comes to a rolling boil, remove it from the heat and place the inner portion of the tamarind and the date sugar in the water. Let simmer together for 5-6 minutes. Let the tamarind soak for about 1 hour and 30 minutes.

Step 4: At this point, the water will have cooled down. Use your fingers to squeeze out the hard tamarind seeds and remove the remaining strings; discard them. Make sure they are cooled off first to avoid getting burned.

Step 5: Place the liquid and remaining pulp in a blender and process until the pulp is fully blended into the water.

Step 6: Run the liquid through a strainer

Step 7: Pour your delicious agua de tamarindo into a pitcher, add the rest of the water, and refrigerate until cold.

Note:

Optional: Add a splash of lime juice for a little extra freshness to your drink.

Drink about 12oz of this twice a day. Children drink 8oz cups.

1. Clean the colon
2. Work to cleanse the blood of toxins
3. While removing chemicals
4. Establish new foundation
5. Repeat through lifestyle changes

Additional Remedies:

Eat Every Two Hours

This is not ideal when we think of what may be sustainable but is something to practice more often than not when working to teach the body how to control its impulses and regulate itself. Dr. Block, a physician from the Block Center in Dallas-Fort Worth, Texas states that "Blood sugar, or glucose, is the body's primary fuel, and low blood sugar is the most significant problem I find in people with the behavioral symptoms of ADHD". Aggression, nervousness, agitation, and anxiety, are all symptoms of hypoglycemia, otherwise known as "low blood sugar," according to Dr. Block.

A simple way to not allow you blood sugar is to eat very often. The challenge would be to monitor your eating by choosing healthy options and not overeating for your body size or age. You do not have to eat exactly every two hours, but close enough where you essentially plan as if you would have three meals a day but consuming something in between as well. This should make you main meals much smaller but help to avoid a constant triggering of symptoms. Eating every few hours is also very helpful with regular practice of incorporating healthier foods and weaning away from the snacks and junk food items many may crave. This step also help provides additional practice of sitting and decreasing physical activity more often throughout the day.

Artificial Sugars

Foods that are high in artificial sugars release glucose into the blood in excess amounts which directly triggers the release of insulin (a natural hormone in the body) which is responsible for lowering glucose. Trying to lower glucose in the body while flooding it with glucose will eventually lead to insulin dependence (type 1 diabetes) where a person needs to inject themselves with insulin or create insulin resistance where the body does not want to release any more insulin (type 2 diabetes). White Flour also turns into glucose when being digested which should be avoided as well.

New Internal Voice

Our internal voices are often responsible for us procrastinating and also feeling unmotivated to completing tasks we have. If you have an internal voice that is demanding, use this time to practice generating a softer voice that is more comforting. You can work on this by whenever you hear a demanding voice, you focus on ignoring them until a softer, or more kind voice asks you to do something or reminds you. Imagine something you have to do in the near future and generate a kind, nurturing voice you want as your reminder/alert that will remind you of all the wonderful things that will come of you completing your task. If a loud, demanding, obnoxious voice comes in to remind you, kindly ignore it and invite in that kind, nurturing voice to help you get back onto your path.

We don't always complete things while under pressure. We must be kind and patient with ourselves. Practice this more regularly will help practice patience which by itself can drastically reduce many of the symptoms associated with ADHD.

Magnesium

This mineral helps calm the nerve in the body. A main reason why many people promote CBD Oils and products for conditions like ADHD is, that CBD Oils are almost pure magnesium. The calming effect a steady consumption of magnesium can have will greatly benefit someone with ADHD.

Common Sources Of Magnesium: Avocados, Bananas, Chickpeas, Tamarind, Basil, Dill, Ginger, Oregano, Thyme, Butternut Squash, Brazil Nuts, Okra, Leafy Green Vegetables, Nopal, CBD (cannabidiol) products, Nettle leaf, Horsetail, Red Clover, Sage

Fatty Acids

The main hype around fatty acids is that they are good for the brain. But what does this mean? It means that fatty acids (Omega-3, Omega-6, and Omega-9) all help the brain cells function better. They provide an additional support for brain cells to do their job without leading to feelings of exhaustion or mental burnout. Avoiding these additional issues along with common symptoms of ADHD can help provide relief while also supporting the brain connect those very important signals necessary for the body to continue to re-wire itself.

Common Sources of Fatty Acids: Brazil Nuts, Walnuts, Kola Nuts, Avocados, Bananas, Sea Vegetables (Nori, Wakame, Hijiki, Sea Moss, Bladderwrack), Coconut, Coconut Oil, Olive Oil, Grapeseed Oil, Avocado Oil, Mushrooms, Quinoa, Wild Rice.

Back Pain

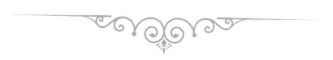

About 80% of Americans have back pain. The majority of these are lower back pain. Surgery has become the primary method for treating back pain, although this does not always appear to be the best option. Many surgeries can lead to more pain than you had before including general surgery complications, infections, and/or nerve damage.

"Most people with back pain have a problem with short, tight, rigid back muscles, and it can be relieved by improved posture while sitting, standing, and working; regular aerobic exercise; stretching; and exercises to strengthen the back muscles", says Dr. Hochschuler, M.D., orthopedic surgeon from Plano, Texas.

Remedies:

Chiropractor

Make sure to schedule a few sessions with a local chiropractor if you are having back pain. A chiropractor can and will provide necessary alignments to specific areas and also encourage or advise you to specific things to do. A chiropractor will also help you avoid certain things such as yoga if it will complicate the pain you are experiencing.

Sit Down (Don't Lean Back)

One of the main reasons we have back pain, particularly lower back pain, is leaning backwards while sitting. When you lean back while sitting it flattens the lower area of the back which deprives it of its natural curve. This adds an additional amount of stress on not only the spine, but the ligaments, and disks. Sitting like this, puts added weight on the buttocks which can pull and apply unnecessary pressure to the sciatic nerve where you can develop sciatica and shooting pains down each your legs.

Tips For Improving Posture:

- Sit while lifting your breastbone.
  - o Will help relieve tension from the pelvis and hips. You want to "lengthen" the space between your belly button and upper chest. You simply raise your chest upwards while also tilting the hips towards your back to help promote the natural curvature of the spine.

- Align your head, first
  - o The rest of your body will follow the motion of your head. This extra weight will drive your spine either forward or backward. You want to position the head in a neutral position to avoid the spine leaning towards one way. Doing this will help alleviate some of the muscles in the back that are getting overused and want to relax.

- Driving
  - o If you drive a lot, you most likely have back pain. The way car seats are designed to have your knees higher than your hips places an incredible amount of pressure onto your back. To minimize this from happening, you want to adjust your car seat so that your knees and hips are at least at the same level. You essentially want to drive in the same position that you sit (when sitting correctly). If your seat does not adjust much, consider sitting on a folded towel or small pillow. The last adjustment to make is making sure your steering wheel is not too far forward that you have to reach for it. This can cause you to round your back which does not promote healthy posture.

Ways To Sleep:

On Your Back

When we lay down on our side, our heads go forward, our shoulders hunch as well, and our backs become limited with how they can stretch. Ideally, we want to sleep on our left side most of the time to help promote proper digestion, but only if our posture is correct to begin with. Laying down on our backs allows all areas of the back feel slight pressure while being able to relax. It is recommended that you sleep with a thin pillow to prevent the neck from being pushed too far in one direction which can hinder your posture. If you have a feather pillow, remove about 1/3 of the feathers and close the pillow back up and adjust to where your head and neck feel most comfortable.

Depending on the type of mattress you have, improvements can vary. If you have a slight pain tolerance, try sleeping on a wooden board for a few days. Place a thick blanket (folded) or quilt down to help cover most of the board you will lay down on. Place your pillow slightly off the top of the board to help keep your head from tilting downward. You may also place a folded towel in the small of your back to help alleviate any feelings of pain. You want a board that is longer than your spine is and is flat as possible. Using a board to sleep on will help at the least, identify spots in need for correction or adjustment.

On Your Stomach

This sleeping method is ideal for those with sciatica. Sciatic pains stem from overstretching of the ligaments and muscles that press down on the sciatic nerves. Laying on your stomach allows these muscles to relax and can help reduce pain as your posture begins to adjust. It is recommended to place a pillow under your stomach to help the body maintain its natural curve.

Pillow Between Knees

Placing a pillow between your knees can be incredibly helpful for reducing back pain, especially the lower back. When our knees touch when we sleep on our side, our hips tend to arc over in the direction you are sleeping and place stress on your ligaments while you sleep. Sleeping should be the main relief period for our backs. Aligning the hips which hold up the torso when up is essential for reducing back pain and promoting better posture. Placing something such as a water bottle, towel, or foam roller before exercise can help keep your spine align when exercising and further promote a healthy posture.

Strengthen Your Core

When our core is weak or needing to carry a larger load, this places tremendous stress on the lower back, as well as the joints, muscles, tendons, and ligaments. Many chiropractors will initially recommend specific core exercises for what your back needs. The connection between back health and core health cannot be ignored. You will want to have a more even core that is stronger so that it can at least withstand any issues it's currently dealing with. Strengthening your core will in turn, strengthen your back and you will feel relief. You can benefit from doing a colon cleanse, avoiding processed sugars and fats which accumulate around the waistline, and doing regular exercises to strengthen your core. You may benefit from getting a personal trainer or looking up exercises that you can do on your own. A yoga or Pilates class can be a great addition for you as well.

Stretching

Many of us would not have the pains we experience if we would stretch more often. A few minutes a day of stretching will help get blood flow going in addition to aligning the spine and skeletal systems. You do want to develop a routine that meets and is designed for your specific needs. Full-body stretches are best as they incorporate more of the body so that the body can become more aligned, rather than focusing on specific areas. There are two specific stretches to do that may help with your back pain.

- Sit upright in a chair. Place your arms slightly in front of you and lean over until your palms touch the ground. If your palms cannot touch the ground, just stretch where your feel comfortable. You may also stretch to each side if you are able to as well.

- This stretch can be difficult for some so do not overextend yourself. For this stretch, lie down on a bed or comfortable bench. Lie on your stomach with your hips touching the edge of the bed or bench. Your upper body should be completely off as you place your hands down for balance. Slowly start walking your hands in front of you until you are completely laying down while your back stretches. You may rest on your elbows if needed as well and can rest on your hands as you tuck your chin to your chest to duplicate the cat and cow yoga poses to stretch other areas of your back.

Yoga

Strengthening the core muscles drastically help align the spine and loosen any tightness in the back. Slow gradual movements, while controlling the breath, helps to "unlock" many of the tighter areas in the back (and the body). Long, extensive stretching will loosen the muscles and ligaments in the body and promote a much healthier posture. Various positions can target the back more, but all Yoga poses use the full body to complete and will help alleviate pains you may have.

Ice and heat

If there's any areas of swelling, place an ice pack or bag of ice on the area and massage the spot for about 6-8 minutes at a time. repeat this every few hours while awake. After a day or two of using ice, switch to applying heat to the same area. Do this by taking a small towel and place it in warm water. Wring out the water after a few minutes and flatten out the towel. Lay down onto your stomach and place the towel across the painful area on your back. You will want to also place a pillow or towel under your hips and ankles to relief tension in the back.

Foam Roller

Sometimes we just need to apply to pressure on the lower back to help provide relief. We're often sitting or standing. A foam roller helps provide a neutral space where our spine is stretched out, but not holding up the rest of our bodies. Steady pressure to specific parts of the back can help provide insight on where specifically your back needs relief, loosening up the muscles will help provide initial relief as the lower back muscles can get tense throughout the day. You do want to test out if your body can handle using a foam roller first before using it regularly to avoid further damage.

Gravity Inversion

This form of therapy involves turning yourself upside down. You strap yourself to a device which slowly tilts back and allows you to hang upside down. We're more often than not standing upright or laying down in a neutral position. Positioning yourself upside down for about 30 minutes a day should provide relief to areas that are typically neglected or do not get enough rest.

Caution: speak to a chiropractor or specialist if you have disk issues or glaucoma to not contribute to symptoms of these conditions.

Tai Chi

Slow, fluid movements will always be best for the back as they provide an opportunity to detect where pain may be but also the severity of the pain without making it worse. Takes practice and discipline but Tai Chi movements in a class or first thing in the daytime can help reduce pain while making your body aware of any areas or positions you want to avoid for your back pain.

White Willow Bark (Herb)

This herb is commonly referred to as "Nature's Aspirin". This herb is often found in capsule form and has an active ingredient called salicylate which provides Aspirin with its anti-inflammatory properties. Caution: those with severe heartburn or ulcers should do without this herb for now to not irritate these conditions.

Clean The Kidneys

The kidneys are located with the top part of the lower back. The kidneys help to regulate blood flow and filter out toxins in the body. When their workload gets too demanding, they will fill up more often and press against your lower back. This can make you hunch forward and lead to lower back pain. Preventing the kidneys from being overworked is best achieved by keeping them clean. Doing this by not consuming toxins is best, but you want to target this area exclusively feel free to follow any of the following methods (with several week gaps in between if you incorporate all of them).

To be consumed in tea form:

1. Stinging Nettle (1 teaspoon of dried herb, ½ teaspoon powder per 8oz water)
2. Hydrangea Root (tea 4-8 oz cup 2-3 times daily)
3. Palo Azul (Kidneywood) (tea 8oz no more than two glasses a day)
4. *Sambong Tea

Sambong tea preparation:

- gather fresh Sambong leaves, cut in small pieces

- wash with fresh water

- boil a 1/2 cup of Sambong leaves to a liter of water

- let it seep for 10 minutes

- remove from heat

- drink while warm 4 glasses a day for best results.

- helps with fluid retention, great for kidneys

Sample Two-Day Kidney Flush:

This will not flush them out entirely. You can have many health complications if you flush your kidneys entirely as you will lose many things vital to your health. You want to keep the kidneys hydrated while you filter out the toxins within the body. You can do this routine somewhat regularly to promote clean kidney health while limiting other snacks and items that are detrimental to our health during this time.

Day 1:

Breakfast: Fruit Juice consisting of, 1/2 cup of berries, 2 key limes (juiced), 2 teaspoons of fresh ginger, 1 cup of watermelon, and 1 cup of Kale.

Lunch: Smoothie of 1 cup walnut or hemp milk, 1/2 cup of brazil nuts, 1/2 cup dandelion leaves, 1/4 cup berries, 1/2 apple, and 1 tablespoon hemp seeds

Dinner: Large mixed-greens salad with 1/2 cup of garbanzo beans, topped with 1/2 cup grapes and 1/4 cup nuts

Day 2:

Breakfast: Smoothie of 1 cup walnut milk, 1 frozen banana, 1/2 cup kale, 1/2 cup blueberries, and 2 teaspoons of sea moss and bladderwrack power

Lunch: 2 cups of quinoa rice topped with 1 cup fresh fruit and 2 tablespoons hemp or sesame seeds

Dinner: Large mixed-greens salad, w/ 1/2 cup garbanzo beans, topped with 1/2 cup cooked parsley and a drizzle of fresh key lime juice plus 4 ounces each unsweetened cherry juice and orange juice

Bad Breath (halitosis)

Bad smell from our breath comes from what we eat. Anything that contains excess bacteria or ferments in the body and leaves behind waste will lead to bad breath. Oral health is essential to our health as this is the area in which we consume items. We just want to avoid masking (or covering up) the issue that is present by doing things like chewing gum or using mouthwash. Our breath does not have to smell like anything; it should just not smell foul. We do want to avoid masking the issue by consuming scents and focus more on what can rid the body of the issue to not need to take anything for this specific issue.

Remedies:

Tongue Scraping

Using a tongue scraper will help remove any excess material left behind from eating. Even if you eat very healthy, materials can always be left behind in some form. If they are not scraped from the tongue, they will begin to fester and can accumulate toxins and bacteria. Tongue scraping should be a daily habit to do upon awakening.

From experience, the best tongue scrapers are the U-shapes ones that you hold both sides with each hand. These cover the most area and take minimal effort to use, unlike the smaller plastic ones which you have to scrape repeatedly and may lead to you pressing down too hard and accidentally cutting your tongue. A silver tongue scraper is very beneficial as the silver material sends off ions which help kill bacteria on contact. If silver is too much for you based upon its taste, try a copper one instead.

Caution: You want to avoid pressing down too hard where you can cut your tongue or scrap it enough that it begins to bleed. This can turn into an open wound that can lead to infection.

Brush and Floss

If you do not brush your teeth and floss often, food particles can build up and create plaque which will irritate the gums and cause damage to the teeth.

Chlorophyll

Chlorophyll is essentially the "blood" of plants. What iron is to our blood, chlorophyll is to plants. This substance helps the digestive tract work properly. Much of the odor that may come from our mouths, is accumulated waste from foods that weren't digested properly. Chlorophyll helps break down waste and support healthy digestion. Natural foods (plants) are best to achieve this but plants high in chlorophyll can be taken in capsule form as well. It is safe for an adult to take three 500-700mg capsules a day before or after each meal to support proper digestion. Doing this more often than not (not daily) is best to help deodorize the digestive tract and colon.

Common sources of chlorophyll: Callaloo, Dandelion, Lettuces, Turnip Greens, Wild Arugula, Watercress, Nopales (Mexican Cactus)

Oil Pulling

Swishing around raw coconut oil in your mouth for about 10-12 minutes a day upon awakening will help remove many of the toxins in our mouth, but also provide some natural freshness to this area as well. Take about ½ tablespoon of raw coconut oil (from a glass jar) and swish around your mouth for about 10-12 minutes before spitting it out. You want to avoid eating before doing this. Also, you want to spit this into your trash or into a small napkin before placing it into the trash. Do not spit this into your sink as it can clog up your pipes in your sink.

Delete The Meat

Consuming animal flesh ferments in the digestive tract. This produces a foul odor that comes through the respiratory system and out of the mouth. Deli meats such as pepperoni, salami, and pastrami (among others), contain a heavy amount of oil which leave behind oils in the mouth that contribute to bad smelling breath. Meats ferment in the digestive tract regardless of what kinds of sauce or flavors you add to them. This fermented (and decaying) flesh of animal will produce odors that cannot be covered up completely with some kind of mint, chewing gum, or mouthwash.

"Cut The Cheese"

Cheese is already fermented and begins to become rancid the moment it touches your gut. This substance takes several hours to digest and contributes to foul smells that may come from the digestive tract.

Caffeine

Caffeine dehydrates the mouth and causes acidity to accumulate. Most commonly found in commercial coffee, processed foods, and foods high in artificial sugars.

Drink More Water

Drinking water can help move along bacteria left behind in the mouth from eating. Not consuming drinks such as coffee, soda, alcohol, or sugary drinks, helps to reduce plaque in the mouth and the digestive walls. It can be helpful to swish around water for a few moments after eating or during the day when you cannot brush your teeth to help remove any excess bacteria.

Cloves (herb)

Cloves can be sucked on or swished around the mouth with water in powdered form to help kill excess bacteria. Now, you want to not consume anything that contains excess bacteria, but as you transition to a healthier lifestyle, cloves can help begin to remove bacteria that has been accumulating in your mouth.

Other Herbs To Incorporate

Ginger, Sage, and Fennel are good options for tea to help freshmen your breath. You can add about 1 teaspoon of each herb to a cup of boiling water and drinking after each meal will help keep your breath from smelling foul, in addition to the other steps outlined here.

Tooth Powder

Unlike traditional toothpaste, tooth powders dissolve easier and can get into crevices to provide a deeper clean. Even using something such as baking soda can help reach those hard-to-get areas in the mouth.

Miswak

Brushing your teeth with a miswak stick can help reduce bacteria in the mouth. No toothpaste is needed, only water. You can chew or lightly brush your teeth directly.

Cleansing Smoothie

This smoothie helps to cleanse the body of toxins, hydrate the body, and fight against bad breath.

1 cup of soft-jelly coconut water

½ cup strawberries

½ apple

1 key lime (juiced)

1 tablespoon of coconut oil

1 handful of greens

1 teaspoon of sea moss and bladderwrack powder

Blend together and add water as needed to get desires consistency.

Bed Wetting (Enuresis)

Bed-wetting is actually a condition known as, "Enuresis", which is an overproduction of urine produced largely at night. This condition is often seen as a nuisance for parents and caregivers where blame is placed on a child. Although children are the most common ones with this condition, they are not alone, and this condition should not be stigmatized as a "child problem".

There are many contributing factors to this condition that should be examined. Factors such as, the reasons why excess urine is being built up during the evening hours, slow physical development, and the inability to recognize that the bladder is full during sleep. In this section, we will review contributing factors to this condition and ways to treat this condition yourself.

Remedies:

Don't Blame or Praise

No one does this on purpose, even though they may appreciate the attention they receive. It is important to remember they do not choose to wet their bed on purpose. They should not also be praised for this activity either, so it does not continue. Simply clean up and change their sheets or sleeping location without saying a word. Patience and support will do more than anything else to help motivate the person especially a child.

Rearrange Bedroom (if applicable)

If you have the space, make some room for the person to change their own sheets. They may not do so as effectively as a parent or caregiver, but providing space for them to change their own sheets can help to greatly reduce psychological stress the endure when someone else is aware of what has happened. Shame, guilt, and worry can increase dramatically during these moments and can be avoided by providing a space for them to be able to change their own sheets.

Limit Fluids In The Evening

Hydration is important but work to even reduce the amount of water consumed at night. A person has the entire day to hydrate so don't try to do this later in the day.

Try To Use Bathroom Before Bed

Even if a person does not feel they need to use the bathroom before bed, they can still try. This can either trigger them to go, initiate the process so they're aware after they lay down, or confirm they do not have to go and can get some restful sleep. The key is to not force anything to avoid any damage or straining the body. Take a few minutes to try before bed and at the minimum, use this time to help begin to relax and power down before bed which will be a good habit to maintain after this is no longer an issue.

Avoid Caffeine

Caffeine is a diuretic which induces urination. Caffeine irritates the bladder and stimulates muscle contractions more frequently. You want to avoid consuming sodas, coffee, chocolate, and over-the-counter products such as Excedrin, Midol, and Anacin, as they all contain caffeine. The more you make efforts towards decreasing your caffeine intake, the more noticeable improvements you should notice.

Train Bladder Muscles

First, examine if the person goes to the bathroom regularly during the day. If so, having them practice bladder exercises during the day can be helpful for them at night. If a person goes to the bathroom frequently during the day, have them drink more liquids than they normally do and upon feeling the sensation to use the bathroom, have them practice holding in their urine until almost the last moment. Doing this will help train the body to remain alert and identify when they will need to go. So, when they are asleep in bed, their body will be triggered to wake up, where they can then go to the bathroom and not wet their bed.

If a person does not go to the bathroom frequently during the day, providing them with more liquids during the day will help as well along with the same exercise; it just may be more difficult to fight their temptation to immediately go to the bathroom. Having a person who does not urinate often practice sitting still as they consume liquids will help them increase their awareness also.

Note: If a child or adult urinates very often, please get checked for Diabetes and review the "Diabetes" section in this text. The word diabetes comes from the Greek word "Siphon" which means "to pass through" and the Latin word for "mellitus" which means "honeyed or sweet". So, *a sweet and honeyed liquid passing through* the body often is a clear sign of diabetes.

Trauma Assessment

Bedwetting is often a sign of some form of trauma. In some cases, this can be a sign that someone was sexually abused as well. It would benefit assessing these areas as well to help promote the use of coping skills in a therapeutic setting.

Belching/Burping (Aerophagia)

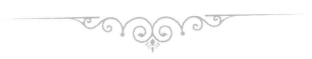

Belching or "burping" is a condition called "aerophagia" which means "to swallow air". Our gastrointestinal tract holds about a cup of air at all times. Throughout the day, we tend to take air in and breath air out. When this is disrupted, the body pushes some of this air out to make way for leaning air by belching/burping.

Remedies:

Eat Slower

Those that open their mouths frequently when eating by eating fast, are more likely to belch. When we eat quickly, we swallow small pockets of air. This is proceeded by closing our mouths to chew and swallow food. These traps the small pockets of air that we just swallowed and leads to the body working to immediately push this out, leading to belching. It is best to eat small amounts at a time but at a slower rate while breathing through the nose. This will eliminate consuming small pockets of air through the mouth, and most likely lead to you eating less after feeling more nourished as opposed to overeating and feeling a need to lay back and belch afterwards.

Avoid Foods With High Air Content

In addition to carbonated beverages (soft drinks), it is equally important to avoid items such as beer, ice cream, omelets, and whipped cream. Not only are these not healthy for you, but they contain tiny air sacs similar to those in soda and create pockets of air when being swallowed and digested.

Stop Chewing Gum

The more we chew gum, the more we swallow. Reducing how many times a day we swallow will reduce those tiny sacs of air we send to our digestive tract.

Ginger Tea

Ginger is great at providing anti-inflammatory properties to the body. inflammation-producing foods are the main culprit in causing the body to belch repeatedly. Ginger can help break down some of the inflammation to help the body avoid the need to belch.

My Personal Remedy:

- 1 teaspoon of cloves
- Finely grained peel of a Seville or sour orange
- Boiling water

Place cloves and orange peel into a cup as you boil water. Pour boiling water into cup and let steep for about 10 minutes. Drink this 2-3 times a day until belching stops.

Binge-Eating

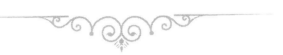

As much as we feel we have control of our urges, Binge-Eating is a disorder that stems from a combination of emotional eating and consuming foods that create cravings. To reduce these temptations, we must remove our cravings, while working to process out feelings and emotions in the moment, without succumbing to the pressure we feel towards eating certain foods. Emotions are fluid and are always changing. Think of an emotion as energy in motion. You would not want to be persuaded simply off of any emotion. We want to acknowledge what emotion we are experiencing as it connects to some area of our life without attaching it to specific foods.

As stated earlier in this text, we have two brains: one in our head, and one in our gut. The gut is the brain responsible for craving foods. Although it sends signals to our primary brain in our heads which influences its decisions, it is crucial to clean the gut to begin.

Remedies:

Cleaning The Gut

(please start by referring to the earlier section on Angina where I go over details on how to clean to colon.)

Meet Your Cravings Head On

Much of our cravings boil down to mineral deficiencies. We often meet these deficiencies short-term by consuming items detrimental to our health and then rely upon them in addition to the sugars attached to them which keep us addicted. Below are the most common deficiencies and cravings we tend to be strongly attached to and foods to each instead.

Cravings For Chocolate and Sugary Foods

Minerals The Are Deficient: Carbon, Chromium, Phosphorus, and Sulfur

Sources To Meet Mineral Needs: Raw fruits, Nuts, and Seeds

Craving For Processed Breads, Non-approved Pastas, and Grains

Minerals The Are Deficient: Carbon, Oxygen, Hydrogen, Nitrogen (and hydration)

Sources To Meet Mineral Needs: Spring Water, Leafy Greens, Fresh Fruit, Fresh Air

Craving For Oily Foods, Salty Foods, Alcohol

Minerals The Are Deficient: Calcium, Chlorophyll, Silicon, Carbon, Hydrogen (and sunlight)

Sources To Meet Mineral Needs: Green Foods, Vegetable Juices, Fruit Smoothies, Spring Water, Direct Sunlight

Meditation

The daily practice is about increasing your awareness. Although it is recommended to practice Meditation for overall health and wellness, this practice can and should be used specifically for increasing awareness skills for this condition. Daily Meditation practice helps alleviate the body of feeling that something is missing. Being present is needed when feeling an uncontrollable urge for anything. Practicing Meditation will help you focus on eating while you are eating. This may sound strange, but we are often preoccupied with other things such as TV, conversations, our cell phones, or some other distraction. Being able to focus solely on eating while you eat will serve you very well with working to overcome this condition.

Cook/Eat While Calm

If we cook while stressed or angry, these emotions can play out in the energy produced by the foods we are consuming. Besides just misplacing items or not being fully mindful of how we're coking which can impact that taste, the mind-body connection that takes place when stressed or frustrated will disrupt this pattern and not provide adequate nourishment to the body. You may eat and not feel like finishing your meal or feel something is creating discomfort when digesting (yes, even if it's raw vegetables). This is a result of the energy exchange you created when cooking while stressed or frustrated. Try waiting until you are not stress or frustrated before cooking. If time is limited, try cooking on low heat so it will take longer to cook, and you can use this time to settle down and relax.

...Or Eat Raw

The reduced tension of having to cook meals, do dishes, and prepare a plate or bowl can help redirect your cravings and restructure your relationship with food. Consuming fresh fruits and vegetables will help you become healthier and get many of the minerals and nutrients your body may have been missing. In addition to this, you will train your gut and brain to eat to live, not live to eat. You will develop better habits around what you eat and when you eat, with intention.

Parasite Cleanse

This is not a fun experience and can be traumatic to many. But, if you are up for it and want to complete a parasite cleanse, it is encouraged.

Parasites are in many of the common foods people eat. Foods such as animal flesh, dairy products, many cruciferous vegetables, and many processed or refined sugars and carbohydrates. These parasites set up shop in the body and tuck themselves away. They feed off of waste materials. It is best to starve these parasites by not consuming what they feed off of and through developing a fasting regimen. There are many herbal cleanses that should come with specific protocols available for purchase online and in person. Seek out those created and made by an herbalist or holistic health practitioner as they will have a set intention when putting together herbal compounds made for removing parasites from the body. They will list out a protocol to follow as opposed purchasing a commercial product that likely contains artificial ingredients and harmful chemicals.

Bites and Stings

These types of hindrances are almost inevitable in life. But when they do happen, we want to remain prepared and work to avoid infection.

Types of Bites

For Small Insect Bites

Baking Soda – dissolve 1 teaspoon in a glass of water. Dip a cloth into the solution and place directly onto the bite mark for about 15-20 minutes.

Epsom Salt – dissolve 1 teaspoon in 1 quart of hot water. Let chill, then apply by also dipping a cloth into the solution and place directly onto bite mark for about 12-15 minutes.

Make sure to identify the attacker to identify if more treatments will be needed.

Ticks

The insects can transmit Lyme Disease which can set forth various illnesses such as fatigue, headaches, joint pain, muscle aches, and fevers. These insects are more present from the spring to the fall seasons, mostly in wooded or high grass areas.

To know if ticks are in the area, tie a piece of white flannel to a string and drag it through the grass. If ticks are present, they will cling to the cloth, and you should spend time elsewhere. You want to leave as little exposed skin as you can if ticks are present. Before going to bed make sure to skin your body, bed, and covers for ticks.

If you notice a tick on your skin, don't try to scratch it off or pull it away. Get some tweezers and slowly pull it off. Ripping it out the skin can leave behind materials from the tick and set the stage for infection.

First sign of Lyme Disease is a bulls-eye rash accompanied with a fever. It could take one to two weeks to notice symptoms after initial bite. You want to keep an eye on an area that you feel you were bitten. Aside from treating the rash and fever with natural remedies such as Fasting and applying aid to the bite as outlined for other bites in this section, please seek medical attention as they will have materials on hand to prevent disease from spreading. After initial diagnosis and treatment from medical professional, continue to treat this condition holistically.

My Recommendations For Holistic Treatments Go As Followed:

1. Fasting regularly
2. Removing all low fiber products, dairy, and processed foods from diet
3. Colon cleanse
4. Load up on iron rich herbs to help clean out toxins in the blood
5. Maintain lifestyle and use herbs beneficial for treating specific condition

Spiders

If you get bitten by a spider, you want to do the following:

- Wash the wound and disinfect with antiseptic
- Apply an ice pack to slow down absorption of the venom
- Neutralize some of the venom by moistening the bite with water.

Dogs and Cat Bites

Anyone is susceptible for getting bit by a dog or cat. If this happens you want to do the following:

- Wash the affected area
- Control bleeding. Do this by covering wound with a thick gauze pad or cloth, thoroughly rinse your hand and press it against the pad or cloth. Add ice against pad and elevate the wound above the heart area.
- Bandage the wound. Cover the bite with a sterile bandage or cloth and then tie or tape loosely in place.
- Reduce Pain. Keep elevated and consume anti-inflammatory foods while healing.
- Treat Wound. Apply a poultice and clean area to reduce further infection.

Remedies for Bites:

Plantain (Weed not the fruit)

This plant will help take the itchiness out of any sting or bite. It is a weed that is loaded with tannins (natural chemicals that help tighten the skin and surrounding tissues) that help reduce inflammation and itchiness around the affected area. The weed grows all over but is abundant in areas that are damp and shady. Grows about 6-18 inches tall and has deep purple veins from top to bottom. From the summertime until the fall, this plant sprouts green, pipe cleaner-like flower spikes.

You can chew this plant if you get bitten by a bee or mosquito. Take the leaves, rinse them off and chew them as you place a handful of the leaves directly on the bite to instant relief. You may also rub the leaves together after you rinse them off until they create a "juice" which you can apply to the infected area.

For dog bites, you want to first scrub the affected area with soap and water thoroughly. Place a handful of rinsed leaves into a blender and add a few drops of warm water and continue to blend together. Put mixture directly over the affected area, then place a gauze pad over the mixture followed by a heat source such as a hot water bottle or heated pad over the gauze. Apply heat for 20-30 minutes and change the poultice about three times a day.

If the dog bite is on a limb, soak in cooled plantain herb tea for about 10-15 minutes in a cooled area. To make tea, take ¼ cup of dried plantain leaves to a quart of boiled water and let steep for 20-30 minutes.

Bentonite Clay

After a bite such as a dog bite has healed you still want to reduce infection. Do this by preparing a poultice of bentonite clay by taking 2 tablespoons of clay, and slowly add water to make a paste. Cover the bite with the paste, cover paste with gauze, and tape down the gauze to keep it in place. Leave this on for 30 minutes and repeat twice a day and you should feel relief within four days.

*If this clay is unavailable to you in the moment, follow same instructions but use mud instead. Take dirt from ground and mix well with water first to avoid using mud that contains excess bacteria so you will avoid infection. Once you can get to your Bentonite Clay, wash off mud and apply instructions as stated above.

Olive Leaf

This herb helps to reduce inflammation and swelling when present in addition to their many other benefits. These are easily found in capsule form and should take as recommended on label. For tea, take about 1-2 teaspoons of dried herb, add to cup and boil water. Pour boiling water over herb and let steep for about 10 minutes. Remove herb from water and let cool for another r10 minutes before consuming.

Remedies For Stings:

Jellyfish Sting

Urine therapy is the primary recommendation if you are stung by a jellyfish. The acidic pH (potential Hydrogen) in urine works to dissolve the venom that a jellyfish injects when it stings. You can urinate directly onto the bite, or onto a towel and massage it in.

Bee, Wasp, Hornet, and Yellow Jacket Stings

You want to first remain calm so that you can remove the singer. Best approach can be to scrape the stinger out so that you can properly wash the area afterwards. After removing stinger, wash out with water followed by applying Baking Soda or Epsom Salt (mixing well with water) to place over the bite for 15-20 minutes. Applying heat immediately can help a sting as well. You can take something like a hair dryer and aim it directly at your sting to reduce lingering pain.

Other Helpful Tips:

Wear Lighter Colors

I'm sure we've all been told that we will attract bees if we were yellow, but most bugs prefer dark colors according to Dr. Raffensperger, professor emeritus of etymology at Cornell University in Ithaca, New York. Beekeepers generally wear white or khaki-colored clothing for this reason.

Isoamyl Acetate ("isopentyl acetate")

This chemical is often in many sprays, lotions, and creams. Bananas contain *isoamyl acetate*. This is the same compound that triggers a bee's alarm pheromone. While bees' alarm pheromone isn't just isoamyl acetate (there are over 40 other compounds as well), it is however, the main active compound. Many lotions, shampoos, body wash, and sunburn sprays contain isoamyl acetate. If you use something that contains this chemical, bees will be in your area and may choose to attack upon your response to them. Start by staying safe by properly hydrating so you won't rely heavily on lotions and creams. There are many natural lotions, creams, and sprays, but it is more important to avoid anything that has isoamyl acetate in it (in general – but particularly anything used on the skin). If bees don't immediately attack, you may attract other bugs and insects as well if you don't avoid this chemical.

Watch Your Scent

Wearing perfume, aftershave, cologne, or any other fragrance can and may confuse an insect by believing that you or something you have on is a nectar-bearing flower and will remain in your area.

Painting

Many of the paints used for painting on canvases contain a turpentine (or are used afterwards to help paint dry quicker) which repels stinging insects.

Run!

As a last (maybe your first) resort, just run away. Try to not run around at random and avoid open fields as many insects reside there. Try running towards a space that has lower cut grass or towards any large tree where the branches and leaves are up high. Most likely an insect will rest on the base of the tree and leave you alone as you can get away. Make sure to not have on much fragrance if you will be outside. You may need to wash it off in the midst of running away so insects lose your scent.

Black Eye

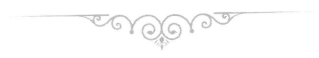

Let's start by acknowledging that black eyes aren't actually "black". They're darker in color but appear more rainbow-like than not. This coloration comes from the fact that are blood is darker until it hits the air from an open wound where it appears red. Since our blood is darker and the skin surrounding the eye is thin, the blood beneath the surface fills in the space under and around the eye where it appears to have this discoloration. Whether you were punched in that area, accidently fell, or ran into something. The body will respond accordingly as needed.

Remedies:

Ice Pack

Probably the most common remedy we reference when thinking treatment for black eyes. This is best to help reduce the initial inflammation around the eye. Use for about 10 minutes every 2 hours after injury. Wrap ice in a plastic bag surround by towel or wrap in a towel before having it placed directly on the affected area.

"Green Ice"

Parsley has been used to reduce bruising and inflammation. Parsley helps blood vessels become narrower which helps provide the benefits mentioned above. Take about 1 cup of Parsley and 2 tablespoons of water and mix together in a blender. Place this mixture into an ice cube tray and place into freezer until they are completely frozen. Wrap an ice cube in a soft cloth and apply directly over your eye socket and bruise for 15-20 minutes at least twice a day.

Arnica Cream

Make your own Arnica Salve to apply to area. If you know an herbalist, you should be able to find Arnica Salve to purchase to use during this time.

My Personal Arnica Salve Recipe:

- You need to infuse your carrier oil with Arnica and St. John's Wort herbs. Place your dried herbs in a sterile (boil before using) glass jar. I use 1 cup of Arnica and 2 tablespoons of St. John's Wort.

- Next, add the carrier oils. I use 1 cup of olive oil and 1 cup of coconut oil.

- Now you will need to infuse the oil. There are several ways to infuse oils with herbs.

- Solar Infusion Method: this is considered to be the best method. To solar infuse your oil, simply place your jar of oil and herbs in the sun for at least 4 weeks. Swoosh the jar occasionally. This makes the best oil but clearly takes much time to complete.

- Slow Cooker Method: to use a slow cooker, place a towel in the bottom of your slow cooker and set you jar of oils and herbs in it. Fill the cooker halfway with water and set to warm or low for 8-10 hours. Gently swoosh the jar occasionally until finished.

- Double Boiler Method: to use the double boiler method, place your jar of oil and herbs into a pot filled with water. Warm the jar over low heat for at least an hour. Then lower the heat (the longer the time the better). Gently swoosh around the jar every 10 minutes or so.

- Once your oil is infused with the and St. John's Wort, it is time to strain the herbs out of the oil. I place a metal strainer with unbleached mullein cloths on top of s glass dish, then pour the oils and herbs onto it.

- Allow the oils to drain through the herbs and cloths, dripping into the container. Don't be impatient during this step. It will take time.

- Typically, I end up with about 1 1/2 cups of infused oil.

- Most will add an essential oil but feel free to skip this step for now. It is now more important to pour the oil into your storage container(s). I use glass jars, but some prefer plastic or tin. The oil will be hot, so proceed with caution.

- Allow the jars to cool. It will form into a nice salve rather quickly.

- Apply the cooled salve to affected area and rub in gently. Wash off after a few hours to avoid any contamination.

Bladder Infection

The bladder's main role in the body is to hold onto urine, while stretching the muscle walls around it, for urine to be released from the body, while also filtering blood within the body. When this process is hindered, it is due to some sort of infection. Infections for the bladder come in the form of excess bacteria in the walls of the bladder, or in the blood. Cleaning these two areas are needed to remove a bladder infection completely. If you do not act on this condition, your bladder infection can turn into a kidney infection.

Remedies:

Water

Drinking close to your bodyweight in ounces a day will promote regular filtration in the body and help the bladder function. Eating more fruits and vegetables that have a high-water content will help provide small, easily absorbed doses of water to help maintain hydration.

Blueberry Juice

Blueberries are very beneficial for the bladder since they are anti-inflammatory and help to kill bacteria within the walls of the bladder. Using a juicer, juice enough blueberries to produce 24 ounces that you can drink daily. This is to be consumed in three 8-ounce servings through the day. Do not use any sweetened brands or purchase any processed blueberry juice. Blueberries need to be the only ingredient. Artificial sugars and preservative being added will not help you receive the most benefits of this juice.

Zinc

The body uses zinc to breakdown bacteria in the body and helps strengthen and support the immune system cells.

Common foods abundant in zinc include: chickpeas, mushrooms, zucchini, squash, okra, Brazil nuts, and walnuts.

Nettle (herb)

A histamine is a natural compound released by cells in the body to help relieve the muscles and tension in the body as it works to break down inflammation. This herb will help begin to break down inflammation caused by this infection.

Red Raspberry (herb)

This herb helps to relax the bladder muscles and relive tension. This herb can also help fight urinary tract infections as well.

My Person Herbal Remedy for Bladder Infections:

Ingredients: Uva Ursi, Dandelion Root, Blue Vervain

Put 1-2 teaspoons of each herb into a cup. Pour boiling water over herbs and let steep for about 10-15 minutes. Strain out herbs and drink an 8-ounce cup twice a day.

If you can combine into a tincture, use 1 ounce of each herb and take ½ teaspoon of mixture three times a day.

Note: if you see any blood in your urine, seek medical attention first before trying any remedies mentioned in this section.

Blisters

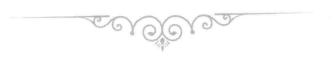

Ablister is a small area of broken cells that are now leaking fluid and have accumulated amongst the underlying muscle tissue, pressing against the outer layer of skin. We tend to want to break open a lister to remove the fluid, but this will not remove the issue; most likely it will worsen it as more fluid will make its way there, but now you will have an open wound that can become infected much easier. A blister is a signal to your body that it's had enough physical activity, or that it is repeatedly using a specific spot on your body where you can make adjustments. It's best to leave it alone an incorporate the remedies outlined in this section.

Remedies:

Lavender Essential Oil

Using lavender essential oil, (not the fragrance or perfume) directly on the skin, will help repair skin cells around the blister. Use a few drops of this oil 2-3 times a day until you notice improvement.

Horse Chestnut (herb)

This herb works to reduce the fluid that is inside of a blister. Get this herb in a tincture form and ass 1 teaspoon of this tincture to 1 cup of cool water. Then soak a small cloth in this liquid and place it over your blister for 20-25 minutes. Do this 2-3 times a day until your blister no longer has any fluid in it and you can move around easier.

Dandelion (herb)

Using this sap from this plant can help provide faster healing for a blister. You want to take dandelions (that have not been sprayed with pesticides) and split their stems. A white "milky" juice should be squeeze out or scraped out of these stems. There may not only be small amounts in each stem, so be patient. Apply this juice directly onto your lister and cover with a bandage. Apply only once a day until blister heals.

Calendula (herb)

Use this herb if your blister has broken open already. You can purchase a calendula oil or tincture. Combine 1 part of tincture with 10 parts of distilled water and apply 1-2 times a day with a bandage until the lister is healed.

Note: the blisters mentioned in this section are for blisters due to physical activity or excessive walking or standing. Not for blisters that come from burns. If you have a burn that begins to ooze yellow materials, it is probably infection, and you should seek medical attention.

Leave The Blister Covering On

If you decide to pop your blister, do not remove the layer of skin around it. This is an additional layer of protection. We feel the urge to remove this skin after we've drained the fluid out but leave this on as we do not want to expose the tender part of the skin where the blister was.

Give It Air

No matter what your approach is, all blisters need air to heal completely. Try to keep it in the air whenever possible in between changing cloths or during a certain part of the day.

Blister Prevention Steps:

Use new socks when wearing new shoes

This may seem unnecessary, but the friction from worn-out socks against newer shoes can promote blisters from reoccurring.

Get insoles for your shoes

Having the correct supports in place can make a huge difference, especially if your current shoes are not helpful with avoiding blisters.

Powder your shoes daily

Applying baby powder to your feet prior to putting on socks will allow your socks to glide easier over your foot and not irritate blisters. Powdering the inside of your shoes will help create the same gliding effect as your feet won't rub very hard against your shoes and help reduce your chances of developing blisters.

My Personal Remedy:

1 tablespoon of Olive Oil

4 drops of Oregano Oil

Crushed onion juice – crush about ½ white or yellow onion until you get 2-3 teaspoons of liquid from it – you may use a juicer as well.

Take all ingredients and mix together well. Gently apply to blister by rubbing onto area. Let air dry and then wash off after about 8-10 minutes if wet.

Body Odor

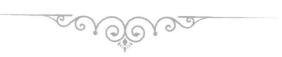

To put things simply, body odor either comes from not washing the outside of our body, or not cleaning the inside of our body. As dirt and sweat accumulates, this creates a layer of waste on the outside of our bodies. On one hand, this layer helps prevent harmful bacteria from getting in immediately. On the other hand, this layer is waste that we are carrying around with us that is not needed and should be washed off.

The intestines are where food and waste materials are collected and broken down within the body. When this area is backed up with items that decay (animal flesh, dairy, sugary-processed foods, and artificial chemicals) this area becomes a literal cemetery of decay and produces a strong aroma that makes its way out of the body through defecation, urination, or the sweat glands. If you left a trash bag outside for a few days, even if the bag was closed shut, the decaying materials inside will give off a strong aroma. We must keep this area of our bodies clean at all times; not just to avoid smelling foul, but for our overall health and longevity.

Remedies:

Chlorophyll

Chlorophyll (a natural chemical in plants) helps the body properly digest what we consume (along with fiber). Making digestion easier will break down items better and help to eliminate toxins from the body quicker. When you have enough chlorophyll in your system, the less odor you will produce.

Common sources of chlorophyll: Callaloo, Dandelion, Lettuces, Turnip Greens, Wild Arugula, Watercress, Nopales (Mexican Cactus)

Dry Brushing

Sometimes when we wash ourselves, we just allow water to mostly run over our bodies. This can be done during the week as we can simply rinse off, but dry brushing helps to remove leftover dried skin cells and provide the body with a much deeper clean. You can purchase a bristle dry skin brush and use it to scrub gently in small circles before taking a shower. You want to scrub yourself while still dry. The discomfort will pass after a few minutes as you work head to toe.

Deodorant

You want to avoid using deodorants to begin with as they contain many chemicals that produce toxins as they enter the bloodstream through the skin. You may choose a simpler option in which you can cut a key lime in half and rub the insides on your armpits and then pat to dry. There are other forms of deodorant you can easily make on your own listed in this section.

Natural Deodorant Recipe #1

Ingredients:

- 1 Key Lime (cut in half)
- 1-2 teaspoons of Coconut Oil

Instructions:

• Rub key lime on your underarms and pat to remove liquid from running down.

• Massage in with a small amount of coconut oil. If you feel a slight burning sensation when you apply your key limes, wash off with water and use less next time.

Natural Deodorant Recipe #2

Ingredients:

- ½ cup of Coconut Oil
- 1 tablespoon of Sea Moss Gel
- ½ cup of Shea Butter
- 1 tablespoon of Key Lime Juice

Instructions:

• Mix all ingredients together and store in a glass airtight container overnight.

• Mix well together before each use.

• Use 1 teaspoon of mixture and massage in and pat to dry.

Avoid Odor Producing Foods:

Making sure to avoid any foods that decay or contain chemicals is best. Removing foods high in oils as well, since they can stick to the walls of the intestines and accumulate bacteria over time.

Main foods to avoid: sugary-processed foods, alcohol, chocolate, dairy, canola or vegetable oil, processed meats, green tea and black tea.

Wear Natural Fabrics

Cotton fabrics absorb perspiration (sweat) better than synthetic materials. The absorbed sweat is then free to evaporate from the fabric, resulting in less odor.

Air It Out

Spend some time outside where natural air is flowing. Go to a beach or park and wear some "breathable" clothing where any smelly areas of the body can air out. If it's your feet, sit down and relax somewhere with your shoes off. If your armpits smell, wear a sleeveless shirt and let the air pass through.

Wash You're A**!

Making sure you properly wash yourself is necessary. Avoid putting on lotions, shampoos, soaps, body wash, etc. within the first few minutes of cleaning your body. Let the water rinse all over first as you wipe and scrub each section.

Boils

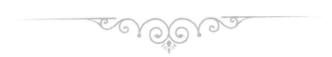

A boil is a bacterial infection on the face, armpit, foot, or groin area caused by a pore or hair follicle being blocked by dead skin cells and other debris. The white blood cells in the body that work to protect these areas and stimulate the immune system, end up dying in the process and create a larger amount of pus and inflammation in the body which leads to swelling and pain.

The main culprit in the development of a boil is, too much (artificial) sugar in the system, particularly in the blood stream. We tend to only associate high sugar in the body to diabetes or high blood pressure. Although those are true in one light, a boil often comes first as the sugar begins to build up in the body and the body works to push it out through the skin cells (hair follicles) and is unsuccessful. What happens when you get a boil is that the gastrointestinal system begins to push out excess bacteria (formed by artificial sugars) which gets into the bloodstream and promotes a skin infection.

Remedies:

Hot Compression

"Bacteria cannot live where there's an adequate blood supply" says Dr. Bennett, N.D., naturopathic and homeopathic physician from Victoria, British Columbia. Using a hot compress on a boil will bring blood flow to the area and diminish the bacteria that is present.

You will want to soak a washcloth in hot water (not enough to burn), wring it out, and then place it onto your boil for 20 minutes at least twice a day. If you've already drained the pus, soak a washcloth in hot water and follow the same steps listed but for only 10 minutes twice a day, followed by the same method using ice-cold water for 10 minutes. Do this hot-cold cycle three time a day if you can for best results.

Echinacea (herb)

Get a tincture of echinacea and apply one tablespoon of this orally three times a day until boil is gone.

Oil of Oregano

Oil of Oregano contains: carvacrol, the main active compound in oregano oil, and a type of antioxidant called a *phenol*. Also, oregano oil contains *thymol*, which helps protect against toxins and fight fungal infections.

One way to use oil of oregano is to add 2-3 drops to water or juice and drink the mixture. However, people should be careful to use oil of oregano and not oregano essential oil. The latter is much stronger and not generally safe to consume.

Kinkeliba / "See-haw" ("leaf of life" herb)

This African her helps kill bacteria that has built up which has contributed to these types of growths. Drink 2-3 teaspoons of this herb in boiled water (cooled off) twice a day following other steps outlined in this section.

Clean the Skin Around Boil

Keeping the skin around the boil clean is a must, especially if it has already been popped or opened. After draining the boil, immediately wash the skin around the boil to prevent excess contamination and chances for infection.

Don't Touch Your Cysts

Boils are usually cysts that have become infected. If you begin touching and messing around with a cyst, a boil will most likely begin to form. Your best bet is that if you have a cyst, just leave it alone when not treating it.

Breast Discomfort

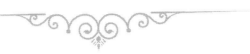

When women have breasts that become lumpy, cystic, or painful, partially around the time of their period, doctors classify this as "fibrocystic breast disease". Do not be alarmed with the word *disease*. Any condition in which the body does not feel at ease is a dis-ease. We must work to not promote disease and contributing to these conditions. What typically occurs to create any breast discomfort is that the natural cycles in the body go through reproductive hormones, which trigger cell growth in the milk-production glands, which then require blood and several other body fluids to fill these areas. The nerve fibers and issues end up feeling more worked than normal and cause pain and discomfort.

Remedies:

Reduce The Excess Estrogen

High-fat diets increase the estrogen levels in the body. This will contribute to the buildup of pain due to additional fluids passing through and around the cellular tissues which can create lumps.

Removing the following foods will be the most helpful when experiencing breast discomfort:

Processed meats, salt, artificial sugars, white (and bleached) flours, soy, high sugar processed foods, and heavier starches that turn into sugar such as potatoes and cruciferous vegetables.

Increase Your Fiber

Fiber begins to push excess estrogen out of the body. Being able to contribute to breaking down estrogen for its removal, helps significantly decrease the workload the body has to do by itself. High-fiber foods contain a natural chemical known as "indole-3-cabinol" which helped estrogen from binding with breast tissues. It is recommended for women to aim towards 21-25 grams of fiber a day, while men aim between 30-38 grams of fiber a day.

Common sources of Fiber: garbanzo beans, lentils, brussels sprouts, sweet potatoes, avocado, pears, sunflower seeds, flax seeds, hazelnuts, apples and berries (high pectin fruits) and onions.

Load up on Iodine

Iodine helps to block out estrogen from sticking to receptors in the breast. Kelp and wakame are very good sources of iodine that you can use in their natural form or as a seasoning. The popular sea vegetable Se Moss also has a very high iodine content and can be consumed in gel, paste, or dried form, or in a capsule after being made into a powder.

Common sources of iodine: Sea Moss and Elderberries as well as many sea plants such as Hijiki, Dulse, Nori, and Bladderwrack.

Cut The Caffeine

Caffeine can contribute to cellular disruption due to depleting the body of oxygen. This substance makes it harder for the cells to communicate and repair themselves as needed, which can continue or add to pains and discomfort.

Massage

A gentle massage can help boost the circulation in the breasts. Using your fingertips, gently massage the areas you feel are in most need. Massage in small, circular motions for a few minutes a day.

Cold Water

Some relief can be achieved by dipping hands in cold water and then cupping the breasts. This can stimulate areas that may have otherwise been asleep, while making it easier to identify any tender spots that you should be aware of.

Get Off "The Pill"

Whenever we say "the pill" most adults immediately know which pill we are referring to, the contraceptive, birth control pill. This pill contains estrogen which should be avoided during this time. Practice other ways of safe sex when feeling any discomfort in or around the breasts.

Check Your Bra Size

Much discomfort can be connected to the size or type of bra you may wear. Many may wear the same bra size without noticing the actual size of their breasts and if they've gotten any smaller or larger over time. It is recommended to not wear a bra to allow the body to work on relaxing as much as possible so it can heal from any discomfort.

Emotional Blockages

The breasts symbolize nurturing. When the body is not being nurtured properly, the breasts are aware of this. Identifying any nurturing role(s) that are being unfulfilled is necessary to explore in order to eliminate many dietary adjustments that may not be required.

Bronchitis

This condition starts out the same as any other cold, stuffy nose and sore throat. But this virus travels further down the respiratory system to the mucous lining of the bronchial tubes which block out air from the windpipe, leading to frequent coughing.

Remedies:

Astragalus (herb)

This plant is an expectorant which means it helps you cough up mucus. Just coughing repeatedly may only send air out of your bronchial tubes and continue to irritate your symptoms. Each time you cough, you should want to expel mucus. This herb can be taken in tea form (about 1 teaspoon per 8-10 ounces of water), in capsule form (600mg capsule), one capsule three times a day, or in tincture form (use 6-8 drops in distilled water) once a day.

Thyme (herb)

Aside from using thyme in tea form, this herb can be very helpful when used as an essential oil in a vaporizer. You want to pour water into the vaporizer that produces warm (not cool) mist. Add 5-6 drops of thyme essential oil and allow the vaporizer to spread the scent into the air. The smell of thyme being sent into the air will help you begin to breathe easier, but also work to warm the air you are breathing so that you can expel mucus from your respiratory system much easier.

Water

Drinking water will help thin some of the mucus. Make sure to drink as needed and aim towards close to half of your body weigh tin ounces until you begin to feel symptoms decrease.

Avoid Dairy

Not that dairy is healthy to begin with, but consuming this substance will essentially clog the breathing tubes as they are being consumed. The excess bacteria allowed in dairy products are not helpful to consume which will only add more issues to this condition.

Cayenne Pepper

Most hot or spicy ingredients can help break apart mucus for it to be discharged from the body. Cayenne pepper is spicy and is an expectorant which helps flush out mucus. Cayenne is very versatile and can be used in a variety of ways, making it easy to incorporate into your diet and lifestyle.

My Personal Remedy For Respiratory Issues:

- Mix together the following herbs (in equal parts): mullein leaf (or mullein flowers), elderberry, dandelion root, guaco, and wild cherry bark.
- Take 1 tablespoon of mixed herbs and place into strainer, then place strainer into cup that hold at least 12 ounces of water.
- Boil spring water and pour into cup (about 8-10oz)
- Let cool and drink twice a day (you can re-use herbs twice each day)

Bruises

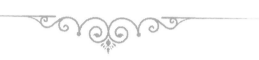

Bruises are broken blood vessels underneath the skin. They can come from a hit, fall, mineral deficiencies, or from constant pressure using certain muscle groups. Most likely, you will know where a bruise came from. If not, and they appear almost at random, then you will want to focus more on the nutritional advice in this section.

Remedies:

Reduce Physical Activity

If you have several bruises or a certain bruise that has been lingering around, you will want to reduce how physically active you are to allow it to heal. You may have gotten it from playing a certain sport, an accident, or from exercising. You will still want the bruise to heal fast regardless, where reducing physical activity will help promote healing in those area(s).

Hydrotherapy

Start by soaking a washcloth in warm water. Then soak another washcloth in cold water. Wring out both washcloths and put the warm washcloth on the bruise for about 3 minutes. Take off the warm washcloth and place the cold washcloth onto the bruise for 30-45 seconds. Repeat this process four times (re-soak cloth after each use). The warm water will help to bring the blood vessels closer to the affected area, while the cold washcloth will push the blood vessels away. This "pumping" motion of having the blood vessels go back and forth will help filter out many of the damaged blood vessels that are present and help reduce the bruise from being visible and heal quicker.

Aromatherapy

Essential oils such as lavender and juniper can help increase circulation and speed up healing. Add a few drops of these oils to a spray or humidifier in your room.

Citrus and Fruits

Citrus and fruits that taste bitter such as, oranges, prickly pears, soursop, and key limes, are rich in flavonoids which help strengthen the blood vessels. They will work to aid the damaged blood vessels that are present from a bruise. Even the white part of these fruits should be consumed as they provide additional flavonoids you can enjoy while helping to heal your bruise(s).

Parsley Ice Cubes

Similar to one of the remedies for a black eye mentioned earlier in this text, making parsley ice cubes can help reduce how long you have a bruise. Simply take some parsley and add a small amount to each cube space in an ice cube tray. Follow this with adding water to fill up each space and place into the freezer to make ice cubes. Wrap a cube (or several) in a cloth and hold on the bruised area to help reduce the severity of the bruise and work to alleviate the pain.

Iron

You want to feed a positive, strong blood flow when working to heal from a bruise. Blood flow to an area that is bruised, allows the body to clean out waste materials and damaged blood and skin cells. Iron is a mineral in the body that transports nutrients, other minerals, and phytonutrients throughout the body so they can get to where they need in order to fulfill their main tasks and obligations. The body may already have enough of these materials that it can borrow them to send to the bruised area in order to promote the healing process until the body is nourished again through diet and lifestyle. As opposed to having to add all of the steps described in this section at a slower rate (as materials don't get where they need to go in a decent amount of time) which will prolong the healing process.

The body uses iron to create a protein (hemoglobin) that's in the red blood cells and carries oxygen to the cells in the body, as well as creates myoglobin, which is a protein that provides oxygen to the muscles. Without iron, nothing we consume really gets to where we need them to go and will create deficiencies that lead to illness. The inability to promote the production of red blood cells that iron provides for us, will reduce the bones' ability to produce bone marrow which sends off these red blood cells into the bloodstream and help to create our immune systems.

Common Sources of Iron: quinoa, wild rice (not black rice), chickpeas/garbanzo beans, kale, dandelion grains, nuts (particularly walnuts), hemp seeds, dates, dried apricots, watercress.

Iron Rich Herbs: sarsaparilla, burdock (and root), guaco, conconsa, chainey root, monkey ladder, chickweed, yellowdock, Lily of the valley, lam's quarters, anamu.

Items That Rob You Of Iron:

- Chocolates
- Cow's milk / "dairy"
- Coffee (yes, even de-caffeinated and weight loss coffee too)
- Sodas
- Yeast
- White flours
- Artificial sugars and food dyes
- Foods high in oxalic acids ("oxalates") such as cauliflower, broccoli, spinach, soy, potatoes, dates, raspberries, navy beans, cashews, and baked potatoes with skin (baked potatoes, French fries, etc.). Oxalates deplete and interfere with iron absorption. You want to increase your iron intake when consuming these items.
- Losing blood. This can happen during women's cycles by not replacing and replenishing iron lost.

Arnica Cream

Make your own Arnica Salve to apply to area. If you know an herbalist, you should be able to find Arnica Salve to purchase to use during this time.

My Personal Arnica Salve Recipe:

You need to infuse your carrier oil with Arnica and St. John's Wort herbs. Place your dried herbs in a sterile (boil before using) glass jar. I use 1 cup of Arnica and 2 tablespoons of St. John's Wort.

Next, add the carrier oils. I use 1 cup of olive oil and 1 cup of coconut oil.

Now you will need to infuse the oil. There are several ways to infuse oils with herbs.

Solar Infusion Method: this is considered to be the best method. To solar infuse your oil, simply place your jar of oil and herbs in the sun for at least 4 weeks. Swoosh the jar occasionally. This makes the best oil but clearly takes much time to complete.

Slow Cooker Method: to use a slow cooker, place a towel in the bottom of your slow cooker and set you jar of oils and herbs in it. Fill the cooker halfway with water and set to warm or low for 8-10 hours. Gently swoosh the jar occasionally until finished.

Double Boiler Method: to use the double boiler method, place your jar of oil and herbs into a pot filled with water. Warm the jar over low heat for at least an hour. Then lower the heat (the longer the time the better). Gently swoosh around the jar every 10 minutes or so.

Once your oil is infused with the Arnica and St. John's Wort, it is time to strain the herbs out of the oil. I place a metal strainer with unbleached mullein cloths on top of s glass dish, then pour the oils and herbs onto it.

Allow the oils to drain through the herbs and cloths, dripping into the container. Don't be impatient during this step. It will take time.

Typically, I end up with about 1 1/2 cups of infused oil.

Most will add an essential oil but feel free to skip this step for now. It is now more important to pour the oil into your storage container(s). I use glass jars but some prefer plastic or tin. The oil will be hot, so proceed with caution.

Allow the jars to cool. It will form into a nice salve rather quickly.

Apply the cooled salve to affected area and rub in gently. Wash off after a few hours to avoid any contamination.

Bunions

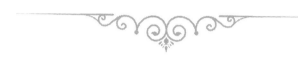

When the joint connected to one of the bones in the foot becomes inflamed from constant pressure, the foot forms a swollen, painful "knob" on the side of the foot (or by the toe joint) that is inflamed. Wearing certain shoes that are tight or those that rub against the toes (which can alter their alignment) are the main ways the foot begins to form a bunion.

Remedies:

Stretching (the big toe)

This is very important due to the main area of bunions being formed comes from the big toe pressing against (or over) the other toe(s). stretching the toe is not the same as stretching the muscles attached to it but stretching it regularly will promote healthy alignment and will remain helpful as a preventative measure. Get an extra-strength (thick) rubber band and wrap around each big toe. Keep your heels together and slowly pull your feet apart to make a "v" shape. Hold in place as you feel your big toes stretch for about 5-10 seconds at a time, and slowly return to the start position. Repeat this 10-20 times a day or as much as you can without much discomfort.

Ice

Place a few ice cubes into a plastic bag and wrap with a small washcloth. Apply directly to area for 10 minutes and then take off for 10 minutes. Repeat this process at least three times a day (replace ice cubes as needed) until you begin to feel better or immediately after you feel any flare ups.

Massage

Put some massage oil onto the affected area and gently massage around the bunion. It will help to also massage other areas of the foot as well, especially around the ankle (even the calf) to help promote circulation.

Hydrotherapy

To help continue to improve circulation, incorporate a hot-and-cold foot bath. Fill two large basins, one with warm water and one with ice-cold water. Place your feet first in the cold basin for 30 seconds, and then immediately place your feet into the warm water for about 2 minutes. Repeat at least three times a day to keep the blood vessels active and stimulated. Massaging your legs regularly will remain crucial to reducing your chances of severe symptoms.

Burns

1st and 2nd degree burn – small burn that does not break the skin or does so minimally. These tend to swell and turn white when you apply pressure (1st degree) or a lower layer of skin, are thicker, very painful, and cause the skin to turn red and swollen (2nd degree).

3rd degree burn – medical emergency. These burns go through deeper layers of the skin and damage the deeper tissues of the skin leaving them white or charred.

First and second-degree burns are what we will focus on in this section as they can be healed and treated with a variety of remedies. Third-degree burns should be handled and managed by a health care professional with available resources needed. However, if a first or second-degree burn cover close to or more than 10% of the body, it should be treated as a third-degree burn as infection can spread and can require additional treatment.

Remedies:

Cold Water

Once your burn occurs, you will want to run cold water over it for about 15-20 minutes. Do not use ice cold water or ice as it can make the burn worse. If your burn is a contact burn, you can immediately begin soaking in cold water. If your burn is from grease or some hot liquid, remove any clothing or material that's near the burn, wash any remnants of liquid off, then begin to soak under cold water.

Lavender Essential Oil

Combine two ounces of distilled water and 25 drops of lavender essential oil into a glass spray bottle. Store the bottle in a cool, dry dark space. When ready to use, shake the bottle a bit and spray directly onto the burn. Do not use on broken skin.

Note: the darker the bottle, the better it will preserve the mixture.

Cover Your Burn

Make sure to cover your burn with a gauze pad or clean cloth to avoid damaging or irritating the burn. This is best practice to helping the burn heal on its on as well.

Leave Your Blisters Alone

When you have blisters around your burn, these are essentially the body's self-made band-aids that serve as an additional layer or protection. Leave them alone and treat them as a part of the whole burn.

Vitamin-E Oil

This oil can help prevent burns from having visible scars. As much as I don't specifically wish to promote any artificial versions of vitamins, eating foods high in vitamin-E will take much longer to heal you wound as opposed to you putting this form of oil directly onto the area it is intended for.

Aloe Vera

Has long been used to speed up recovery for 1st and 2nd degree burns. You can find this plant at most local markets or grocery stores. You want to slice this plant open with a knife, squeeze or scoop out all of the transparent pulp, and then apply directly on the skin covering the burn. You can let this settle in before washing off after about an hour. You can do this as often as you want, and this method is recommended over purchasing any commercial products that contain many other ingredients.

Calendula

This flower contains many anti-inflammatory properties that can help heal and bring down swelling. You may find many skin care products that contain Calendula, but you will want to either drink this in tea form often or make a compress to place onto the burn. For tea, about 2 teaspoons of this herb twice a day would be recommended. Or boil 1 tablespoon of this plant, strain, and after being cooled off, soak a small towel or cloth in the water and then let soak directly over the burn. Leave it on for about 10-15 minutes before letting it dry and then repeating 2-3 times a day. This flower is particularly helpful for 2nd degree burns as it helps promote the formation of blood vessels that work to repair the affected area.

Bursitis (and Tendonitis)

*B*ursitis is inflammation that provides padding between a muscle and the bony projection of a joint such as a knee, elbow, hip, or shoulder. We have about 150 of these areas within the body to help assist with mobility when being physically active. When they become inflamed, this is when bursitis is formed.

Tendonitis is inflammation of a tendon that connects the muscle to the bone.

The main cause of both of these similar conditions is, sudden overuse. We often have a regular schedule that our body adjusts to. When we suddenly use an area of the body more than usual, this contributes to the development of one or both of these conditions.

Remedies:

Ice

Using ice to soothe these inflamed areas is best practice for the first 24-hours. An ice massage can help reduce the inflammation and help prevent some of the irritableness of these conditions. Using a bag of frozen vegetables such as peas or carrots can help as well since their shapes can feel like smaller ice cubes but do not shrink in size like ice cubes do. You can plan to regularly massage the area with ice for about 5-10 minutes and then remove for 5-10 minutes. You don't want to leave this on too long so that the area becomes numb because then it can be hard to determine if any of the symptoms are going away.

Fatty Acids

Omega-3 is a fatty acid to focus on if you have bursitis or tendonitis. Dr. Edwards, M.D., a physician form Fresno, California states that, "A person who gets omega-3 fatty acids in adequate amounts will not get bursitis or tendonitis as readily."

Common Sources of Fatty Acids: Brazil Nuts, Walnuts, Kola Nuts, Avocados, Bananas, Sea Vegetables (Nori, Wakame, Hijiki, Sea Moss, Bladderwrack), Coconut, Coconut Oil, Olive Oil, Grapeseed Oil, Avocado Oil, Mushrooms, Quinoa, Wild Rice.

Rest

Anytime you can rest, will not make the condition worse. Rest whenever possible and do not attempt to work through the pain as often as you can.

Gently Move The Area

Eventually you will want to move the area that is in pain to detect when recovery is achieved. Start by gently moving the area by stretching, moving slowly around in a pool or hot tub.

Calluses (and Corns)

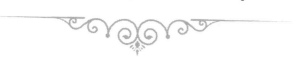

Calluses protect the body from excess pressure. They are formed by dead skin cells that accumulate from pressure and form a bump. When these bumps for a hard cover, they create what we call "corns". These can be formed mostly on the hands and feet. Due to additional pressure, we have on our feet, we tend to develop corns on our feet and calluses on our hands even though both can be formed in either place.

Remedies:

Don't Become A Surgeon

Do not make attempts to use any tools to cut or tear off layers of calluses or corns. This will literally open up these areas to unwanted, harmful bacteria and may actually increase the size of a callus or a corn as they body will want to create a protection layer over it which will make it larger. You can also injure yourself by using any sharp tools you are not familiar with using.

Callus File

When you notice a callus begin to form you want to avoid touching it. Once a callus has made its mark and is settled in, you should begin to gently use a callus file (or pumice stone) to lights scrub against the callus to help remove some of the outer layers of the callus and help work towards healing the area. Make sure to wash the area with warm water and then cover after to avoid bacteria from getting in. remove covering at night so the area can air itself out.

Chamomile Tea

This is a common herbal tea but can also be helpful for developing calluses that begin to form. You can soak your callus in chamomile tea. It will work to soothe and soften the harder skin. Take 2 tablespoons of Chamomile herb (and its parts) and add to a small pot of boiling water. Let cool and pour into a container that is large enough to soak your callus. If it's one of both of your feet, pouring the tea into a foot massager would be best, but a bowl or large plastic container can be suitable enough. If it is on your hand, a bowl or smaller container would be best.

Calendula (herb)

Use this on a corn or callus that is hard. It is needed to heal harder skin in order to accurately treat the area. Put calendula oil or calendula salve onto the area and cover with a bandage. Do this twice a day, but you may have to reapply this moisturizer following any exercise.

Custom Shoe Insoles

This can reduce some of the pressure applied to the foot when dealing with a corn. They will work to redistribute your weight so there is less added pressure to certain areas of the foot as well.

Cancer (general)

When cancer is present you want to be very specific due to which form it is (i.e. prostate cancer, thyroid cancer, breast cancer, etc.) to be most effective and not contribute to it spreading. This section will review general things to remain mindful of upon a cancer diagnosis or warning sign(s). To begin, we must understand that we all have cancerous cells within our bodies all of the time. These cancer cells help to kill of various items in the body and also help to promote balance and homeostasis in the body. However, if we feed these cancerous cells and they stick around longer than normal, they will leech off of other cells and when those cells replicate as all cells do while we are alive, we develop a condition known as "abnormal cell growth", otherwise known as, *cancer*.

Also, it is important to note that different cells fight different types of cancer. For example, one way the immune system fights cancer is by sending out a special form of white blood cells called T cells: The T cells see cancer as "foreign" cells that don't belong in the body. The T cells attack and try to destroy the cancerous cells.

Nature provides protection against natural causes of cancer, but human-made causes are problematic for the body to address because they exist outside the normal development and patterns of life. The radiation, pollution, and chemicals we consume in processed foods challenge the homeostasis in the body which causes mental and physical stressors that adversely affect our biology and genes.

Cancer develops in 3 stages (1. initiation, 2. promotion, and 3. progression).

1. Once u absorb or consume carcinogens, they make their way into the bloodstream and store themselves into fat cells. Consuming fatty foods overworks the liver which prevents these carcinogens from being removed from the body.

2. Inability to remove carcinogens from the body replicates cells which promote maintaining those carcinogens and leads to tumors growing or spreading in the body.

3. After removing a tumor or growth without cleansing the cells promotes further cell reproduction to sustain the body's cellular needs which leads to the progression of cancer cells spreading through the rest of the body away from the initial location of cancer cells.

Nutrition controls the expression and replication of mutated cells. What u consume:

1. limits the initiation stage, 2. controls and regulates the promotion stage, and 3. works to eliminating cancerous cells in the progression stage.

The human immune system is designed to protect against viruses, macrophages, and antibodies. Consuming plants provides protection against these pathogens. Phytonutrients in plants help protect the body from viruses, macrophages, and antibodies. Ridding the body of cancer involves limiting cancer "promoters" while increasing "anti-promoters". Promoters include processed foods (which create nutritional imbalances) exposed to radioactive materials, viruses, bacteria, and stress. Anti-promoters include foods without exposure to radioactive materials, viruses and bacteria. Nutritional imbalances serve as promoters, while a balanced nutrition serves as an anti-promoter.

Cancer cells also need sugar to thrive. When u consume sugar, the "beta-cells" in the body produce insulin. By consuming sugar excessively this creates an overproduction of insulin in the body and u will feel immune to the effects cancer is causing the body. This is why people are often shocked to learn that they have had cancer for several months although they would have noticed the side effects earlier if they did not consume much sugar.

Remedies:

Guinea Hen Weed (herb)

Used to reverse cancer, reduce muscle spasms and fever, relaxes nerves, relives pain, lowers blood-sugar levels, and treats bacterial, fungal, and virus infections. This is NOT a form of Marijuana. It is a Jamaican Herb. Guinea Hen Weed Tea several times per week can directly help reduce symptoms of lymphoma.

Blessed Thistle (herb)

High in iron, increases circulation and oxygen delivery to the brain, supports heart and liver functioning. Supports the gallbladder (improves digestion / improves appetite) and can increase/enrich milk in nursing mothers. This herb also helps remove toxins, acids, and mucus to assist in cleansing the inside of cells.

Caution: for pregnant/nursing women. Best to be used prior to pregnancy.

Rhubarb Root (herb)

Used to regulate the digestive tract to treat digestive issues that include: diarrhea, constipation, stomach pain, and acid reflux. Rhubarb Root softens stools to ease bowel movements and reduce pain from hemorrhoids Also used to treat kidney stones and kidney disease, removes acids and mucus – intracellularly cleanses the cells.

Mullein (herb)

Used as an expectorant to remove mucus from the respiratory tract, including the lungs. Can be used in tea form as you can use the flowers or the leaves of this plant.

Sea Moss

Helps provide an abundance of minerals that the body needs to remain in good health. Can help remove any deficiencies a person may have which has contributed to their cancer diagnosis.

Vitamin-C

Vitamin-C helps to improve a stressed immune system that is fighting an infection. It plays a major role in helping the body to protect itself. What we refer to as Vitamin C is a water-soluble nutrient and powerful antioxidant that help form and maintain connective tissues, including the bones, blood vessels, and the skin. This nutrient can help reduce symptoms of allergic reactions and inflammation which will help to avoid any prolonging issues. Vitamin-C also is responsible for manufacturing the adrenal hormones which are needed to combat the stress the body goes through when trying to heal from a disease or illness.

Common Sources of Vitamin-C: Black Currants, Bell Peppers (red and green), Papaya, Spring Onions, Strawberries, Cantaloupe, Mango, Oranges, Watercress, Raspberries, and Tomatoes

Rattlesnake

The rattlesnake (dried) and meat has been used in some cultures to treat various cancers; primarily the Asian Sand Viper and the South American Rattlesnake (RDB) according to researchers at the Jinnah University for Women in Pakistan, and the Red Diamondback Rattlesnake in Arizona, USA, according to researchers at Wright State University in Ohio, USA, who've researched snake venom being a treatment for various illness including cancer.

Researchers at the Jinnah University for Women in Pakistan have researched proteins such as, "eristostatin" and "contortrostatin" that have been found in the venoms of Asian sand viper and South American rattlesnake respectively have the ability to fight against cancers. "Mambalgins" (from the venom of black mamba) are believed to have analgesic and anti-inflammatory effects as well which can prevent cancer from spreading.

Lycopene

A pigment called lycopene works to block free radicals that damage cells and help stimulate the immune system. Both of these benefits provide what someone needs who is battling prostate cancer. Dr. Robert Roundtree, M.D., co-founder of the Helios Health Center in Boulder, Colorado prescribes 1 teaspoon a day of tomato paste for his patients with prostate cancer. The reason he does this is because the pigment lycopene is abundant in tomatoes. Dr. Roundtree notes that, "Lycopene has more potent antioxidant properties than beta-carotene, and it has anti-cancer properties." Oxidative stress (imbalance of free radicals) remains the primary cause of depleting lycopene from the body.

Common Sources of Lycopene: tomatoes, watermelon, papaya, pink guava, and pink grapefruit.

Soursop

According to the National Institute of Health (NIH), soursop fruit, leaves, and extract inhibits the proliferation of PC-3 human cancer cells. Traditional uses of soursop have been used to treat bacterial and fungal infections, as it possesses anthelmintic, antihypertensive, anti-inflammatory, and anticancer activities. In the NIH study, they found that soursop seeds induce apoptosis, helping to inhibit colorectal cancer cells and breast cancer cells. Also, that soursop leaves inhibited prostate cancer cells and colon cancer cells.

You can find soursop extract to take topically, and soursop leaves which you can make into a tea. The soursop fruit can be found at. Local markets but prices can vary where it is expensive in some areas.

Tea Tree Oil (extract)

This extract causes "mitochondrial superoxide production" and "apoptosis" which promotes compounds that induce tumor regression which can help prevent tumors from growing or spreading.

Cannabidiol (CBD) Products

Research indicates the CBD may have potential for the treatment of cancer, including the symptoms and signs associated with cancer and its treatment. Preclinical research suggests CBD may address many of the pathways involved in the pathogenesis of cancers.

Selenium

This mineral helps control free radicals in the body that damage cells and DNA which triggers the formation of cancer and many other conditions. In a research study, researchers found that hundreds of men who took 20-miligrams of selenium cut the incidence of prostate cancer by 60%. Dr. Michael Schachter, M.D., director of the Schachter Center for Complementary Medicine in Sufern, New York treats his patients for prostate cancer with 400-600 micrograms of selenium daily.

Common sources of Selenium: brazil nuts, walnuts, chickpeas/garbanzo beans, kola nuts, dandelion greens, and nettle, and alfalfa. Recommended to consume about 400 micrograms a day. You may also plan to purchase a tasteless, odorless, liquid form of selenium by the brand Aqua Sel where you take 1-2 drops per day (or no more than 190mg daily).

Fatty Acids

Fatty acids contain an abundance of nutrients that work to control the development of cells. All forms of cancer are conditions in which cell growth and development out of control. Essential fatty acids (omega-3, omega-6, omega-9) help repair the cellular damage that has taken place over the years from consuming too many artificial sugars.

Common Sources of Fatty Acids: (Brazil Nuts, Walnuts, Kola Nuts, Avocados, Bananas, Sea Vegetables (Nori, Wakame, Hijiki, Sea Moss, Bladderwrack), Coconut, Coconut Oil, Olive Oil, Grapeseed Oil, Avocado Oil, Mushrooms, Quinoa, Wild Rice.

Items To Cut

Items listed in this section are geared towards avoiding the development of prostate cancer in the first place. However, removing these items will help to reduce the chances of this condition form spreading as well.

Saturated fats – these weaken the immune system and increase your risk of prostate cancer. Red meat, dairy products, and processed foods are the main items with these types of fat.

Stress Reduction Activities

You can place a eucalyptus plant in your shower (hang it behind the shower head or possibly on a window). When the steam interacts with the eucalyptus it will reduce stress, create mental clarity, improve "dendrite" interactions in the brain, and also act as an anti-inflammatory and help with respiratory health. RELAX and get enough sleep. Engaging in physically stimulating exercises such as, working out, yoga, clenching fists, and buying things like a weighted-blanket can all directly help with relaxation. You can also use things like lavender oil and drinking lavender tea to help enhance sleep quality. There is much research conducted on how conditions such as cancer impact and disrupt the digestive system and the bowels which make absorbing nutrients challenging and can include the development of Irritable bowel Syndrome (IBS).

Douglas A. Drossman, M.D., professor of psychiatry with the division of digestive diseases and co-director of the UNC Center for Functional Gastrointestinal and motility Disorders at the University of North Carolina at Chapel Hill School of Medicine, states that "There's a very good connection between stress and an irritable bowel." He adds that we do not want to become stressed simply because we have IBS and create a cycle of symptoms and stress. It is best to recognize early symptoms, acknowledge that this has happened before and will pass, and understand that you will not die because you are having a bowel issue. Anything you do to help relax will help you decrease overall symptoms. Try to become more still, meditation, or even self-hypnosis can help to become calmer.

Colon Cleanse

Clean the colon. You will need to do this regardless of your condition but specifically for clearing the system in the body that gets rid of waste materials (which you will have more of with a cancer diagnosis).

Clean the colon using some or all of the following: Ginger, Cascara Sagrada, Rhubarb Root, Prodijiosa and Blessed Thistle. Drink as a tea daily. All herbs should come with instructions, and these are safe to mix together. Caution: these herbs can be very bitter. This is not a cause for concern and does not mean these herbs are spoiled or contaminated in any way.

For Adults:

(for children, cut dosages in half to 1/3 the amount listed)

Colon Cleanse Tea: 1 teaspoon of Cascara Sagrada, ½ teaspoons of Black Walnut, and 1 teaspoon of Rhubarb Root for about 10-12oz of tea. This tea is very bitter. But you want this tea to be bitter so that it can break down what is not needed in the body. If this tea is too difficult for you to adjust to, you can always search for these herbs or colon cleanses available in capsule form. You will want to try this tea prior to fasting to identify which option will be best for you during your liquid fast. Cleaning the colon is vital for survival. The Colon is a part of the gut which is essentially our 2nd brain. It holds onto leftover waste and materials that create inflammation in the body and directly trigger many symptoms of disease. Without a clean colon, the body cannot function well as a whole.

Duration: 5-6 consecutive days at a time. Do for 5 days then take at least 2 days off.

Ingredients:

Cascara Sagrada (1 teaspoon)

Black Walnut hull (1/2 teaspoon)

Rhubarb Root (1 teaspoon)

Prodijiosa (1 teaspoon) – if applicable/available to you.

Water 8oz (boiling)

*You can do any combination of these herbs or take individually for this cleanse. You do not need every ingredient, but this cleanse works best when including all herbs mentioned above.

This cleanse is probably the most important to our health. The colon is essentially our second brain and is a part of the large intestine which works to remove waste from the body. The colon is responsible for holding a temporary storage of feces, but also reabsorbing water and minerals necessary to our health.

Iron

You will want to load up on your iron-rich items during your healing/restoration period. Iron from plants (Iron-phosphate and Iron-fluorine) are essential to the body, as opposed to iron-oxide which comes from heavier metals and does not assimilate in a manner with the body that can help promote healing within the blood. As you have a steady blood flow to this area (and the rest of the body), it is crucial to strengthening the quality of this flow so that the body does not have to work as hard to send blood to where it's most needed in the body. Many prescriptions and pharmaceuticals contain a higher amount of iron-oxide and can lead to several side effects and other conditions.

Iron is the mineral that helps transport nutrients in the body to wherever they need to go or are most needed. Keeping these passageways clear is best for absorbing nutrients, vitamins, and minerals, and helping the body identify what is waste and not needed. We must consume enough iron, but also not consume what robs us of iron which are processed foods and items difficult to digest as we send blood to the colon to help create additional mucus that pushes waste material through the digestive tract. Even if you consume 100% of everything that the body needs, if you do not consume enough iron regularly, these vitamins, nutrients, and minerals will not get to their destinations, and you will continue to show signs and symptoms of illness.

Common sources of Iron: Quinoa, Wild Rice (not black rice), Chickpeas/Garbanzo Beans, Kale, Nuts (particularly Walnuts), Hemp Seeds, Dates, Dried Apricots, Watercress

Common Herbs for Iron: Sarsaparilla, Burdock (and root), Guaco, Chainey Root, Monkey Ladder, Chickweed, Yellowdock.

Canker Sores

Canker sores are caused by salt and stress. Excess salt creates small deposits that build up in the body, and with the added moisture in the mouth, this begins to create and ulcer (an open sore) which inevitably turns into a canker sore. Canker sores are known as "aphthous ulcers" to doctors in the medical field.

As mentioned in other sections in this text, stress create salt molecules within the body as well. A nucleus of an atom can only hold 2 electrons in the 1st valance and 8 in the remainder valances (outer layers). When we get stressed (heat rises) this causes the sodium (Na) molecules in the body to throw electrons off as they lose energy. This makes it unstable and causes it to create a bond with whatever is compatible with it in its current state (this is called "Covalent Bonding"). In this case the sodium molecule is now compatible with chloride (Cl) molecule because chloride produces "free" electrons to the body.

Now you have Na + Cl which is "NaCl" which creates Sodium Chloride aka "Salt".

Remedies:

Zinc

A canker sore is a wound. Wounds heal faster when there's adequate zinc in the body according to Beverly Yates, N.D., physician and director of the Natural Health Care Group located in Seattle, Washington. Loading up on this necessary mineral will help relieve you of your canker sore.

Common Sources of Zinc: hemp seeds, wild rice, quinoa, avocados, chickpeas, mushrooms, zucchini, squash, okra, Brazil nuts, and walnuts.

Iron

Women tend to get more canker sores than men on average. This is directly contributed to low iron. Lack of iron means there is not a strong blood flow. Without a strong blood flow, toxins cannot move out regularly and with the added moisture within the mouth, canker sores begin to develop.

Common sources of Iron: Quinoa, Wild Rice (not black rice), Chickpeas/Garbanzo Beans, Kale, Dandelion Greens, Prunes, Nuts (particularly Walnuts), Hemp Seeds, Dates, Dried Apricots, Watercress

Common Herbs for Iron: Sarsaparilla, Burdock (and root), Guaco, Chainey Root, Monkey Ladder, Chickweed, Yellowdock.

Natural Toothpaste

Using baking soda or some form of natural toothpaste is best to avoid consuming chemicals which can further irritate this condition.

Miswak Brush

Brushing your teeth with a miswak stick can help reduce bacteria in the mouth. No toothpaste is needed, only water. You can chew or lightly brush your teeth directly.

Tea Bags

Chamomile contains "tannins" which are natural chemicals that work to relieve pain. Place this herb into a tea bag and let sit in your mouth against your canker sore for about 10 minutes. Remove tea bag and rinse your mouth out with water. Repeat three times a day.

Avoiding Irritants

The amino acid known as arginine can irritate and even contribute to causing many canker sores. This amino acid is in many natural and unnatural food items. Avoid the following when you have a canker sore: coffee, citrus fruits, walnuts, chocolate, and strawberries.

Carpel Tunnel Syndrome

We use hands for just about everything. The issue of Carpel Tunnel come about when there is repeated use of particular muscles and joints in the hard more so than others. It's essentially accumulated trauma from repetitious movements with the hands. When the inflammation remains present to protect the joints and are then repeatedly used while inflammation is present, this is when Carpel Tunnel syndrome begins to settle in. Carpel Tunnel is like trying to weave through traffic during rush hour.

Remedies:

Circular Movement

Whenever you have a joint issue, it's best to move in circular motions. Once you feel a tingling sensation, it's best to stop what you are doing and begin to move your hands and fingers in circular motions. You want to keep circulation flowing well during moments you feel pain settling in so that you can rest immediately after. If you choose to "work through the pain", you will have to deal with pain while you rest.

Keep Your Hands High

Our hands pretty much never reach above our hears unless we are reaching for something, or when we exercise or play a sport where this happens very briefly. A lot of the blood flow to the hands are downward. We want to reduce this by raising our hands up so flow can work away from our hands when resting. Feel free to sit back in a seat and put your hands behind your head as you relax. Take a few minutes whenever possible to keep your hands up to relive the tension your hand must feel.

Exercise Regularly

As you exercise and strengthen the connecting muscles and tissues around the hands, the more you will reduce your symptoms. It is important to do simple exercises to not irritate the area, but exercise will remain best for preventative action to treat carpel tunnel.

Willow Bark (herb)

This herb is a natural pain reliver. It contains a chemical known as *salicylate*, which is an active ingredient in aspirin that's used for headaches but can help reduce other pains as well. Drink one to two (measuring cups) every 6 hours until you feel better. You can make tea with 2 teaspoons for every 10-12 ounces of water. Make a batch of it in advance if you choose. For carpal tunnel syndrome it would benefit you to soak your hands in tea or a compress after water has cooled off.

Sea Moss

Besides being abundant in many of the minerals we need to fulfill out cellular needs, Sea Moss is particularly high in potassium-chloride which help to break down inflammation. You can consume this in gel or paste form for best results. Can take a few tablespoons a day or add to a drink or make as a tea.

Iron

You will want to load up on your iron-rich items during your healing/restoration period. Iron from plants (Iron-fluorine) is essential to the body, as opposed to iron-oxide which comes from heavier metals and does not assimilate in a manner with the body that can help promote healing within the blood. As you have a steady blood flow to this area (and the rest of the body), it is crucial to strengthening the quality of this flow so that the body does not have to work as hard to send blood to where it's most needed in the body. Many prescriptions and pharmaceuticals contain a higher amount of iron-oxide and can lead to other related health issues you want to avoid. Boosting your iron levels will promote much needed blood flow that has remained stagnate from the constant inflammation in and around the joints that have developed into this condition.

Common sources of Iron: *Quinoa, Wild Rice (not black rice), Chickpeas/Garbanzo Beans, Kale, Dandelion Greens, Prunes, Nuts (particularly Walnuts), Hemp Seeds, Dates, Dried Apricots, Watercress*

Common Herbs for Iron: *Sarsaparilla, Burdock (and root), Guaco, Chainey Root, Monkey Ladder, Chickweed, Yellowdock.*

Cataracts

This condition is formed when one off the lenses in the eye becomes "cloudy". Many opt for surgery which goes in to remove the clouded lens. The main cause of cataracts is nutritional deficiencies. If you were deficient before and went in for surgery to remove that clouded lens, it won't be long before another lens is clouded. You want to remove this from happening by meeting your nutritional needs. Doctors may wish to prescribe various supplements such as vitamin-A or vitamin-c due to their antioxidant properties. However, the primary minerals that are deficient are, selenium and zinc. Selenium works to prevent cell deterioration and Zinc helps the immune system detect and remove weaker cells from the body.

Remedies:

Selenium and Zinc

As stated above, Selenium and Zinc play two crucial roles in the body. We must work to meet these needs whether or not cataracts are present.

Common Selenium sources: brazil nuts, walnuts, chickpeas/garbanzo beans, kola nuts, dandelion greens, and nettle, and alfalfa. Recommended to consume about 400 micrograms a day.

**Consuming zinc along with copper will provide an additional boost towards improvements for his condition. You can drink water from a copper vessel to receive adequate copper daily. Recommended to consume about 30mg a day.

Sulfur

Sulfur is another mineral that has been a main contributor to cataract development and vision difficulties. The nutrient sulfur is considered one of the most important elements for good vision says Dr. Grossman, O.D., optometrist, acupuncturist, and co-director of the Integral Health Center in New Paltz, New York.

Common Sulfur sources: walnuts, chickpeas/garbanzo beans, tomatoes, dandelion greens, kale, apples, onions, watermelon, turnip greens, and avocados.

Remove High Fat and Fried Foods

These foods increase the production of free radicals in the body which are responsible for damaging immune cells and interrupting the communication of cells in the body. these items will not only greatly contribute to cataract development but remain detrimental to overall health as well.

Manuka Honey

Manuka honey is produced by bees that pollinate the flowers found on a manuka bush; a kind of tea tree. The form of honey originates from parts of Australia, New Zealand, and Honduras. Traditionally used to heal wounds, sore throats, and to prevent tooth decay. However, this honey has become more commonly known to treat acne, prevent ulcers, and treat eye deficits.

This form of honey is much different from traditional honey as it comes from a different source and provides additional benefits. Manuka honey is an antioxidant, and antibacterial substance. It contains a compound (omega-3 fatty acid) known as, dihydroxyacetone (DHA) which are found in the manuka flowers. DHA increases mitochondrial activity while reducing inflammation in the eyes, helping promote overall eye health. This compound studied by registered dietitian, Bailey Flora, RD, notes the amount of DHA present in manuka honey. Flora states, "it's about 100 times higher than other traditional honey."

There are many ways to use manuka honey for the eyes. Boiling the comb itself in distilled water, using as an eye wash, or as eye drops. Follow directions on label, but typically it is available in eye drop form in which you can place 3-4 drops directly into each eye daily. You should see noticeable changes within or after 4-5 weeks.

Note: like any other honey, manuka honey does contain a high amount of sugar made from fructose and glucose. So, you will want to remain mindful of this if you have diabetes, liver disease, heart disease, or want to avoid consuming excess calories.

My Personal Remedy:

(this is just an eye rinse. It will help moisturize the eyes but will not cure or solve issues regarding cataracts)

Mix 1 tablespoon or eyebright herb

Mix 1 tablespoon of blue vervain herb

Boil 4 cups of distilled or spring water

Add herbs to boil, let cool for 10-15 minutes (or until completely cool)

Strain herbs and place water in the refrigerator.

Take a small cup, tincture tube or handful and pour gently into your eyes one at a time.

Move your eyes in close wise, counterclockwise, diagonal, up and down, side to side motions while keeping your eye lids closed to rinse your eyes.

You may also drink this mixture but will need to make several more servings and may not directly go right for washing out your eyes.

(Note: make sure no small pieces are in the water as even the smallest piece can irritate your eye).

Chapped Lips

The lips are covered with tissue called epithelial tissue which is the same type of sensitive tissue that lines your digestive tract. This tissue can only take so much damage until something has a negative impact on it. Our lips being on the outside of our body causes it to adjust and adapt more than our digestive tissues but are also more visible for us to see any issue such as chapped lips.

Remedies:

Proper Hydration

Anytime the body is not adequately hydrated, areas will become drier by default. Not only drinking about half of your body weight in ounces (ex. if you weigh 100lbs, drink 50oz) but consuming foods that provide water is necessary. Melons, berries, tomatoes, and cucumbers are only a few items that should regularly be in your diet. Consuming items that provide hydration can help wash away and also neutralize the erosive acids that remain in the body from eating things detrimental to our health.

Calcium, Magnesium, and Fatty Acids

Calcium works to help hold the cells together. However, cells can't absorb calcium with fatty acids, and calcium by itself can be harmful and needs Magnesium to help stimulate digestion within the body so the cells know what to absorb and what to not absorb. These three working in tandem is ideal for cellular health, but specifically for the form of tissue the lips (and digestive tract) are made of.

Common Calcium sources: sea moss, kale, okra, dandelion greens, turnip greens, lettuce, papaya, and oranges.

Common Magnesium sources: quinoa, brazil nuts, hemp milk, CBD products (specifically CBD oil).

Common Fatty Acids: hemp seeds, avocados, avocado oil, walnut oil, grapeseed oil, and walnuts.

Water

Remain hydrated with water to help reduce skin issues. If lips are chapped or beginning to feel tighter, make sure to sip hot water lightly to help the skin tissues to relax and hold onto moisture. Drinking some form of herbal tea is recommended daily to provide a warm liquid in addition to the many benefits herbal teas provide the body.

My Person Lip Balm Recipe:

1 tablespoon of Shea Butter

1 teaspoon of coconut oil

Take 2 carnauba leaves and set them to dry. When the leaves begin to dry, the wax will begin to form on the outside of the leaf. Scrape this off and use a knife to cut open the inside of the leaf where you can scrape more of the wax out. 1 carnauba leaf should produce about 2g (0.07oz) of wax.

Slowly mix all ingredients together and let settle in the refrigerator for about 1 hour. This substance will start to harden a bit but will form a substance you are familiar with if you've used lip balm before.

Gently apply this mixture to your lips periodically throughout the day as needed.

Chronic Fatigue Syndrome

Most doctors and health professionals will attribute chronic fatigue to stress or working too much. But we all know many people who work all of the time and under a lot of stress that do not report fatigue as often. Rather than this condition being called, "Chronic Fatigue Syndrome", this condition I would present a term or phrase that describes addressing what is needed for the mitochondria in the body and working to boost the energy in the body. Something such as "mitochondria impairment syndrome" would effectively help label this condition better.

The mitochondria in each and every cell controls the energy. When the energy of the cells is low, chronic fatigue syndrome settles in. mitochondria produce energy in the form of a natural chemical known as, "adenosine triphosphate" (ATP) which powers all of the functions within the body. In order to regain power back into the body and work help the body of experiencing constant fatigue, we must help the body produce more ATP. Chronic Fatigue Syndrome boils down to a combination of the following:

Nutritional deficiencies

Hormone deficiencies

Poor immunity

Disordered sleep

The remedies in this section will identify natural ways to boost ATP and help you increase your natural energy levels.

Remedies:

Magnesium

This mineral is primarily responsible for muscle and nerve function and helping the digestive system function properly. It supplies the energy production within the body. Without it, low energy is all that can be produced.

Common Magnesium Sources: avocado, chickpeas, tamarind, basil, dill, ginger, oregano, thyme, any *CBD (cannabidiol) products are helpful. (CBD Oils are almost pure magnesium.), nettle leaf, horsetail, red clover, sage, and nopal.

*To test the purity of a CBD Oil, send to a lab for testing or you should feel a steady decline in needing to rely on this substance after your need has been met regularly.

Potassium and Aspartate (and more Magnesium)

The mitochondria in the body requires a nutrient known as aspartate to produce energy. This nutrient has to combine with Potassium and Magnesium in order to become charged and ready to work. Aspartame is made of the two naturally occurring amino acids, phenylalanine and aspartic acid, which are also components of proteins in our body and in food. When the minerals, potassium and magnesium are present in the body, this interaction can occur. Most doctors and nutritionists often target the magnesium deficiency which only partially helps provide relief but does not and cannot result in long-lasting change.

Common Potassium Sources: squash, zucchini, bananas, avocado, dried apricots, and herbs such as, guaco (also high in iron), conconsa (has the highest concentration of potassium phosphate), lily of the valley (rich in iron fluorine and Potassium phosphate).

Common Aspartate Sources: avocado, asparagus, molasses

Iodine (addressing the thyroid)

Common conditions that impact the Thyroid are Hypothyroidism (underactive thyroid – doesn't produce enough hormones) and Hyperthyroidism (overactive thyroid – produces too many hormones). The thyroid functions off of Iodine just like the bones thrive when having enough calcium. You will want to include many items such as Sea Moss and Elderberries as well as many sea plants such as Hijiki, Dulse, Nori, and Bladderwrack.

Note: If you have Hypothyroidism, you will want to incorporate more Bladderwrack into your diet. This plant is often found in products that contain Sea Moss but can be consumed in capsule or powder form. If you have Hyperthyroidism, you will want to consume as herb named, Bugleweed often in tea form.

Common sources of iodine: Sea Moss and Elderberries as well as many sea plants such as Hijiki, Dulse, Nori, and Bladderwrack.

Hypothyroid Smoothie:

- Large handful of watercress

- 2 apples

- 1 key lime (juiced)

Hyperthyroid Smoothie:

- 2-3 green apples

- 4-5 large dandelion leaves

- 1 handful of cilantro

- 1 key lime (juiced)

**Both of these smoothies are not a "cure" but a way to help deter many of the symptoms associated with each form of Thyroidism. They help the body begin to function well in preparation of additional dietary adjustments that can and should be implemented in a timely manner.

Drink This Tea (daily): Tamarind Juice, Ginger, and Key Lime (juice).

This tea can help cleanse out unnecessary waste materials while promoting a natural way of balancing hormones within the body.

Sunlight

Aside from absorbing vitamin-d, (which is an essential fat-soluble nutrient) getting direct sunlight can promote the healthy producing of natural hormones and chemicals within the body and help to reduce triggers that come from being deficient in these key hormones and chemicals. It is generally recommended to get 15-30 minutes of direct sunlight when the sun is at its highest point around noontime. But get in the sun whenever possible, even if you have to take a few minutes in the morning before you start your day, or briefly during a break while at work or school.

Lemon Balm and Valerian (herb)

Taking these herbs together at night can help promote a deeper sleep. Getting these in a tincture form may be best as liquids are absorbed better by our bodies and can be taken quicker than making tea. Follow the instructions on the label, but typically consume around 160-480mg of Valerian and 80-240mg of Lemon Balm together at night. Dosage will depend on your age, weight, and size which should be noted on the product labels. For tea, take about ½ tablespoon of each herb per 10-12oz of water. Placed dried herbs into a cup, boil water separately, then pour water onto herbs and let steep. Strain out herbs after letting cool off and enjoy.

Avoid Animal Products Altogether

Many forms of animal flesh (particularly red meats) are loaded with antibiotics, growth hormones, and steroids. Consuming these items complicates the digestive process, which places additional stress on not only the liver, but the gallbladder, and pancreas, among other organs. Dairy also contains a high amount of fat and sugars which are difficult to digest as well.

Zinc

This mineral helps regulate hormones in the body. When zinc is low in males, they can fail to produce enough hormones that promote fertility. It is recommended to consume about 30 milligrams of zinc daily for a few months to increase fertility.

Common Sources of Zinc: chickpeas, mushrooms, zucchini, squash, okra, Brazil nuts, and walnuts.

Antioxidants and Vitamin E

These nutrients help to deactivate free radicals which are responsible for destroying the cells. These both also protect the pituitary gland which controls and regulates the hormones being produced in the body. An issue with the pituitary gland directly decreases testosterone production in the body. Doctors will notify patients of this as the get closer to the age of 75. Most of the time doctors will not mention this due to life expectancy age currently around the age of 78 in the USA and will focus on other areas regarding health.

Natural Sources of Antioxidants: blueberries, onions, lettuce, squash, tomatoes, grapeseed extract, and herbs that you can use the flower, root, and leaves for as they contain polyphenolics (compounds that produce antioxidant activity).

Natural Sources of Vitamin-E: red bell pepper, mango, avocado, sunflower seeds, brazil nuts, turnip greens, blackberry, black currants, olives, and butternut squash.

Apply Pressure to Your Adrenal Glands (Qigong)

Whenever you stimulate the adrenal glands in the body (which are responsible for regulating blood pressure as well as the body's response to stress) it will create awareness for the body to adequately address its needs involving blood pressure, stress, metabolism, and the immune system among other things. Whenever you are stressed, the adrenal glands pump out hormones they irritate and overstimulate the heart muscle where it begins to race, flutter, or skip a beat.

Start by making a closed fist with both hands and place them behind your back (knuckles facing your lower back). Your hands should be pressing against your lower back (right near your kidneys) just above your waist, but below the ribs. Slowly rub your hands against this area up and down until the area is warmer. Do this for about 2-3 minutes each time at least twice a day.

Cold Sores

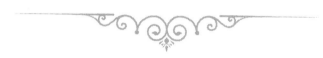

Cold Sores are tiny white blisters that are located in the mouth and around the lips. Unfortunately, having cold sores, means you have *oral herpes*. Unlike the widely known Herpes 1 and Herpes 2 virus, this form of herpes can go away over time without interfering much with it. These sores typically come up when a person is battling a cold or flu since the immune system compromised by staying busy fighting off an illness and gets overwhelmed, in which the body sends additional white-blood cells which contributes to an outbreak resulting in cold sores.

Remedies:

Lysine

This substance is an amino acid. When a virus looks to spread, it reproduces itself by combing with the amino acid *arginine*. However, when a cell is already occupied by another amino acid (Lysine), the virus does not have a place to call home and can die off if the conditions are right. Many doctors will provide an artificial form of Lysine to take but there are natural forms if it as well. The important part when taking a natural approach is consuming what's helpful, while avoiding what's not (in the moment). So, in the case of oral herpes (cold sore) you will want to load up on your Lysine while avoiding your Arginine consumption.

Common Lysine Sources (consume): quinoa, olives, wild blueberries, grapes.

Arginine Sources (avoid): walnuts, brazil nuts, zucchini, and seeds (stay away from consuming too many seeds – many foods that contain seeds can be consumed, but the seeds should be removed for now).

Ice

Viruses do not do well in a cold environment says William Payne, D.D.S., dentist in McPherson, Kansas. Once you detect a cold sore, cover the area with an ice cube wrapped in a napkin or washcloth. Hold it in place (as long as it's comfortable) for about 15 minutes, then take a break for 30 minutes. Repeat this 2-3 times a day.

Astragalus (herb)

This herb helps to boost the immune system and kill off viruses (pretty convenient for cold sores). This herb is most potent in capsule or tincture form. A typical dosage can span from 9-30g a day in tincture form and two 80mg capsules a day in capsule form for no more than 6 weeks at a time.

Lemon Balm (herb)

This herb used as an ointment can help soothe the area and prevent flareups. You can easily find this herb in most herb shops. Mix 1-2 teaspoons in with boiling water. Let cool off and drink 1-2 ten-ounce glasses a day.

Calcium, Magnesium, and Zinc

These minerals help build the immune system and strengthen the epithermal tissues the lips are made of, and the inside of your mouth. As new cells are able to be produced in these areas, any dead or weaker cells will go away quicker as they are replaced. This will promote faster healing for this condition.

Common Sources of Calcium: sea moss, kale, okra, dandelion greens, turnip greens, lettuce, papaya, and oranges.

Common sources of magnesium: avocado, chickpeas, tamarind, basil, dill, ginger, oregano, thyme, any *CBD (cannabidiol), nettle leaf, horsetail, red clover, sage, and nopal.

*CBD oils are almost pure magnesium. To test the purity of CBD oil, send to a lab for testing such as Eurofins Laboratory in Pennsylvania and Texas. To know if it is helpful, you should feel a steady decline in needing to rely upon this substance after this need has been met more often.

Common Sources of Zinc: chickpeas, mushrooms, zucchini, squash, okra, Brazil nuts, and walnuts.

Replace Toothbrush

To avoid any future flareups or reinfecting yourself, get a new toothbrush. Once you notice getting a cold sore, it is recommended to throw your current toothbrush away. For future reference, a moist environment like your bathroom is the perfect setting for a virus like oral herpes (cold cores) to accumulate. Try putting your toothbrush in a dryer area within your bathroom. Place your toothbrush in a bathroom that does not have a bathtub/shower if applicable.

Colds and Flu

To be brief, there is no remedy or recovery for a cold or the flu. Simply because, a cold or the flu IS the remedy and recovery. These conditions work to promote cleansing by pushing out excess waste. We've been programmed to always rely upon a "take something" remedy which only stifles the body's efforts to eliminate waste. However, most people have maintained unhealthy bodies and unhealthy habits which have contributed to these conditions being sought out by the body often. Although these conditions themselves are healing, remedies for these conditions are meant to pass these illnesses much easier with less discomfort so that the condition does not reach its highest levels or result in being a more chronic illness or death.

The main reason there's no "cure" for the common cold is the fact that there are almost 200 different viruses responsible for a variety of colds based on their severity, length of time to overcome, point of arrival in the body, and many other variables that take place when developing the symptoms of a common cold. Providing a "cure" would mean we prevent toxins and waste from leaving the body; whereas toxins and waste remaining in the body would promote sickness as we cycle back to where we started.

Remedies in this section will work to promote ways of opening up the many channels within the body responsible for elimination to help pass through these conditions with minimum discomfort.

Remedies:

Fasting

All forms of Fasting can help reduce inflammation within the body. besides expelling things like mucus, Fasting helps promote the elimination/detoxifying organs in the body to remove excess waste and contribute to the body locating and removing inflammation in the body and help alleviate many of the symptoms of Arthritis. You can learn much more about Fasting in my book entitled, *Fasting: A Guide To Health And Wellness*, which comes with descriptions of different forms of Fasting, recipes, and plans to stick to.

Clean The Respiratory System

The respiratory system is not only responsible for passing oxygen around the body and helping blood flow to remain constant, but it's your very own cooling system within the body. The body on average is about 98.6 degrees Fahrenheit and needs to have a cooler current running through it regularly to prevent the temperature from immediately rising. Keeping the respiratory system clean will help the body remain cool which helps to reduce any fever, make it easier to expel any excess mucus, cough up phlegm, and make it easier to consume items that will help you overcome your cold or flu.

Echinacea (herb)

This herb is helpful for relieving upper-respiratory issues. Echinacea works to boost the production of disease-fighting immune cells such as, leukocytes, and phagocytes. Although this herb can be consumed in tea form, it is recommended to take in capsule or tincture form to promote the most disease-fighting immune cells. A daily dose of 175-225mg two to three times a day is recommended.

*Note: due to this herb boosting the production of immune cells, their life span can be greatly diminished if used regularly. It is best (and strongly recommended) to only use this herb for a week or so followed by an immediate break for a week or two.

Licorice Root (herb)

This herb can help soothe irritated throats and relieve coughing. Take 2-4 pieces of this root and steep in boiling water for about 10 minutes. Strain herb and drink this tea twice a day.

Maitake Mushrooms

These mushrooms which are mostly added to soups, contain a high number of poly-saccharides which stimulate the immune system by releasing infection-fighting components such as macrophages and t-cells, which are stem cells which come from bone marrow to help fight cancer. The moment you feel a cold coming on, take 20mg of a standardized liquid of maitake mushroom to help deter symptoms from increasing suddenly.

Zinc

An added boost of zinc can help reduce symptoms of a cold or flu to just a few days rather than it is lingering on for an extended period of time. Taking a zinc supplement isn't ideal and tastes very bitter but can help in more sudden cases of a strong cold or flu. Take more 40mg of zinc from a supplement can lead to nausea, dizziness, heart burn, and vomiting in some cases.

Common Zinc Sources: chickpeas, mushrooms, zucchini, squash, okra, Brazil nuts, and walnuts.

Go For A Walk

It is always best to stimulate circulation in the body. If it is colder out, you do want to dress warm to not worsen your symptoms.

Liquids

Eating many foods can irritate the throat and respiratory system which you want to avoid while sick. Drinking room-temperature or warm water will help soothe the respiratory system and help to dissolve any excess mucus. Herbal teas are best but warm water will also remain helpful.

Gargle Salt Water

Make time to gargle some salt water a few times throughout the day. Mix 1 teaspoons of salt with 8-ounces of warm spring or distilled water. Gargling this mix can help break down some of the mucus in the body.

My Personal Remedy For Removing Colds and The Flu:

- Mix together the following herbs (in equal parts): mullein leaf (or mullein flowers), elderberry, dandelion root, guaco, and wild cherry bark.
- Take 1 tablespoon of mixed herbs and place into strainer, then place strainer into cup that hold at least 12 ounces of water.
- Boil spring water and pour into cup (about 8-10oz)
- Let cool and drink twice a day (you can re-use herbs twice each day)

Colic

If you're not familiar with the term "colic" it is generally describing the condition where an infant around 4-6 weeks old to 3-4 months old will cry excessively for hours a day. This condition is more severe for infants 4-6 weeks old than it is for those 3-4 months old. The child may scream at random, and when feeding or changing diapers, and pull and tug at their clothes around their abdomen with the appearance that they are in physical pain. The remedies in this section address ways to help reduce the severity of symptoms followed by relieving many of the signs associated with Colic, while remaining safe for children within the age ranges mentioned above.

Remedies:

"Colic Carry"

This is a carrying technique where you extend your forearm with you palm up and place the baby on your arm with their chest down, with their head in your hand and their les on either side of your elbow. Place them in this position and walk slowly around your house to help relieve many of their symptoms.

Burping

Sometimes babies can have more gas than others and trigger their crying and signs of discomfort. We want to reduce this feeling through not allowing a child to consume items that cause constipation and congestions (dairy products, processed foods, and animal flesh). But other times, it is important to focus on how a baby is sitting during feeding times as this can impact how they digest foods and can cause them to feel "backed up". When bottle-feeding it is recommended to burp after every ounce if needed.

Turn Onto Side (when changing)

When changing a diaper, you will want to turn your baby onto their side while you wipe as opposed to holding their legs in the air to prevent any leftover crevasses to wipe. Sometimes they may appear clean but there still may be materials that are hidden. Turning them onto their side and wiping will help clean better, and also keep any unnecessary pressure off of their necks and torso. This method will help to also avoid restricting the air passageways momentarily which will help avoid colic.

Cow's Milk Is For Infant Cows

Cow's milk is lactic acid which creates additional waste and bacteria into the body. this substance will create unnecessary congestion. Chairman of the department of pediatrics at Indiana University School of Medicine states, "I firmly believe that milk in the mother's diet is a frequent cause of colic in breastfed babies. I strongly recommend mothers start by eliminating milk from their diets and see what happens". If not able to breastfeed, hemp milk, coconut milk, and walnut milk is recommended in addition to a healthier, inflammation-free diet best achieved through plant-based meals and snacks.

Wrap Your Baby

Holding or swaddling you child has a calming effect on them. Do that often to prevent long sessions of crying and irritableness. Use a backpack or something to hold your baby comfortably while your arms remain free to do other things.

Use Vacuums

Although not heavily researched, the sound of a vacuum has a calming effect on a child. Try using a vacuum instead of a broom whenever possible. Some parents will record or play the sound of a vacuum while doing other tasks. If your baby requires constant attention, it is a good practice to wear a front pack where you can hold them comfortably in front on your chest while you vacuum, and your child should go to sleep much easier.

Warmth

Placing a warm towel, warm bottle wrapped in a towel, or heated pad set on low can help a baby relax and feel mor comfortable. Place any of these items onto their stomach (not warm enough so they can get burned) to provide any stomach relief.

Swinging

Repetitive motion is good for a colicky baby. A small swing or bringing to the park when showing signs of being colicky can help calm your baby and reduce their crying.

Soak Towel In Herbs

Soaking a towel in herbs is great way of consuming benefits of herbs without having to drink or eat them. There are many herbs such as mullein, lavender, eucalyptus, and rosemary that provide calming effects upon consumption. Soak a towel in with a few teaspoons of any or all of these herbs and place the towel directly on your baby. Towel can be placed on their stomach or on their back as they lay down. You can squeeze out any excess before to avoid having much runoff. Do this while relaxing and inhaling the aroma produced by these herbs and promote a space for your child to naturally relax and calm their nerves.

Conjunctivitis

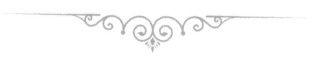

Conjunctivitis (commonly referred to as "Pinkeye") is when there's inflammation in the *conjunctiva*, which is the membrane that lines the inside of the eyelids that covers the white part of the eye. There are three forms of this condition: (1) viral, (2) allergies, or (3) bacterial. No matter which one you have come in contact with, symptoms and treatment will generally be the same. This condition feels like there's small grains of sand in your eyes that won't come out, along with a yellow-ish discharge that forms a crust around your eye lids.

Remedies:

Keep The Eyes Clean

Make sure to begin by wiping the crust that forms around the eyes away so there's less bacteria for this condition to attach itself to. make sure to dip a cotton ball or cotton swam ("q-tip") in warm water to clean the eyelids as well.

Ice

If your eyes are itching with great discomfort, place an ice cube wrapped in a towel on each eye to help reduce the itching. Place an ice cube on each eye for about 5-10 minutes and then remove for 10 minutes. Repeat at least 2-3 times a day. Make sure you do not use the same ice cube for each eye because you can spread this condition. You want to start over after each use.

Chamomile (herb)

Use this herb to create a compress to help reduce inflammation. Use this herb to make some tea (about 1 tablespoon of herb added to cup of boiling water) and lightly place a small towel in warm tea. Stake towel and squeeze out any excess fluid and place towel on your eye(s) (either together at same time or each individually). Do this treatment for about 4-5 minutes and then wipe eye clear. Repeat 3-4 times a day.

Reflexology

Pressing on certain pressure points on your feet can help send energy to the eyes and work to relief symptoms of conjunctivitis. Using your thumb, firmly press on the bottom, side, and top of each of your big toes, second toes, and third toes. Focus on the areas that surround each of these toes. If any particular spot is sensitive, continue to press lightly and increase firmness on those areas.

Other reflexology points to focus on:

- BL1 – the inner corner of the eye, just above the tear duct.
- BL10 – about ½ inch below the base of the skull on the back of the neck.
- GB1 – the lateral end, closest to the ear, or each eye
- L14 – in the web between the thumb and index finger (at the highest point of the muscle when the thumb and index finger are close together.
- LV2 – in the web between the first and second toes (starting with the big toe).
- ST44 – in between the 2nd and 3rd toes about ½ inch above where they both meet.
- TB23 – is in the lateral end of each eyebrow.

Take your time and look up these pressure points and work to gently apply pressure to these areas as instructed and remain patient.

Chinese Herbal Formula

I cannot say I am knowledgeable of the exact ingredients due to this formula being made and prepared many different ways, but a traditional herbal formula called, *Ming Mu Di Huang Wan* which translates to "Brighten The Eyes" has been effective with treating specific conditions connected to conjunctivitis.

Cold Compress

Coldness can help to reduce responses that may be triggered by allergies during this time. Allergies can be triggered easier when working through conjunctivitis and lead to itching and irritation.

Fill up a bowl with ice cubes and water. Soak a medium-sized washcloth in the bowl. Remove the cloth from the water and squeeze out any excess water. Fold the cloth evenly and place over both of your eyes at the same time. This will help reduce redness and your eyes from being itchy.

Constipation

One, soft bowel movement a day is healthy. Anything less, signals signs of constipation in the body. When the system in the body becomes "backed up" this is often due to having too much waste to process and eliminated at once, or when the digestive system is not functioning properly. When either of these instances occur, toxins from this waste material are sent and absorbed into the bloodstream which can lead to innumerable health issues and complications; this is also why those who suffer from constipation, often have blood in their stools. It is important to note that simply purchasing laxatives will not solve this issue. Laxatives can force your bowels to become overworked within a small timeframe and can seriously (and sometimes permanently) damage your digestive tract). This can deplete your body of energy and also necessary minerals it needs to function well.

Although it can remain helpful to incorporate the remedies that will be described in this section, make sure you find out if you are constipated first. This is a condition that consistently impacts the body. it's not just a feeling of discomfort, bloated for a brief period of time, or minor pains in your abdominal area. These may occur, but determining if you are actually constipated should include all of the following:

- Difficulty emptying the bowels
- Hardened stools
- High level of restriction when you do go to the bathroom

Remedies:

Adequate Consumption

Although it is a must to remove these toxins and waste materials, it is more important to stop consuming that which creates additional waste. Leaving alone the processed foods, meats (which take about 2hrs to digest), the heavy starches (potatoes, white flours), and the dairy products, are enough to significantly reduce your current signs and symptoms you may be experiencing. If you eat several times a day, it is time to consume fewer, but more (nutritionally) fulfilling meals. Consuming items that are healthier such as fresh fruits and vegetables, grains, nuts, and seeds, will provide your body with more of what it needs to feel fulfilled and help you consume less often.

Load Up On Your Fiber

Fiber helps promote ease of digestion because it absorbs a lot of water and helps create softer stools, which promote eliminating larger quantities of waste easier. The American Dietetic Association recommends 20-35 grams of fiber daily. This may sound like a lot but, ½ cup of leafy green vegetables can provide about 5g, a small apple is about 3g, and consuming grains like quinoa can provide up to 8g per cup. Just these three items together and you are almost at your daily recommended amount in addition to any other foods you consume that have fiber.

Common sources of Fiber: garbanzo beans, lentils, brussels sprouts, sweet potatoes, avocado, pears, sunflower seeds, flax seeds, hazelnuts, apples and berries (high pectin fruits) and onions.

Walking

Regular exercise helps the body maintain healthier circulation which will help support healthier digestions and reduce constipation.

Relax

When the body is stressed or tense, it can trigger a "fight or flight" response, which causes the body to tense up and pause itself. This also pauses the bowels as well temporarily. Introduce yourself to some mindfulness or other relaxing practice more often to avoid difficulties.

Review Your Supplements and Medications

If you are currently (or have a longer history of) taking any supplements or medications, you should review the listed side effects. Many will state that it *may cause constipation* and should be addressed appropriately.

Use The Right Oils

Canola oil, soy, or "vegetable" oils do not digest well. These substances remain intact and create a very difficult task for the body to digest and search for any nutrients to hold into. Due to these substances remaining almost intact when digesting, they contribute to clogging up the intestinal walls and make digesting anything more difficult afterwards. Try grapeseed oil or avocado oil when cooking and use olive oil and walnut oil on dryer foods like salads.

Water

Drinking 6-8 cup of water a day (about 64oz) is generally recommended. Due to increasing you consumption of fiber during this time, it is more essential to meet this requirement since fiber will absorb water and you will not want to feel dehydrated.

Prune Juice

Prune juice will help stimulate the intestinal tract. Stick to two 8oz glasses a day mixed with 8oz of water until you begin to have more bowel movements. Once this occurs, cut your intake to 4oz of prune juice and 4oz of water for a few days. Then stop completely to avoid any bowel issues and due to the need not being there anymore.

Cascara Sagrada (herb)

This is the primary herb used in many colon cleanses, detoxes, and recipes to help contribute to cleaning the colon. This herb has laxative properties but helps to also strengthen the bowels without irritating them like laxatives do. Take this herb in the evening before bedtime to help promote a healthy bowel movement by the time you wake up. You can drink this herb as a tea (about 2tsp per 8oz of water) or in capsule form (about 450mg size). Drink the tea once a day or take one 450mg capsule a day; do not do both. If you drink the tea, drink for 5 days and then take 2 days off, then repeat for about one month before taking a longer break of a few weeks or more. If you take the capsule, do so for only 3-4 weeks before taking a longer time off as well.

Note: this herb is highly recommended over another commonly used herb called "Triphala" due to Triphala being very low in pH level (3.2) and can contribute to damaging the liver by interrupting proper function of a liver enzyme known as *cytochrome P450* which helps keep the liver cells metabolism healthy.

Magnesium

Being deficient in this mineral lowers the energy in the body which can contribute to digestive muscles relaxing and slow down digestion.

Common sources of magnesium: Avocados, Bananas, Chickpeas, Tamarind, Basil, Dill, Ginger, Oregano, Thyme, Butternut Squash, Brazil Nuts, Pumpkin Seeds, Chia Seeds, Black Beans, Edamame, Kidney Beans, Okra, Leafy Green Vegetables, Nopal, Nettle leaf, horsetail, red clover, sage, and *CBD (Cannabinol) products.

Coughing

We cough when we irritate the airways in the body. Everyone may take a deep breath and cough, but when the coughing continues, this is when the body is telling that there are irritating substances getting in the way. This form of coughing that typically involves mucus buildup that has accumulated is a signal that there are excess toxins in the system. We must first work on breaking down this mucus, so it does not remain in the respiratory tract. Then, promote the natural function of the respiratory system without any hindrances to help reduce and remove the body's response of coughing.

Remedies:

(Note: do not do every remedy listed here. If you incorporate any herbal remedies, choose one before moving onto another one. Do not do more than one at the same time).

Slippery Elm (herb)

This herb helps to reduce coughing by soothing the throat. Helping reduce how irritated the throat feels helps to reduce the body from feeling triggered to cough. To use this herb as a tea, add 1-2 tablespoons to a small pot of water until the water begins to boil. Strain out herb and drink 10oz of tea twice a day. This herb can also be found as a lozenge where you can take 5-6 lozenges per day.

Ginger (herb)

Ginger is a natural anti-inflammatory and helps reduce a painful throat. For tea, take one cut of ginger (about the size of your fingertip) and add to cup (8-10oz) of boiling water. Let cool and drink 2-3 times a day. You may add fresh ginger to your meals to as well. Ginger is a good herb to consume to help identify if you have strep throat or not. If your throat pain continues after not coughing anymore, this is an indicator of having strep throat.

Water

Whenever you have a cough, cold, or flu, you lose fluids from coughing up mucus, sweating, and the body perspiring more. Remaining hydrated is necessary at this time. work towards consuming at least 64 ounces of water a day to help calm your coughing and moisturize the respiratory system.

Mullein Leaf (or flowers)

The herb is used to relieve soreness in the throat and reduce coughing. Helps to kill excess bacteria and break apart mucus. This is best used in tea form by adding 1-2tsp of herb to a cup while boiling water. Pour boiling water into cup and let cool. Strain out herb and drink twice a day.

Blow Your Nose

Blowing your nose can help get rid of mucus before it travels down to your throat. This can help reduce discomfort and help relieve many of your symptoms.

Humidifier

Turning on a humidifier while you're in a room for an extended period of time can help reduce your coughing and help moisten the air enough to prevent you from having any dryness in the nose, mouth, or throat.

Eat Smaller Meals

It can be in your best interest in eating smaller amount throughout the day rather than a few larger meals so the throat can remain at ease for longer periods of time. The repetitiveness of swallowing bits of food from a larger meal can irritate parts of your throat can trigger coughing, which can also increase your chance of choking. Eating smaller meals during the day can help you not overwork your respiratory tract and also help the body digest items easier to avoid feeling bloated or "stuffed".

My Personal Recipe:

- Add one teaspoon of Slippery Elm powder (or liquid) to 2 cups of hot water. Stir in ½ tablespoon of date sugar slowly.
- Let cool and drink once a day

Cuts (and Scrapes)

We've all had cuts and scrapes before. Often these come from accidents at various points in our lives, but are common, nonetheless. The site of blood often causes panic where we respond by quickly covering up these wounds. Covering wounds is, however, the final step you can learn to take when naturally aiding and treating your wounds.

Note: If you have a wound that is bleeding and does not stop after 10 minutes, your wound is deep enough to see the muscle or bone, is more than an inch long, or have several cuts or scrapes and is hard to cover all of them, you should see a doctor.

Remedies:

Remain Calm

This is the first thing to do whenever you have a cut or scrape. These accidents can be shocking to the body, so you want to relax. Start by taking some deep breaths and acknowledging that the

Apply Pressure

Apply direct pressure to your wound to help decrease blood from escaping and to reduce infection. You want to use a clean cloth but can use your fingers if no cloth is available. If applying pressure does not slow down your bleeding, elevate the area to heart level or above to reduce the blood pressure to the area.

Calendula (herb)

This herb has many benefits it provides, but specifically helps prevent infections from cuts or scrapes when used as a spray. After washing off your cut or scrape, use a non-alcoholic Calendula spray to cover the wound. Apply this 3-4 times a day and lightly bandage the area. You want to protect your wound by lightly covering it, but you want free flowing air to reach this area so that this spray can dry. You can completely cover the area, with a plastic wrap or cloth, but want to avoid covering too tight to not cut off circulation.

My Personal Essential Oil Remedy:

- Take three drops of Lavender essential oil, three drop of Frankincense essential oil, one drop of Myrrh essential oil, and one ounce of Jojoba essential oil and slowly mix together.
- Gently apply to your cut or scrape (after washing it off) and allow to dry on its own.
- Lavender oil helps to reduce the pain, frankincense and myrrh help to calm the body, and Jojoba helps to speed up the healing and hold these oils together.

Dandruff

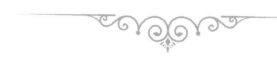

Dandruff is a skin issue, not a hair issue. Most common recommendations try to treat the hair, but the skin follicles are where dandruff comes from. More specifically, the itchiness that derives from Dandruff is due to a substance called *sebum* which come from the glands in the scalp which over accumulates due to the scalp becoming excessively dry. Shampoos and hair conditioners may provide some help to address the symptoms but will not accurately address the condition itself.

Note: If you try remedies for several weeks and no sign of change, you may have a yeast infection or hormonal imbalances. Addressing those first are highly recommended by referring to those sections within this book.

Remedies:

Brush Your Scalp

By only putting on oils, shampoos, or conditioners and washing the scalp, these essentially cover the scalp and often leads to more buildup of dandruff. You want to shower often but brush your scalp; don't just wash your hair. You can begin by gently using your fingers to rub your scalp, but also use a soft brush to apply pressure directly to your hair follicles and brush of any remaining debris as you incorporate more natural remedies.

Thyme (herb)

Boil 4 tablespoons of dried thyme in 2 cups of water for about 10 minutes. Strain out the herb and allow it to cool. Pour half of this mixture over your clean, damp hair, covering the entire scalp. Massage in gently and do not rinse off. Use the remainder of this mixture in a few days.

Eucalyptus (herb)

Take 4 teaspoons of dried eucalyptus leaves into a quart of water. Leave until mixture comes to a boil. Remove from heat, and cover, while letting steep for one hour. Strain liquid into a bottle once it's cooled off. After you take a shower, pour this mixture onto your hair and massage in gently. Do not rinse this out; let it dry on its own. Use this mixture daily.

Olive Oil

Using oils on the scalp regularly can lead to more issues, but occasionally using oils can help reduce many of the symptoms associated with dandruff. Start off by wetting your hair, then apply a few ounces of olive oil directly to your scalp with a brush or cotton ball. Apply to each section of the scalp separately and then place a shower cap over your head to leave on for about 30 minutes. Then rinse.

Onion and Coconut Oil

To do this you want to begin by taking a few medium-sized red onions and chopping them into small pieces/chunks. Begin frying them in grapeseed or walnut oil. Once they begin to turn black (and start to float), turn off the flame, cool and strain out the onions. Take the "juice" from the onions and mix together with coconut oil (enough to fill a contain or bottle you'll be storing this mixture in. Let sit for a few hours or overnight. Apply the mixture to your hair and scalp by gently massaging in. Do this daily to help reduce your dandruff. Make sure to wash/rinse your hair thoroughly after letting mixture settle into your hair for about 30-40 minutes.

Soursop

This fruit is great for treating numerous hair problems such as, split ends, dandruff, grey hair, and head lice. Soursop is more commonly associate with its anti-cancer properties, but you can use this to help with hair issues as well. Besides just eating this fruit, you can also juice it or make a tea from the leaves of this fruit and use as a hair rinse.

Take a small handful of the soursop leaves and add them to 3 cups of boiling water. Let them boil and then steep until cooled off. Strain out the herb and drink this tea 1-2 times a day.

Mexican Marigold (flower) and Tea Tree Oil

3-4 dried marigold flowers

10-12 drops of tea tree oil

1 cup of distilled water

Step 1: Dry the marigold flowers. Crush the petals to make a paste (you can also purchase marigold flower powder).

Step 2: Add the marigold powder to a teaspoon of water and proceed to add 10-12 drops of tea tree oil to it. Mix together well.

(Note: it is extremely important to dilute it, or it can damage the scalp.)

Step 3: Add 1 cup of warm water to this paste-like mixture or marigold flowers and tea tree oil to make sure it rinses out well.

Step 4: After you're done washing your hair, pour the hair rinse on your scalp and gently rub into your scalp.

Step 5: Let it sit for 3-5 minutes

Step 6: Now, rinse your hair with warm water. You will not need to shampoo or use other products afterwards.

Make sure that you use this hair rinse at least once or twice a week to see an improvement in your hair health.

Zinc

Dr. Pratima Raicher, an Ayuvedic practitioner in New York City, recommends 15-20mg of zinc daily to help balance the oils on the scalp and relieve any dryness.

Common Sources of Zinc: chickpeas, mushrooms, zucchini, squash, okra, Brazil nuts, and walnuts.

Batana Oil

This oil, native to Honduras, is extracted from the nuts of the American Palm Tree by the indigenous Miskito Indian tribes. Miskito people are commonly referred to as "Tawira" which means "the people of beautiful hair" which they credit to their regular use of batana oil. Traditionally used for hair and skin treatment as this oil is known for rejuvenating hair, repairing damaged hair, clearing out grey or white hairs, promoting hair growth, as well as moisturizing the hair and skin. You can lather on as much as you want (without wasting) directly onto your hair and directly onto your scalp and skin. Let it settle in for about 20-30 minutes and then wash out with warm water a few times a week or as often as your able to.

My Personal Remedy:

Mix 2-3 drops of rosemary essential oil with 1 tablespoon of avocado oil. Massage mixture into scalp once a day for 1-2 minutes. Lightly rinse out afterward.

Depression

Dr. Jonathan Zuess, M.D., psychiatrist at the Good Samaritan Regional Medical Center on Phoenix, Arizona, USA, refers to depression as, *"a cold of the soul"*. He describes depression as a condition that can be brief and requires an active response and treatment but does not have to remain a part of oneself permanently.

To begin, let's first address how the physical body, and the mental mind are not separate entities. Mental health and physical are not separate. However, treatments can be applied differently, but we must keep in mind is that millions of people unnecessarily suffer painful mental health symptoms due to untreated nutrient deficiencies, hormonal imbalance, blood sugar swings, and excess inflammation.

Depression is a complexed diagnosis. Simply feeling sad or down does not mean depression is present. We often have many emotions and a consistent combination of them can lead to the condition of depression.

Depression DSM-5 Diagnostic Criteria:

The DSM-5 outlines the following criterion to make a diagnosis of depression. The individual must be experiencing five or more symptoms during the same 2-week period and at least one of the symptoms should be either (1) depressed mood or (2) loss of interest or pleasure.

1. Depressed mood most of the day, nearly every day.

2. Markedly diminished interest or pleasure in all, or almost all, activities most of the day, nearly every day.

3. Significant weight loss when not dieting or weight gain, or sudden decrease or increase in appetite nearly every day.

4. A slowing down of thought and a reduction of physical movement (observable by others, not merely subjective feelings of restlessness or being slowed down).

5. Fatigue or loss of energy nearly every day.

6. Feelings of worthlessness or excessive or inappropriate guilt nearly every day.

7. Diminished ability to think or concentrate or indecisiveness nearly every day.

8. Recurrent thoughts of death, recurrent suicide ideation without a specific plan, or a suicide attempt or a specific plan for committing suicide.

To receive a diagnosis of depression, these symptoms must cause the individual clinically significant distress or impairment in social, occupational, or other important areas of functioning. The symptoms must also not be a result of substance abuse or another medical condition.

Note: Nearly every diagnosis in the DSM-5 shares one common criteria: "organic causes of the symptoms must be ruled out". The recommendations made in this section will address meeting the organic/natural ways to help reduce symptoms of within this condition.

Remedies:

Avoid Self-Diagnosis

Our minds are not in the healthiest space when we are experiencing depression. Yes, we can simply refer to the diagnosis listed in this section and confirm what we feel is accurate, but it is important to meet with a professional as there are many assessments that can provide more clarity to our current situation. We may agree with all parts of the criteria listed for depression when we are alone. Seek out a mental health provider and work to provide more clarity to what is going on and connect with helpful services.

Go To Therapy!

A therapeutic relationship can at times be the only remedy needed. Having a therapeutic relationship with someone who can provide structure and support on treating your signs and symptoms is vital. Being able to peel back the layers of your life and examine without judgment will help dissolve your symptoms as you work to create, establish, and fine-tune healthy coping skills. Regular assessments can be reviewed as perspective-taking can take place in this therapeutic setting as you work towards exploring all areas of self-identified growth. You will also be able to learn more about a depression diagnosis and have access to more valid information that you can remain mindful of.

Mineral Deficiencies

When the body is deficient in a wide variety of minerals, leaving the body malnourished, the receptors in not only the body, but the brain become impaired. This will set forth the stage of neurotransmitters (which deliver and transport information to the cells), to send along incomplete messages left to interpretation by the brain. This can trigger headaches, fatigue, decreased awareness, poor decision-making, and thoughts of self-doubt, lack of confidence, and loss of interest in daily tasks. The primary minerals in the body are: calcium, chloride, magnesium, phosphorus, potassium, sodium, sulfur, iron, and zinc. These have vital roles within the body that control and regulate our energy levels. Working to keep these mineral needs met is crucial when working to keep the body and mind healthy.

A whole food, plant-based diet is recommended for achieving a high-mineral diet. The variety of minerals that are able to be regularly consumed without causing hinderance on the body that takes place on a whole food, plant-based diet, helps meet many of the mineral deficiencies that may be present. This dietary regimen encourages the regular consumption of juices, smoothies, and herbal teas that also provide an abundance of minerals necessary in the body. Begin by introducing a variety of items to feel fulfilled without sticking directly to any script. Have fun and remain flexible with getting healthier. For the foods that contain some of the highest mineral content, I'd recommend referencing the Dr. Sebi Nutritional Guide that can be downloaded for free by doing a simple online search.

Get Creative

Essentially, the opposite of *depression* is *expression*. Identifying ways to express yourself that promote joy and cheerfulness can help decrease many symptoms associated with a depression diagnosis. We're often taken away with what provides us the most joy and cheer by working various jobs, family responsibilities, and activities of daily life. It is crucial to make time for activities that provide you joy even if it appears to disrupt the daily activities and tasks you may have. Most likely, you will experience a "new-found" energy source which will make accomplishing many of your daily tasks much easier, and help work through other difficulties with more ease, resulting in a decrease in the severity of your current symptoms.

Get Out More

Being in the same place most of the time (especially if you're alone) is often the foundation for depression symptoms to settle in. Regular stimulation helps produce the natural neurotransmitters that make us feel good; most notably the neurotransmitter *serotonin*. Work to avoid remaining stagnant whether it's at home, work, or another setting you spend longer periods of time in.

Socialize

You do not necessarily need to go out with friends to socialize. Simply acknowledging other people as you encounter them is a great way to work away from your typical symptoms due to you placing yourself outside of your normal comfort zone and bringing your awareness to something else that will keep you stimulated, even for brief moment of time. Go to a local restaurant, sporting game, park, or just go for a walk and make it a point for you to increase socializing. Maybe start off with setting a small goal of saying "hi" to one or more people, or even planning to have a small conversation with someone. These regular encounters we can create will remain helpful towards working away from that negative perception we may have of ourselves if depression is present.

You can perhaps keep a frequent schedule of being out more by going to the gym, walking around your neighborhood, or meet this need through some other job/volunteer service in your community such as coaching a sport, helping organize various food pantries or soup kitchens, or attending local youth or performance-related activities.

Create A Regular Schedule

When your inner world appears chaotic and difficult to manage, having a regular schedule can help regain some control and maintain order in your life. You don't want to be too strict on your schedule or develop a regular routine that does not allow much time for yourself or flexibility.

Forgive Yourself

Knowing you have an internal battle that challenges you, try to not hold any grudge towards yourself and work on laughing at the smaller accidents or inconveniences that would normally disrupt your day. We will always feel just about anything throughout the day, so work on making more room for letting go of the feelings you don't want to remain present when you can. Don't immediately blame yourself when something does not go as planned.

Sleep

Adequate sleep is necessary not only when dealing with symptoms of depression, but not getting enough quality sleep can strongly trigger many of the individual symptoms of depression and set the tone for your day. You want to avoid this by getting quality sleep when you can, but also making sure you do not oversleep so the body does not feel more tired and desire to remain stagnant.

Make Someone Else Feel Good

Helping another person feel better will help you walk away feeling better also. Planning to do a good deed you know someone will appreciate, or giving a compliment to a stranger can make someone else feel good and you as well as a result.

Anticipate Enthusiasm

Work to identify and establish at least one activity that you can look forward expecting to do that you are enthusiastic about. It may be something as small as sitting down and reading a book on your day off, or as large as planning a weekend getaway. Something to look forward to will become necessary when working to alleviate yourself of depression.

Avoid Alcohol

Alcohol disrupts the central nervous system. This slows down the functioning of the body and can greatly trigger many of the symptoms of depression.

St. John's Wort (herb)

This herb taken in liquid form is easy to consume and can help naturally boost the *serotonin* (the happy/feel-good neurotransmitter") in the body. Take about 300mg of standard extract of this herb three times a day with each meal. You may slowly increase your dosage but do not exceed 900mg regularly. Overconsuming this herbal extract can become harmful to the body so the recommended dosage listed above is low and may take some time before you notice direct benefits. Simply give it time and work on applying anything you find helpful with working effectively on dealing with depression.

Note: St. John's Wort flower essence can be a very beneficial as well. You can drop 4-6 drops of this essence under your tongue 3-4 times a day.

Valerian Root (herb)

This herb can be used for best results. Taking 150-300 milligrams of this herb can help the nerves relax in the body, promote stillness, help you fall asleep faster and improve sleep quality. This herb can help combat some of the symptoms associated with depression.

Damiana (herb)

This herb is known for boosting libido and sexual organs but can help increase testosterone which can be decreased when coping with symptoms of depression. Drink this herb as a tea twice a day. Take 2 teaspoons and make as a 10-12-ounce tea twice a day for best results.

Sunlight

Aside from absorbing vitamin-d, (which is an essential fat-soluble nutrient) getting direct sunlight can promote the healthy producing of natural hormones and chemicals within the body and help to reduce triggers that come from being deficient in these key hormones and chemicals. It is generally recommended to get 15-30 minutes of direct sunlight when the sun is at its highest point around noontime. But get in the sun whenever possible, even if you have to take a few minutes in the morning before you start your day, or briefly during a break while at work or school.

Movement Is Medicine

Daily exercise should be looked at as a requirement for those who experience depression. Not that this is an additional task but viewed as more of being an activity to avoid being stagnant. It's not necessary to develop a body-building schedule or spend all of your free time at the gym. Simply going for a walk for 20-30 minutes a day can be very beneficial to alleviating symptoms of depression. Keith W. Johnsgard, Ph.D., professor emeritus of psychology at San Jose State University in California, USA states that, "the changes in brain chemistry provoked by exercise appear to parallel those of the major antidepressant drugs".

Music

We have all most likely listened to music when feeling down or upset. Music has the ability to not only provide connection and understanding but help improve our mood and feelings of well-being.

"Magnet Therapy" Acupressure

Magnet therapy involves taping magnets over certain acupressure points for 4-8 hours at a time. Some points to place magnets to help alleviate depression (according to Rosa Schnyder, an acupuncturist in Tucson, Arizona, USA) are listed here:

- LI4 – located on the top of the hand, between the thumb and index finger at the highest spot on the muscle when these two fingers are closed together.
- LV3 – located on the top of each foot between the first and second toes, about two inches from the web between these two toes, closer to the body.
  - o *It is recommended for women to use the hand point on the right side (LI4) and the foot point on the left (LV3); men to use the left-hand point (LI4) and right foot point (LV3).*
- Schnyder states, "These points calm the mind and settle the spirit". Schnyder recommends using magnets between 400-800 gauss (unit of measurement), taping them to the body with first-aid tape and leaving them on for a large portion of the day.

o   Make sure to not be very active when using these magnets to avoid sweating, and to allow the body to relax as these magnets can apply constant pressure.

Dopamine, Serotonin, Endorphins, and Oxytocin

These are some of the "feel good" chemicals that we often hear of. You want to get these releases through natural methods and not through pharmaceuticals or unhealthy habits. When these chemicals are released, we feel a temporary release from things such as stress, anger, frustration, or sadness.

<u>**Dopamine**</u> has a role in the following functions:

-    Learning and attention, mood, movement, heart rate, kidney function, blood vessel function, sleep, pain processing, and lactation.

Neurons in the region at the base of the brain produce dopamine in a two-step process. First, the amino acid *tyrosine* is converted into another amino acid, called *L-dopa*. Then L-dopa undergoes another change, as enzymes turn it into dopamine. Dr. Miller recommends 00-1,000-milligrams of tyrosine early in the day on an empty stomach.

Common Sources of Tyrosine: avocado, bananas, sesame seeds, oranges, peaches, okra, tomato, wild rice.

*note: sticking to recommendation to consume on an empty stomach, it would serve you best to consume some of these items listed in juice form shortly after awakening.

<u>**Serotonin**</u> has a role in the following functions:

-    Memory, fear, stress response, digestion, addiction, sexuality, sleep, breathing, and body temperature.

Neurons in the brain take amino acids and once the combination of amino acids needed to produce *tryptophan*, serotonin is release. Vitamin-B6 (Pyridoxine) is known to utilize tryptophan to produce serotonin. Pyridoxine is compound composed of hydrogen, oxygen, and nitrogen. It is known for animals to be able to use B6 to utilize the amino acid known as tryptophan which creates melatonin and serotonin to balance hormones, appetite, sleep, mood, and pain. Also helps increase the body's utilization from Vitamin-B3 which is needed to energize metabolism and DNA production.

Common sources of pyridoxine: avocado, carrots, bananas, peas, lentils, spinach, chickpeas, acorn squash, quinoa, sunflower seeds, brussels sprouts, oranges, pistachios.

<u>**Endorphins**</u> are "natural painkillers" in the body. They can be produced by doing many of the activities already described in this section. Exercise, music, acupuncture, and laughter are the most common. Others include sex, meditation, and the use of ultraviolet lights.

Oxytocin is a hormone produced by a section of the brain (hypothalamus). As it is released into the bloodstream, it promotes deep relaxation and feelings of well-being. Primarily produced to help facilitate childbirth, this hormone helps to reduce stress. Again, exercise and physical activity helps boost the production of this hormone. However, there's been many studies that test the saliva from those after being physically active in groups, which show a greater production of this hormone. Playing sports, martial arts training, etc. all contribute much more to producing oxytocin as compared to doing individual activities. Research has also shown that even activities such as singing in a group, can produce higher levels of oxytocin in addition to physical touch through activities such as sex, massage, cuddling, and giving hugs.

Psychedelics (caution)

There are various forms of psychedelics which range from mushrooms which contain psilocybin which is the compound found in "magic mushrooms", to *mescaline* which is the active compound in the peyote cactus which is known to produce psychedelic effects. There is still much research to be conducted on psychedelics, so you want to do so under guidance of a shaman or experiences healer. There is evidence of psychedelics working to encourage the growth of new connections between neurons in the brain. This ability of the brain to make new connections is called *plasticity*. Brain plasticity involves the ability of the nervous system to change its activity in response to intrinsic or extrinsic stimuli by reorganizing its structure, functions, or connections, which impact how the brain functions and responds during challenges such as mental health. States such as Oregon and Colorado have allowed psychedelics to be use medically under assisted adult use, where other states such as California, Michigan, Minnesota, Washington, and Massachusetts, have several cities where psychedelics are decriminalized under possession.

Dermatitis (and Eczema)

Dermatitis is a skin rash that results in red, itchy, swollen, or scaly skin areas. There are several forms of dermatitis: (1) Irritant Contact, (2) Allergic Contact, (3) Photo Contact, (4) Nummular, (5) Seborrheic, (6) Hand, (7) Perioral, and (8) Atopic. The most common form that lingers more than the rest and is more visible is, *Atopic*, otherwise known as Eczema. Dermatologists often can identify which form of rash you have, but more often than not decide if their preferred treatment involves a topical cream, or other form of treatment; they pretty much always choose the cream.

What happens with any of these conditions is that the organisms that are living on the skin have remained on the skin for a while now. But something has caused the skin to become unhealthy, and the newly formed skin cells begin to have a negative reaction with these organisms as they fight to identify who belongs there. As the skin remains weak, the rash will settle in, and symptoms will continue. They may be maintained by using a certain topical creams and moisturizers, but these will not solve the issue at hand. The recommendations in this section will work to show you how to naturally solve the issue and continue to take promote healthy skin to help ward off any future infections or issues that may impact the skin.

Remedies:

Selenium

This mineral is very crucial when it comes to our skin care and our body's immune system protection against infections that can turn into a rash such as dermatitis. Selenium combines with several other substances in the body to form a compound known as "glutathione peroxidase", which allow your immune system to sample organisms that are inhabiting (but not yet overgrowing) on the outer layer of the skin. This not only reduces any overgrowth which creates dermatitis, but also allows the immune system to respond accordingly and destroy any organisms that may be harmful to the body.

Common Selenium sources: brazil nuts, walnuts, chickpeas/garbanzo beans, kola nuts, dandelion greens, and nettle, and alfalfa. Recommended to consume about 400 micrograms a day. You may also plan to purchase a tasteless, odorless, liquid form of selenium by the brand Aqua Sel where you take 1-2 drops per day (or no more than 190mg daily).

Fatty Acids

The typical fatty acids we hear about such as omega-3, omega-6, and omega-9 help reduce inflammation in the body and can ease dermatitis.

Common sources of fatty acids: (Brazil Nuts, Walnuts, Kola Nuts, Avocados, Bananas, Sea Vegetables (Nori, Wakame, Hijiki, Sea Moss, Bladderwrack), Coconut, Coconut Oil (do not cook), Olive Oil (do not cook), Grapeseed Oil, Avocado Oil, Walnut Oil, Mushrooms, Quinoa, and Wild Rice.

Foods (Allergies)

Most often, dermatitis is triggered and maintained by food allergies. There are specific foods you may be allergic to that you can stay away from, but sometimes it's the ingredients within the foods that you may be allergic to also. It's often best practice to not only avoid specific foods you know you're allergic to, but avoiding items within the same food group to reduce potential triggers and fine-tune your search of what may be helpful to avoid. Most common food allergies come from dairy products, wheat, white sugars, white flours, citrus fruits, corn, soy, peanut better, chocolate, coffee, and alcohol. It is best to avoid these products in general but making it a priority when you experience any skin issues or dryness.

There's a blood test recommended by Bradley Bongiovanni, N.D., naturopathic physician from Cambridge, MA, USA, called the "IgG (immunoglobulin G) Test" that can help identify foods that can trigger an allergic reaction for your body. This test takes a snapshot of how the antibodies in the body interact with your immune system to provide a particular response to things like allergies. Noticing any deficiencies of higher levels of antibodies, this test can identify what can be harmful to the body and what the body may need protection from, so it does not get triggered by allergies.

Meditation

The practice of meditation is to help provide clarity to the mind and reduce stress. Stress can cause and contribute to dermatitis, particularly eczema. Meditation will also allow the mind and the body to relieve any stress it has accumulated in the day. Take about 15 minutes to sit somewhere comfortably where there are no interruptions and control your breathing. Allow your thoughts to come to you and pass or pick out a mantra you want to try to focus on that will help you remain focused on meditating. There are also many guided meditations you can follow along with as well.

Horsetail (herb)

This herb can be used as a compress to help alleviate symptoms and decrease discomfort for dermatitis. Take 1 teaspoon of this (dried) herb and put into 1 cup of water to boil for about 10-15 minutes. Let cool after removing from the heat but identifying when it's still warm enough to before removing and apply to your skin. Immerse a clean towel into the boiled water, then squeeze out any excess liquid. Wrap the towel around the inflamed area and cover with a larger, dry towel. Keep this area wrapped for 10 minutes at a time before rinsing off. Repeat at least two times a day. After each treatment, apply a few drops of avocado oil and gently rub over the inflamed area.

Hua Tuo (Cream)

Located in many Asian markets, this cream is often recommended for skin issues. It works to reduce swelling and irritation of the skin. The specific ingredients may vary by product and store but is often made by hand and sold in individual Asian markets. Hua Tuo was a Chinese physician and surgeon who is best known for being the first to successfully use anesthesia during surgery using the hemp plant. Tuo created various products to help assist him when performing surgery to the body. Prior to many of Tuo's creations, performing surgery was an aggressive and violent process due to the pain inflicted upon the victim. Tuo expanded into other fields such as hydrotherapy and helped to pioneer acupuncture treatments. His methods and process of making his cream to relieve skin irritation and dermatitis have been passed down and are still in use today, although specific ingredients may vary.

Batana Oil

This oil, native to Honduras, is extracted from the nuts of the American Palm Tree by the indigenous Miskito Indian tribes. Miskito people are commonly referred to as "Tawira" which means "the people of beautiful hair" which they credit to their regular use of batana oil. This oil is also very beneficial for the skin as well. Helps to clear up imbalances and smoothen the skin (you just have to rinse it off afterwards). Traditionally used for hair and skin treatment as this oil is known for rejuvenating hair, repairing damaged hair, clearing out grey or white hairs, promoting hair growth, as well as moisturizing the hair and skin. You can lather on as much as you want (without wasting) directly onto your hair and directly onto your scalp and anywhere on your skin. Let it settle in for about 20-30 minutes and then wash out or rinse off with warm water a few times a week or as often as your able to.

Hemp Seed Oil

Hemp seed oil is suitable for all skin types. It is particularly beneficial for those with dry or mature skin. Make sure to not have on any makeup as it can be runny. But, to remove makeup, wash hands thoroughly before applying a bit of hemp seed oil onto your fingertips and apply to areas you wish to clean. Massage this oil into your scalp and leave in for about 10 minutes before rinsing out with cool water. Hemp seed oil helps to hydrate the skin and regulate the skin's oil production. Skin dryness is actually a sign that the skin may attempts to overproduce oil which in turn, can stimulate acne and other issues you want to avoid. You can use this oil if you have oily hair or skin, but also if you have area of dry hair or skin.

Shea Butter

Shea butter is great for evening out and moisturizing the skin. In various parts of Africa, a child will be scrubbed with shea butter daily (their entire body) for the first few months of their life to serve as a protection for the skin to help reduce chances of various illnesses. Shea butter can be found in stores, but you want to get it without the added chemicals and artificial ingredients for best results.

My Personal Remedy:

(You can increase the amount of shea butter, nopales, and batana oil to your desired texture. All other ingredients remain the same).

Shave off thorns or nopales and peel off skin. You can use one large or 2 medium sized nopales pads. Large should be considered larger than the size of your opened hand. Blend together or place into food processor.

Add 2oz of burdock root to boiling water. Cook for 8-10 minutes, then let steep until cooled off.

Add nopales, burdock (tea), ½ cup shea butter, 8 drops of chamomile oil, and add a small scoop or batana oil and mix together thoroughly. Apply as much as you feel is needed directly onto skin twice a day.

Diabetes (Type-1)

Type-1 diabetes is an autoimmune disease. The immune system mistakenly identifies part of the body as being an outside invader, and proceeds to attack itself with antibodies, specifically the pancreas organ. Type-1 diabetes is when the immune system destroys insulin-making cells. Insulin is a hormone that helps cells in the body use glucose for energy. The pancreas is responsible for producing the hormone *insulin*, which sends blood sugar in the form of glucose out of the bloodstream and into the cells in the body. When there is not enough insulin being produced by the pancreas (due to getting attacked by antibodies), those with type-1 diabetes take insulin injections to make up for their lack of insulin production. This often creates a lifelong dependence on injections, especially since type-1 diabetes can be formed from a young age.

Tests Completed For Type-Diagnosis:

Type-1 diabetes is diagnosed with a series of tests, and you are diagnosed with diabetes on the basis of the following criteria:

Fasting blood sugar > 126 mg/dL on two separate tests. You cannot eat or drink anything but water from 8 to 9 hours prior to the time of getting your test done.

Random blood sugar > 200 mg/dL, along with symptoms of diabetes. It helps in assessing how well the disease is being managed.

Haemoglobin A1c > 6.5 on two separate tests. It tells your average level of blood sugar over the past 2 to 3 months. It's also called HbA1c, glycated haemoglobin test, and glycohemoglobin.

Although these are similar criteria to those of Type 2 diabetes, at times there can be delayed diagnosis of Type 1 diabetes. It is usually when you have a prolonged illness.

Remedies:

No Dairy (Ever)

Dr Jonathan Wright, M.D., who works as a physician and director of the Tahoma Clinic in Kent, Washington, USA, has stated that, "If the genes for Type-1 diabetes are in your family, meaning that any relative has had the disease, you are putting your children at risk for developing Type-1 diabetes by feeding them cow's milk instead of breast feeding". Now, it is understandable that there are various views on breastfeeding as opposed to providing cow's milk, but this condition does not appear overnight. The consistent consumption of cow's product and dairy products from birth onward, are the main contributor to developing type-1 diabetes, especially from a young age. Dairy products outlined here does not only include that one glass of milk. It includes everything from chocolate to ice cream, to cream cheese, to butter, to products such as instant mashed potatoes and chewing gum which have lower traces of this substance.

In a Finland study, researchers viewed the blood specimens from over 100 children who were recently diagnosed with type-1 diabetes. In every child, researchers found high levels of an antibody that is found within a protein in cow's milk. Researchers later found that the sequence of amino acids (chemical building blocks of protein) of the proteins in cow's milk were the exact same sequence of amino acids in the insulin-producing cells of the pancreas. What this means is that the cow's milk interferes with the pancreas being able to produce insulin for the body and creates an environment where the body thinks it is getting what it needs without being able to absorb it. So, it continues to (mistakenly) attack any source that is producing insulin, which happens to be the pancreas and will either prolong type-1 diabetes, worsen symptoms, or create this condition for those who do not have it. This study showed how diabetes is not simply an autoimmune disease as we typically view autoimmune disease created from the body's response to outside invaders or bacteria, but cow's milk provides an allergic response between the cells of the pancreas and the amino acids in cow's milk which results in these two "cancelling out" one another, destroying the natural cells within the pancreas.

A follow-up study to this Finland study was conducted by Italian scientists to test the validity of the Finland study. In Italy, cow milk consumption is typically much higher in northern Italy than in the south. These Italian scientists found a direct correlation where the higher the consumption of milk, leads to a higher chance of developing type-1 diabetes. Removing all dairy products from diet will stop the destruction of insulin-producing cells within the pancreas, which will directly help those with type-1 diabetes decrease their dependence on insulin injections in addition to the amount of insulin they may need per day. Those who do not have type-1 diabetes. Removing all dairy products from diet will further remove this condition from being a part of their lifestyle.

No More Gluten

Gluten provides no essential nutrients. It is a protein found in wheat, oats, barley, certain breads, cakes, soy products, white pastas, and various vegetarian or vegan "meats". Gluten is most associated with celiac disease, which is an autoimmune disease that damages the intestines. Although gluten is more associated with celiac disease, the immune system establishing the norm of attacking an organ in the body will make the immune system become more easily compromised and easier to be persuaded to attack other organs such as the pancreas which is the norm for type-1 diabetes. We want to avoid gluten items as they cause unnecessary damage to our bodies with no essential nutrients in them. Gluten will create additional work for our immune systems that we can do without so that we can ward off other potential illnesses and symptoms of disease.

Essentially, if gluten triggers one autoimmune disease, it will trigger another. When working to avoiding diseases such as type-1 diabetes, we must eliminate any and all contributing factors. Fortunately, there are many foods, cookbooks, and labels on items that signify they are "gluten-free".

No Refined Sugars

Refined sugars are in many junk foods, but they are often "hidden" in many soft drinks as well. Refined sugars rapidly spike blood glucose, and soda, fruit juice and other sugary beverages are the worst culprits. These forms of sugar enter the bloodstream rapidly and can cause extreme elevations in blood glucose.

Exercise

According to Eric P. Durak, director of Medical Health Fitness in Santa Barbara, California, USA, people with type-1 diabetes who exercise 35-40 minutes 3-4 days a week may be able to cut their insulin needs by 20-25%. Reducing daily insulin needs means fewer shots and less wear on the injection sites. A well-balanced exercise routine is encouraged to avoid remaining stagnant. A routine that consists of some light cardio, some strength training, and some endurance training in addition to regular stretching.

Smaller Meals More Often

Whenever we eat or drink anything, our pancreas produces insulin. Eating 3 meals a day will only provide the body with three opportunities to produce insulin. Eating more often (not overeating) will provide more opportunities that the body can respond and adapt to as you work on healing. Plan ahead some meals and break them into smaller amounts. Or choose to still have 3 meals a day but make them smaller while incorporating a few small (healthy) snacks or drinks during the day.

Note: Fasting does have it benefits with cutting down inflammation, but it is more of a risk for those with type-1 diabetes. Fasting would be more beneficial short-term and long-term for those with type-2 diabetes.

Thiamin (Vitamin-B1)

Many how have both, type-1 and type-2 diabetes are thiamin deficient, according to researchers at Warwick University in Coventry, England. Thiamin directly affects carbohydrate metabolism which is needed to regulate sugar levels.

Common Sources of Thiamin ("Vitamin B1"): asparagus, peas, oranges, clementines, lemons, sunflower seeds, sesame seeds, pecans, Brazil nuts, lentils, pecans.

Ivy Gourd (herb) (coccinia indica)

This herb is used a lot in Ayurvedic remedies for diabetes. It is believed to contain insulin-mimetic properties (essentially mimics the function of insulin) which can help reduce the need for injections for those with type-1 diabetes.

Holy Basil (herb)

This herb helps to nourish the pancreas and lower blood sugar levels. Also helps to decrease inflammation which can reduce aches, pains, and swelling for those with type-1 diabetes.

Jamun (java plum)

According to the National Institutes of Health (NIH) there was a study of 50 participants with diabetes who ingested 10 grams of jamun seed powder for 90 days experienced a 30% reduction in fasting blood glucose levels. Caution: consuming too much of this fruit or powder can lower blood pressure so make sure to follow recommended amounts on ingredient labels.

Diabetes (Type-2)

Type-2 diabetes is developed when the body becomes impaired with how it regulates and distributes sugars that are consumed. The underlying cause of Type-2 diabetes is insulin resistance. Insulin resistance is directly caused by excessive amount of fat within cells that were not intended to store large quantities of fat. Type 2 diabetes starts with insulin resistance. This means your body cannot use insulin efficiently. That stimulates your pancreas to produce more insulin until it can no longer keep up with demand. Insulin production decreases, which leads to high blood sugar.

It is important to note that sugars from fruit and artificial sugars are not the same nor processed the same. There are simple sugars and there are complex sugars. The simple sugars contain only about 1-2 sugar molecules whereas the complex sugars have about 3-4 sugar molecules. Both come from carbohydrates which are turned to glucose (blood sugar) in the body and are used as energy. These sugars are all found naturally in fruits, vegetables, and certain grains, but are also added to dairy products and many processed foods. They do, however, differ in their chemical structures (the way your body digests and metabolizes them and how they affect your health). The deciding factor of who develops type-2 diabetes is when the body begins to refuse to accept more sugar deliveries, which sends the excess sugar into the bloodstream. High blood sugar is identified in the initial assessment, later to be referred to as type-2 diabetes.

There are several different forms of sugar our bodies must remain aware of which are listed below:

Simple Sugars (monosaccharides)

Glucose: Fruits and vegetables are natural sources of glucose. It's also commonly found in syrups, candy, honey, sports drinks, and desserts.

Fructose: The primary natural dietary source of fructose is fruit, which is why fructose is commonly referred to as "fruit sugar". This sugar is commonly made into a chemical and added to junk foods.

Galactose: This sugar most commonly promoted as being in milk products, but is abundant in various fungi, avocados, mushrooms, beans, dates, bell peppers, tomatoes, and watermelon, among others.

Complex sugars (disaccharides)

Sucrose (glucose + fructose): Most often called "table sugar" is a sweetener derived from sugarcane or beets. It's added to foods during processing but occurs naturally in fruits and vegetables.

Lactose (glucose + galactose): Also known as milk sugar, lactose is found in milk and milk products.

Maltose (glucose + glucose): Maltose is found in malt beverages, such as beer and malt liquors.

As you may assume, we can do without many of the Complex Sugars when we are getting enough Simple Sugars in our diets. We do need glucose to survive which is produced by carbohydrates, but many of the other sugars listed above (especially when they are coming from artificial sources) are referred to as refined sugars which serve no benefit to the human body. If it sounds difficult to understand how a person can live primarily on one type of simple sugar, keep in mind how often most people consume the other sugars unnecessarily, and how we must simplify what we eat to get the most nutrients in our diets through eating more naturally. And if you haven't realized it by now, that fruits do NOT cause diabetes, nor do they have to be avoided whether you have type-1 or type-2 diabetes. The important piece is to monitor your consumption of fruits if you are consuming a high amount of artificial or processed sugars. You will want to remove these artificial and processed sugars from your diet and getting not only your sugar from natural sources, but the rest of your diet from natural sources so you can work on reversing this condition of type-2 diabetes.

Type 2 diabetes is usually diagnosed using the **glycated hemoglobin (A1C) test**. This blood test indicates your average blood sugar level for the past two to three months. Results are interpreted as follows:

Below 5.7% is normal.

5.7% to 6.4% is diagnosed as prediabetes.

6.5% or higher on two separate tests indicates diabetes.

Random blood sugar test. Blood sugar values are expressed in milligrams of sugar per deciliter (mg/dL) or millimoles of sugar per liter (mmol/L) of blood. Regardless of when you last ate, a level of 200 mg/dL (11.1 mmol/L) or higher suggests diabetes, especially if you also have symptoms of diabetes, such as frequent urination and extreme thirst.

Fasting blood sugar test. A blood sample is taken after you haven't eaten overnight. Results are interpreted as follows:

-   Less than 100 mg/dL (5.6 mmol/L) is considered healthy.
-   100 to 125 mg/dL (5.6 to 6.9 mmol/L) is diagnosed as prediabetes.
-   26 mg/dL (7 mmol/L) or higher on two separate tests is diagnosed as diabetes.

Oral glucose tolerance test. This test is less commonly used than the others, except during pregnancy. You'll need to not eat for a certain amount of time and then drink a sugary liquid at your health care provider's office. Blood sugar levels then are tested periodically for two hours.

Results are interpreted as follows:

-   Less than 140 mg/dL (7.8 mmol/L) after two hours is considered healthy.
-   140 to 199 mg/dL (7.8 mmol/L and 11.0 mmol/L) is diagnosed as prediabetes.
-   200 mg/dL (11.1 mmol/L) or higher after two hours suggests diabetes.

Remedies:

Remove White Flour and White Sugar

Items that contain white flour or white sugar contain excess gluten that gets sent into the bloodstream. This is the worst-case scenario for a person with type-2 diabetes as blood sugar levels will skyrocket quickly. These items are typically referred to as "refined foods". The white breads, cookies, and chips are sugar's first cousin. They are not absorbed by the body and are almost immediately sent directly into the bloodstream.

No Refined Sugars

Refined sugars are in many junk foods, but they are often "hidden" in many soft drinks as well. Refined sugars rapidly spike blood glucose, and soda, fruit juice and other sugary beverages are the worst culprits. These forms of sugar enter the bloodstream rapidly and can cause extreme elevations in blood glucose.

No Hydrogenated Oils

These include vegetable oil, soybean oil, cottonseed oil and canola oil. Because these oils are processed, treated at very high temperatures, and combined with bleaching agents and artificial dyes, consuming them has been linked to many health concerns, including diabetes. Use olive oil, avocado oil, hemp seed oil, sesame oil, or grapeseed oil instead.

Minimize Your Sodium Intake

Excess sodium can often increase chances of high blood pressure. If you already have diabetes, this will quickly worsen symptoms. If you do not have diabetes, consuming excess sodium can increase the likelihood of developing diabetes. You want to generally aim towards consuming less than 2,400mg a day of sodium; this is about the amount of sodium in 1 teaspoon of salt. This may seem restrictive, but making an estimate of no more than 800mg per meal can be a rule to stick to.

Fiber

High-fiber foods tend to be more filling than most foods, so you end up eating less. Consuming a high amount of fiber (25-35 grams a day) will help reduce blood sugar levels. Fiber slows the absorption of fats and carbohydrates which helps the body properly maintain a healthy glucose-insulin relationship.

Common sources of Fiber: garbanzo beans, lentils, brussels sprouts, sweet potatoes, avocado, pears, sunflower seeds, flax seeds, hazelnuts, apples and berries (high pectin fruits) and onions.

Magnesium

How the body digests, metabolizes, and processes energy, rely upon magnesium. If this mineral is low, this will make these functions not operate normally and the body will just work towards keeping things regulated as long as it cans before more severe issues present themselves. Low magnesium leads to insulin resistance and blood sugar problems.

Common sources of magnesium: Avocados, Bananas, Chickpeas, Tamarind, Basil, Dill, Ginger, Oregano, Thyme, Butternut Squash, Brazil Nuts, Pumpkin Seeds, Chia Seeds, Black Beans, Edamame, Kidney Beans, Okra, Leafy Green Vegetables, Nopal, Nettle leaf, horsetail, red clover, sage.

Also any CBD (cannabidiol) products are helpful. CBD Oils are almost pure magnesium.

To test the purity of a CBD Oil, send to a lab for testing or you should feel a steady decline in needing to rely on this substance after your need has been met regularly.

Chromium

This mineral is only needed in trace amounts, but it supports normal insulin sensitivity and promotes healthy fat and carbohydrate digestion. It is recommended that men have between 30-35 mcg of chromium a day, while women have between 20-25 mcg a day (increasing to 30 mcg a day while pregnant and 45 mcg a day while breastfeeding).

Common Sources of Chromium: green beans, lettuce, peas, carrots, orange juice, grape juice, tomato juice, apples, Brazil nuts, dried fruits, broccoli

Bilberry (herb)

This herb helps shrink the thickened capillaries (blood vessels the transport nutrients and oxygen from the blood into the cells). When the bloodstream filled with sugars, this results in decreased kidney function, nervous system damage, and various pains in areas like the hands and the feet from capillary damage. Those with type-2 diabetes have capillaries that slowly expand. Bilberry works to shrink the capillaries back to normal size (when there's not excess sugar in the bloodstream and the body). The flavonoids in this herb also work to heal the capillaries.

Use 80mg-100mg of this herb (extract) daily and within a few months, in addition to following other recommendations outlined in this section.

Bitter Melon

Researchers at the Gyeongsang National University School of Medicine, Jinju, Republic of Korea found that bitter melon helped lower glucose levels for those with type-2 diabetes. You can eat this melon, but most commonly added to a soup or juice this fruit.

Jamun (java plum)

According to the National Institutes of Health (NIH) there was a study of 50 participants with diabetes who ingested 10 grams of jamun seed powder for 90 days experienced a 30% reduction in fasting blood glucose levels. Caution: consuming too much of this fruit or powder can lower blood pressure so make sure to follow recommended amounts on ingredient labels.

Nopal (prickly pear cactus)

This plant has a ton of fiber which can help to regulate blood sugar levels. This is particularly helpful for those with type-2 diabetes.

Wild Yam (herb)

Also known as: colic root, American yam, four-leaf yam

No this is not some sort of potato. This is an herb used for a variety of reasons. This herb is able to assist the body with being able to keep blood sugar within the normal range. A typical daily dosage is between 1,500mg – 3,000mg. Instructions should be listed on the bottle. For tea, use about 1-2 teaspoons per cup daily.

Fatty Acids

Essential fatty acids (omega-3, omega-6, omega-9) help repair the cellular damage that has taken place over the years from consuming too many artificial sugars.

Common Fatty Acid Sources: (Brazil Nuts, Walnuts, Kola Nuts, Avocados, Bananas, Sea Vegetables (Nori, Wakame, Hijiki, Sea Moss, Bladderwrack), Coconut, Coconut Oil, Olive Oil, Grapeseed Oil, Avocado Oil, Mushrooms, Quinoa, Wild Rice.

Cinnamon

This spice improved blood sugar levels and benefits insulin resistance.

Fenugreek

This seed is rich in fiber and can help slow down how quickly the body breaks down sugars which benefit glucose and insulin regulation.

Exercise

When muscles are fit and well-conditioned, it takes less energy for the body to move sugar out of the bloodstream and into the cells. It is best to find any form of exercise you find most enjoyable that is not too difficult for you to do on your own. It's recommended to do about 15-20 minutes of exercise in the morning and at night. This may sound a bit challenging to add to your daily regimen, but starting off with simple exercises such as walking, and yoga can help the time pass by much easier until you're ready for other forms of exercise and training routines. Make sure to practice slower, controlled movements and take you time in between any sets you do to also make the time more manageable. It has been recommended to commit to a goal of burning 1,000 calories a week to help track your progress and set a standard each week to word towards.

Caution: If you immediately incorporate weight-training into your schedule, do so every other day to avoid feeling fatigued upon being more active.

Eat The Rainbow

Consuming a wide variety of colors from natural sources will provide you with an abundant amount of nutrients, antioxidants, and essential minerals. These foods from whole food sources also provide the body with fiber, help stabilize blood sugar levels, and controlling high blood pressure.

Stress Reduction: Develop A Mantra

When the body feels stressed, the adrenal glands will pump out excess cortisol which is a hormone that hinders the ability that insulin has available to clear the blood of sugar. Those with diabetes, this leaves excess sugar in the bloodstream and worsens the symptoms you may experience. Taking deep breaths and exhaling can help tremendously with reducing stress.

The mantra "haaa" is often used in various breathing exercise or during activities such as yoga. Dr. Virander Sodhi, M.D., N.D., naturopathic physician and director of the American School of Ayurvedic Sciences in Bellevue, Washington, USA states, "At a funeral, for example, everyone is spontaneously taking deep breaths and sighing 'Ha-a-a-a'. It's a natural way to release sorrow and other stress-caused negative emotions". Incorporate this practice into your daily life. Start with the "ha-a-a-a-a" chant with each exhale and move onto developing your own mantra that you feel is helpful.

Acupressure

Within acupressure, it is believed that the body's "chi" or energy flows through the body in currents called meridians. Stimulating these spots along the currents in the body can aide and facilitate healing. There are specific spots (acupressure points) that can provide relief to areas impacted by particular conditions. Below are specific points to apply gently, but steady pressure to in order to help provide additional relief for type-2 diabetes:

SP6 – is located above the bulge of the anklebone on the inside of your leg.

KI3 – located between the anklebone and the back of your ankle (in the hollow area behind the ankle).

KI6 – directly below the inside of the ankle bone.

CV4 – below the navel, running vertically down the middle of your body directly through the navel.

CV12 – on the same line on your navel but located slightly above the navel but to the edge of your sternum.

LI11 – on the outside of your elbow. Slightly bend your elbow to locate this point.

LU5 – located on the inside of your elbow on the outer edge of the bicep muscle.

LI4 – is in the web between you're your thumb and index finger at the highest point of the muscle that protrudes when the thumb and index finger are close together.

LU9 – is located on the wrist closest to your palm.

ST44 – this point is on the top of your foot between the 2nd and third toe about ½ inch above where the toes connect with the rest of the foot.

Start by searching for images of these locations. Then, gently apply pressure in small circular or round motions with your hands or fingers to these areas for a few minutes several times per day. As you get more comfortable with these areas, your pressure can become firmer.

Diaper Rash

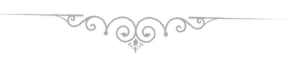

Having a diaper rash is most common for babies within the first 2-3 years of their life. The two main causes are, bowel movements, and urine. Nearly all diaper rashes go away within a few days, but these issues can linger for a longer period of time. When these issues linger, this can create future skin issues such as eczema and sensitive skin.

Remedies:

Breastfeeding Over Bottle Feeding

Babies who are breastfed are less likely to experience diaper rashes than bottle-fed babies. Serving sizes and bowel movements are often more difficult to track when feeding from a bottle. Babies who drink breastmilk absorb essential minerals at a quicker rate and feel fulfilled more easily. Most formula given to babies for bottle feeding often contain an assortment of chemicals which are pushed through the digestive system at a faster rate and increase the frequency of bowel movements; leakage from the bowels and urinary system can occur more often as well as a result of consuming chemicals.

Turn Onto Side (when changing)

When changing a diaper, you will want to turn your baby onto their side while you wipe as opposed to holding their legs in the air to prevent any leftover crevasses to wipe. Sometimes they may appear clean but there still may be materials that are hidden. Turning them onto their side and wiping will help clean better, and also keep any unnecessary pressure off of their necks and torso.

More Air

You can take off the diaper and lay your baby chest down (face turned to one side), on top of a towel or waterproof surface. Keep your eye on them but leave them alone for a few minutes at a time.

Soak In Water

It will help to soak additionally in water rather than always air dry. After changing your baby's diaper, they can soak in a tub or basin of room temperature water for several minutes. This can help assist with keeping this area clean and also help keep them calm.

Avoid Alcohol Wipes

Using wipes that contain alcohol can irritate the skin. An irritable baby will move around more or scratch and when this is mixed with any amount of urine or feces, this will promote a rash or create an infection. You will want to use any alcohol-free brands to begin and/or cotton balls dipped in natural oils when wiping clean to prevent a rash from spreading. You may also choose to get a spray bottle filled with warm water to rinse a baby's bottom to help cover the area without applying too much direct pressure to the area.

Blow Dry Clean

Wiping this area with a towel can also scratch and irritate the area where a rash can develop, especially if they have sensitive skin. Linda Jonides who works as a Nurse practitioner in Ann Arbor, Michigan, USA recommends using a blow dryer set on its lowest setting to avoid creating any abrasions to the skin while it is wet. Work to avoid using cornstarch or baby powder because they can develop into breathing problems in smaller children and infants.

pH Balancing (ph = "potential Hydrogen")

When there is urine and feces present, in a diaper rash, this raises the pH in the affected area. We typically associate a high pH in health as we want to avoid acidity, but a high pH in certain areas is not helpful. For example, if the pH of the digestive juices in your body were raised, the digestive system may not function properly, and this would lead to many health complications. What we want is to neutralize any area in need, particularly the outside of the body. Having your infant consume a few ounces of fruit juice such as blueberries or blackberries a day will help leave a semi-acidic residue in the urine and help to (internally) lower the pH from where it is and help reduce the irritation.

(Ex. we tend to hear of pH regarding the levels of health. Anything above a 7 on the pH (alkaline vs acidic scale) is considered "alkaline; anything below is considered acidic in its nature. Having urine and feces on the exterior of the skin may bring the pH (hypothetically) up to a 10 on the pH scale. Blueberries (although very healthy) have a pH generally between 6.5-7.5 and blackberries tend to have pH around 4-7, these items can essentially bring the pH down a bit while not consuming very acidic and unhealthy items that can create additional health issues.

Note: both blueberries and blackberries have a pH of about 8.5 once digested but can still remain lower than the hypothetical "10" the body is at by having urine and feces present on the skin.

Coconut Oil

Simply apply a thin layer of organic, cold-pressed coconut oil to your baby's rash-afflicted area. This natural barrier helps lock in moisture while providing gentle relief.

Aloe Vera

Is a natural anti-inflammatory. According to the National Center for Complimentary and Integrative Health, applying aloe vera to the skin can help people with acne, herpes simplex, psoriasis, and other conditions affecting the skin. It is typically well-tolerated. But, as with any new remedy, it's important to do a skin patch test before application, especially if you have sensitive skin. Some commercial aloe products may also have added fragrance or other chemicals that can irritate the skin, so be sure to read the label(s).

You can find this plant at most local markets or grocery stores. You want to slice this plant open with a knife, squeeze or scoop out all of the transparent pulp, and then apply directly on the skin covering the affected are(s). You can let this settle in before washing off after about an hour. You can do this as often as you want.

Chamomile Spray

Boil two cups of chamomile herb in water. Strain herb and let cool, then add to a spray bottle. Spray the affected area and gently rub in. Wash off after air drying.

Diarrhea

Diarrhea is one of the many defense mechanisms. If you've experienced diarrhea, you may have ingested something very toxic to the body such as harmful bacteria or possible it can be a parasite that your body is working to get rid of. If you've consumed something toxic to the body, the body will try to expel this immediately which comes shortly after it hits the digestive tract and is broken down with the digestive juices that help digest and break down materials in the gut. This may feel unpleasant and uncomfortable, but you do not want to absorb a toxic substance you have consumed. You want it out as soon as possible, and this is a good sign. If the body is working to get rid of a parasite, try to not think much about what's going on and good riddance to your parasite(s).

In addition to the unpleasantness of this condition, the fear of having an accident, stress, and the constant "holding in" an anticipated bowel movement, are all other contributing factors to work on eliminating by remaining proactive with some of the recommendations covered in this section.

Remedies:

Remove The Dairy

William Y. Chey, M.D., reports that, "a leading cause of diarrhea in this country is lactose intolerance". Now, the common argument against lactose intolerance is that us humans, cannot be tolerant of a substance that is designed for another animal, and we have a reaction in the form of lactose intolerance. All of the symptoms leading to diarrhea are promoted by consuming dairy. From an upset stomach, to congestion, to unstable (non-consistent) bowel movements. These early warning signs are promoted from consuming dairy, and removing these items helps to not only reduce the likelihood of diarrhea from occurring but decrease the severity or how long this condition is present.

Remain Hydrated

This may sound odd, given diarrhea is a liquid substance coming from the body, and you wouldn't want to contribute to this condition. But we often lose water whenever we have a bowel movement whether diarrhea is present or not. However, when diarrhea is present, we do lose more water from our bodies and can become dehydrated quickly. We want to avoid this by drinking water as often as possible, while consuming more water-filled fruits and vegetables (ex. berries, melons, cucumbers).

When working to remain hydrated, check your urine color often which should be pale/light yellow upon awakening and can be clearer throughout the day.

Avoid Foods That Take Longer To Digest

Many foods that take longer to digest (more than 40 minutes) should be avoided in general due to the additional work placed on the digestive organs, but more specific foods such as beans, pasta, cabbage, apples, potatoes, bananas, corn, soft drinks, oats, and white bread (and white flour) should be avoided because they either take longer to digest, or contain poorly absorbed carbohydrates which can irritate the gut and the condition of diarrhea.

Slippery Elm (herb)

This herb helps to soothe the colon and can calm diarrhea. Larger quantities of this herb (as compared to other herbs) of needed to help more immediately to help with diarrhea but this herb is very safe. These are often found in capsule form, but the best wat to consume this is to use powder, or open 2-3 capsules (sized ~370mg) and mix the powder with water slowly until it makes a gel-like paste. You want to continue to repeat this 2-3 capsules at a time until you have enough to take about 1 tablespoon of this paste. You may mix with a banana or soft fruit to consume the paste easier. You want to do this daily until this condition begins to decrease.

Fiber

You want to increase your fiber intake to help pass stools more easily and more often. As you remain hydrated, the added fiber will help repair the areas impacted the most by diarrhea and eventually lead to passing regular stools hopefully sooner rather than later. You want to avoid loading up on fiber excessively because you may feel congested long after this condition is no longer present. Simply start by increasing your normal fiber intake and monitor how you are feeling. You want to fall within the normal range daily at minimum which is between 21-25g per day for women, and between 30-38g a day for men.

Common sources of Fiber: garbanzo beans, lentils, brussels sprouts, sweet potatoes, avocado, pears, sunflower seeds, flax seeds, hazelnuts, apples and berries (high pectin fruits) and onions.

Cinnamon

Cinnamon has antimicrobial, demulcent (soothing), and astringent (tissue-tightening) properties to help fight infections, tighten tissue, and stop diarrhea. Combine with some homemade applesauce for best results.

Nutmeg

When consumed in small dosages, nutmeg can help with digestions and reducing flatulence which reduces the chances of diarrhea.

Go For Plain/Bland Foods

Bananas, rice or grains by themselves, will be most helpful. Many will have boiled potatoes, but we want to avoid stuffing our bodies to prevent this condition as it can start up again right after. Can have soups and homemade broths but want to avoid any artificial ingredients.

Chinese Herbal Remedy For Diarrhea

6 grams of lotus seeds (lian zi)

3 grams of Euryale (qian shi)

3 grams of dried ginger (gan jiiang)

6 grams of dioscorea (shan yao)

9 grams of poria (fu ling)

3 grams of codonopsis (dang shen)

2 red dates (hong zao)

Mix all of these together in a pot and cook with a grain such as quinoa to help deter diarrhea. Chinese practices often recommend this serving to be added to congee (boiled rice pudding), but we are looking to avoid as many starches as possible when trying to holistically treat a condition such as a virus.

My Personal Homemade Broth Recipe

Ingredients:

½ Cup Okra

2 Chopped Red Onions

1 Full Butternut Squash (cut into cubes)

1.5 Cups of Dandelion Greens

Add 3 Cups of Spring Water (add more as needed)

Step 1: Cook ingredients until boil, simmer for 1-hour, stirring ingredients every 10 minutes.

Step 2: Add seasonings about 5-7 minutes before completing cooking time.

Seasonings: ½ teaspoon of Sea Salt, 1 teaspoon of Dried Basil, ½ teaspoon of Dried Oregano, add Thyme and Cayenne Pepper powder to taste.

Step 3: Add to blender and blend until desired texture is achieved (blend to avoid any pieces left in mixture).

Note: Cut Up Veggies For Soup Ahead Of Time

Step 4: Strain out all ingredients for broth. Or you may choose to blend together to make a liquid soup that can help soothe your stomach.

Diverticulosis

This condition is created when the smaller areas of the colon walls begin to pop out between the group of muscles that surround the colon, and form diverticula, which are small pouches that line the digestive tract. When these pouches are created, this will make digesting items more challenging and present a host of issues within the digestive system. These pouches can become inflamed and will irritate the digestive lining and can often lead to developing a "leaky gut". Fortunately, this condition is not an indicator or develop into cancer.

Remedies:

Fiber

Adequate fiber intake lessons the pressure within the digestive tract and will alleviate symptoms. Fiber to give certain foods "bulk", they are often very small, and the muscles have to squeeze extra hard in order to pass a stool in which they now become overworked. Reduce the internal work of the digestive system by balancing your fiber intake. Typical recommendations for fiber are around 21-25g a day for women and between 30-38g a day for men.

Common sources of Fiber: garbanzo beans, lentils, brussels sprouts, sweet potatoes, avocado, pears, sunflower seeds, flax seeds, hazelnuts, apples and berries (high pectin fruits) and onions.

Slippery Elm (herb)

This herb helps to soothe and strengthen the digestive tract which can reduce current symptoms but also prevent future hidden symptoms that have not yet been on display. About 2,800-3,000mg of this herb a day will remain helpful in either powder or capsule form.

Avoid The Smaller Seeds

Seeds in items such as strawberries, tomatoes, cucumbers, and others, can get caught in some of these open sacs within the wall of the digestive tract and can contribute to creating inflammation.

See A Gastroenterologist

If you've had reoccurring symptoms or have been diagnosed with diverticulosis, it would be helpful to see a gastroenterologist. These are doctors who specialize in digestive disorders. The end goal may be to simply improve the digestive system by increasing fiber intake and remaining hydrated, by a gastroenterologist can provide insight on any additional complications or identify issues attached to your condition. These specialists can help with other issues such as abdominal pain or give notice if hospitalization is needed.

Homemade "Laxative" Remedy

Mix ½ cup of applesauce (blend up a few cup apples while slowly adding water until you reach desired texture) with 1/3 cup of prune juice. Put into refrigerator and take 2-3 tablespoons a day after your last meal of the day followed by drinking a full glass of spring water (8-10oz).

Liquid Diet or Fast

You will want to drink any variety of fruit or vegetable juices. This helps ensure you get enough nutrients while having something easy to digest. Identify which items you may need to stay away from for now before making or purchasing juices or drinks. If you wish to embark on a lengthier protocol, I wrote a book entitled, *A 21 Day Liquid Fast* which is available on my website and retailers such as Amazon. This book includes shopping lists and recipes for juices, smoothies, teas, and soups that you can make into liquid form. Start by incorporating small juices into your daily regimen before making any long-term adjustments.

Exercise

Being physically active releases *endorphins* in the brain, which are the body's natural pain relievers. Exercising can help alleviate the pains due to diverticulitis. Start with low to medium impact exercises to reduce the chance of creating any additional aches or pains.

Iti s recommended for adults to get at least 2.5 hours of moderately intense physical activity per week. The America Heart Association (AHA) suggests that you do any of the following moderately intense activities:

- Brisk walking (at least 2.5 miles per hour)

- Cycling (slower than 10 miles per hour)

- Water aerobics

- Dancing

- Gardening

- Tennis

- Pickleball or racquet sports

Berberine

This is an alkaloid found in several plants such as Oregon Grape, Coptis (Chinese goldthread), and barberry, among others. This alkaloid is anti-inflammatory with the ability to help fortify cells within the intestinal walls. Berberine increases the production of *butyrate*, which is a short-chain fatty acid that improves the expression of tight junctions such as the seal that's between two cells in membrane tissue. This helps create a filtering system that prevents the digestive tract from leaking, while regulating nutrient absorption. When areas like that are disrupted, there's increased rates of triggering inflammation, disease, and circulation.

Boswellia (herb)

Due to providing anti-inflammatory and anti-oxidative properties for the intestinal tract, this herb can be very beneficial for diverticulitis. Boswellia contains two active compounds (incensole acetate and incesole) which can help suppress symptoms of diverticulitis. The pro-inflammatory known as, cytokine, is often overexpressed in those who have diverticulitis, which Boswellia also helps to suppress.

In a 2020 pilot study published in the *Drugs In Context* (peer-reviewed Journal Database), Boswellia and curcumin were provided for patients with SUDD (symptomatic uncomplicated diverticulitis disease). After 30 days of this treatment, 77% of participants reported lower pain intensity, and 88% reported symptom relief within the first 10 days.

Dizziness

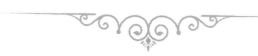

Dizziness displays a balance issue. Not just in the physical sense of balance, but more often than not, there is an unbalanced communication in the brain. Poor blood circulation, blood pressure, inner-ear issues, or side effects from medications are the most common contributors to dizziness, aside from any head trauma or injury. Dizziness can disappear on its own but can often have long-term consequences or lingering effects on our health which we want to avoid.

Remedies:

Stop Moving and Sit Down

This is the safest method of preventing injury and helps to allow the blood flow to stabilize. If you are moving while dizzy, you can bump into something or fall over, and your blood flow will continue to remain irregulated. Sitting down makes it easier to focus on your breath to calm and relax your body as best as you can while assessing for any other potential issues.

Touch Something

When you are dizzy, it can be difficult to identify when you feel better enough until it eventually stops. Placing your hand on something like a chair or table nearby can help you track when you are starting to become less dizzy. You know that these objects are not moving and placing your hand on them can help you remain connected to them as you work to stabilize yourself. When you feel as still as the object you are touching, you should be close to moving around once again.

Remain Hydrated

Even mild dehydration can cause a reduction in blood pressure and result in dizziness. You want to remain hydrated by consuming about half of your current bodyweight in ounces and work to retain fluids in the body by "eating your water" by regularly consuming foods filled with water (ex. tomatoes, cucumbers, melons, berries).

Be Cautious In Your Bathroom

From the slick, flat surfaces, to the sharp corners and hard materials such as the tub, the bathroom is not the ideal place to be if you frequently get dizzy. You want to be as careful as possible whenever in a bathroom. Also, whenever you bathe or shower the blood vessels dilate and can trigger a sudden drop in blood pressure. If you move too quickly during this time period, dizziness can appear by the time you're ready to step out of your bathtub.

Check Your Blood Sugar Levels

When blood sugar is low, dizziness can settle in more often than not. Not eating enough can contribute to dizziness, while eating can cause dizziness in others. To determine what may be causing your hunger-related dizziness, it is important to check your blood sugar levels.

Normal blood glucose levels for adults, without diabetes, is 90 to 110 mg/dL.

A blood sugar level less than 140 mg/dL (7.8 mmol/L) is within normal range.

A reading of more than 200 mg/dL (11.1 mmol/L) after two hours indicates diabetes.

A reading between 140 and 199 mg/dL (7.8 mmol/L and 11.0 mmol/L) indicates pre-diabetes.

Normal Blood Sugar Levels (For Adults)

While Fasting: less than 100

Before Meal: 70-130

1-2 hours After Eating: less than 180

Bedtime: 100-140

Ginger (herb)

Dizziness most common symptoms is nausea. Ginger's anti-inflammatory properties can help ease nausea and alleviate the severity of symptoms connected to feeling dizzy. This herb can be eaten, taken in capsule form, or made into a tea.

Licorice (herb)

Not to be confused with the candy, this herb helps to retain sodium that's already in the body. We often don't want to retain sodium as it can make its way into the bloodstream, however, low sodium in the body can immediately cause dizziness. We want to avoid artificial versions of sodium in the form of unnatural sugars; while retaining the sodium we have in our bodies to avoid feeling dizzy. This herb can be taken in tea form or capsule. You do want to track your potassium levels and monitor you blood pressure to avoid blood pressure from getting too high while taking this herb regularly. Follow instructions that come with instructions on labels but avoid consuming more than 100mg a day on average.

Quick Tip: if you boil pieces of hickory, walnuts, and pecan roots, this extracts nutrients such as sodium where you can use this water for meals or to drink after it cools off to boost your sodium intake.

Glucose

This is the sugar the body uses for energy and can increased simply by eating more fruits. You want to accompany an increased consumption of fruit with and increase in fiber intake to promote smooth digestion, in addition to removing simple carbohydrates such as white sugar and white flour which turns into sugar as it's being digested. Essentially, you want to increase your energy levels (glucose) while not wasting energy on digesting various substances such as simple carbs to help avoid feeling dizzy. We burn calories whenever we consume anything. Burning extra calories (from heavier digestion) while running low on things like sodium and glucose can trigger more frequent symptoms or feelings of dizziness.

Indigestible Fiber

Consuming too much indigestible fiber can clog the lymph nodes in the body and cause dizziness. These are most common in foods high in estrogen such as soy. You will want to track your fiber consumption and possibly decrease temporarily to track any relief. You want to fall within the normal range daily at minimum which is between 21-25g per day for women, and between 30-38g a day for men.

Common sources of Fiber: garbanzo beans, lentils, brussels sprouts, sweet potatoes, avocado, pears, sunflower seeds, flax seeds, hazelnuts, apples and berries (high pectin fruits) and onions.

Acupressure

There is a specific pressure point located on the wrist that can provide significant relief for contributing factors of dizziness such as nausea and vertigo. Dr. Dozer, M.D., president and chief executive officer of the California Institute of Integrative Medicine in Calistoga, recommends applying pressure to the PE7 point on the body for relief. This point is located on the inside of the wrist, in the center about a ½ inch below the wrist crease. Use your thumb to apply light, but steady pressure to this area for about five minutes. Rub around this area with you palm in circles after a short break when the five minutes are completed.

Dry Eyes

Dry eyes can occur for numerous reasons, but it all boils down to the eyes not producing enough tears in order to keep the eyes moist. The main effort is to restore moisture in the eyes. Whenever we blink our eyes, we create a layer of water, oil, and mucus around the eye to keep it moist while cleaning any bacteria that may be present. As we get older, our tear glands begin to not produce as much of this combination of tears, oil, and mucus, and contribute to the eyes drying up. Women who deal with menopause notice these changes due to hormonal shifts drying up secretions in the body which include the fluids in and around the eyes. Other primary contributing factors include redness, burning, itching, sensitivity to light, and general environmental factors.

Remedies:

Warm Compress

The warmth can help stimulate tear flow by soothing the passageways that tears flow from. Soak a small towel in warm water and then squeeze out all liquid until it does not drip. Place warm towel directly onto your eyelids (eyes closed) for about 5-10 minutes about 2-3 times a day.

Proper Hydration

Anytime the body is not adequately hydrated, areas will become drier by default; the eyes, which require a lot of moisture will experience this when the body is not hydrated. Not only drinking about half of your body weight in ounces (ex. if you weigh 100lbs, drink 50oz) but consuming foods that provide water is necessary. Melons, berries, tomatoes, and cucumbers are only a few items that should regularly be in your diet. Consuming items that provide hydration can help wash away and also neutralize the erosive acids that remain in the body from eating things detrimental to our health.

Remove Your Contact Lenses

If you are having eye dryness, the last thing you want is to add another layer that prevents the eye *fluids* from being produced or absorbed completely. When you do not need your contact lenses it is best to not use them. If you rely upon contact lenses, you will want to incorporate several of the other remedies and recommendations listed in this section.

Primrose Oil or Black Currant Seed Oil

Both of these oils contain a specific fatty acid known as, *gamma-linolenic acid (GLA)* which can increase tear production. Primrose Oil is typically used in the evening while Black Currant Seed Oil can be taken at any time. Either oil can be consumed by mouth. A daily amount of about 1,500mg a day of either oil is recommended.

Potassium

This mineral helps maintain regular amounts of fluids in the body. Dr. Grossman, O.D., optometrist, licensed acupuncturist, and co-director of the Integral Health Center Rye in New Paltz, New York, USA, states that his patients with dry eyes are typically low in potassium.

Common Potassium Sources: squash, zucchini, bananas, avocado, dried apricots, and herbs such as, guaco (also high in iron), conconsa (has the highest concentration of potassium phosphate), lily of the valley (rich in iron fluorine and Potassium phosphate).

Avoid Artificial Sugars and Sweeteners

These foods should be avoided at minimum, but these foods deplete the body of potassium and dry the tear ducts in the body. These items interfere with the body metabolizing of fatty acids such as *gamma-linolenic acid (GLA)* which contribute to dry eyes.

Practice Blinking During Screentime

When we are looking at screen such as a computer, laptop, television, or cell phone, we often focus on what we are doing and by default, do not blink as often. Forcing the eyes to remain open for extended periods of time, will cause the tears and oils in the eyes to dry up and increase how dry the eyes are. Remain mindful of when you may be looking at a screen for an extended period of time so that you can remember to blink. Practice blinking frequently without forcing this upon yourself so that you can avoid not blinking during these moments and keep a steady flow of fluids around to moisturize your eyes.

My Personal Remedy:

Mix 1 tablespoon or eyebright herb

Mix 1 tablespoon of blue vervain herb

Boil 4 cups of distilled or spring water

Add herbs to boil, let cool for 10-15 minutes (or until completely cool)

Strain herbs and place water in the refrigerator.

Take a small cup, tincture tube or handful and pour gently into your eyes one at a time.

Move your eyes in close wise, counterclockwise, diagonal, up and down, side to side motions while keeping your eye lids closed to rinse your eyes.

You may also drink this mixture but will need to make several more servings and may not directly go right for washing out your eyes.

(Note: make sure no small pieces are in the water as even the smallest piece can irritate your eye).

Dry Mouth

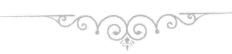

This condition is not just a result of lacking adequate hydration; more often than not this is the condition known as xerostomia which is when salivary glands in the mouth are not producing enough saliva. Having a dry mouth more of a short-term issue, while xerostomia is an underlying issue that is starting to regularly display itself in the form of having a dry mouth. If you have regular moments where you experience having a dry mouth, you may have xerostomia.

Note: dry mouth is often a side effect to treatments such as chemotherapy and radiation, medications, and connected to many other conditions. If you have another condition, having a dry mouth may just happen more frequently due to the other condition and not be xerostomia. Xerostomia is a condition that more so is present when no other lingering ailments or conditions are present.

Remedies:

Stop Chewing Gum

Chewing stimulates the salivary glands. This additional workload for the salivary glands will cause these glands to run dry more often than not. We do not want out salivary glands to produce additional saliva when we are not eating. This can and will make swallowing food more difficult and require a drink of some sort to be consumed while eating, which will reduce nutritional absorption, which can lead to other contributing factors related to dry mouth or other conditions.

Proper Hydration

Not only drinking about half of your body weight in ounces (ex. if you weigh 100lbs, drink 50oz) but consuming foods that provide water is necessary. Melons, berries, tomatoes, and cucumbers are only a few items that should regularly be in your diet. Consuming items that provide hydration can help wash away and also neutralize the erosive acids that remain in the body from eating things detrimental to our health.

Avoid Irritants (Salty or Spicy Items)

These items can cause pain when dry mouth or xerostomia are present. Even natural items such as homemade orange juice, cayenne pepper, foods high in sodium, or adding salt or sea salt to foods can cause pain in the mouth, particularly the tongue, teeth, or even the jawbone. Foods high in salt contribute to dehydrating the body internally and will contribute to areas such as the mouth being drier.

Use Natural Toothpaste

Using something as simple as baking soda or coconut oil can help alleviate symptoms and keep the mouth clean to promote proper hydration. Dr. Peterson, D.D.S., dentist from Gering, Nebraska, USA, who has over 25 years of practice recommends not using traditional toothpastes that contain the foaming agent known as sodium lauryl sulfate because they can irritate gum tissue. When we irritate gum tissue, this triggers the saliva glands to turn on again and an deplete the salivary glands in the mouth and lead to dry mouth. In addition to using a more natural toothpaste, you want to replace your toothbrush frequently, and brush diligently.

Breathe Through Your Nose

Breathing through your mouth is not necessary and does not provide adequate oxygen to the lungs and respiratory system as compared to "nose-breathing". Practice taking a few moments every day to take deep breaths through your nose. This can be applied as a form of meditation but can be performed while you are on your way to work, school, or just during your normal routine. I would highly recommend the book entitled, *Breath: The New Science of a Lost Art*, by James Nestor who covers an array of health benefits from nose-breathing, and the many conditions that are connected to breathing through the mouth.

Oil Pulling

Take 1-2 tablespoons of coconut oil or sesame oil and swish it around your mouth for about 10-15 minutes. Using this natural method for treating dry mouth works because the oil cleans out the mouth while coating and soothing irritated spots.

Slippery Elm and Marshmallow Root (herbs)

These herbs contain *mucilage*, a substance that helps to coat the tongue, mouth, and throat, and keeps moisture locked in your mouth.

Slippery Elm: Dr. Pamela Jeanne, N.D., naturopathic doctor in Gresham, Oregon states, "Slippery elm is a wonderful herb that helps relieve the symptoms of acid indigestion" and recommends taking one capsule of this herb before each meal for best results.

Slippery Elm or Marshmallow Root: Take ½ teaspoon of herb (dried herb can deteriorate quickly after picked so powder form is useful as well) into a cup of war, water. Let cool for 15 minutes then stir together. After drinking this do not eat for at least 30-minutes to 1-hour to allow this herb to make contact with your intestines uninterrupted. Do this every other day.

My Personal Remedy: Mouth Wash

- Blend 1 cup of warm water with ¼ teaspoon baking soda and ⅛ teaspoon salt.
- Swish in your mouth for a few seconds, then rinse out with water.
- Repeat every three hours.

Dry Skin

When the skin is dry, there is often not enough moisture, hydration, or oils in the body. Although loading up on these items is a necessary step, we must also work internally to address these issues as well. Not washing with hot water, using clean soap, and using lotions or moisturizers will not be enough to completely overcome this issue.

Remedies:

Hydration

Remaining hydrated has a role in just about every condition so it's best to start here. Not only consuming several glasses of water a day but accompanying this with fresh fruits and vegetables will help tremendously. However, it should be noted, that is you are dehydrated, you will notice improvements, but if you are only partially dehydrated and have dry skin, drinking an excess amount of water may not be helpful. You want to essentially check off the hydration box as a starting point when addressing dry skin.

Soak Yourself In Water

After addressing your internal hydration, it is important to focus your intention on the external part of your body, the skin itself. You want to soak your skin (entire body if your able to) in lukewarm water for about 15 minutes a day. You should follow this by bathing in cooler water once a day. Depending on activity level, it is not necessary to shower 2-3 times a day. It would be best to shower once a day and soak once a day until your skin becomes less dry because additional amount of cool or hot water on the skin when showering or bathing, several times a day, can irritate the skin and contribute to this condition.

Natural Soap

There are too many brand names and items to list that fall under the category of "natural soap". You simply want to search for soaps that have minimal ingredients and come from natural sources, not a long list of chemicals. Also, when using soap, follow the advice/recommendation of Dr. Pearlstein, M.D., assistant clinical director of dermatology at Mount Sinai School of Medicine of New York in New York City, who states, "If it's not dirty, don't wash it". This recommendation is not saying to avoid any areas, but using soap on every area of your body daily can do more harm than good. Yes, we want our entire bodies to be clean, but targeting the areas in need are more important while the rest of the body can be rinsed only for now to help target specific areas where your skin is dry. If you are using soap that contain many chemicals, applying these daily over the entire body will increase your consumption of chemicals and contribute to your condition.

Humidify The Air

In colder climates and during the winter season, the humidity in the air decreases about 10%. This contributes to dry skin and can be avoided by using a humidifier in certain areas of your home or office. It can help to close the door of wherever you decide to place a humidifier to help trap in some of the humidity and not have to leave it on as long as you would have to by placing it in a more open space.

Spay On Mist

Spraying on direct areas of dry skin can help alleviate symptoms. It is recommended of putting a few drops of an essential oil (about 10 drops into a spray bottle) such as jojoba oil, lavender, or chamomile to help provide additional benefits to the body while working to overcome this condition. You want to spray onto skin at least three times a day but as often as needed to begin determining how severe the issue may be. Make sure to not spray into your eyes and airy dry whenever possible.

Black Currant Oil

Consuming about 1,000 – 2,000mg of this oil daily can provide a rich source of fatty acids which are crucial for healthy skin.

Batana Oil

This oil, native to Honduras, is extracted from the nuts of the American Palm Tree by the indigenous Miskito Indian tribes. Miskito people are commonly referred to as "Tawira" which means "the people of beautiful hair" which they credit to their regular use of batana oil. Traditionally used for hair and skin treatment as this oil is known for rejuvenating hair, repairing damaged hair, clearing out grey or white hairs, promoting hair growth, as well as moisturizing the hair and skin. You can lather on as much as you want (without wasting) directly onto your hair and directly onto your scalp and skin. Let it settle in for about 20-30 minutes and then wash out with warm water a few times a week or as often as your able to.

Sea Moss

You may use this sea vegetable in gel form as a scrub to brush and clean your skin with. Consuming this regularly in addition to not consuming items detrimental to your health, can provide the body will additional nutrients and minerals that can help strengthen and repair drier skin.

My Personal Remedy:

Take equal parts of the following herbs: marshmallow root and fennel seeds.

Mix together and add to water to boil for 20 minutes.

Add 2 teaspoons of plantain leaves and let water simmer for another 20 minutes.

Turn off the heat and let cool for 10-15 minutes.

Strain out all herbs and parts.

Make enough of this mixture to be able to drink 1 quart of this tea daily.

Ear Ache

To begin, "Ear Ache" is usually one word (earache) but for the purpose of this book being a guide to help with various condition, I thought "earache" may be mispronounced as it's not a word we're often seeing spelled out. So, I used "Ear Ache" to help easily identify this and label this condition to help not skip over it in case it mispronounced or assumed to be some other condition we're not familiar with.

An earache is usually formed due to some form of infection. Earaches are most common in children as their ears are still developing and various pains can come with this outside of any infection. Tooth pain can also "travel" to the ears and contribute to these types of conditions. There are tubes (eustachian tubes) that go from the back of the throat all the way to the middle part of our ears. Clogged tubes are the most common cause of earaches. During the day our heads are mostly held upright in addition to when we eat in which these tubes open slightly to allow air in when we swallow. At night while resting, our heads are not regularly upright which make it more difficult for these tubes to drain and they get clogged. When they cannot drain easily, this air located by the middle part of the ear closes and creates a vacuum-like motion where it sucks the air inward to properly close to prevent any bacteria or debris in. As you sleep, these tubes remain closed off and become clogged. This is when you begin to feel pain settle in and experience a reduction in hearing.

Remedies:

Mullein (herb)

This herb is mostly used for cleaning the respiratory system but also helps to soothe the skin in the ear when used as an oil as well reduce pain and inflammation. Use mullein flower oil by adding some oil to a cotton ball and gently wiping on infection or swollen area or add 2-3 drops directly in the ear every four hours until pain and/or swelling begins to decrease. Caution: do not use liquids in your ear if you think your eardrum may be punctured or ruptured.

Echinacea (herb)

You can find a liquid form of this herb. Based upon which parts of this herb are used (leaf, flower, or root) the recommended dosage can change. Be sure to follow recommended dosage with any product you may purchase and follow instructions. Caution: do not use liquids in your ear if you think your eardrum may be punctured or ruptured.

Lavender Essential Oil

This oil will help the body relax which is necessary when battling an irritating, and sensitive condition. Fill a bowl with a cup of boiling water and add 3-5 drops of lavender essential oil. Wrap your hair up in a "tent" position (wrap your hair by wrapping a towel around your head until the top is completely covered). Slowly lean over the bowl (making sure to not burn yourself from the steam) and take allow, controlled breathes for about 5-10 minutes. If at any point you feel dizzy or unbalanced, make sure to stop.

Allergies

Anyone who is allergic to specific foods are more likely to have ear infections. This is due to the excess inflammation that remains present around the throat, ear, and nasal passages when allergies are being displayed. Most common food allergies are dairy, wheat, corn, peanuts, oranges, butter, refined sugar, and various fruit juices. If you feel congested, cough, or your skin itches after eating any of these items, you most likely have an allergy. Just removing these items form your diet can remove stronger allergic reactions and also contribute to decreasing your likelihood of having an ear infection.

Colloidal Silver

In his bestselling book, *The pH Miracle: Balance Your Diet, Reclaim Your Health*, by Dr. Robert O. Young, Ph.D., he states ,"Eye or ear problems, including cataracts, glaucoma, redness, blurred vision, poor eyesight, ringing in the ears, earaches, soreness or swelling of the ears, eardrum damage, hardness of hearing, and (in rare cases) loss of hearing: Use 1 drop of colloidal silver topically (directly in the eye or ear) 3 times a day."

Qi Gong Massage

Using a technique from Traditional Chinese Medicine can help work towards improving the healing process of an earache. You want to make a "V" with your index and middle fingers pressing flatly on both sides of your ear (middle finger in front of your ear and other finger behind the ear). Starting at the bottom, move your fingers up while pressing firmly, the release pressure as you slide your fingers back down to the bottom of your ear. Do the movement repeatedly (at least 30 times) to help stimulate circulation and promote lymph drainage. The lymph drainage is responsible for moving fluids around the body and help begin to reduce any excess inflammation in the body. inflammation in the ear can decrease as a result of doing this practice regularly.

Don't Aggravate The Condition

Do not prolong how long your earache is present. Work to not pick at it or constantly rub it. You may feel tempted to touch to track how large the swelling may be, but remind yourself, every time you touch this area, the more often it will remain stimulated and will remain present. Do not squeeze your earache as it will not only be painful, but in some cases, it can break open and your treatment will have to change and will likely take longer to heal. You also want to avoid things such as tight-fitting hats, or doing activities such as swimming which can irritate your earache.

Steam Onions

Cut into small chunks, a few onions and place them into a pot of boiling water. Place a lid on top and steam for about 10-12 minutes. Strain out the onions and pour the leftover contents into a bottle. Use a dropper to pour 3-4 drops a day into your ear to help provide relief.

*if you do not want to pour this liquid directly into your ear, you can bake an onion in the oven for about 25-minutes. Bake on medium temperature until it begins to start coming apart on its own. Take it out and place in a hand towel and hold it to your ear for 30-35minutes. This will help draw out some inflammation causing the ear to be in pain.

"Sweet Oil"

This oil is easy to find and is often made from olive oil and almond oil. Follow instructions on label but you can either drop in a few drops directly into your ear, or massage into the skin in and around the ear daily until pain decreases.

Earwax (build-up)

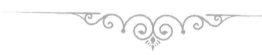

Earwax is a vacuum cleaner for bacteria while also being a lubricant for our ears. Having earwax is essential for keeping our harmful debris which protects our ear canals. However, sometimes earwax can build up more than needed which calls for some form of intervention before it clogs the ear canal and end up causing more harm than not to this area of the body.

Remedies:

Olive Oil

This multipurpose oil can also be used to treat earwax buildup. Start by laying down on your side so that your ear in need is facing up (ex. left ear needs help, lay on your right side). Slowly drop 2-3 drops of olive oil into your ear and allow the oil to roll down into your ear canal. Continue to lay on your side for about 10-15 minutes as this will allow the wax in your ear to loosen so it can be removed. Wax you can visibly see can be guided out as if softens, while earwax that is deeper in your ear canal can begin to loosen as it will naturally begin to be removed/expelled from the body. If your earwax is more internal, you should begin to notice improvements with your hearing in a few days to help track progress and know the oil is helping.

Increase Good Fat, Decrease Bad Fat

This is a general recommendation to follow outside of having excess ear wax but can help speed up your healing process. Eating foods with saturated, hydrogenated, or trans fats can not only increase the amount of inflammation in the body, but these "bad fats" directly help create thicker earwax says Dr. Haas, M.D., director of the Preventative Medical Center of Marin in San Rafael, California, USA. Decreasing the consumption of "bad fats" while consuming the "good fats" found in omega-3, omega-6, and omega-9, will provide adequate nourishment we need in the form of not only fatty acids, but the oils we need to help keep areas like our ears lubricated enough to cleanse out unnecessary waste.

Common Sources of Fatty Acids: Brazil Nuts, Walnuts, Kola Nuts, Avocados, Bananas, Sea Vegetables (Nori, Wakame, Hijiki, Sea Moss, Bladderwrack), Coconut, Coconut Oil (do not cook), Olive Oil (do not cook), Grapeseed Oil, Avocado Oil, Walnut Oil, Mushrooms, Quinoa, and Wild Rice.

Note: Black Currant Seed Oil is also a great alternative to using besides the recommended fish oil(s) that a doctor may prescribe. Take about 1,000 milligrams of this oil.

Onions

Onions have many benefits for the ears as stated in previous section about earaches. A simple remedy to see how much of an issue may be present, is to cut a small piece of an onion and place it in your ear overnight. Cut a piece that won't get lost or be hard to remove, but large enough to stay put. If you do not notice progress after a few days, then you will want to pursue additional remedies.

Mullein (herb)

This herb is mostly used for cleaning the respiratory system but also helps to soothe the skin in the ear when used as an oil as well reduce pain and inflammation. Use mullein flower oil by adding some oil to a cotton ball and gently wiping on infection or swollen area or add 2-3 drops directly in the ear every four hours until pain and/or swelling begins to decrease. Caution: do not use liquids in your ear if you think your eardrum may be punctured or ruptured.

"Sweet Oil"

This oil is easy to find and is often made from olive oil and almond oil. Follow instructions on label but you can either drop in a few drops directly into your ear, or massage into the skin in and around the ear daily until there's less earwax buildup and/or until any pain decreases

Emphysema
(Chronic Obstructive Pulmonary Disease - COPD)

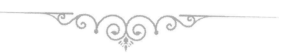

This condition is a degenerative disease which develops gradually over many years of regular exposure to toxins. The warning signs of this condition remain present long before an official diagnosis of emphysema. Coughing excessively, inability to take deep breaths, shortness of breath, wheezing, chest tightness, and coughing that produces excess mucus, are all of the most common symptoms of COPD.

Emphysema is a more extensive form of bronchitis. If you refer to the bronchitis section in this book, you will find helpful tips that will work for this condition also. This condition more is more or less the end result of regular loss of lung function. Now, it can be difficult to restore lung function to where it was once before, but when treating Emphysema (COPD), we want to maximize the lung function we have currently, while working to limit causing disruption, in addition to achieving an end result of optimal lung function. An overarching theme with approaching ways to treat Emphysema, is working to make sure that this condition does not get suddenly worse and develop into pneumonia.

Remedies:

Stop Smoking

This includes everything you may inhale from recreationally smoking; cigarettes, marijuana, cigars, vaping, or other form of smoke. It is never too late to stop smoking and this is often a difficult process for many to do. Smoking fills up the lungs and irritate the respiratory system. Starting first with educating yourself on the many benefits of not smoking is a great way to set reminder for yourself to stay motivated with this goal.

Avoid Allergens

If you are someone who has allergies, start by first reviewing the allergies section in this book to work on reducing symptoms. Next, it is important to completely avoid anything you are allergic to in order to prevent any breathing difficulties.

Exercise

You want to use exercise to tone the muscles in your upper extremities (neck, shoulder, and chest areas). This includes, but is not limited to, cardiovascular exercises such as walking, and light jogging. You want exercises that help you train these muscles while maintaining a steady breath flow in and out. Swimming is a very helpful exercise for those with COPD due to the humidity which supports healthy breathing. Simply going for more frequent walks every day will help you use your lungs more and help decrease your symptoms as well as build up your tolerance when/if you are "out of breath".

Smaller Meals, More Often

Eating several large meals a day will restrict your breathing in some capacity as you have to swallow and have less frequent breaths during meals. You want to maintain a regular breathing pattern and can do this easier throughout the day by having smaller meals and snacks during the day. Making smaller meals and having some small (healthy) snacks will help you not only complete your eating quicker but allow your body to return back to its normal breathing pattern for longer periods of time during the day. Eating larger meals causes the body to send things such as blood and oxygen towards other parts of the body and away from where these are most needed for someone who has COPD which are the lungs and respiratory system.

Works Towards Having a Leaner Physique

Anyone who gains a lot of weight of maintains a larger mass for their body size (ex. taking Body Mass Index (BMI) into account, their bodies retain more fluids. Not just water, but digestible liquids, lymphatic fluids, and waste. This creates additional constraints for the lungs to breath given they have to provide for a larger mass, while being weighed down (literally) which can limit the lungs' ability to maximize its space when inhaling (or exhaling). You will want to monitor and decrease your overall size and a leaner physique so you have a more even weight distribution and can alleviate how much work the lungs are required to do.

Diaphragmic Breathing

Steady, repetitious breathing is best. Babies will do this naturally as you can view their belly go in and out with each breath. Breathing from your core is best achieved by breathing through the nose. For diaphragmic breathing, you should notice your belly going out with each inhale and going back in with each exhale. This steady form of breathing can help the body feel more relaxed and also hold onto more air with each breath. A common practice to help get accustomed is attempting to exhale longer than you inhale. Try inhaling for about 3-4 seconds followed by exhaling for 6-8 seconds. Controlling your breath is the goal you are practicing here. Once you are able to control your breath, diaphragmic breathing becomes easier to do without much effort.

Don't Isolate Yourself

Although you may feel limitations around being in social settings or being able to do certain things. You want to avoid withdrawing completely from your normal activities because it can make your condition worse. Your withdrawal may prevent you from testing your typical limits as you work towards progress, which can slow your progress down. Continue to go out as needed and just remain mindful of your condition. Continue to live your life and communicate with those you spend your time with so that they are aware.

Avoid Sprays

Spraying chemicals into the air such as deodorant, air fresheners, or some form of cologne or perfume may become more hazardous to your condition. "You don't need to add to your respiratory problems by inhaling unknown substances" according to the American Lung Association.

Magnesium

This mineral is responsible for maintaining normal muscle functioning and contractions. It is recommended to consume 300-500 milligrams a day, divided into three doses or an equal amount three times a day. Dr. Lombardi, M.D., pulmonary specialist in Belmont, California states that, "It (magnesium) cam strengthen the skeletal muscles involved in breathing and relax the bronchi, the tubes leading to the lungs".

Common sources of magnesium: avocado, chickpeas, tamarind, basil, dill, ginger, oregano, thyme, any "CBD (cannabidiol) products are helpful.

*Magnesium Sources: avocado, chickpeas, tamarind, basil, dill, ginger, oregano, thyme, any *CBD (cannabidiol) products, nettle leaf, horsetail, red clover, sage, and nopal.*

*CBD oils are almost pure magnesium. To test the purity of CBD oil, send to a lab for testing such as Eurofins Laboratory in Pennsylvania and Texas. To know if it is helpful, you should feel a steady decline in needing to rely upon this substance after this need has been met more often.

Carotenes

Carotenes are what are known as phytonutrients ("plant chemicals") that provide anti-oxidant benefits that protect the lungs from damage. Great sources of carotenes come in the form of dark, leafy green vegetables, and highly colored foods such as red, orange, and yellow peppers, and various kinds of squash.

Homemade Cough Syrup

To avoid the many chemicals which can trigger additional reactions within the respiratory system, making your own cough syrup will help soothe the areas that are triggered and can help decrease symptoms as well.

Recipe:

1 cup of elderberries

2 tablespoons of ginger root powder

3.5 cups of distilled water

¾ cup of agave (for taste)

Add elderberries and ginger root powder to boiling water. Let simmer for about an hour, until about half of the water has evaporated. Then let sit and cool for about 15-minutes. Store in a mason jar or container and mix in agave. Have 1-2 tablespoons daily.

Mullein, Red Clover, and Ley Lime Tea

For this recipe, take 2 teaspoons of mullein leaf (or mullein flowers), 2 teaspoons of red clover, and 1 key lime to juice. Add mixture to boiling water and let steep for about 15-minutes or until cooled off. Drink 1-2 times a day to provide relief and help keep the respiratory system clean.

My Personal Remedy:

(in additional to more strict plant-based dietary restrictions)

No condition typically has a "take this remedy". However, there have been many symptoms drastically reduced for those with COPD when consuming the following recipe.

2 teaspoons of mullein

2 teaspoons of burdock root

1 teaspoon of nettle

1 teaspoon of tila

1-2 pieces of star anise

Boil 4 cups of water and add herbs. Simmer on low for about 15-20 minutes. Strain herbs and let cool off. Drink 2-3 times a day.

Endometriosis

Endometriosis is a condition where the cells of the uterine lining (endometrium) begin to grow in other parts of the pelvic area, such as the cervix, ovaries, bowel, or bladder. These cells group together and respond to hormones by bleeding every period, becoming inflamed, and eventually scar the tissues in this area of the body. This leads to frequent pain and severe cramps which can impact fertility. Medical doctors often prescribe powerful pharmaceutical drugs that stop menstruation which disrupt your entire system, particularly the reproductive system and its organs. Following these methods do not allow the body to flow as it is intended to. Issues will slowly pile up and reversing the condition will not seem to be possible.

What needs to be understood is that endometriosis is simply an allergy-stressed immune system response to what is going on with the hormones in the body. In other words, the hormones are being disrupted which creates an additional workload for the immune system which comes unannounced similar to how an allergy can trigger sneezing or coughing. As each period/cycle comes, this continues to further disrupt the hormones and only adds to the issue that is present and often leads to many other issues that remain undiagnosed. Like many other conditions, the restrains that are getting in the way of the immune system functioning properly is the approach to revering/removing this condition from the body.

Remedies:

What You Eat

This entire section could be dedicated to diet as the lifestyle change is the "fix/cure". But start with addressing this will be the main remedy to remain mindful of during each and every step of working on reversing this condition. This does not involve a "take this" remedy.

Removing foods detrimental to your health, and involve hormonal imbalances are necessary. Removing meats, all forms of dairy, soft drinks, sodas, coffee, alcohol, and highly processed items such as ketchup or salad dressings.

Cut Out Refined Carbs

"Sugar and white flour weaken the immune system and rob the body of energy" says Dr. Metzger, M.D., Ph.D., medical director of Helena Women's Health in San Francisco, California, and Palo Alto, California. When excess sugars and white flour are consumed, this creates an enormous workload on the digestive system and due to their toxicity, the immune system t-cells respond by treating this as a foreign invader. The body can do without the additional immune response which can be better served focusing on other areas of the body and avoid accumulating waste within the body.

Essential Minerals

Those with endometriosis have higher needs due to constantly repair and strengthen the immune system. When we consume the minerals that are most present in the body, we become more fulfilled and the white blood cells and other components of the immune system can increase in their intensity. This will help prevent the body from getting sick and begin to decrease the intensity and frequency of some of the major symptoms of endometriosis. Our immune system is comprised of mineral produced from our bones. Focusing on these minerals is essential.

Most Common Minerals In the Bones: (in alphabetic order)

Boron, Calcium, Chromium, Iron, Magnesium, Manganese, Potassium, Phosphorus, Selenium, Silicon, Sulfur, Zinc.

Getting these minerals from natural sources will be best. There are apps such as Chronometer which can help you keep track of these levels on a daily basis.

Common sources of Boron: raisins, peaches, prune juice, grape juice, avocadoes, legumes, dried apricots.

Common sources of Calcium: sea moss, kale, okra, dandelion greens, turnip greens, lettuce, papaya, and oranges.

Common Sources of Chromium: green beans, orange juice, grape juice, tomato juice, apples, Brazil nuts, dried fruits, broccoli

Common sources of Iron: Quinoa, Wild Rice (not black rice), Chickpeas/Garbanzo Beans, Kale, Nuts (particularly Walnuts), Hemp Seeds, Dates, Dried Apricots, Watercress, Sarsaparilla, Burdock (and root), Guaco, Chainey Root, Monkey Ladder, Chickweed, Yellowdock.

Common Sources of Magnesium: Avocado, Chickpeas, Tamarind, Basil, Dill, Ginger, Oregano, Thyme, Nettle Leaf, Horsetail (herb), Red Clover, Sage, Nopal, and almost any CBD (cannabidiol) products are helpful. CBD Oils are almost pure magnesium.

To test the purity of a CBD Oil, send to a lab for testing or you should feel a steady decline in needing to rely on this substance after your need has been met regularly.

Common sources of manganese: quinoa, fonio, spelt, walnuts, sunflower seeds, sesame seeds, and hemp seeds.

Common sources of potassium: squash, zucchini, bananas, avocado, dried apricots, and herbs such as, guaco (also high in iron), conconsa (has the highest concentration of potassium phosphate), lily of the valley (rich in iron fluorine and Potassium phosphate).

Common sources of phosphorus: sunflower seeds, pumpkin seeds, Brazil nuts, quinoa, walnuts, pecans, hazelnuts, chickpeas, lentils, amaranth, adzuki (red) beans.

Common sources of Selenium: brazil nuts, walnuts, chickpeas/garbanzo beans, kola nuts, dandelion greens, and nettle, and alfalfa. Recommended to consume about 400 micrograms a day.

Common sources of silicon: horsetail, bananas, almonds, Kenyen beans, red lentils, spinach, dried fruits.

Common Sources of Sulfur: leafy green vegetables, (dried) peaches, onions, watercress, chickpeas, walnuts,

Common Sources of Zinc: chickpeas, mushrooms, zucchini, squash, okra, Brazil nuts, and walnuts.

Fatty Acids

Dr. Metzger states that, "The omega-3 and omega-6 fatty acids, found primarily in raw nuts, seeds, and oils, help create hormone-like chemicals in the body called series-1 prostaglandins, which relax muscles and blood vessels, thus reducing menstrual cramps".

Omega-3 and Omega-6 natural sources: Brazil Nuts, Walnuts, Kola Nuts, Avocados, Bananas, Sea Vegetables (Nori, Wakame, Hijiki, Sea Moss, Bladderwrack), Coconut, Coconut Oil (do not cook), Olive Oil (do not cook), Grapeseed Oil, Avocado Oil, Walnut Oil, Mushrooms, Quinoa, and Wild Rice.

Grapeseed Extract

This extract is very potent and can help kill candida overgrowth, which is a yeastlike parasitic fungus that triggers many symptoms of endometriosis such as fatigue, headaches, joint pain, stomach pain, constipation, and directly impacts the reproductive organs. Make sure to follow instructions on label when consuming.

Eyesight

Eye issues can vary but all impact vision in some way. Some difficulties such as glaucoma can present a blurred/cloudy vision, while other issues can present sensitivity to light, or more common issues such as being dry or excessive tearing, among others. All of these issues will impact vision in some form as we use our eyes to see.

What must be examined is that healing eye issues, is a form of therapy. There are specific parts of the body to help cleanse over time in order to properly address what is impacting the eyes. Cleaning the colon is a practice to incorporate with any condition, but when addressing the eyes, emphasis must be placed on the pancreas.

The role of the pancreas is to absorb and send "enzymes" into the intestines for the proper ingestion of foods. The pancreas manufactures insulin which it secrets into the blood stream. Insulin is essential for the proper utilization of sugar in the body.

The pancreas is a sensitive organ, easily damaged by the acidity of modern life. It is known for producing hormones, like insulin, also critical for optimizing digestion and creating alkaline conditions in the gut. The pancreas can actually 'taste' sugar, but the response is not always so sweet.

The sponge-like pancreas is 6 inches long, and sits behind your stomach, in front of the kidneys. Alkalizing juices flow from the pancreas into the intestine, neutralizing stomach acids (to protect gut lining), and creating optimal conditions for digestion.

The pancreas also manages blood sugar levels. Certain foods (sweet or starchy) trigger insulin release, making cells absorb nutrients and store leftover energy (as fat). The pancreas also produces the 'opposite' hormone, glucagon, to release fat for energy, when no food is available. Refined sugar, and artificial sweeteners, stress and inflame the pancreas. Super-concentrated refined sugars create 'panic' because the pancreas must prevent blood sugar from getting too high. Large portions of food, eating late at night and processed food all create pancreatic stress and inflammation.

When the pancreas becomes inflamed it enters a vicious cycle of acidity, mucous and impaired digestion. The pancreas shares ducts (tubes just 1mm wide) with the gallbladder, and if they become inflamed, and blocked, the fluids stagnate. Reduced bile flow (from the gallbladder) also impairs liver detox and leads to gallstones.

Feeling stressed reduces digestion, even more, impacting nutrient absorption. We need to feel calm to stimulate the (parasympathetic) nervous system to initiate digestion. When fine ducts, capillaries, or tubules are inflamed they get blocked, and delicate cell membranes produce mucus to fend off an acid attack. This begins a cycle of impaired eyesight.

Remedies:

Portion Sizes

You will want to cut down portion sizes of your meals until you are at least plant-based at minimum. Reducing your portion sizes will help the body (particularly the pancreas) have less work to do when working to absorb and organize essential minerals and nutrients. This helps promote the elimination of waste that may be present in the body.

Hydration

There are many fluids involved in our eyes functioning properly. Keeping the body properly hydrated is necessary in order for the eyes to also be hydrated adequately enough to not promote any hindrances. Best foods for hydration are foods with high water content such as cucumbers, melons, coconut, berries, oranges, peppers, lettuce, and tomatoes. Fruit smoothies and green juices daily are highly recommended as well. Distilled spring water is primary form of drink as well to remain adequately hydrated.

Tamarind

Tamarind naturally produces anti-inflammatory chemicals (TNF alpha and polysaccharides) that work to protect the pancreas from inflammation. The seeds from the Tamarind fruit help boost the production of new cells in the pancreas also. Helping to heal the pancreas and protect it will serve to help begin working to improve eyesight and delay/avoid any further damage.

How to make Tamarind Juice ("agua de tamarindo ")

(from 21 Day Liquid Fast, by Bryan McAskill)

15 dried tamarind pods

2 quarts water, divided

1/2 – 3/4 cup date sugar

Step 1: bring half the water to a boil in a large pot over high heat.

Step 2: While you are waiting for the water to boil, prepare the tamarind pods. Remove the brittle outer shell and pull off as many strings as you can. Discard the shell and strings.

Step 3: After the water comes to a rolling boil, remove it from the heat and place the inner portion of the tamarind and the sugar in the water. Let the tamarind soak for about 1 hour and 30 minutes.

Step 4: At this point, the water will have cooled down. Use your fingers to squeeze out the hard tamarind seeds and remove the remaining strings; discard them.

Step 5: Place the liquid and remaining pulp in a blender and process until the pulp is fully blended into the water.

Step 6: Run the liquid through a strainer

Step 7: Pour your delicious agua de tamarindo into a pitcher, add the rest of the water, and refrigerate until cold.

Diuretic Teas

A "diuretic" is when you consume something that helps increase the passing or urine. Through the urine, we can help expel many items we do not need in our bodies, as well as stimulate regular activity from the pancreas. Many items can fall into this category but the simplest way that put the least amount of work on the digestion system are using natural herbs in the form of tea. Below is a brief list of common herbs to incorporate (not all together) into your daily lifestyle with the intention of cleansing the pancreas and providing additional protection.

Chaparral (helps also cleanse the lymphatic system)

Nettle (reduces inflammation)

Nopal (blood sugar control)

Cuachalalate (relieves stomach issues and helps break down harmful bacteria)

Sarsaparilla (very high iron content to help provide steady blood flow to organs)

Dandelion Root (high in iron and helps pancreas digest and process fats).

Burdock Root (helps purify the blood, and increase urine flow)

Purslane (inhibits pancreatic lipase – reduces work by pancreas of processing fats and sugars)

Yellowdock (reduces inflammation and can serve as a laxative)

Sea Moss (provide many essential minerals and help expel excess mucus from the body)

**Note: By addressing the root issues of disease (acidity and mucus) you can restore optimal function to the entire body. Reducing inflammation increases nutrient absorption, allowing organs to repair cellular damage.

Pancreatic-Support Smoothie

This smoothie is full of minerals and anti-inflammatory ingredients, to provide you with pancreatic support.

Ingredients:

2 cups Stomach Relief Herbal Tea (Cuachalalate herb)

1 tablespoon tamarind pulp

1 seeded cucumber

1 fistful of watercress or wild arugula

Juice of one key lime

Instructions:

-   Boil two cups distilled water and add 1 ½ tablespoons of Cuachalalate herb.
-   Simmer for about 15 minutes. Strain and allow to cool.
-   Blend the tea with the rest of the ingredients in a high-speed blender.

You have to be able to go to the restroom when working on cleansing the pancreas. We have to set our intention on cleaning the pancreas, and by default, cleaning the intestines. If the state of the intestines and pancreas are acidic, the eyes will suffer. Problems with the eyes are directly related to the pancreas which is why diabetics have eye problems.

Exercise

Exercise that is somewhat rigorous that induce sweat. Regular exercise promotes deeper breathing. Deep breathing is simultaneously responsible for more oxygen getting into the cells and activating the lymphatic system, which causes the cells to cleanse themselves. So, as we sweat, unnecessary oils are expelled from the body as well as toxins.

There have been reports that regular exercise can reduce the risk of age-related macular degeneration (AMD) by up to 70%. AMD is a degenerative eye disease in which the light-sensitive cells in the back of the eye, an area called the macula, stop working. It is the leading cause of severe vision loss in people over age 60.

This disease is divided into two types: "wet" AMD and "dry" AMD.

In dry AMD, patients get deposits in the macula called drusen. Dry AMD is the more common of the two types of AMD; it can lead to wet AMD.

In wet AMD, there is a growth of abnormal blood vessels underneath the macula; the blood vessels leak into the retina.

Give Up Smoking

Smoking cigarettes has long been known to cause heart disease and lung cancer; however, many people don't realize that smoking can also lead to vision loss. Smoking increases the risk of age-related macular degeneration, glaucoma, diabetic retinopathy, and dry eye syndrome. Work to stay away from thoughts of "quitting" smoking and more towards "giving up" smoking. Quitting is easy and often a one-step process. This is not the case when working away from smoking cigarettes regularly. Adopt the mindset of giving up smoking as you take steps towards decreasing this habit.

"20/20/20" Rule For Screentime

The 20/20/20 Rule applies to taking breaks while you are viewing a screen. For every 20 minutes you are looking at a screen, take a 20 second break, while looking at something (approx.) 20 feet away. What this does is reduce the eyes from straining and helping to avoid fatigue.

Colloidal Silver

In his bestselling book, *The pH Miracle: Balance Your Diet, Reclaim Your Health*, by Dr. Robert O. Young, Ph.D., he states ,"Eye or ear problems, including cataracts, glaucoma, redness, blurred vision, poor eyesight, ringing in the ears, earaches, soreness or swelling of the ears, eardrum damage, hardness of hearing, and (in rare cases) loss of hearing: Use 1 drop of colloidal silver topically (directly in the eye or ear) 3 times a day."

Eyebright (herb)

Eyebright, also known as "Euphrasia" is an herb that can be consumed in tea form or used to wash the eyes. Helps to reduce inflammation in the eye caused by blepharitis and conjunctivitis.

Eyesight Smoothie

(this smoothie is used to adequately hydrate the body while breaking down inflammation and including healthy fats to reduce work on the pancreas of breaking down these substances)

Ingredients:

1 1/2 cups mango

1 ripe burro banana

1 tablespoon coconut oil

1 cup approved greens (amaranth, wild arugula, etc.)

1 cup homemade walnut milk

Instructions:

1. Blend all the ingredients together in a high-speed blender.
2. If the mix is too thick, add a splash of spring water until the desired consistency is reached.
3. Enjoy.

Fennel

This herb made as a tincture can be used as a daily eye drop to help moisturize your eyes and keeping them hydrated. You can purchase fennel eye drops online and at many local herbal stores.

Manuka Honey

Manuka honey is produced by bees that pollinate the flowers found on a manuka bush, a kind of tea tree. The form of honey originates from parts of Australia, New Zealand, and Honduras. Traditionally used to heal wounds, sore throats, and to prevent tooth decay. However, this honey has become more commonly known to treat acne, prevent ulcers, and treat eye deficits.

This form of honey is much different from traditional honey as it comes from a different source and provides additional benefits. Manuka honey is an antioxidant, and antibacterial substance. It contains a compound (omega-3 fatty acid) known as, dihydroxyacetone (DHA) which are found in the manuka flowers. DHA increases mitochondrial activity while reducing inflammation in the eyes, helping promote overall eye health. This compound studied by registered dietitian, Bailey Flora, RD, notes the amount of DHA present in manuka honey. Flora states, "it's about 100 times higher than other traditional honey."

There are many ways to use manuka honey for the eyes. Boiling the comb itself in distilled water, using as an eye wash, or as eye drops. Follow directions on label, but typically it is available in eye drop form in which you can place 3-4 drops directly into each eye daily. You should see noticeable changes within or after 4-5 weeks.

Note: like any other honey, manuka honey does contain a high amount of sugar made from fructose and glucose. So, you will want to remain mindful of this if you have diabetes, liver disease, heart disease, or want to avoid consuming excess calories.

Eyestrain

We use our eyes for the majority of the day besides when we are asleep. When dealing with this condition, you may notice having difficulty reading, trouble seeing things further away, or blurred vision. When forced to be used excessively, the eyes can become more strained. We want to not contribute to our eyes being strained, as well as not needing to strain our eyes in order to see.

Remedies:

Reduce Screen Time

When we are looking at a screen for several hours a day, this can worsen this condition. Our eyes are not designed to look directly at a screen and focus our eyes in various directions in front of an illuminated background. Technology has become a larger part of our lives, so our intention behind avoiding screen time whenever possible also must be given higher priority in our daily lives than in the past. You can track your time on apps of how much you use each app in your phone if you find yourself spending longer periods of time on your phone, tablet, watching television, or computer than usual. If you have a block of time, you can set a timer to track how long you've been looking at a screen as well.

Rest Your Eyes

Just reducing your screen time unfortunately won't be enough. We need to balance out our time by resting our eyes for a few hours a day. We don't necessarily need to take a nap or go to sleep to rest our eyes as well can simply limit our activity by spending time in solitude and relaxation. We should spend a few moments each day closing our eyes while limiting how much they have to focus on things when our eyes are open.

Lighting

You want to make sure you can adequately see, but it is important to remain mindful of the quality of lighting where you are. Having low (or very bright) lighting can cause you to strain your eyes more. Sometimes the solution is just a new lightbulb but other times you want to make sure that you have adequate lighting for what you are trying to do. If you are reading, you want to be able to clearly see the pages you are viewing, but if you are trying to relax by drinking tea or spend time in solitude, low lighting may be best to help you relax. You should also darken your screens to reduce the brightness that can irritate the eyes.

Interrupt Yourself

If you have a job or career or work a lot while being in front of a screen, it is recommended to interrupt how long you work straight through and take more frequent breaks. You do not always have to take a complete break, as you can do something else, but want to shift your focus away from your screen temporarily as often as possible while still remaining productive.

Eyebright (herb)

This tea can be consumed several times a day but taken as needed. There are more present variables in place outside of just drinking this herb. For eyestrain, you can make some tea with this herb, let cool, and soak a small towel in the tea. Lightly squeeze and rinse off the towel, close your eyes, and place the towel on your closed eyelids for about 10-15 minutes. This can help reduce many symptoms of eyestrain, especially any lingering pains. Do not worry if some of this tea gets into your eyes; just make sure it is not too warm before placing onto your closed eyelids. Take about 1 tablespoon of herb and add to a small pot of water to boil. Once water begins boiling, you can pour into cup and then strain out herb completely before placing onto towel.

Blue Light Blocking Glasses

These are eyeglasses that help block out the blue light that comes from screens. We often look at things like our phones and televisions as second nature. This time adds up over time. We can be intentional with our screentime by wearing these glasses to help avoid straining our eyes.

Fennel

This herb made as a tincture can be used as a daily eye drop to help moisturize your eyes and keeping them hydrated. You can purchase fennel eye drops online and at many local herbal stores.

Fatigue

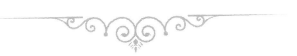

This condition is NOT a disease, although symptoms of this condition often remain present in many lives. Symptoms such as headaches, pains, tiredness, and irritability are the most common we associate with this condition. Fatigue is not considered a disease because it does not show up in any diagnostic test however, the signs and symptoms that are clear to see are areas to be addressed collectively together. As there are numerous symptoms of fatigue, addressing each one individually would take an extended period of time to properly address; time that you or someone else may not have in this lifetime. We must address that which is directly contributing to reducing our energy levels and overloading our bodies, while also placing our awareness onto what we can add to our lifestyles to help promote healthy ways of processing, absorbing, and expressing our energy.

Energy is often a vague term when we are referring to our bodies. When discussing "energy" within the body, it refers to what is stored in each cell in order to do the work (fulfill role) required to promote the body's (each system) capacity of functioning properly.

Most people remain under-fueled by an unhealthy diet and overload the body with poor habits to the point where the body can no longer manage to work to complete the regular tasks and responsibilities in life. Energy is inscribed into every one of our cells. We need these inscriptions to serve as directions to fulfill our needs which allows this energy to flow throughout our bodies in which fatigue is no longer present.

Recommendations in this section are geared towards addressing ways to decrease commonalities of all symptoms associated with fatigue. If certain symptoms are more present, visit other sections of this book that address them or do additional research around those areas to effectively address your primary challenges. Fatigue can signal a need to manage your lifestyle better or can be a sickness coming on. You want to address it early on to avoid the beginning stages of disease.

Remedies:

Stop Smoking (cigarettes)

Smoking cigarettes reduces the amount of available oxygen in the body. This will force the body to slow down and feel tired (fatigued). Nicotine in cigarettes is a stimulant and the temporary withdrawals create additional tiredness.

Cut Out Caffeine

Caffeine makes you feel like you have energy that is not really there. You're basically running on an empty tank until you "crash". Part of crashing is caffeine withdrawal combined with the fact that caffeine interrupts oxygen delivery to the brain. You want to stay away from anything that contains caffeine such as coffee, sodas, and artificial energy drinks.

L-Carnitine

This amino acid is most often prescribed in a pharmaceutical capsule and promoted by medical doctors as something to take to "feel young". However, given that this is a book on natural remedies, and the fact that amino acids come from plants, getting L-Carnitine can come from numerous sources. What we know about what we call "L-Carnitine" is that it is responsible for transporting nutritional fuel into the mitochondria which stores energy into each of our cells. Without this essential amino acid, the body won't have enough energy stored in order to produce or fulfill many of our daily tasks. If our cells are having difficulty storing and producing enough energy, then the rest of our body will follow along, leading to a condition such as fatigue.

Dr. Mukta Agrawal, dietician and technical director at Inlife Healthcare in India, specializes in diabetes and cardiac care, has stated that "Approximately 54% to 86% of dietary L-carnitine is absorbed in the small intestine and then enters the bloodstream. Even L-carnitine lack diets have little effect on the body's total carnitine content as the kidneys conserve carnitine very efficiently." Typically, those who follow a plant-based lifestyle would not consume L-Carnitine in abundance and closer towards remaining deficient than others. However, this specific amino acid is conserved well when consumed and the body can do without more often than not, especially when other essential minerals and nutritional needs are being met regularly. Not much is needed, but when consumed, remain mindful of when the body will appreciate and be able to use L-Carnitine as needed to help restore the energy levels in the cells and eventually the body as a whole.

Common Sources of L-Carnitine Can Be Found In: Avocado, brazil nuts, garbanzo beans, oranges, orange juice, apples, pears, peaches, tomato, and grapes.

Magnesium

Magnesium is responsible for regulating the nerves in the body (among other responsibilities). Whenever you are low on magnesium, the response your body will give will mimic many of the symptoms attributed to fatigue. Too little magnesium in the body does not allow the system to charge the muscles and nerves for optimum performance. Magnesium also helps stimulate digestion within the body, so the cells know what to absorb and what to not absorb. Reducing this workload on the body will tremendously help reduce many of the symptoms associated with fatigue.

Common Sources Of Magnesium: Avocado, Chickpeas, Tamarind, Basil, Dill, Ginger, Oregano, Thyme, Nettle Leaf, Horsetail (herb), Red Clover, Sage, Nopal, and almost any CBD (cannabidiol) products are helpful. CBD Oils are almost pure magnesium.

*To test the purity of a CBD Oil, send to a lab for testing or you should feel a steady decline in needing to rely on this substance after your need has been met regularly.

Glutamate

This amino acid helps to stabilize blood sugar and protects the brain. If you are experiencing fatigue in the form of mental fatigue, this is an area you want to gear your focus. When we have sharp decreases in blood sugar, our brain can be hindered and result in more frequent headaches and tiredness.

Common Sources of Glutamate: Papaya, Kale, Garbanzo Beans, Bananas, Onions, Tomatoes, and Mushrooms.

Omega-3 Fatty Acids

Fatty acids help protect the brain from deteriorating and stores fat that it uses for energy. Loading up on omega-3 fatty acids will help to alleviate any mental fatigue that may be present when dealing with fatigue.

Common Sources of Omega-3: Walnuts, Brazil Nuts, Avocados, Hemp Seeds, Hemp Milk, Walnut Oil, Olive Oil, and Sea Vegetable such as Nori, Hijiki, Bladderwrack, Kelp, and Dulse.

Hydration

One of the main reasons people feel fatigued is that they do not drink enough water. The word "feel" is underlined in the previous sentence because many of feel fatigued but are not actually fatigued. They associate the feeling to the actual condition. Making sure you are adequately hydrated can determine if you are actually fatigued or just feeling like you are. Drinking enough water and consuming foods high in water will help you remain hydrated.

Berries, melons, leafy green vegetables, coconut, coconut water, cucumbers, tomatoes, and oranges are some of the most common hydrating foods to consume more often than not.

Digestion

We want to reduce how much our digestive system has to work in order to avoid feeling many symptoms connected to fatigue. We must eliminate any item that takes a long time to digest. Meats, dairy, and processed foods, especially those with a high sugar content, take the longest to digest (one or more hours) as compared to fruits, vegetables, nuts, beans, and grains which take almost half the time.

Stimulating Colors

What we view has a considerable impact on our energy and overall well-being. From what we wear as clothes to colors that surround us. Although darker colors can be more soothing for many, we want to do away with them temporarily while adding more medium tones and brighter tones to add variety. Begin by cleaning up any clutter in your home, at your work desk, or anywhere else you spend most of your time. work to eliminate some of the whites, blacks, and darker blues as these colors can appear redundant throughout the day and also drain your energy. You can easily replace items such as picture frames, notebooks, and other accessories, with more "warmer" colors such as red, orange, yellow.

Incorporating colors such as lighter blues and green can also stimulate higher energy levels. You don't have to do a complete overhaul of everything and can mostly focus on removing clutter and adding things that promote energy. A plant with bright flowers, or even a picture of a sunset can be enough to begin charging your energy. Note: if you identify as being more of an "extrovert" you may want to choose more soft blues and greens as colors as yellow, red, and orange may make you become overstimulated and add to your symptoms of fatigue later on.

Scents

If you're able to, keep a bowl of oranges or a few key limes nearby. The aroma of these in close proximity can stimulate "wakefulness" just by inhaling their aroma. An orange as a snack and key lime water will also help reduce many feelings of fatigue as well. A small herb plant such as rosemary or thyme can help throughout the day by picking off a small amount and smelling it.

Sleep

If you are feeling fatigued, you want to be able to make time to rest in both, quality, and quantity. You want to avoid oversleeping or making attempts to "catch up" on sleep, but you do want to rest as much as you can for a short-term time period to help accurately assess the severity of your symptoms. If you never take a moment to rest, your symptoms will linger. Use sleep as a temporary reset as you begin making necessary adjustments to address your condition. Our bodies adjust to routines so making sure to go to bed around the same time will be important. Creating a bedtime routine that includes, avoiding screentime, some form of breathing exercise, and any activity that helps you to calm and power down.

Exercise

Pamela Smith, R.D., nutritionist in Orlando, Florida, USA, states that, "A brisk 10-minute walk can energize you for 2 hours". Walking can be done almost anywhere and can incorporated into your daily schedule. Adding onto walking more, developing an exercise routine is a healthy way of relieving stress, reducing headaches, and plan ahead when you will use your energy. Slowly building up to an exercise routine is important also as exercising can contribute to your feeling more tired. Start stretching and practice warming up as a foundation and then add on more specific exercises and tailor it to your goals that you develop over time. After building up to developing a regular routine and/or exercise schedule, you will begin feeling more energized due to exercising more often.

Resolve Problems

Whether it's a family disagreement or problem at work, it will benefit you to put your efforts towards resolving them. Additional energy spent on worrying or remaining frustrated will only add to you feeling fatigued. It is best to address whatever the issue is at minimum to have a common understanding to help dissolve the issue. If a problem can be resolved completely, great! If not, then at least working towards dissolving any issues can help you begin to feel more relieved than you were previously.

Learn To Say No

Many tend to want to be helpful and contribute as much as they can, but this can create additional responsibilities and increase how often you experience symptoms of fatigue. Commit to your primary obligations and learn to say "no" to additional things at least temporarily.

Fever

A "fever" by definition is essentially anything that keeps your body consistently above its normal temperature of 98.6°F. Typical temperatures can remain around 100°F and can go up to 103°F before hospitalization may occur. Experiencing a fever is more of a warning sign that something is not functioning well within the body that requires attention. Although you may know what the issue is, sometimes the body clears up the issue itself while you are experiencing a fever. The mechanics of how a fever occurs is rather simple. The brain tells the body to move blood from the surface of your skin to the interior parts of your body to serve as a support and filter out any toxins the body wants to remove. As the blood moves away from the skin, the body loses less heat and causes your temperature to rise. The skin occasionally feeling colder is just the blood moving away from the surface and presents as "cold chills" when experiencing a fever.

Remedies:

Don't Create More Work For The Body

We're all aware of various soups and personal remedies that can be helpful, but you want to work on not complicating your condition if you have a fever. It is important to keep in mind that a fever is not the illness itself but is a symptom of some form of illness. You may not know what illness is present or what's needed so it is best to simplify and not fight against the fever by doing anything you can think of. Do not overburden your body at this time and make that your mindset as you follow many of the other steps listed in this section.

Hydration/Liquids

When the body begins to remain hot, it perspires (sweats) more to cool down. As this happens, there is less water in the body that will need to be replaced. As a response the body eventually turns off the sweat ducts to avoid becoming dehydrated, but this can make your condition linger on. You want to drink water and consume foods high in water content (fresh fruits and vegetables). Eating can be a challenge at this time, so it is recommended to consume these items in the form of a juice or smoothie. These are easy to make as your energy will be low.

Herbal Tea

Not only will drinking herbal tea to your hydration, but the herbs come with additional benefits to provide relief when working through a fever. There are many herbs that you can use such as mullein, thyme, linden flower, elderberry, dandelion, and many more. Search for the benefits of any herb you intend to use and keep things simple. Use about 1 teaspoon for each cup of water. Strain out your herbs after allowing them to steep and cool off and then enjoy.

Ice Cubes

If you feel too nauseated to drink liquids, you can always make ice cubes to suck on. This will help with avoiding feelings of dehydration and keep your awareness sharp during this time. I recommend making a fruit juice or smoothie and pouring mixture into an ice cube tray so that you're able to consume many essential minerals.

Wet Compress

We may feel temporary relieve using a cold compress, but ironically a warm compress can help the body recover more during a fever, says Dr. Eleonore Blaurock-Busch, Ph.D., an associate lab director, at King James Medical Laboratory and Trace Minerals International, both locations in Cleveland, Ohio, USA. You want to wet a small towel in warm water, then wring out water to avoid dripping, and place directly onto your forehead. If your temperature rises, replace compress with a cooler one. If not, it can benefit you to also place a warm compress around your wrists and ankle as well.

Sponge Yourself

The skin sending off more heat than it normally does can irritate the skin and the sweat glands. Although you can use a sponge slowly to wash all over your body, it is necessary to focus on the areas that send off the most heat. Areas such as the armpits, the groin, and the head. You want to wring out water from your sponge and wipe each of these areas also to avoid any irritation or allow harmful bacteria to build up which can trigger a fever also.

Dress For The "Occasion"

Avoid wearing heavier clothing (no matter how comfortable you may feel) and remove additional layers that are not needed. This includes thick sweaters, slippers, robes, and anything else you can do without to allow the body to help you excess body heat evaporate into the air and not remain trapped within your clothes. If you have a chill add one extra layer at a time to avoiding wearing too many layers which can prolong your condition.

Steam Some Herbs

You can take some herbs such as eucalyptus, oregano, thyme, ginger, and add some lime and elderberry to a pot of boiling water to steam them. The aroma in the air is similar to aromatherapy, but with the added heat to help the steam reach deeper areas of the respiratory system and (potentially) help unclog any areas in need to help promote fuller breaths. You can even take this mixture and drink as a tea twice a day.

Feverfew (herb)

This herb contains natural compounds known as sesquiterpene lactones which have anti-inflammatory properties similar to aspirin's according to Dr. Alexander Mauskop, M.D., director of the New York Headache Center in New York City. You want to take 125 milligrams daily of this herb in capsule form. Ingredient will be on label but look to make sure the botanical name on the label says Tanacetum parthenium to make sure it's the actual herb and not a knock-off product.

Ginger (herb)

This herb is a "grounding" herb which help the body and mind relax. Put 1 teaspoon of fresh grated ginger into a 16–24-ounce thermos of hot water and sip throughout the day. Don't attempt to finish the drink in one sitting; work to make it last all day by just sipping.

Avoiding Monosodium glutamate (MSG) and Aspartame

MSG is a food additive that has scientifically been proven to trigger migraines. However, this additive dies not always show up as MSG or monosodium glutamate on ingredient labels. Other names that are used instead are, "hydrolyzed protein", "yeast nutrient", or "natural flavoring".

Aspartame (aspartic acid) another artificial sweetener has the same addictive quality as MSG and lead to migraines and headaches.

The following ingredients ALWAYS contain MSG:

Monosodium glutamate, Hydrolyzed protein, Sodium caseinate, Yeast extract, Yeast nutrient, Maltodextrins, Autolyzed yeast, Textured protein, Calcium caseinate, Yeast food, Hydrolyzed oat flour

The following ingredients OFTEN contain MSG:

Malt extract, Malt flavoring, Bouillon, Barley malt, Broth, Stock, Flavoring(s), Natural flavoring(s), Natural beef flavoring, Natural chicken flavoring, Natural pork flavoring, Food seasonings

Fiber and Water

Most headaches can be from feeling constipated or dehydration. Dr. David Simon, M.D., medical director of the Chopra Center for Well-Being in La Jolla, California states, "I've been surprised to see that a very high percentage of my patients with migraines are constipated and the improving their regulatory helps reduce their headaches."

You will want to consume properly hydrated (consuming half your bodyweight in ounces of water and increasing intake of fresh water-filled fruits and vegetables) while keeping up with your daily fiber intake (21-25g per day for women, and between 30-38g a day for men).

Common sources of Fiber: garbanzo beans, lentils, brussels sprouts, sweet potatoes, avocado, pears, sunflower seeds, flax seeds, hazelnuts, apples and berries (high pectin fruits) and onions.

Tyramine

The chemical "tyramine" is strongly linked to migraines and headaches according to Dr. Lawrence Robbins, M.D., director of the Robbins Headache Clinic in Northbrook, Illinois.

Common Sources of Tyramine (avoid during headache):

Smoked, cured, aged, and packaged meat

Herring, caviar, and smoked fish

Vinegar

Pickled and fermented foods

Aged cheeses

Products high in yeast (doughnuts, coffee cakes, and breads)

Chocolate

Artificial sugars (any sugar not from fruits)

Citrus fruits (when consumed in large amounts)

Figs

Sour cream and yogurt

Lima beans, navy beans, and peas

MSG

Caffeine

Alcoholic beverages (especially red wine)

Meditation

Slowing down the inner workings of the body will help alleviate the tension that often triggers and contributes to headaches. Simply close your eyes and gently inhale and exhale while remaining observant on your breath.

Simple Herbal Remedies For Reducing Fever:

Feverfew (herb) and Elderberry Tea – take about 1 teaspoon of each ingredient and boil together in a cup of water. Make sure to strain out herbs (which you can re-use once more) prior to consuming. You may drink this tea every few hours.

Yarrow (herb) Tea – take 1-2 teaspoons of this herb to use as tea. Place herb into cup and fill cup with boiling water. Let steep until almost completely cooled off. You may also drink this tea every few hours.

Note: start with one of either of the options listed above; not both. You may enjoy one more than the other or just have certain herbs more readily available. But try one before moving onto the other to avoid any sign of caution. It can be best to stick with one option throughout as every person may respond a bit differently or progress may be slower, but you'd want your body to know what to expect and build in a steady routine.

Fibroids

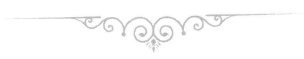

Fibroids are (non-cancerous) masses that grow from the wall of the uterus. They can vary in size, and you can have one or many. Sizes can vary from a small dot to the size of a grapefruit. These growths may not present any direct symptoms but can often be detected by issues such as heavy menstrual bleeding, bleeding between periods, abdomen pain, frequent urination, and sometimes, lower back pain.

About 25%-50% of all women develop fibroids and many end up getting hysterectomies (surgery to remove the uterus or womb). Many do not make any dietary or lifestyle changes and as their fibroids grow, the need for surgery becomes more present; although this does not have to be the case in many situations as you'll learn more about in this section.

It is recommended that if surgery is mentioned as an option in the near future, one should commit to waiting about three months while they stick to natural recommendations outlined in this section and revisiting the need for surgery.

Remedies:

Acupressure

As stated in several other sections in this text, Tradition Chinese Medicine (TCM) works to address the *chi*, or life force energy that's runs throughout the body by means of consuming natural foods, herbs, physical movement, and pressure points in the body to promote healing and remove any stagnation. There are specific acupressure points to help release flow in the blood and liver that may be contributing to the creation of fibroids as well as them remaining stagnant.

- CV4 – is essentially located in the "middle" of the body; between the pubic bone and navel cavity.

- LV3 – located on the upper part of the foot, between the bones of the big toe and second toe.

- LV14 – in the space between the ribs; located two ribs below from where the nipples are on the body.

- SP6 – about three finger-widths above the inside of the ankle just on the side of the shinbone.

- SP10 – just inside the knee, about 2 ½ inches above the kneecap in the fleshy part of the knee bulge.

To stimulate each of these points, start by sitting in a chair and move from point to point in circular motions with your thumb in a clockwise motion in and around the area for about one minute at a time. apply pressure towards the center of each point where it is slightly painful but not enough where you want to stop. It is recommended to work each point at least twice a day for at least three months. By the end of three months, along with ither recommendations listed in this section, your doctor should report fibroids shrinking in size. If many completely dissolved, or are confirmed to begin shrinking, continue these routines to help prevent future fibroid growth(s).

Eliminate Estrogen From Diet

Estrogen feeds fibroids this is why fibroids often vanish during menopause due to estrogen levels decrease. Foods that are high in the hormone estrogen include, red meats, poultry, soy products, dairy products, and also eggs which contain the synthetic form of estrogen that is routinely fed to animals that are grown for the market. It is also recommended to avoid alcohol, caffeine, cigarettes, and refined sugars as they interfere with healing this condition as they overwork the liver. I would also recommend avoiding anything white, which includes, white flour, white sugar, white (animal milk), and items such as potatoes, cauliflower, etc., as these items are more than not a hybrid which rob us of many essential minerals, but they lead to stagnation and trigger fibroid growth.

Fiber Intake

You may already consume enough fiber daily, so there may not be a need to necessarily increase your fiber intake. But, making sure you keep an eye on your fiber intake will be necessary part of working towards reducing this condition. Fiber helps assist the liver with excreting any excess estrogen in the body. It is recommended for women to aim towards 21-25 grams of fiber a day, while men aim between 30-38 grams of fiber a day.

Common sources of Fiber: garbanzo beans, lentils, brussels sprouts, sweet potatoes, avocado, pears, sunflower seeds, flax seeds, hazelnuts, apples and berries (high pectin fruits) and onions.

Magnesium

Increasing your magnesium intake will always benefit you as it is a vital mineral the body uses for just about everything, and you cannot consume too much. Specifically for fibroids, magnesium helps relax the muscle walls of the uterus that have remained stagnant and allows for a fresh flow of blood into the area. This not only helps to begin cleansing the area of waste materials but helps to reinvigorate the area to avoid remaining stagnant which promote repair where needed.

Common sources of magnesium: avocado, chickpeas, tamarind, basil, dill, ginger, oregano, thyme, red clover, nopal, sage, and any *CBD (cannabidiol) products are helpful.

*CBD oils are almost pure magnesium. To test the purity of CBD oil, send to a lab for testing such as Eurofins Laboratory in Pennsylvania and Texas. To know if it is helpful, you should feel a steady decline in needing to rely upon this substance after this need has been met more often.

Iron

You will want to load up on your iron-rich items during your healing/restoration period. Iron from plants (Iron-fluorine) is essential to the body, as opposed to iron-oxide which comes from heavier metals and does not assimilate in a manner with the body that can help promote healing within the blood. As you have a steady blood flow to this area (and the rest of the body), it is crucial to strengthening the quality of this flow so that the body does not have to work as hard to send blood to where it's most needed in the body. Many prescriptions and pharmaceuticals contain a higher amount of iron-oxide and can lead to several side effects and other conditions.

Common sources of Iron: Quinoa, Wild Rice (not black rice), Chickpeas/Garbanzo Beans, Kale, Nuts (particularly Walnuts), Hemp Seeds, Dates, Dried Apricots, Watercress

Common Herbs for Iron: Sarsaparilla, Burdock (and root), Guaco, Chainey Root, Monkey Ladder, Chickweed, Yellowdock.

Ditch The Dairy

As stated in other sections in this text, dairy from cow's milk adds excess mucus production in the body and exposes it to additional bacteria. Most dairy products are filled with additives that create addictions and are often hidden with how ingredients are listed and labeled. One of the main addictive ingredients is *casein*, which releases "casomorphins", which is a substance very similar (chemically) to opioids. These casomorphins can attach themselves to the same receptors in our brains as drugs such as heroin and other narcotics, resulting in a small hit of dopamine (the "feel good" chemical in our brains). What these items also do is make iron absorption more challenging in which nutrients do not get to their destinations in a reasonable time frame and triggers additional symptoms. Low energy then results in less physical activity. Remaining stagnant after consuming loads of bacteria feeds the growths associated with fibroids.

Try setting a goal to go 7-10 days or longer where you can avoid common items such as milk, chocolate, yogurt, and ice cream, while remaining mindful of items such as baked goods, snack foods and others that contain dairy components such as casein, caseinate, lactose, sodium caseinate, or whey. If you're not sure if something contains dairy, do your best to avoid it and do without.

Fibromyalgia

Those with fibromyalgia often experience fatigue, sore muscles, sleep difficulties, and racing thoughts on a daily basis. Although there are many contributing factors to these symptoms, the core of this condition is directly caused by a malfunctioning hypothalamus, which is a part of the brain that is responsible for regulating and controlling the hormones in the body and directly (or indirectly) interacts with almost every part of the body. From leaving the muscles fatigued and tens due to restricting supply of nutrients, to interrupting the typical role of the immune system, to sending neurotransmitters to the brain to promote digestion, the hypothalamus has a role in all of the contributing factors of fibromyalgia. This malfunctioning hypothalamus greatly increases the body's levels of a neuropeptide known as "substance P" which acts as a neurotransmitter and sends mixed signals throughout the body and increases sensitivity to pain. Substance P is comprised of amino acids which typically serve to repair parts of the body as needed, but since those with fibromyalgia have irregular sleep patterns, and sleep is the space where our bodies do the majority of their healing and repair, the body never gets a chance to properly repair, and the symptoms become deeper and require more attention in the form of more severe symptoms over time.

General protocol for this condition:

- Treat deficiencies of thyroid, adrenal, or testicular hormones
- Herbs and routines that promote and induce sleep
- Lower your blood pressure to reduce workload of hypothalamus
- More frequent parasitic cleansing herbs to reduce infections or bacteria buildup
- Load up on essential minerals to address additional deficiencies

Note: these steps are all in addition to removing hormones from diet in the form of meat, dairy, and soy, conducting a colon cleanse, working to purify the blood, removing all processed foods, and achieving adequate hydration on a daily basis.

Remedies:

Lemon Balm and Valerian (herbs)

Taking these herbs together at night can help promote a deeper sleep. Getting these in a tincture form may be best as liquids are absorbed better by our bodies and can be taken quicker than making tea. Follow the instructions on the label, but typically consume around 160-480mg of Valerian and 80-240mg of Lemon Balm together at night. Dosage will depend on your age, weight, and size which should be noted on the product labels. For tea, take about ½ tablespoon of each herb per 10-12oz of water. Placed dried herbs into a cup, boil water separately, then pour water onto herbs and let steep. Strain out herbs after letting cool off and enjoy.

Magnesium

The mineral relaxes the muscles to relax. This does not mean you will become weak, but when the muscles are not relaxed, they tend to spasm and require more blood to be sent to those areas which creates additional work for the body and contributes to symptoms. Most magnesium in foods is lost due to processing so it is important to take note of what you're consuming that has magnesium. It is generally recommended that 400mg of magnesium be consumed daily. This may sound like a lot but just about most people are deficient in magnesium and experience at least minor symptoms of those such as the ones connected to fibromyalgia.

*Common sources of magnesium: avocado, chickpeas, tamarind, basil, dill, ginger, oregano, thyme, red clover, nopal, sage, and any *CBD (cannabidiol) products are helpful.*

*CBD oils are almost pure magnesium. To test the purity of CBD oil, send to a lab for testing such as Eurofins Laboratory in Pennsylvania and Texas. To know if it is helpful, you should feel a steady decline in needing to rely upon this substance after this need has been met more often.

Note: You do want to avoid supplemental magnesium due to them promoting and causing diarrhea. You do not want to trade one problem for another one. If you experience some type of diarrhea, it is best to decrease your dosage/intake for a few days until you notice positive changes.

Deep Tissue Massages

Just about every city or town has a local place that provides massages and are licensed to conduct deep tissue massages. My recommendation is to invest in this service to help relax the body while working to promote tissue regeneration and repair and improve circulation in the body. If you do not feel you can financially afford this service and have ongoing documentation from your doctor stating you have fibromyalgia, it would be in your best interest to request a referral from your doctor and request any assistance they can provide.

Foam Roller

Getting a foam roller can be helpful but can at times be too severe on certain areas. Use a foam roller to identify your weaker or more sensitive areas and work on massaging these areas yourself. Press down with your fingertips (not to hard where they won't slide over your skin or clothing) and start making about 5-10 circular motions around your most sensitive areas. You can do this in almost any area of your body. If this creates more pain or soreness, you may be applying too much pressure or for too long and work on adjusting accordingly.

Minerals

You definitely want to accurately assess your current diet and remove anything that does not help you. Removing meat and dairy will take hours a day off of your digestive system, while removing processed foods will help not create additional deficiencies in the body. The body is made of minerals, so this is what you want to replenish. Items such as sea moss, bladderwrack, fresh fruits and vegetables, natural grains, and herbs you can incorporate are what you want your diet and lifestyle to consist of.

Fasting

Fasting is a foundational piece to any healthy lifestyle. Whether a particular fasting regimen is implemented, or a person ends up fasting by default after feeling regularly fulfilled with essential minerals from their diet and lifestyle. there are many fasting methods and routines to follow but something to become more familiar with is intermittent fasting where you schedule a specific time block (could be anywhere from 8hrs-12hrs or less) where you eat and only consuming liquids outside of those hours. I go over many fasting routine and regimens to follow in my book entitled, *Fasting: A Guide To Health And Wellness.*

Colon Cleanse

Clean the colon. You will NEED to do this regardless of your condition but specifically for fibromyalgia. Clean the colon using some or all of the following: Ginger, Cascara Sagrada, Rhubarb Root, Prodijiosa and Blessed Thistle. Drink as a tea daily. All herbs should come with instructions, and these are safe to mix together. Caution: these herbs can be very bitter. This is not a cause for concern and does not mean these herbs are spoiled or contaminated in any way.

For Adults:

(for children, cut dosages in half to 1/3 the amount listed)

Colon Cleanse Tea: 1 teaspoon of Cascara Sagrada, ½ teaspoons of Black Walnut, and 1 teaspoon of Rhubarb Root for about 10-12oz of tea. This tea is very bitter. But you want this tea to be bitter so that it can break down what is not needed in the body. If this tea is too difficult for you to adjust to, you can always search for these herbs or colon cleanses available in capsule form. You will want to try this tea prior to fasting to identify which option will be best for you during your liquid fast. Cleaning the Colon is vital for survival. The Colon is a part of the gut which is essentially our 2nd brain. It holds onto leftover waste and materials that create inflammation in the body and directly trigger many symptoms of disease. Without a clean colon, the body cannot function well as a whole.

Duration: 5-6 consecutive days at a time. Do for 5 days then take at least 2 days off.

Ingredients:

Cascara Sagrada (1 teaspoon)

Black Walnut hull (1/2 teaspoon)

Rhubarb Root (1 teaspoon)

Prodijiosa (1 teaspoon) – if applicable/available to you.

Water 8oz (boiling)

*You can do any combination of these herbs or take individually for this cleanse. You do not need every ingredient, but this cleanse works best when including all herbs mentioned above.

This cleanse is probably the most important to our health. The colon is essentially our second brain and is a part of the large intestine which works to remove waste from the body. The colon is responsible for holding a temporary storage of feces, but also reabsorbing water and minerals necessary to our health.

And Iron-Fluorine-Phosphate Not Iron-Oxide

Load up on the right type of iron (Iron Phosphate and Iron-Fluorine) which come from plants, not (Iron Oxide) which comes from metals which are in many medications and products advertised as containing Iron. Much of the muscle soreness and blood flow is attributed to low iron levels, so many doctors will prescribe "iron-pills", but these do not contain the iron that is needed. And much of the low iron in the body can be traced to poor diets that send blood flow to all areas of the body as it tries to remove toxins and digest unrecognizable materials. Just stopping the consumptions of items, the body does not recognize is often all that is needed to reduce this issue from continuing, however, the body will need to replace what has been lost, which can be achieved through consuming natural plants that are high in iron (phosphate).

Common Iron-Phosphate Herbs: Sarsaprilla, Flor de Manita, Burdock Root, Red Clover, Hombre Grande, Blue Vervain, Contribo, Guaco.

Common Iron-Phosphate Foods: Wild Rice, Dandelion Greens, Prickly Pear, Soursop.

Iodine (addressing the thyroid)

Common conditions that impact the Thyroid are Hypothyroidism (underactive thyroid – doesn't produce enough hormones) and Hyperthyroidism (overactive thyroid – produces too many hormones). The thyroid functions off of Iodine just like the bones thrive when having enough calcium. You will want to include many items such as Sea Moss and Elderberries as well as many sea plants such as Hijiki, Dulse, Nori, and Bladderwrack.

Note: If you have Hypothyroidism, you will want to incorporate more Bladderwrack into your diet. This plant is often found in products that contain Sea Moss but can be consumed in capsule or powder form. If you have Hyperthyroidism, you will want to consume as herb named, Bugleweed often in tea form.

Hypothyroid Smoothie:

- Large handful of watercress

- 2 apples

- 1 key lime (juiced)

Hyperthyroid Smoothie:

- 2-3 green apples

- 4-5 large dandelion leaves

- 1 handful of cilantros

- 1 key lime (juiced)

**Both of these smoothies are not a "cure" but a way to help deter many of the symptoms associated with each form of Thyroidism. They help the body begin to function well in preparation of additional dietary adjustments that can and should be implemented in a timely manner.

Drink This Tea (daily): Tamarind Juice, Ginger, and Key Lime (juice).

This tea can help cleanse out unnecessary waste materials while promoting a natural way of balancing hormones within the body.

How To Get Rid Of Fibroid Tumors? (If applicable)

Mucous membrane has been compromised (broken down) in the reproductive organ and it accumulates small fibroid tumors along the walls of the body there. Doctors try to cut it out, but there is no knife that can separate this fibroid from the walls of your uterus; the doctor is going to cut into you now. If the doctor doesn't cut all the way into you, they're going to have to leave some in there.

You need something that is consistent with removing things from the wall of the intestines, which is potassium phosphate, and iron. These enter the blood in which the blood travels everywhere in the body. This is how you get rid of fibroid tumors.

If you have a fibroid tumor, you will need one herb specifically to address this issue (in addition to the many recommendations listed in this section): Lily of the Valley. It has two active ingredients when most plants have only one. 1) Iron Fluorine 2) Potassium Phosphate. It will also assist with removing Uterine Fibroid tumors and cysts.

Yarrow is another, powerful herb for this issue if it applies to you. Yarrow and Lily of the Valley are helpful to those who don't have fibroid tumors as well.

Flatulence

Flatulence is a natural part of digestion caused by gas-producing bacteria within the digestive tract, when diet is healthy this gas-producing bacteria is almost non-existent. Many choose to take artificial supplements to help breakdown their gas, but this does not solve the issue and often leads to other complications. When this gas-producing bacteria is destroyed, other bacteria (like yeast) can take their place and generate additional toxins in the body. Better overall digestive functioning is both, the short-term and long-term goal of removing the issue of flatulence.

Remedies:

Remove Gas-Producing Items

Most people are very sensitive to artificial sugars and proteins; many just chose to accept flatulence as a side effect rather than viewing it as a warning sign. Work on eliminating the following items listed below until you can identify what you may be the most sensitive to. I recommend continuing to remove all of the items listed below even after you've identified your sensitivities.

Dairy – we cannot be tolerant of a substance made for another species, although many appear to have a higher tolerance than most. The additives in cow's milk such as sugars and even bacteria increase digestive difficulties and lead to flatulence.

Artificial Fruit Juices – these are fruit juices that are not created by simply juicing the fruit(s) themselves. These contain an excess of fructose sugar that does not metabolize easily and disrupts digestion.

Artificial Sweeteners – items such as Xylitol and sorbitol which are found in many baked goods and candy, can increase flatulence.

Wheat – the substance we refer to as "gluten" can trigger a digestive sensitivity and prolong digestive enzymes from being produced.

Beans, Cabbage, Brussel Sprouts, Cauliflower – these items also contain a carbohydrate named, raffinose, which is known for increasing gas production by interfering with bowel movements.

Ginger

This herb helps stimulate digestion while relaxing the muscles of the digestive tract, so food spends less time sitting in the intestines. You may take about 250mg with each meal or just work to incorporate as a staple in your daily regimen.

Fennel Seeds

Dr. Pamela Sky Jeanne, N.D., naturopathic doctor from Gresham, Oregon, USA states that, "Chewing on fennel seeds after a meal is an excellent way to relieve flatulence". The oils that are in the fennel seeds help aid the digestive process. Chew on about 5-10 seeds a few at a time and swallow them after to continue to send these helpful materials to the gut and digestive tract.

Chlorophyll (from plants!)

There are chlorophyll supplements that you can take as needed after following instructions. But I'd like to recommend getting chlorophyll from plants, particularly leafy greens. Dandelion Greens, lettuce, kale, and just about any other leafy green vegetable you can name, is a good source of chlorophyll. Working in more leafy greens immediately will help begin to decrease flatulence and help clean up waste materials in the digestive system.

Common sources of chlorophyll: Callaloo, Dandelion, Lettuces, Turnip Greens, Wild Arugula, Watercress, Nopales (Mexican Cactus)

Eat Smaller Meals

Sometimes our intestines are just backed up from digesting items frequently, that it begins to push back which forces any air sacs to flatulate. Avoid overeating and preparing large meals. Try to save leftovers for the next day to help save time or donate to someone in need. This can help to avoid any unnecessary flatulence that may feel is a norm for your body.

Flu

Influenza ("The Flu") can appear at random most times unless you're in direct contact with someone who was experiencing the flu. This condition is a virus that has several types which all vary in symptoms, which is why the term "flu" is very a very broad term used to describe what's going on in the body. The four types of flu are listed as, A, B, C, and D.

Influenza A is the most common one that is experienced that most people tend to attract during the winter and colder months. Anytime there's an epidemic or symptoms seem difficult to predict, this is Influenza A.

Influenza B is a less severe form of the flu that can be categorized by different strains. Unlike other forms of the flu which can be spread amongst humans and wildlife, Influenza B specifically only impacts humans.

Influenza C primarily impacts the respiratory system but does not lead to epidemics and are not a type of flu that medical doctors recommend getting vaccines for.

Influenza D is a type of flu that affects cattle and wildlife.

Due to the changing nature of the flu and having several types, the common symptoms throughout have been grouped together and are just referred to as "flu". Although this places a blanket over this condition altogether, there are specific ways of understanding which form of influenza you have so that you can best treat it. This begins by reviewing the names given to specific strains. If there is a strain being advertised or promoted, it is simple to search up the name. If not, you can identify which type (A, B, C, D) the strain is and its origin. This will shed light on methods and treatment you may seek out in order to reduce the severity of your symptoms and/or preventing any anticipated symptoms that have yet to be on display.

Every strain of Influenza is categorized by listing out the following:

- The antigenic type (A, B, C, D)

- The host of origin (ex. swine, chicken, equine, etc). There is no host of origin for types that have human origin.

- Geographical Origin (ex. Taiwan, Denver, etc).

- Strain Number (ex. 1, 2, 15, 7, etc).

- Year of Collection (ex. 2003, 1841, 2029, etc).

Examples of Naming A Flu Virus

Ex. 1 – Duck. Avian influenza. A(H1N1)

Ex. 2 – Human. Seasonal influenza. A(H3N2)

Sample Name: A/Sydney/05/97/H3N2

A ← Virus Type / Sydney ← Place of Origin / 05 ← Strain Number / 97 ← Year Isolated / (H3N2) ← Virus Subtype

Remedies:

(Note: This remedies section will not go over specific remedies for each type of influenza. This section will focus on what to incorporate to reduce the severity of symptoms as well as the symptoms that are common throughout each type of influenza).

Water

Drinking enough water will be essential when working through this condition. It is typically recommended to drink about half of your body weight in ounces (ex. you weigh 200lbs, drink 100oz….you weight 100lbs, drink 50oz), but you will want to aim for slightly higher than this amount to help flush out excess waste, replace any lost from increase perspiration, and help curb your hunger as you most likely aren't (and shouldn't be) consuming much food while working through this condition.

Hydrotherapy

Aside from consuming enough water, it is important to applying water to the outside of your body can be just as helpful. Many have done parts of the routine that will listed below, but it is important to provide structure and order when following through with this method.

Step 1: Take a warmer to hot bath for 5 minutes

Step 2: Get out of shower and dry yourself off.

Step 3: place a towel in cold water, wring it out, and wrap it around your body from your armpits to your groin. Leave towel in place for at least 20 minutes. To avoid getting chilled, place a wool blanket or covering over yourself as well.

Do this routine 1-2 times a day until your symptoms are minimal.

No dairy

This substance should not be consumed in general to avoid health complications but, dairy items increase mucus production, which makes the nasal congestion caused by the flu even worse, according to Dr. Mark Stengler, N.D., naturopathic physician in San Diego, California, USA. The body will likely waste immune cells on digesting for a longer period of time to break down the dairy, which could've been better served fighting against this virus.

Ginger (herb)

Ginger helps a variety of ailments that cover many involved with influenza. Ginger can help relieve nasal congestion, improve blood flow, reduce pain and muscle aches, and relieve a sore throat. Drinking a few cups of ginger tea during the day can drastically reduce your symptoms. It is recommended to make this tea from scratch and avoiding any artificial brand-name teas. Cut a 3-5 inch piece of fresh ginger and boil in 2 cups of water for about 5-10 minutes. Let steep then strain out when you are ready to drink. Make this tea several times a day.

Avoid (Only) Fighting Your Fever

A fever stimulates and acts as an internal alarm for your immune system to respond. Although a fever is one of the main symptoms of a fever we do not wish to experience, simply removing or reducing your fever will not result in your flu going away. If you were to eliminate your fever, you could actually prolong your flu as the body will not treat your condition with as much urgency. You do, however, want to avoid your fever from getting worse and decrease the severity of it.

Simple Remedies For Reducing Fever:

Feverfew (herb) and Elderberry Tea – take about 1 teaspoon of each ingredient and boil together in a cup of water. Make sure to strain out herbs (which you can re-use once more) prior to consuming. You may drink this tea every few hours.

Yarrow (herb) Tea – take 1-2 teaspoons of this herb to use as tea. Place herb into cup and fill cup with boiling water. Let steep until almost completely cooled off. You may also drink this tea every few hours.

Note: start with one of either of the options listed above; not both. You may enjoy one more than the other or just have certain herbs more readily available. But try one before moving onto the other to avoid any sign of caution. It can be best to stick with one option throughout as every person may respond a bit differently or progress may be slower, but you'd want your body to know what to expect and build in a steady routine.

Steam

Coughing is a primary symptom when influenza is present within the body. To help alleviate this symptom, we must expel excess mucous from the body. At times, mucous can sit still deeper within the respiratory system and linger around, keeping the influenza virus present. To avoid this, you want the mucus to remain moist which you can do by having a humidifier or steamer running nearby while you are sick. For relaxation and further cleansing properties, add a few drops of an essential oil such as thyme, rosemary, or lavender.

Salt Water For Sore (or Scratchy) Throat

This irritating part of the flu can make the flu feel worse and also linger after the flu has worked its way out of your system. You want to treat this as soon as possible but also to prevent any future damage that may occur from coughing excessively. Dissolve about 1 teaspoon of sea salt in a cup of warm water. Sip slowly and gargle a few times. Make sure to not drink this mixture as the sodium content can provide a sudden shock to your body and is not necessary.

Fresh Air

Whenever possible take a few minutes to breathe in some fresh air. You may step outdoors or just open a window. The room you are staying in the majority of the time while sick, make sure it has access to fresh air. Just be mindful of not having a draft of wind coming in as it can contribute to your symptoms and experiencing any chills.

My Personal Remedy For Influenza:

6-8oz of tomato juice (non-processed)

Juice of 2 key limes

¼ teaspoon of Cayenne Pepper (powder)

3-4 drops of Cat's Claw (herb) from a tincture.

Mix together all listed ingredients and place into a blender. Add ice cubes and blend together. Ice cubes are added in order to make this mixture easier to consume as the taste is strong. Sip on this drink slowly twice a day to reduce your symptoms and help promote recovery from this condition.

Food Allergies

What we are told about food allergies is that, if you consume something and have some irritable response (mostly skin, respiratory, and/or digestive issue) within an hour of consuming a certain item, that you are allergic to it and should never consume it. As an initial starting point, this item should not be consumed to eliminate further irritation, but the body's specific reaction or trigger is what must be addressed. Some go the route of exploring what specifically in particular foods while others just restrict these foods from their diets altogether.

What deserves more attention is the actual process of what happens when someone has a food allergy. The immune system is alerted just how it is when for other allergies such as pollen and produces an antibody that causes a release of histamine which is one of the many chemicals that trigger allergy responses from the body. This reaction occurs when food allergens (typically undigested proteins and waste materials that pass into the bloodstream through a gut wall that has been made permeable ("leaky") due to many dietary factors, which results in an inflammatory response, where the production of many antibodies are sent out to attach themselves to the allergens and work to break them down. This process is all that occurs when a food allergy response occurs. This also signifies that MOST people have food allergies, and not just a small percentage of people, and not mostly in younger children as typically reported. What has happened, is that only the most severe reactions are reported or considered to be a food allergy. In addition, many symptoms that appear to be irritating the skin, digestive system, or respiratory system, are actually not specifically targeting those areas as food allergies can impact any system, tissue, or organ in the body.

The main aspect of food allergies that is most commonly ignored is the fact that the allergic reaction is not specifically tied only to the presentation that is displayed when one experiences a food allergy. These allergies, or rather the presentation of the bodily response, are simply signifying that something is wrong and need to be healed and/or restored within the body. Certain systems may need to be cleaned, or particular organs may be backed up which sends of much quicker and stronger signals that are present during allergic reactions.

We feel as though we "graduate" from more acute and specific symptoms, to more severe and complicated symptoms and/or diseases. We treat these as if they are separate from one another. This includes both, those who have experienced a food allergy, and those who are not aware an allergic response has taken place, as stated earlier in this section. Not addressing the initial warning signs (allergies) will often lead to additional work on the body. Simply avoiding this by not consuming items you have an allergic response to does not mean an issue is still not present. You may think you have avoided an underlying issue by not eating items you feel allergic to, but later go onto develop any variety of illness, condition, or disease.

To summarize, we all (at least most of us at some point in our lives) have some form of food allergy that over time, can be minimized, corrected, or eliminated altogether.

Remedies:

Food Journal

Writing down what you consume on a daily basis can help determine what may be causing any sort of reaction. This is also a great way to redirect and make more positive changes to your diet as well. Most people eat generally the same things week after week. If there's an issue present in your body (whether you're aware of it or not) you can be essentially adding tax or accruing interest by eating the same items all of the time. After a while you may start writing down certain ingredients you consume and look at a deeper level what may be contributing to any issues. Eliminate or at least take a break from any item on your list to see if you feel any better or notice any changes. Rather than just restrict yourself, use this as an opportunity to add more variety to your diet and lifestyle.

Fruits (eat by themselves)

Many that are allergic to fruit will tend to avoid all fruits. What is most helpful when this is the case is to try eating one fruit at a time. Not eating a bowl of different fruits one at time, but eating a bowl of only grapes, or a small container of just blueberries, or watermelon. You want to isolate the fruit you eat to help identify which ones are causing these reactions. This does not mean you cannot have a variety throughout the day but avoid doing this in one sitting.

"Vitamin-C"

What we refer to as Vitamin C is a water-soluble nutrient and powerful antioxidant that help form and maintain connective tissues, including the bones, blood vessels, and the skin.

This nutrient can help reduce symptoms of allergic reactions and inflammation which will help to avoid any prolonging issues. Vitamin C also is responsible for manufacturing the adrenal hormones which are needed to combat the stress the body goes through when an allergic reaction takes place.

Common Sources of Vitamin-C: Black Currants, Bell Peppers (red and green), Papaya, Spring Onions, Strawberries, Cantaloupe, Mango, Oranges, Watercress, Raspberries, and Tomatoes.

Sulphur

This mineral works to prevent inflammatory responses in the body. This is an essential part of decreasing the severity and frequency of things like food allergies and allergic responses.

Common Sources of Sulphur: Chickpeas, Walnuts, Brazil Nuts, Spelt, Kamut, Fonio, and Quinoa.

Digestive Enzymes

Many allergies involving food are often triggered when there's a deficiency in stomach acid needed to digest. There's a host of reasons why stomach acid may be deficient, but this eventually leads to a deficiency of food-digesting enzymes that are produced by the pancreas.

This is a primary reason many who experience food allergies are told they are at risk of developing diabetes. Replacing these enzymes is achieved from reducing the workload on the digestive system. Removing the foods that take hours to digest (meats, dairy, processed sugars, (typical) potatoes, etc) is the first and most crucial step. Then keeping the digestive tract clean by consuming more items that naturally promote cleansing properties such as fresh produce and herbs. After a more regular routine is created, it is then important to identify more specific ways to meet your needs depending on if you're feeling congested, notice any imbalances, or work towards achieving a steadier flow of healthier stools upon going to the bathroom.

Malabsorption

The process of malabsorption involves the body not absorbing many nutrients. This is the common theme of having a "leaky gut". Many times, malabsorption is a signal that you are allergic to certain items since the body will pass things through quicker to avoid an allergic response. If you notice foods not being absorbed (ex. Seeing pieces of it in your stool) then you may have a leaky gut or some intestinal issue as a result of a food allergy. To increase absorption of nutrients and minerals you will want to do the following:

Keep your colon clean. This may involve a colon cleanse, Fasting, or just eating minimally a diet high in fiber, and low in protein and processed items.

Chlorophyll

Chlorophyll is essentially the "blood" of plants. What iron is to our blood, chlorophyll is to plants. This substance helps the digestive tract work properly. Much of the odor that may come from our mouths, is accumulated waste from foods that weren't digested properly. Chlorophyll helps break down waste and support healthy digestion. Natural foods (plants) are best to achieve this but plants high in chlorophyll can be taken in capsule form as well. It is safe for an adult to take three 500-700mg capsules a day before or after each meal to support proper digestion. Doing this more often than not (not daily) is best to help deodorize the digestive tract and colon.

Common sources of chlorophyll: Callaloo, Dandelion, Lettuces, Turnip Greens, Wild Arugula, Watercress, Nopales (Mexican Cactus)

Iron

Iron is a mineral that transports nutrients. Think of iron as your body's personal delivery service that takes nutrients and minerals where they are needed. When deficiencies are present, the body will be more aware of this and essentially "crave" certain foods that are higher in these minerals and nutrients. You can help by consuming items high in iron more regularly to help push along these nutrients and minerals.

Common Sources of Iron: quinoa, wild rice (not black rice), chickpeas/garbanzo beans, kale, nuts (particularly walnuts), hemp seeds, dates, dried apricots, prunes, watercress

Iron Rich Herbs: sarsaparilla, burdock (and root), guaco, chainey root, monkey ladder, chickweed, yellowdock

Food Poisoning

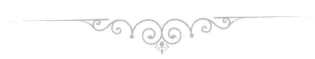

We often associate food poisoning with undercooked items or foods that are not prepared properly. Ironically enough, we do not associate food poisoning with the chemicals and toxins that are in many items we may eat. The most common form of food poisoning comes from undercooked meat but can also come from improperly washed fruits and vegetables, leaving certain foods in the sun, bacteria that comes from packaging/processing, and other items that harbor microscopic organisms and bacteria that can trigger potentially life-threatening causes of food poisoning.

Not all cases of food poisoning reach the extreme levels. Minor issues such as dizziness, headache, stomach cramps, and diarrhea can happen as well. We may feel these issues are short-lived and go back to our regular routines, but the body still needs to clean out waste materials, heal any damaged areas, and work to avoid this process form occurring again. Whether it's minor or severe, these situations are still food poisoning.

Common Signs You Have Parasites:

Hearing loss, face paralysis, rapid or slowed heartbeat, hot and/or swollen joints, insomnia, and flu-like symptoms (headache, fever, fatigue, chills, sore throat, muscle aches).

Remedies:

Hydration

Getting food poisoning can mimic the flu virus. Food Poisoning can be viewed as a "food virus" similar to the flu as many symptoms will be the same. The main difference is that this condition is directly connected to the food(s) you ate which you are most likely aware of as symptoms begin to be on display. Just like the flu, hydration is a must. A person can lose a lot of fluids through throwing up, diarrhea, and/or sweating. Eating may be difficult at this time (even soft foods) so it is difficult to begin with water and clear liquids that will help you. Incorporating fresh fruit or vegetable juices is important also, just be cautious on any specific items that may cause discomfort and look to choose items with a higher water-content than others.

Avoid Antacids

These products that are commonly used for heartburn can reduce the digestive acids in your stomach which will weaken your body's defense against bacteria. Bacteria has a good chance of multiplying when Antacids are consumed which will prolong symptoms. You want to avoid this altogether and you can do this by choosing to avoid a product many people get thinking it is helpful for when they are sick, particularly when working through food poisoning.

Replenish Electrolytes

You lose electrolytes by vomiting and through diarrhea – specifically potassium, sodium, and glucose. The term "electrolyte" is often given to commercially prepared products like Gatorade, Powerade, and artificial supplements so much that most people believe these are the only sources for these minerals. There are many foods that contain potassium, sodium, and glucose, but eating solid foods are not recommended at this time.

A simple solution to replenishing and restoring electrolytes goes as followed:

Blend or juice a fruit of your choosing (for potassium)

Add ½ teaspoon of date sugar or agave (for glucose)

Add a pinch or two of sea salt (for sodium)

Mix all of this together well and drink a few times a day.

Parasites

Parasites are in many of the common foods people eat. Foods such as animal flesh, dairy products, and many processed or refined sugars and carbohydrates. These parasites set up shop in the body and tuck themselves away. They feed off of waste materials. It is best to starve these parasites by not consuming what they feed off of and through developing a fasting regimen.

There are many herbal parasite cleanses that should come with a specific protocol available for purchase. Seek out those created and made by an herbalist or holistic health practitioner as they will have a set intention when putting together herbal compounds made for removing parasites from the body and will list out a protocol to follow as opposed to purchasing a commercial product that likely contains artificial ingredients and harmful chemicals.

Anti-parasite Smoothie

½ large papaya with seeds

4-5 dates

2 bananas

½ key lime (juiced)

1 cup of distilled water

Blend together and enjoy.

<u>Anti-parasite Tea</u>

1 teaspoon of Wormwood

1/2 teaspoon of black walnut hull

½ teaspoon of myrrh

2 thumb-sized pieces of bitter melon

Boil 3 cups of water and add ingredients to a cup. Pour boiling water into cup and let steep for 12-15 minutes. Strain herbs and let cool. Drink twice a day until symptoms decrease.

Coconut Oil

Take one tablespoon of coconut oil daily during a parasitic cleanse. Coconut oil will balance the bacteria in the gut and assist the liver during this process.

Slowly Reintroduce Foods

The moment many of us feel better, we tend to try to go back to our regular schedule and eating habits. It is much better to slowly introduce foods. Stating with foods that dissolve easily such as tomatoes, grapes, cucumbers (peel off the skin), melons, and berries. Then eventually working your way back up to more semi-solid foods such as nuts, apples (without the skin first), and some grains. From there you can slowly begin preparing more complete meals. If you introduce solid foods or more than your body is prepared for, your digestive system can experience damage, feel congested, and feel many symptoms you do not want to go through such as headaches or dizziness.

Don't Interfere

As the body works through this issue, don't begin experimenting and adding a ton of materials, from various herbal concoctions to pharmaceutical meds, to artificial supplements. Let it run its course and you will recover sooner rather than later. Keep everything simple and let nature run its course.

Food Poisoning (Prevention Steps)

- Wash your hands with warm water all the way up to the wrists before preparing foods. If you have any cut or damage on your hands or fingers, make sure to wear gloves when preparing foods. It is good practice to wear gloves whenever you're preparing foods you need to do anything more than chop or cut into smaller pieces.

- Heat or chill raw foods. Bacteria cannot multiply above 150°F or below 40°F.

- Avoid leaving food at room temperature for more than two hours. We may get distracted or forget about a meal we made and left to cool off and chose to eat it but take the time to reheat on the stove or countertop to help reduce the chances of any bacteria. While letting your food cool, it is good practice to do your dishes, clean up your kitchen area so that you do not get distracted and remain aware of when your food is cooled off enough to eat after cooking.

- Avoid taste-testing often while you cook. You may get closer towards getting the taste how you want it, but it may be your last complete meal for a while as you increase your risk of food poisoning.

- Use different cutting boards for different items. You do not want to slice fresh fruit and then place your raw vegetables on top of the leftover fruit juice while cutting them. (same goes for not letting "juice" from meats drip onto other foods you plan to prepare, although it is recommended to avoid eating meats and eggs to avoid food poisoning altogether).

- Clean your countertops before and after you prepare your foods and cook to help wash away even minor bacteria.

- Replace your cleaning sponges often and wipe down counters with paper towels.

- Immediately refrigerate leftovers even if they are warm to avoid leaving them out for too long. Cool down larger stews or soups faster by refrigerating in smaller portions.

- If it does not spell right or taste right, just do without to remain safe.

Foot Aches

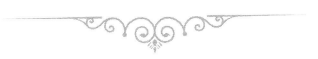

Each foot consists of 26 bones, 33 joints, 107 ligaments, 19 muscles, and various tendons that keep all of these together. There is a lot of pressure applied to the foot daily. Our feet remain intact and are extremely durable. However, a lot can go wrong with our feet if we do not properly take care of them as there is room for innumerable things that could go wrong since the foot is made up of so many parts.

Remedies:

Elevate

No matter what type of foot ache you have, make sure to elevate your foot to decrease and slow down blood flow to the area to help relieve additional pressure. While keeping your foot elevated at around a 45-degree angle, begin moving your toes often to stimulate circulation. We often have waste materials or inflammation that can become stagnant whereas elevating our feet can help reduce this from happening as well. Elevate your feet for at least 20 minutes a day.

Salt Bath

Warm water mixed with 1-2 tablespoons of Epsom salt typically help reduce many aches and pains. You do not want to rely upon treatments such as this one but can be handy for more short-term relief so that you don't develop any prolonged or more severe symptoms.

Running Water (Hot & Cold)

To help "kickstart" or reinvigorate circulation, this remedy will help. Sit on the edge of your bathtub and hold your feet under running water; 1-minute warm water, followed by 1-minute cold water. Repeat 2-3 more times for 30 seconds each. If you have a shower attachment that can gently massage your feet while doing this, it is encouraged. Stimulating and promoting circulation is the primary need with any soreness, particularly the feet.

*Note: if you currently have diabetes do NOT do this exercise. Blood flow and capillaries can be hindered during this time. Please go back and read the diabetes section first if you have diabetes in addition to following the other remedies covered in this section.

Foot Massage

You can do this yourself if you do not have a partner or access to a place that offers foot massages. You want to be gentle but work the entire foot, pressing in circular motions, squeezing the toes, and pressing against any tender areas as often as possible. Use some essential oils that you enjoy as well.

Ice

Wrap your feet with a few ice cubes in a wet washcloth, then rub it over your feet and ankles for a few minutes. Ice will help reduce the inflammation in the feet. Pat to dry and let sit for a few minutes elevated after they are dry.

Exercise

Not involving any strenuous activities or heavy weightlifting. But rather, making an effort to regularly exercise your feet and legs to maintain positive circulation. This will help alleviate any future issues and help speed up recovery when needed.

Heel Heights

If you wear heels often look into the height of the heel and adjust accordingly as you can. High heels tighten the calf muscle and can lead to foot fatigue. Wearing lower heels is best but changing them halfway through the day would be a good idea.

Shop For Shoes In The Afternoon

Our feet tend to expand during the day once we get moving. Some people's feet will tighten up and appear smaller and even stiff upon awakening due to sleep. Start by buying shoes in the afternoon to accommodate for your feet expanding. If one foot is larger than the other, make sure the larger foot feels comfortable before purchasing a pair of shoes.

Stretch Your Shoes Often

As we wear our shoes, they can occasionally become accustomed to our foot size. Other times, adding things like insoles can cause shoes to tighten around the toe area. Fill a sock with some sand and push it to the end of the toe area to avoid any tightening and lightly stretch all parts of each shoe to keep them loose.

Warning Signal for Disease

If you have regular foot pain, this can be a sign of a variety of diseases. Without going into too much detail, there are many diseases and conditions that involve lack of blood flow to the extremities, or things such as low or high blood sugar which impacts the areas such as the feet and the nerves. You will want to get checked out by a Podiatrist ("foot doctor") as they'll have direct insight into what may be impacting your foot. Podiatrists diagnose and treat disorders, diseases, and injuries to the feet as well as specialize in areas such as sports medicine, surgery, biomechanics, and generalized foot care. Getting their opinion can help narrow down your search on what may be impacting your feet.

Foot Odor

Foot odor comes from the feet perspiring. Feet perspiring more than needed is due to them working harder than what is necessary. It may be due a need for an arch support, or shoes fitting too tight. Address any underlying issues by treating the entire foot to identify what's needed. Bacteria feeds on any dead skin cells under the socks while trapping in any fumes that are produced, leading to a foul stench. Exercising or being physically active for an extended period of time or wearing shoes that don't allow the feet to breathe will add to foot odor. We don't want to simply become less active to reduce this issue but want to apply frequent remedies to prevent this issue from prolonging or reaching more extreme levels.

Remedies:

Wash Your Feet

Besides showering or just taking a bath, make sure your focus on directly washing your feet – all areas, including in between your toes. You want to wash your entire feet and not just run water over them as this will not properly clean your feet. Get a brush and gently scrub your feet while bathing. If you have difficulty lifting one foot to scrub while showering or bending over, make sure to get some anti-slip grips for your shower floor or install a sturdy handle you can hold onto.

Powder Your Toes

After washing your toes, add some basic foot powder or antifungal spray to limit the foot odor you may smell. Also place a small amount of powder in your shoes when you are not wearing them also to cut odor.

Change Your Socks Often

Our socks absorb everything from sweat to dirt, to bacteria. We must change them daily but if you perspire excessively with little to no physical movement, you may want to change them a few times per day. Purchasing new socks regularly may be a necessity at first prior to reducing your foot odor so prepare ahead of time for additional expenses if needed. Try getting some linen socks to allow more air to pass through freely as well.

Wear Open-Toe Footwear When Appropriate

Allowing your feet to breath is a necessary part of reducing foot odor. You do want your fee to be protected but, wearing sandals or any open-toe footwear will serve you well in the meantime.

Sage (herb)

If you want to soak your feet in warm water and place a small handful of sage leaves in there, this can help kill excess bacteria on your feet. You can also place sage in your shoes or crumbled pieces of sage in your shoes to help eliminate odor. Make sure to remove any stems or pieces that may puncture or poke your feet.

Thyme Essential Oil

Add no more than 3 drops of thyme essential oil to warm water daily. Fill up a foot soaker or large basin that your feet fit comfortably in and fill with warm water and add your thyme essential oil and let soak for about 20 minutes a day.

Dietary Restrictions

You may notice a stronger odor when you consume certain foods. Even healthier foods such as onions, peppers, or various herbs. You want to reduce adding additional odor to what's already there. remain mindful of what you eat and remove items you feel are adding to the issue. Making an effort to remove items that turn quickly into waste such as artificial sugars, refined carbohydrates, animal flesh, and dairy, to help eliminate and avoid any foul-smelling odors coming through your sweat glands in your feet; bacteria that creates odor feeds off of these items.

Fractures

There are six types of fractures: (1) Simple/Stable, (2) Open/Compound, (3) Hairline/Stress, (4) Transverse, (5) Oblique, and (6) Comminuted.

Simple Fracture - The broken ends of the bone line up and are barely out of place.

Open - The skin may be pierced by the bone or by a blow that breaks the skin at the time of the fracture. The bone may or may not be visible in the wound.

Hairline/Stress - a fracture that appears as a narrow crack along the surface of a bone.

Transverse fracture. This type of fracture has a horizontal fracture line.

Oblique fracture. This type of fracture has an angled pattern.

Comminuted fracture. In this type of fracture, the bone shatters into three or more pieces.

A doctor will attempt to immobilize the break with a cast of some sort. A cast is typically used since the arm has some weight to it where you cannot use a splint like you would for a finger that may be fractured. While you have a cast on, you may feel irritated, hot, or itchy where you want to incorporate natural ways to help speed up the recovery process.

Remedies:

"Vitamin-K"

What we refer to as "vitamin k" is actually two forms of intestinal bacteria (lactobacillus acidophilus and Bifidobacterium bifidum) that are formed in the intestinal tract via bacterial synthesis when processing and digesting items. This nutrient during this process turns into a protein called, osteocalcin that aids in building (in this case re-building) the bone. You can find supplements that provide this substance but the primary way to absorb this is to not hinder the bones from absorbing nutrients and minerals that we will review in the rest of this section. The typical dose of supplements with the two forms of bacteria mentioned is about 1 teaspoon.

"Vitamin-D"

This naturally occurring hormone within the body has to remain presently active in order to help the body. Without vitamin D the body cannot absorb calcium which is commonly listed as an active mineral that helps the bones. For the first 4 weeks after your fracture, you should work in at least 400 units of vitamin d (do your research on foods high in vitamin d to identify quantities). It is highly encouraged to sit in direct sunlight for at least 20-30 minutes a day. Sitting in the sunlight allows the body to produce and absorb its own vitamin d.

Calcium

Calcium is the active mineral that is present in the bones within the body. When a long road or highway is built, cement is poured in and around the cross-linked cables. When bones are being built (and re-built) calcium is the "cement".

Common Sources of Calcium: sea moss, kale, okra, dandelion greens, turnip greens, lettuce, papaya, and oranges.

Silicon

This mineral is crucial in assisting recovery as well as maintaining strong bones. Dr. Thomas O'Bryan, D.C., a chiropractor, nutritionist, and director of Omnis Chiropractic Group in Glenview, Illinois has often cited a scientific research study in which laboratory animals with fractures were given the mineral silicon, and their breaks healed completely within 17 days. A group of animals who did not receive silicon, showed little to no healing after 17 days. Dr. O'Bryan recommends 1 milligram a day of silicon.

Common sources of silicon: horsetail, bananas, almonds, Kenyen beans, red lentils, spinach, dried fruits.

Bicycle In A Pool For Lower Body Fractures

Bones begin to grow when they have a good amount of stress due to activity. not grow in size as an infant or growing child but grow in depth and in repair. Make sure you can apply pressure on your legs first, especially if it is a broken hip, hip replacement, or a leg fracture. The bike will hold the majority of your body weight. You want to make sure you are in a shallow end of a pool of water that you can easily get out of or walk out of. Start slow but go for a 5-10 minute bicycle "ride" daily. This will allow your injury to work on repairing itself without adding additional pressure to it which would prolong your injury. As your leg feels stronger, start walking briefly in shallow water. This alone will reduce the amount of time you will spend on crutches.

Note: Wait until your cast is off or you have a set date on when your cast will come off before doing this activity.

Horsetail (herb)

This herb is abundant in the mineral silicon. Drink 2-3 cups a day to get the recommended amount of 1 milligram. For tea, take 2 teaspoons of this dried herb per cup of boiling water. Pour desired amount of water over the herb in a saucepan, boil for about 5 minutes, then let steep for 10-15 minutes. Strain out dried herb and drink when tea is cooled.

Note: do not use horsetail powdered extract as it will dissolve quickly, and you won't absorb this mineral as intended.

Caffeine

Caffeine blocks the body's ability to absorb calcium. You want to avoid drinking this substance especially while trying to heal a broken bone.

Soda

There's a specific ingredient in soda called phosphoric acid. This substance leech's calcium from the bones. Dr. O'Bryan notes that this substance also inhibits the formation of new bones and will either cause fractures or significantly delay the recovery process.

Frostbite

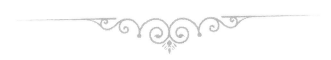

Fluids freeze. Whether you place water in the freezer or you remain in a freezing environ-ment for too long. Frostbite is a medical emergency that occurs when our bodies (which are mostly fluids) stays in the cold for too long. Skin may appear to look like wax, while being numb, or stings and burns. These symptoms alone are reason for an immediate trip to an emergency room. The next stage of frostbite involves blisters on the skin, then turns red, followed by turning purple as the blisters become deeper. The most common treatment for frostbite is, rapid rewarming and painkillers such as ibuprofen. Not that these items should be avoided during this emergency, but you want to heal and recover completely as much as possibly by restoring the body without any dependence on pharmaceutical medications or chemicals. You not only want to recover so that you can return homme but, you want to also promote healing of any damaged tissues to avoid opening you up to future ailments.

Frostbite is the body's way of trying to preserve heat by shutting down circulation to the extremities.

Remedies:

Cayenne Pepper

If you are going to head out in weather than can put you at risk of frostbite, put some cayenne pepper in your shoes. Pamela Fischer, who is the founder and director of the Ohlone Center for Herbal Studies in Concord, California, USA states that, "In third-world countries, this (cayenne pepper) is a much-used folk remedy for stopping frostbite. Cayenne pepper and many other Chile peppers work externally to improve circulation in the body. You can take one size 00 capsule a day filled with cayenne pepper powder but can also mix 1 teaspoon with an equal amount of olive oil and rub this mixture onto your feet before you go out into any extreme cold temperatures.

Note: these remedies are not to take place of any common sense such as dressing warmly by covering the head, ears, face, hands, and feet. If you get wet, you want to get to a warm space and take off any wet items immediately as you replace them with dry items.

Avoid Alcohol

Many who live in colder climates will bring along alcohol as they believe this substance will help them keep warm as they will often sweat when drinking. However, alcohol just creates more heat loss as you perspire which reduces the amount of available warmth your body has, which will contribute to this condition spreading to vulnerable areas.

No Smoking

Smoking any substance will decrease your peripheral circulation and make your extremities more vulnerable to frostbite.

Loose Fitting Clothes

Make sure some of your internal clothing is not tight. You do not want your outer layers of clothing to be loose where you can feel a drift or wind but want items looser to avoid cutting off circulation. When out in the colder temperatures avoid wearing rings or tight jewelry as well.

Always Use The Buddy System

You want someone around to see anything you cannot see or notice, but also to help take care of one another if needed. A call for help that you are not well enough to make can save your life.

Gallstones

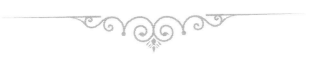

About 500,000 people every year have gallbladder surgery where this organ is removed. Mark Stengler, N.D., a naturopathic physician in San Diego, California, states that, "most of those (gallbladder) surgeries – possibly up to 85 percent – are unnecessary. People could achieve the same results (eliminating pain and the risk of damage to the gallbladder, liver, and pancreas) with alternative remedies." Most surgeries are completed due to gallstones being very large and dangerous, while the majority of these surgeries, these gallstones can be dissolved and prevented through dietary adjustments.

The gallbladder store bile (liquid produced by the liver when digesting fats). When bile becomes too concentrated by sitting in the gallbladder, stones can begin to form. About 80% of these stones are formed due to high cholesterol consumption which additional bile is created by the liver, and about 20% are formed due to calcium salts. Those who are overweight and have a larger frame are more likely to develop gallstones due to the liver working extra to clear out toxins in the body and created additional bile that is sent to the gallbladder. For every pound of fat in your body, you produce about 10 milligrams of cholesterol.

Gallstones start off small but become larger the more they are "fed" with bile and cholesterol, as well as many waste materials in the body. The goal is to not feed the growth/size of these stones while working to dissolve their current size and remaining proactive with avoiding the creation of future stones. Following the recommendations in this section, you should be less likely to developing stones while removing symptoms and any need for surgery (unless your stones are currently massive enough to plan of more immediate surgery.

Remedies:

Low Fat Diet

"The saturated fat in dairy foods, meats, vegetable shortening, coconut oil, palm oil, and hydrogenated oils makes bile more concentrated" says Elizabeth Lipski, a certified clinical nutritionist in Kauai, Hawaii. You want to reduce the bile from becoming sent often from the liver to the gallbladder to reduce the chances of small stones from being created.

Omega-3 Fatty Acid

Although you are decreasing your fat consumption, increasing your omega-3 fatty acid consumption will help make bile more soluble and less likely to create a stone.

Omega-3 Sources: Walnuts, Brazil Nuts, Avocados, Hemp Seeds, Hemp Milk, Walnut Oil, Olive Oil, and Sea Vegetable such as Nori, Hijiki, Bladderwrack, Kelp, and Dulse.

Fiber

Fiber helps digestion which is needed to help the body continue to clear out toxins and unnecessary waste. Dr. Stengler, N.D., a naturopathic physician in San Diego, California notes that the indigestible portions of many whole-food plant-based foods help to remove excess cholesterol from the body also. We do not necessarily absorb every bit of every nutrient provided by what we consume, but unlike many processed food items, plant-based foods help cleanse out additional waste even the indigestible parts. It should be a goal to consume about 5 portions of plant-based foods daily, regardless of any specific dietary regimen you may follow.

Common sources of Fiber: garbanzo beans, lentils, brussels sprouts, sweet potatoes, avocado, pears, sunflower seeds, flax seeds, hazelnuts, apples and berries (high pectin fruits) and onions.

Water

Bile becomes more concentrated when the body is dehydrated. It is recommended to drink about half of your bodyweight in ounces of water daily (ex. if you weight 200lbs, drink 100 ounces of water, if you weigh 100lbs, drink 50 ounces of water).

Remove Artificial Sugars

Regular amounts of artificial sugars which take longer to digest and process than natural sugar, inflames the gallbladder ducts. You want to avoid common "junk foods" and table sugar that is often added to drinks.

Milk Thistle (herb)

This herb helps stimulate the liver which helps reduce the cholesterol levels in the bile that is sent to the gallbladder. It is recommended to take about 600 milligrams of milk thistle extract daily until symptoms and condition is better.

See-Haw (herb)

This herb helps provide an assortment of minerals to the body, is an anti-inflammatory, antibacterial, and helps promote digestion while protecting the gallbladder and liver. While clearing out and breaking down gallstones, the body will become more exposed to many toxins that are in the body. See-haw helps fight against free radicals, slows the aging of premature cells, and even helps lower high blood sugar and high cholesterol. You can drink this herb as a tea.

Place 20g of dried leaves in with 1-liter of water. Once water starts to boil, let it boil for 3-minutes, then remove from heat and let steep for about 20-minutes. Drink 2-3 cups a day for 3 weeks and you should notice significant changes.

My Personal Remedy:

About an hour before you go to bed is the best time to consume this mixture. Take ¼ cup of olive oil, 1/3 cup of key lime juice and mix well together. Drink this mixture and immediately begin drinking a small cup (about 8oz) of Cascara Sagrada herbal tea. Then lie on your right side for about 30 minutes and then go to bed lying on your left side to reduce pressure on the digestive tract. Upon awakening you may find that your stools contain tiny green stones. If you see these tiny green stones, this means you have successfully flushed out small stones beginning to form.

Repeat this routine for only 2-3 days at a time.

*For Cascara Sagrada Tea: take 1 teaspoon of dried herb and place into cup. Boil water and pour into cup, let steep for about 10 minutes, then strain out herb and enjoy.

Gingivitis

Gingivitis is a gum disease. It is typically the first sign of periodontal disease which leads to losing teeth. Like most diseases, gingivitis involves excess inflammation. The gums in the mouth begin to go from light pink to blueish red and will bleed easily.

Remedies:

Correct Teeth Care

Brushing correctly, flossing, and tongue scraping are necessary. You want to brush daily but not too hard and in small circles to help clear out anything hidden within the gum and teeth. Flossing can be completed daily as well as tongue scraping, especially in the morning. You want to scrape away and get rid of any unnecessary materials first thing upon awakening, but also prior to going to sleep so that things like bacteria don't settle in.

Keep 2 Toothbrushes

It is recommended to have 2 toothbrushes, one wet and one dry. The wet brush can be your normal toothbrush that you brush your teeth with while a dry brush can be used to scrub off any excess plaque on the teeth. Be careful not to use the dry brush on your gums as they can puncture your gums and cause them to bleed.

Strengthen The Bones

Treat your teeth with the same care as the rest of your bones. Don't overuse them, not apply a great amount of pressure onto them, and provide the essential minerals that are needed for the bones and skeletal system as a whole. Gingivitis can be viewed as "periodontal osteoporosis"; weakened teeth bones. The 12 primary minerals that make up the bones are (alphabetical order): boron, calcium, chromium, iron, magnesium, manganese, potassium, phosphorus, selenium, silicon, sulfur, and zinc. These are the minerals to incorporate into your lifestyle as much as possible if any gum or tooth issue is present.

Common sources of Boron: raisins, peaches, prune juice, grape juice, avocadoes, legumes, dried apricots.

Common sources of Calcium: sea moss, kale, okra, dandelion greens, turnip greens, lettuce, papaya, and oranges.

Common Sources of Chromium: green beans, orange juice, grape juice, tomato juice, apples, Brazil nuts, dried fruits, broccoli

Common sources of Iron: Quinoa, Wild Rice (not black rice), Chickpeas/Garbanzo Beans, Kale, Nuts (particularly Walnuts), Hemp Seeds, Dates, Dried Apricots, Watercress, Sarsaparilla, Burdock (and root), Guaco, Chainey Root, Monkey Ladder, Chickweed, Yellowdock.

Common Sources of Magnesium: Avocado, Chickpeas, Tamarind, Basil, Dill, Ginger, Oregano, Thyme, Nettle Leaf, Horsetail (herb), Red Clover, Sage, Nopal, and almost any CBD (cannabidiol) products are helpful. CBD Oils are almost pure magnesium.

To test the purity of a CBD Oil, send to a lab for testing or you should feel a steady decline in needing to rely on this substance after your need has been met regularly.

Common sources of manganese: quinoa, fonio, spelt, walnuts, sunflower seeds, sesame seeds, and hemp seeds.

Common sources of potassium: squash, zucchini, bananas, avocado, dried apricots, and herbs such as, guaco (also high in iron), conconsa (has the highest concentration of potassium phosphate), lily of the valley (rich in iron fluorine and Potassium phosphate).

Common sources of phosphorus: sunflower seeds, pumpkin seeds, Brazil nuts, quinoa, walnuts, pecans, hazelnuts, chickpeas, lentils, amaranth, adzuki (red) beans.

Common sources of Selenium: brazil nuts, walnuts, chickpeas/garbanzo beans, kola nuts, dandelion greens, and nettle, and alfalfa. Recommended to consume about 400 micrograms a day.

Common sources of silicon: horsetail, bananas, almonds, Kenyen beans, red lentils, spinach, dried fruits.

Common Sources of Sulfur: leafy green vegetables, (dried) peaches, onions, watercress, chickpeas, walnuts,

Common Sources of Zinc: chickpeas, mushrooms, zucchini, squash, okra, Brazil nuts, and walnuts.

Gum Massage

Take a few moments and massage your gums with your tongue or finger. This can help increase blood and circulation.

Salt

Salt dehydrates the bacteria and germs you want to remove from the teeth and gums. You can rinse your mouth with salt occasionally to help kill bacteria you will be washing or cleaning away. Place 1 teaspoon in a bottle, mix it up, and use as a daily rinse when you notice any signs or symptoms of gingivitis.

Examine Your Lifestyle

Like all sections in this text, dietary adjustments are to be reviewed and implemented. But you do want to review what you are already consuming and link it to how these items may directly impact your teeth and gum health as you work to remove them to not add to your condition. You want to work on removing any unhealthy habits at this time.

Cloves (herb)

Cloves can be sucked on or swished around the mouth with water in powdered form to help kill excess bacteria. Now, you want to not consume anything that contains excess bacteria, but as you transition to a healthier lifestyle, cloves can help begin to remove bacteria that has been accumulating in your mouth.

Glaucoma

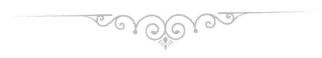

The eyes have several lenses and require constant fluids to be pumped to and from for optimal health. Each eye has its own systems of filtering fluids and removing/protecting the eyes from waste. These filtering systems are essentially the eyes' plumbing system. A specific fluid in the eye called "aqueous humor" helps remove waste materials and bacteria. When the eyes' plumbing system get backed up, this fluid remains stagnant and presses against the optic nerve, damaging the vision, resulting in a "smoky eye" which is referred to as Glaucoma.

Typically, there is no pain or other symptoms present until vision loss occurs. Medical doctors will then work in treatments structured around eye drops and recommended surgery to address what they refer to as "intraocular hypertension" which is pressure on the eyes from fluid not draining.

Now, you are thinking that maybe the "cure" to glaucoma is to simply drain the fluid that is there, correct? Although this would help, it could also impair vision as the other remaining fluids in the eye can get clogged and this condition reoccurs or worsens. We want to reduce the pressure upon the eyes while allowing the eyes' plumbing/drainage system to function properly without sending fluids elsewhere. The recommendations in this section are to promote ways to naturally reduce the pressure being placed upon the eyes, while working to carefully clean the eyes' plumbing system, while also restoring eye health.

Remedies:

Colloidal Silver

In his bestselling book, *The pH Miracle: Balance Your Diet, Reclaim Your Health*, by Dr. Robert O. Young, Ph.D., he states ,"Eye or ear problems, including cataracts, glaucoma, redness, blurred vision, poor eyesight, ringing in the ears, earaches, soreness or swelling of the ears, eardrum damage, hardness of hearing, and (in rare cases) loss of hearing: Use 1 drop of colloidal silver topically (directly in the eye or ear) 3 times a day."

Fatty Acids

A main reason the eyes' plumbing system gets drained is due to inflammation. Inflammation often serves as a protective layer when there are excess bacteria or a wound. However, inflammation does not dissolve on its own. Fatty acids such as omega-3, omega-6, and omega-9 help to decrease inflammation which will decrease the amount of pressure being placed upon the eyes. Dr. Marc Grossman, O.D., an optometrist, acupuncturist, and co-director of the Integral Health Center in Rye and New Paltz, New York, recommends a daily amount of 1,000-1,500 milligrams of fatty acids.

Common Sources of Fatty Acids: Brazil Nuts, Walnuts, Kola Nuts, Avocados, Bananas, Sea Vegetables (Nori, Wakame, Hijiki, Sea Moss, Bladderwrack), Coconut, Coconut Oil (do not cook), Olive Oil (do not cook), Grapeseed Oil, Avocado Oil, Walnut Oil, Mushrooms, Quinoa, and Wild Rice.

Note: Black Currant Seed Oil is also a great alternative to using besides the recommended fish oil(s) that a doctor may prescribe. Take about 1,000 milligrams of this oil.

"Vitamin" B12

Dr. Grossman cites that, "This nutrient can help improve eyesight or prevent it from worsening in glaucoma patients." This nutrient is often prescribed in pill or spray form since doctors will say that B12 does not come from a direct source as calcium or magnesium does besides consuming animals. However, B12 is acquired by animals either directly or indirectly from consuming bacteria. Animals will be force-fed supplements and given untreated (contaminated) water. This is not a desirable way to consume this nutrient. The reason why doctors will recommend animal products, soy, or supplements for B12 is because they can detect it within these substances. However, all plants contain B12. The issue is that this nutrient gets washed off or is lost during production and is not very present on items such as produce so doctors cannot recommend any specific items. When growing your own foods or shopping at local farmer's markets, you will be able to tract an increase in B12 (if you decide to test for any deficiencies before and after shopping locally). Dr. Milton Mills, M.D., an internal Medicine Specialist, from the United Medical Center in Washington, DC, states that, "If we were living in more natural environments, drinking unprocessed water, and eating foods that we dug up out of the ground, because that food would have bacteria on it, it would have B12. There would be B12 in the water. But what do we do? We take our water and process it, throw chlorine in it, we kill all of the bacteria — we have eliminated the natural sources of B12."

We essentially only need about 1 microgram of B12 a day. When we repeatedly do not meet this need, it can become noticeable, but we don't need nearly as much B12 as we do calcium, magnesium, or any other mineral. Since we have worked to kill off any form of bacteria (harmful or helpful) most people remain deficient. If we consume that which is natural and work on eating locally grown produce and growing our own plants (even something small to put in a window at home) we can consume enough B12 and do away with any B12 deficiency (and many others) so that B12 deficiency is no longer a topic of decision.

You will want to go to local markets and farmer's markets in your area where there is a shorter "farm to table" distance where B12 will remain more present in some capacity. Also growing some of your own plants at home or a t a local garden will be best.

"Vitamin" C

In Europe and parts of Asia, what we call "Vitamin C" is an integral part of many treatments for glaucoma. What we call "Vitamin C" is ascorbic acid, a water-soluble, powerful antioxidant that helps the body form and maintain connective tissues in the body, including within the bones, blood vessels, and skin. Dr. Grossman, O.D., has reported that vitamin c helps to decrease excess fluid production in the body, and increase "blood osmolarity" which allows blood to flow out of the eyes. This is to begin reducing the fluid that impacts the eye and help draw attention to this specific need. Now, we always need this antioxidant in our bodies, but making it a priority will help address this condition more directly. Dr. Grossman recommends 1,500 milligrams a day.

Magnesium

This mineral works to relax the muscles. Doing this while having any eye issues will help reduce additional pressure on the eyes. The smooth muscles within the eyes regulate the flow of the fluid aqueous humor which becomes backed up and contributes to this condition. Having more magnesium in the body can help relax these muscles and allow this fluid to flow out of the eyes according to Dr. Grossman, O.D. He recommends 500 milligrams of magnesium a day.

*Magnesium Sources: avocado, chickpeas, tamarind, basil, dill, ginger, oregano, thyme, any *CBD (cannabidiol) products are helpful. (CBD Oils are almost pure magnesium.), nettle leaf, horsetail, red clover, sage, and nopal.*

*To test the purity of a CBD Oil, send to a lab for testing or you should feel a steady decline in needing to rely on this substance after your need has been met regularly.

Marijuana

The cannabinoids found in marijuana reduce the intraocular pressure within the eyes to help decrease the inflammation. As the intraocular pressure decreases, the less bacteria and fluid will make its way to the eyes. A caution for those with glaucoma is to avoid smoking. Marijuana is most commonly consumed by smoking, but make sure to juice the leaves, mix this herb or infuse into foods and drinks. You may also drink this herb in tea form as well.

Reduce You High Blood Pressure

High blood pressure will not only bring more pressure to the arteries connected to the heart and the extremities but will bring more pressure to your eyes as well. You'll want to manage your stress, reduce your sale intake, increase healthy fats while decreasing unhealthy fats, sugars, and starches, while getting essential minerals your body needs. Becoming more physically active and reducing overall size can significantly help reduce high blood pressure in addition to herbs mentioned in the "High Blood Pressure" section earlier in this book.

Meditation

This remedy is almost always overlooked by doctors, physicians, and even holistic practitioners. Meditation is commonly used to reduce stress which can reduce pressure around the eyes, but breath-focused meditation can help reduce dependence on medications specifically prescribed for glaucoma. Dr. John Hull, M.D., an ophthalmologist and co-director of the Prather-Huff Wellness Center in Sugarland, Texas, states, "The person can often stop using glaucoma Medication, with a doctor's approval."

Dr. Hull recommends the following steps to practice Breath-Focused Meditation:

Sit comfortably in a chair upright and close your eyes. Focus your attention on your abdominal muscles and let them relax.

Take deep breaths through the nose. Allow your breaths to be slow and deep.

Keep your attention on your breath – notice your breath flow in and out.

Do this for five to twenty minutes twice a day.

Finally, as you get use to this routine, place emphasis on imagining fluid travel away from your eyes. Don't squeeze or try to make your body do this; just keep your focus on healing the eyes, knowing what they need which is excess fluid to move back away from clogging the eyes.

Manuka Honey

Manuka honey is produced by bees that pollinate the flowers found on a manuka bush, a kind of tea tree. The form of honey originates from parts of Australia, New Zealand, and Honduras. Traditionally used to heal wounds, sore throats, and to prevent tooth decay. However, this honey has become more commonly known to treat acne, prevent ulcers, and treat eye deficits.

This form of honey is much different from traditional honey as it comes from a different source and provides additional benefits. Manuka honey is an antioxidant, and antibacterial substance. It contains a compound (omega-3 fatty acid) known as, dihydroxyacetone (DHA) which are found in the manuka flowers. DHA increases mitochondrial activity while reducing inflammation in the eyes, helping promote overall eye health. This compound studied by registered dietitian, Bailey Flora, RD, notes the amount of DHA present in manuka honey. Flora states, "it's about 100 times higher than other traditional honey."

There are many ways to use manuka honey for the eyes. Boiling the comb itself in distilled water, using as an eye wash, or as eye drops. Follow directions on label, but typically it is available in eye drop form in which you can place 3-4 drops directly into each eye daily. You should see noticeable changes within or after 4-5 weeks.

Note: like any other honey, manuka honey does contain a high amount of sugar made from fructose and glucose. So, you will want to remain mindful of this if you have diabetes, liver disease, heart disease, or want to avoid consuming excess calories.

My Personal Remedy:

In Traditional Chinese Medicine (TCM) the condition of glaucoma (and many other eye conditions) is linked to the liver. Recommendations are made to promote and increase movement of energy within the liver. The liver is responsible for eliminating and filtering waste from the body, among many other things. There are many things that can help begin to breakdown waste in the liver and promote elimination of these waste materials which help the liver become "unclogged" or helps to increase movement within the liver and help reduce stagnation of fluids in the body, particularly the eyes.

Mix together the following (1oz of each tincture):

Bilberry bark

Eyebright

Dandelion

Milk thistle

Mix all together in a large bottle and drink 1 teaspoon twice a day for 3-6 months.

Gout

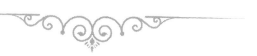

Gout is a very painful form of arthritis (for more information about arthritis, refer to section on Arthritis in this text). Gout involves excess inflammation (in liquid form) but imagine this liquid turning into glass, and then the glass breaking. This is how brittle, stiff, and painful this condition can be. What happens is that small amounts of uric acid (a normal by-product of protein metabolism) begin to turn into small crystals that settle into your joints in your foot; the big toe happens to have the most room and larger joint and is when Gout will form in this toe more often than other areas of the foot. The end result is increased swelling, redness, and pain that can intensify to the point where one cannot walk; this is called Gout.

Remedies:

Cherry Juice (raw)

There's a substance in cherries called "anthocyanocides" that work to lower uric acid levels. It is best to use Wild Cherries or Black Cherries that are seeded. Take a few large handfuls of cherries and begin removing the seeds from all of them. It may help to press down on them to break them apart easily, just be cautious of not losing any juice from the cherries. The seeds are very hard and can damage or get stuck in your blender. After removing the seeds, blend them together with distilled water. Spread out serving but drink full amount each day.

You should aim to eat as many as 70 cherries or about 1-pound of cherries daily. Doing this will help heal the body by reducing symptoms and can help avoid an attack in progress. Dr. Gus Prosch, M.D., a physician in Birmingham, Alabama, USA, notes that, "Old country doctors would tell patients to eat black cherries to stop having gout attacks, and the remedy usually worked." Dr. Jay M. Holder, M.D., D.C., Ph. D., a chiropractor and addiction specialist in Miami, Florida, USA, has stated, "We use this remedy in our clinic, and it works."

Water

Dr. Holder recommends drinking "tremendous amounts of water on a daily basis to flush the uric acid crystals out of your system and dilute the concentration of uric acid." Dr. Holder recommends drinking slightly more than half of your body weight in ounces a day while experiencing gout. You can cut back your consumption of water as your symptoms decrease in severity. Dr. Holder recommends distilled water as well.

Auricular (ear) Therapy

"I don't know of any noninvasive remedy that works as quickly or as well for the pain of gout as ear acupuncture, or auricular therapy" says Dr. Holder. In Traditional Chinese Medicine a person's energy (chi) flows along meridians in the body. when chi is not flowing, particular meridians are in jeopardy and symptoms begin to come to the surface. Acupressure can be achieved by using needles to apply pressure or through the use of fingers applying pressure (acupressure). When you stimulate nerve points, you can unlock the chi energy for particular conditions.

For Auricular Therapy, an electronic stimulator (handheld wand) is used to detect points in your ear where chi is blocked. To use an electronic stimulator/wand, run the wand over your cranial nerve points (research to locate exact areas prior to doing this exercise). When the wand begins to "buzz" apply each point with slight pressure for 30 seconds or until you begin to feel relief. Continue this on other cranial nerve points until you've touched them all.

*Note: you can purchase an electronic stimulator/wand made for the ear for about $150 or more.

Avoid High-Purine Foods

A specific protein located in many foods called purine, turns into uric acid which contributes and triggers gout attacks. Foods such as fish, sardines, mackerel, liver, sweetbreads, gravy, anchovies, asparagus, and too many beans and mushrooms. You want to avoid these items when experiencing gout as they have likely contributed to your condition.

Alcohol

All alcoholic beverages trigger the body to produce uric acid in order to break down these toxic liquids. Beer, wine, and liquor all contain ethyl alcohol, which is the culprit behind uric acid buildup according to Dr. Holder.

Avoid "Pain Relievers"

Over-the-counter pills such as aspirin can inhibit excretion of uric acid and does not do well at fighting inflammation which can make a condition such as gout, worsen.

Grief

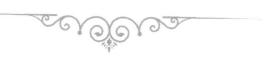

The transition of a loved one can be a difficult emotional experience to navigate through. It is to experience our emotions at this time but work on preparing the body for reducing and releasing the pain in your time of sorrow. If you do not allow your body to feel your emotions, they will be stored in the body as tension, according to Dr. Arthur Samuels, M.D., medical director of the Stress Treatment Center of New Orleans. Tension inevitably plays a role in all physical and emotional disease.

Remedies:

Breathing/Meditation

Meditating on saying goodbye and focusing your intention on holding positive memories, as well as imagining living your life with this person (or people) being present, requires much focus and attention to detail. Many memories will come to your awareness and many racing thoughts. Controlling one part of yourself will help to regain composure and help to works creating balance and harmony within the body. as you inhale and exhale, set your intention on calming your nerves and your thoughts. Imagine opening a space in your body to serve as a filter to allowing your emotions to pass through while transforming these thoughts into loving feelings. Think of the essence you felt when around this person (or people) and commit (even for a short time period) re-creating this feeling for others you encounter as well as breathing in this essence to contribute to helping you heal your pain. At some point, the reality of what happened will settle in and you will be able to practice this more often with ease.

Flower Essences

Flower essences are specifically formulated preparations of specific flowers, created with the intention of healing emotional instability, removing blockages, and regain strength.

"Bleeding Heart" – this flower essence is created to help mend your heart and help process grief and feel closure.

Borage – this remedy helps to feel more uplifted after experiencing sorrow for a consistent amount of time.

Love-Lied-Bleeding – this remedy works to resolve any self-pity. If you feel as though you are a victim and develop "why has this happened to me?" thoughts, this remedy helps to accept this transition and begin to create detachment.

Yerba Santa – unreleased grief stores itself deep within the tissues in the body when it is not processed or released. This can create congestion and respiratory issues. This remedy works to provide relief congestion particularly in the chest.

Cedarwood (essential oil)

This oil help to feel less tense and anxious. Applying and inhaling this essential oil helps the body to ground itself.

Basil (essential oil)

Basil helps to promote concentration which will help serve you well as you want to avoid getting distracted during this time.

Rose Geranium (essential oil)

This common oil helps promote opening the heart chakra and balance the energy in the body.

Cognitive Behavioral Therapy (CBT)

CBT is a therapeutic approach where clients learn to do the following:

- Cope better with difficult life situations
- Positively resolve conflicts in relationships
- Deal with grief more effectively
- Mentally handle emotional stress caused by illness, abuse or physical trauma
- Overcome chronic pain, fatigue and other physical symptoms

The specific steps in Cognitive Behavioral Therapy include:

- Identification of situations or circumstances in your life that lead to trouble

- Awareness of your thoughts and emotions surrounding anger triggers
- Acknowledgement of inaccurate, negative thought patterns
- Relearning of healthier, positive thought patterns

Very few risks are associated with cognitive behavioral therapy, and you will likely explore painful feelings and emotions, but you will do it in a safe, guided manner. Cognitive Behavioral Therapy (CBT) is considered a short-term approach and generally lasts about 10 to 20 sessions depending upon your specific disorder, the severity of your symptoms, the amount of time you've been dealing with symptoms, your rate of progress, your current stress levels, and the amount of support you receive from friends and family. Engaging in CBT will help work to take an assessment of the root of your thoughts to help them dissolve and re-wire your responses to typical triggers, resulting in decreased severity of your expressions.

Psychedelics (caution)

There are various forms of psychedelics which range from mushrooms which contain psilocybin which is the compound found in "magic mushrooms", to *mescaline* which is the active compound in the peyote cactus which is known to produce psychedelic effects. There is still much research to be conducted on psychedelics, so you want to do so under guidance of a shaman or experiences healer. There is evidence of psychedelics working to encourage the growth of new connections between neurons in the brain. This ability of the brain to make new connections is called *plasticity*. Brain plasticity involves the ability of the nervous system to change its activity in response to intrinsic or extrinsic stimuli by reorganizing its structure, functions, or connections, which impact how the brain functions and responds during challenges such as mental health. States such as Oregon and Colorado have allowed psychedelics to be use medically under assisted adult use, where other states such as California, Michigan, Minnesota, Washington, and Massachusetts, have several cities where psychedelics are decriminalized under possession.

Guilt

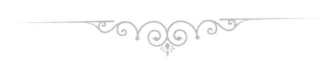

Joan Borysenko, Ph.D., a psychologist and president of Mind/Body Health Sciences in boulder, Colorado, USA states that, "Unhealthy guilt is one of the biggest blocks to healing." Guilt can be a necessary tool in helping to steer yourself in the right direction and help you observe your decision-making. Guilt is your body telling you that you are off track. The goal for eventually overcoming guilt is to release your thoughts and feelings in a way to outgrow this condition so it does not continue to block your growth and creativity.

Remedies:

Consistent Habits

Establishing a routine that you can commit to. This does not have to be every day for the rest of your life but can be minor changes you make that you stick to. Many people feel guilty due to behaviors or what they consume. Start by making a conscious effect to adjust to more beneficial changes for yourself fand others. This may be walking more often or removing a certain food or drink for your lifestyle. It is most important to start somewhere with what you feel you can manage.

Drop The Artificial Sugars

Most "guilt foods" are items that we know are generally unhealthy. Aside from not providing benefits to the body, there are many forms of addictive chemicals in these items. Our brain receptors process what is being consumed, but manufacturers have found creative ways of producing the "happy chemicals" in our brains by finding combinations of ingredients that promote relapsing these natural chemicals through purchasing and consuming their products.

"I believe that people with addictive personalities are sugar-sensitive" says Kathleen DesMaisons. Ph.D., and President and CEO of Radiant Recovery, which is a treatment facility centered around alcoholism, drug addiction, and compulsive behaviors located in Albuquerque, New Mexico, USA.

It is best to remove these artificial sugars from your diet to reduce feelings of guilt when you are eating or drinking. It is easy to eat based off of our emotions so we want to disrupt this from happening so we do not have to process thoughts about it and the after affects which can include weight gain, skin issues, self-doubt, and many others.

Pine (flower essence)

Patricia Kaminski, co-founder and co-director of the Flower Essence Society in Nevada City, California states that Pine flower essence "is the most important remedy for guilt." Kaminski reports that this flower essence help to promote acceptance for self and others.

Mullein (flower essence)

This oil is for those who know they have done something wrong and seek to correct what has happened. This essence helps to come to inner peace about their moral decisions and choices.

Pink Yarrow (flower essence)

Unproductive guilt such as feeling guilty when two other people are mad at one another, or a child who feels guilty due to parents divorcing, pink flower essence is to be used.

Crab Apple (flower essence)

For sexual guilt, this remedy can reduce emotional attachment to these thoughts or feelings. This does not relate to "cheating" and seeking out ways to not feel guilty, but for those who feel impure or those who feel guilty about their sexuality.

Energy Healing

Guilt is associated with feeling that others' needs are more important than your own. Experiencing guilt results in you not as often being able to express what you need to say or do, which creates tension and strain in the throat. To combat this feeling and counteract this pattern of guilt, place your hand (palm down) on the lowest part of your throat (around your collarbone), announce you have something to say, and then say it. Repeat this practice often to release this guilt.

Vetiver (essential oil)

This oil is believed to stabilize the body and promote grounding to help relieve guilt. Vetiver essential oil helps build self-awareness and shift your attention towards self rather than on others. This oil also helps to nourish the kidneys. To use this oil, put one drop over each kidney twice a day. You can inhale this oil when feeling guilty.

*Note: kidneys are located above the waist and about 3 inches from each side of your spine.

Petitgrain (essential oil)

Talking about a situation that created guilt for someone can help to restore the mind and relieve guilt that has remained attached. Place 2-3 drops of this oil in a bath while taking a few moments to process what the guilt is about, and then reach out (or speak out loud to yourself) to speak about the problem that has led to guilt. This oil helps to calm the body to help get the words out that may be difficult to say.

Avoid "Busy" Foods

"Busy" foods are those that are complicated in taste, texture, and/or how they are digested. Carbonated beverages, pickles, citrus foods, vinegar, fermented foods, and refined sugars send a load of signals to and though the body when consumed. Eliminate these items to slow down the signals in the body which will allow less "traffic" being flowed and processed in order to work towards restoring balance and harmony.

Hair Loss

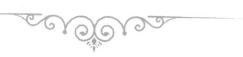

Hair loss is often a hereditary issue that has not been stopped in its tracks until it is too late, or overall appearance is not desirable and is cut off. What only adds to the problem is that most products to prevent hair loss are rip-offs, and most dermatologists often won't work with a person on developing a sound plan on reversing this issue. For men, baldness and hair loss is generally accepted and taken in stride whereas baldness and hair loss in women is often more complicated.

The most common method for addressing hair loss is using the drug Propecia. This drug taken in pill form even has had several research studies reporting results of about 66% effectiveness of reversing and preventing hair loss in men. This drug, (prescribed to me) is also used for prostate issues, works to block the hormone dihydrotestosterone (DHT) which is a by-product of testosterone that shrinks and kill hair follicles. Being able to locate and identify specifically how this drug seeks to prevent hair loss is why it's become to most common "prescription" being recommended by dermatologists and other doctors. What you will learn in this section will involve several natural remedies that work to also block DHT as well as several other substances that damage the hair follicles and their growth.

Remedies:

Batana Oil

The is by far the best remedy for applying directly onto your hair, if you can get it. This oil, native to Honduras, is extracted from the nuts of the American Palm Tree by the indigenous Miskito Indian tribes. Miskito people are commonly referred to as "Tawira" which means "the people of beautiful hair" which they credit to their regular use of batana oil. Traditionally used for hair and skin treatment as this oil is known for rejuvenating hair, repairing damaged hair, clearing out grey or white hairs, promoting hair growth, as well as moisturizing the hair and skin. You can lather on as much as you want (without wasting) directly onto your hair and directly onto your scalp and skin. Let it settle in for about 20-30 minutes and then wash out with warm water a few times a week or as often as your able to.

Saw Palmetto (herb)

As stated in the opening paragraph in this section, this herb works to block DHT. More specifically this herb stops DHT from binding with receptors around the hair follicles to prevent the promotion of hair loss. Take about 160-miligrams, once during the day and once in the evening.

Pygeum and Nettle (herbs)

The herb Pygeum helps to block a substance called 5-alpha-reductase which works to prevent DHT at the source because this substance is what converts testosterone into DHT. Proactively stopping DHT from being produced will avoid any interaction with hair follicles. The herb Nettle is known to enhance the effects of Pygeum. It is recommended to take anywhere from 60 to 500 milligrams a day of Pygeum, along with anywhere from 50 to 100 milligrams of Nettle for best results. Dosage varies due to factors such as height, weight, and gender. Follow instructions on each label.

Zinc

This essential mineral helps cut the activity of 5-alpha-reductase as Pygeum does and helps prevent this substance from interfering with hair follicles it is recommended to take 60 milligrams of zinc daily for 6 months for results.

Common Sources of Zinc: chickpeas, mushrooms, zucchini, squash, okra, Brazil nuts, and walnuts.

*Zinc: 15 milligrams a day within diet is recommended.

Fatty Acids

Fatty acids such as omega-3, omega-6, and omega-9, are crucial for sustaining hair and skin moisture, and promoting hair texture.

Common fatty acid sources: Brazil Nuts, Walnuts, Kola Nuts, Avocados, Bananas, Sea Vegetables (Nori, Wakame, Hijiki, Sea Moss, Bladderwrack), Coconut, Coconut Oil (do not cook), Olive Oil (do not cook), Grapeseed Oil, Black Currant Oil, Avocado Oil, Walnut Oil, Mushrooms, Quinoa, and Wild Rice.

Nettle (herb)

Nettle is one of the oldest recorded remedies used for treating and preventing hair loss. This is primarily due to the high amount of sulfur and silica in nettle, which improves hair health by strengthening the hair shafts. Regularly using nettle when showering can promote hair re-growth and reduce hair loss. Nettle oil is also very effective at relieving a dry, tense scalp, which sometimes contributes to alopecia.

Rosemary Oil

Prevents hair follicles from being starved of a steady blood supply in which they die off prematurely, contributing to hair loss.

Avocado Oil

Massaging avocado oil into your scalp also stimulates blood flow to your hair follicles. Also, good source of healthy fats and fatty acids.

Argan Oil

Is rich in natural phenols (organic compound) that are beneficial to hair follicles. This oil can contribute to hair growth, as well as thicker hair.

Jojoba Oil

Rich in nutrients and capable of moisturizing hair without leaving residue. Helps promote the growth and reproduction of hair cells.

Lavender Oil

In a 2016 study conducted by Moonsung, University in Changwon, Korea, researchers found that, lavender oil applied to lab mice, caused their hair to grow back twice as fast. Their hair also grew back thicker and faster than without the use of lavender oil.

Eucalyptus Oil

Eucalyptus helps to bring down inflammation. Being applied to the scalp, this can bring down inflammation in the scalp and create an ideal environment for promoting hair growth.

Lemongrass Oil

This oil is antibacterial and strengthens hair follicles.

Tea Tree Oil

Helps to unclog hair follicles and nourishes your hair roots.

Avoid Glucose Spikes

Sudden glucose spikes speed up the glycation cycle which process glucose in the body. Advanced glycogen end" ("AGE") is when the body's natural glycogen cycle speeds up which results in symptoms of aging such as greying or white hair, or hair loss. We can easily avoid this first by not consuming carbohydrates by themselves. Carbohydrates break down into sugar already which will send the small intestine into overdrive and will result in spikes of glucose. So, make sure to eat your carbohydrates with other items to help the body process everything. Even healthier items such as dried fruit are high in carbohydrates and should be eaten with other items to avoid glucose spikes. Energy drinks, sugary beverages, and processed foods that contain enriched flours or doughs are to be avoided.

Preventing Hair Loss (For Women)

Much of the research around preventing hair loss and baldness has been studied on male subjects. The remedies mentioned earlier in this section focused on preventing substances such as dihydrotestosterone (DHT) and 5-alpha-reductase, both of which are specific to males due to being centered around testosterone. However, besides blocking substances now known to contribute to hair loss, there are remedies and treatments to consider to begin promoting healthy hair and rejuvenating the scalp to prevent future damage.

Remedies:

Batana Oil

The same information provided in earlier section applies to both, men and women.

Stress Reduction

Constant stress causes the hair follicles to remain at their resting period and decrease its growing potential. Hair is then susceptible to being pulled out easier when brushing or combing your hair, and eventually may grow back at a slower pace, or not at all. In a research study at Harvard University, USA, Dr. Ya-Chieh Hsu, studied underlying mechanisms that link stress and hair loss. Researchers began testing the adrenal glands (where stress hormones are produced) in rodents and found that mild stress increased a chemical called "corticosterone" and reduced hair growth. Researchers also found connections in earlier grey hair as well.

Fenugreek (make your own paste)

Mix ½ teaspoon of fenugreek powder with ¾ cup of unsweetened coconut milk. Whisk together until a paste is formed. Apply this paste gently rubbing it into your scalp. Wrap your scalp with a plastic cap for about 30 minutes and then gently wash out the paste. Do this twice a day for about 2 months to begin seeing noticeable improvements.

Sesame Oil Massage

When stressed, heat in the body collects in the head. Hair roots can become unstable and contribute to hair loss. To keep the skin on the head adequately lubricated, begin rubbing in sesame oil onto the scalp. Take 2-4 teaspoons of sesame oil and dip your fingertips in it as you begin gently massaging the entire scalp. You can do this activity as long as you like but no more than a few minutes but let settle in for about 5 minutes before washing out.

Aromatherapy

A woman named Melanie Von Zabuesnig was diagnosed with alopecia (partial or complete loss of hair) at the age of 7. By the time she turned 32-years-old, this condition had advanced to *alopecia universalis* (total loss of hair, including body hair). Von Zabuesnig began researching how beneficial many essential oils are to hair growth and overall health and began applying her findings by creating her own tinctures and products. She eventually created a formula she applied daily and after several months, she had a full head of soft, new hair where she no longer had to wear a wig.

Von Zabuesnig's Remedy:

Mix the following essential oils in a glass bowl (with wooden utensil, not aluminum):

- 1 tablespoon of Jojoba Oil
- Three drops of Rosemary Oil
- Three drops of Lavender Oil
- One drop of Lemon Balm Oil
- One drop of Atlas Cedarwood Oil

Mix together well and massage mixture into your scalp with your fingertips. Leave on for at least 30 minutes (or overnight). Wash out with shampoo while adding one drop of rosemary oil to each shampoo application. On your final rinse, add one drop of lavender oil and one drop of rosemary oil to a quart of cool water and pour it over your head.

Hangover

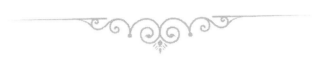

Drinking alcoholic beverages in excess is never recommended due to the many health implications involved. The first of many implications is the combination of a headache, dry mouth, red eyes, and dizziness that we refer to as a *hangover*. Again, drinking in excess is never recommended, but if a hangover or even a partial hangover with less severe symptoms does occur, the remedies in this section will help promote a faster recovery to alleviate this condition.

Note: It is not helpful to use these remedies to begin drinking soon after. If this occurs visit the Substance Abuse and Mental Health Services Administration (SAMHSA) website or use contact below for additional help.

Website: https://www.samhsa.gov/

Phone: 1-800-622-HELP (4357)

TTY: 1-800-487-4889

The National Helpline provides 24-hour free and confidential referrals and information about mental and/or substance use disorders, prevention, treatment, and recovery in English and Spanish.

Remedies:

Bifidus Powder

Bifidus also known as "bifidum" is a helpful form of bacteria that inhabits in the intestines working to fight off harmful bacteria and assists with manufacturing many necessary minerals in the body while helping to promote regular bowel movements. Another benefit of Bifidus powder is that it helps to detoxify a substance known as *acetaldehyde* which is a digestive by-product of alcohol that contributes to many of the symptoms connected to a hangover. Dr. Walter Crinnion, N.D., a naturopathic doctor and director of Healing Naturally in Kirkland,

Washington, USA states that, "The level of acetaldehyde is dramatically lowered when a person takes bifidus after drinking."

Place 1-teaspooon of Bifidus powder in one glass filled with about 10-12 ounces of water and mix together. Drink prior to going to bed after drinking.

Willow Bark (herb)

This herb is a natural pain reliver. It contains a chemical known as *salicylate*, which is an active ingredient in aspirin that's used for headaches. Drink one to two (measuring cups) every 6 hours until you feel better. You can make tea with 2 teaspoons for every 10-12 ounces of water. Make a batch of it in advance if you choose.

Fruit Juice

The fructose sugar in fruits will help burn the alcohol quicker. Juice together a few of your favorite fruits or just an individual fruit and drinks 2-3 glasses a day a few hours in between each glass. Pick fruits high in water content such as melons.

Cucumbers

You can cut into slices to eat, blend together for a quick drink, and even place slices of cucumber on your eyes to relieve any puffiness or soreness in the face. Cucumbers are high in minerals and electrolytes which can help rejuvenate some energy you have to help the body filter out the toxins and avoid feeling fatigued.

Key Lime and Coconut Water

Take 1 key lime and juice it. Mix in well with 10-12 ounces of coconut water. Drink this to promote hydration and absorption of electrolytes that are lost while the body is intoxicated.

*Note: avoid coconut water that comes in an aluminum can or plastic bottle. Get coconut water fresh from the source of a coconut, or in a glass bottle for best results.

Aromatherapy (morning after)

Marjoram is an essential oil to place a drop behind your ear to help reduce headaches.

Frankincense oil helps cool the body to prevent regular sweating. Place one drop of this oil on the skin over your liver (above the upper right side of your abdomen).

My Personal Remedy:

1 handful of Watermelon

2 tablespoons of ginger

2-3 orange slices

3 pieces of cucumber

Blend together and drink twice a day. Increase service size of each and make enough to last for the day. Main purpose of this is to properly hydrate the body upon awakening.

Quick Tips On Avoiding A Hangover:

- Avoid drinking alcohol by consuming water, tea, or other beverage
- Sip slowly. Give the body time to burn off the alcohol (body typically burns alcohol at one ounce per hour).
- Eat first. Drinking after having a full stomach, the body will slow the absorption of alcohol and reduces how quickly alcohol gets to your brain.
- Avoid the "bubbles". Any drink that has bubbles (champagne, rum-and-coke, etc) these bubbles move the alcohol quickly into your bloodstream. The liver attempts to process more at once and the body becomes intoxicated quicker.
- Drink for your size. There's nothing to celebrate about "holding your liquor". A person who weighs 120 pounds should not drink as much as someone who weighs over 200 pounds.

Avoid drinking alcohol in general but follow these steps if you do make this choice. Also, do not make attempts to drink excessively and use these remedies as a "cheat" to avoid symptoms of a hangover. Most likely, you'll only avoid them for a short time period until something more drastic occurs within your body, particularly the liver.

Headaches

A headache can be caused by a variety of reasons. Stress, lack of hydration, irritableness, overthinking, attempting to focus more intensely, and many others. However, many are often born with an untreated deficiency of the natural brain chemical known as serotonin. Serotonin can be depleted in numerous ways such as excessive stress, consumption of processed items filled with chemicals, and lack of direct sunlight. Lack of serotonin in the brain alters the physiology of the blood vessels, which triggers the pain receptors, leading to frequent headaches.

More often than not, medical doctors attribute headaches to being a regular part of our daily lives where they never get treated. "Painkillers" become the norm where the body develops a pain tolerance during this time and eventually relies upon these painkillers, in which the body will experience more severe headaches without the medications and also experience headaches when trying to withdraw from these same medications; this cycle is known as a "rebound headache". We must include more long-term remedies to specifically address the issue while removing that which continues to add to the development of this condition.

Remedies:

Ice

Ice helps to reduce the swollen blood vessels that come from a headache. A reusable ice pack or ice wrapped in a layer of cloth to protect the skin will remain helpful the sooner it is used once a headache begins to form. Apply ice to the head for about 15 minutes followed by a 5-minute break will be helpful without causing damage to the skin.

You may also take one ice cube and place it directly on the back of the neck (above the bone) and let it rest there for a few minutes. Cover ice cube in a towel or cloth and keep it there until there is relief.

Acupressure

The pressure point known as L14 is located between the web of your thumb and forefinger. Applying pressure to this area by using your other hand to gently squeeze both sides of this area in a rhythmic, pumping action will help reduce the severity of your headache.

Note: women who are pregnant should not try this as it can cause premature contractions of the uterus.

Aromatherapy

Begin by diluting an essential oil in water by adding 3-4 drops to a small bowl of water. Dip your fingers in the water and gently massage in the diluted oil onto your temples (side of your head next to your eyes). You may also want to consider dropping in 5-6 drops of your favorite essential oil into a bath.

Deep Breathing

Most headaches are caused by tension. Taking several minutes to take deep breaths can help reduce the tension. Deep breathing can work to calm the body and work towards re-stabilizing itself which is needed when working to alleviating the symptoms associated with a headache.

Do A Body Scan

You can greatly benefit by sitting down for a moment in an upright position, and just focus on resting. Close your eyes and scan the body for tension in other areas that can be contributing to your headache; clenched teeth, clenched fists, hunched shoulders, or any tightness in your chest area are the most common. You can do this while deep breathing also.

Take A Nap

If you're able to take a nap, this can help the body adequately gain some additional rest while limiting how much activity there is in the body so that it can address its needs at this time. When you do wake back up, expect symptoms to initially increase. Use this time to hydrate immediately and eat something easy to digest (preferably fruit) to help maintain the body's functions working in order.

Steam Some Herbs

You can take some herbs such as eucalyptus, oregano, thyme, ginger, and add some lime and elderberry to a pot of boiling water to steam them. The aroma in the air is similar to aromatherapy, but with the added heat to help the steam reach deeper areas of the respiratory system and (potentially) help unclog any areas in need to help promote fuller breaths. You can even take this mixture and drink as a tea twice a day.

Biofeedback

Biofeedback is based on a principle known as "operant conditioning," also known as positive reinforcement. Research has shown positive reinforcement increases the likelihood of a behavior and when a behavior is reinforced repeatedly and consistently over time, the behavior can be learned and retained.

There are three common types of biofeedback therapy:

Thermal biofeedback measures skin temperature.

Electromyography measures muscle tension.

Neurofeedback, or EEG biofeedback focuses on electrical brain activity.

Biofeedback is a method of learning to voluntarily control certain body functions such as heartbeat, blood pressure, and muscle tension with the help of a special machine. This method can help control pain.

During a biofeedback session, your provider places painless sensors on your skin. The sensors measure physiological signals from your body, such as, breathing, heart rate, muscle activity, sweat, muscle movement and tension, using surface electromyography (sEMG), electrical brain activity, using neurofeedback or EEG biofeedback, and skin temperature.

A nearby screen displays the results, which your practitioner will explain. Then your practitioner will suggest strategies to change how your body is functioning. The practitioner may ask you to:

Change how you sit, stand or move: Positioning your body differently may ease muscle tension.

Alter your breathing: Breathing patterns can help calm anxiety.

Release muscles: If you concentrate on relaxing your muscles, it may relieve pain.

Use mindfulness and focus: Thinking about different things can help you control your breathing or slow your heart rate.

Take a test: If you try to solve a math problem or riddle, you can see how stress affects your body's response.

As you try each suggestion, you can watch how it affects the results on the screen in real time. With practice, you can learn to create the same bodily changes without the feedback screen or the practitioner's prompts.

You can search for a local biofeedback practitioner in your area by searching on the following website listed here: www.bcia.org (Biofeedback Certification Institute of America).

White Willow Bark

The bark of the white willow tree contains a natural chemical called, Salicin which is the active ingredient in the common over-the-counter headache relief medication. The bark is taken from the white willow trees that are 2-3 years old.

Dosage(s): Capsules (240mg a day), Liquid/tincture (1-2 milliliter drops a day), Tea (2-3 teaspoon of dried herb to 10-ounces of water).

Arnica (herb)

This herb has many anti-inflammatory properties similar to ibuprofen (Advil). Take this herb and add to boiling water to drink as a tea. Let cool completely and massage gently onto your temples on the sides of your head for relief. Only use about a pea-sized amount to massage onto your temples as too much can cause itchiness or an allergic reaction.

Feverfew (herb)

This herb contains natural compounds known as sesquiterpene lactones which have anti-inflammatory properties similar to aspirin's according to Dr. Alexander Mauskop, M.D., director of the New York Headache Center in New York City. You want to take 125 milligrams daily of this herb in capsule form. Ingredient will be on label but look to make sure the botanical name on the label says Tanacetum parthenium to make sure it's the actual herb and not a knock-off product.

Ginger (herb)

This herb is a "grounding" herb which help the body and mind relax. Put 1 teaspoon of fresh grated ginger into a 16–24-ounce thermos of hot water and sip throughout the day. Don't attempt to finish the drink in one sitting; work to make it last all day by just sipping.

Avoiding Monosodium glutamate (MSG) and Aspartame

MSG is a food additive that has scientifically been proven to trigger migraines. However, this additive dies not always show up as MSG or monosodium glutamate on ingredient labels. Other names that are used instead are, "hydrolyzed protein", "yeast nutrient", or "natural flavoring".

Aspartame (aspartic acid) another artificial sweetener has the same addictive quality as MSG and lead to migraines and headaches.

The following ingredients ALWAYS contain MSG:

Monosodium glutamate, Hydrolyzed protein, Sodium caseinate, Yeast extract, Yeast nutrient, Maltodextrins, Autolyzed yeast, Textured protein, Calcium caseinate, Yeast food, Hydrolyzed oat flour.

The following ingredients OFTEN contain MSG:

Malt extract, Malt flavoring, Bouillon, Barley malt, Broth, Stock, Flavoring(s), Natural flavoring(s), Natural beef flavoring, Natural chicken flavoring, Natural pork flavoring, Food seasonings.

Fiber and Water

Most headaches can be from feeling constipated or dehydration. Dr. David Simon, M.D., medical director of the Chopra Center for Well-Being in La Jolla, California states, "I've been surprised to see that a very high percentage of my patients with migraines are constipated and the improving their regulatory helps reduce their headaches."

You will want to consume properly hydrated (consuming half your bodyweight in ounces of water and increasing intake of fresh water-filled fruits and vegetables) while keeping up with your daily fiber intake (21-25g per day for women, and between 30-38g a day for men).

Common sources of Fiber: garbanzo beans, lentils, brussels sprouts, sweet potatoes, avocado, pears, sunflower seeds, flax seeds, hazelnuts, apples and berries (high pectin fruits) and onions.

Tyramine

The chemical "tyramine" is strongly linked to migraines and headaches according to Dr. Lawrence Robbins, M.D., director of the Robbins Headache Clinic in Northbrook, Illinois.

Common Sources of Tyramine (avoid during headache):

Smoked, cured, aged, and packaged meat, Herring, caviar, and smoked fish, Vinegar, Pickled and fermented foods, Aged cheeses, Products high in yeast (doughnuts, coffee cakes, and breads) Chocolate, Artificial sugars (any sugar not from fruits), Citrus fruits (when consumed in large amounts), Figs, Sour cream and yogurt, Lima beans, navy beans, and peas, MSG, Caffeine, Alcoholic beverages (especially red wine)

Meditation

Slowing down the inner workings of the body will help alleviate the tension that often triggers and contributes to headaches. Simply close your eyes and gently inhale and exhale while remaining observant on your breath.

Laugh

Those who seem to take life very seriously most of the time are often angered very easily and experience stress more often which led to more frequent headaches. Try to find something to laugh about when you have a headache to help reduce the tension in the body, but also seek opportunities to laugh whenever you begin to feel any tightness or tension in the body to avoid having headaches.

Exercise

No specific routines or form or exercise; just get moving. Movement is a great way to release stress and reduce tension in the body.

Stand Tall and Sit Straight

Don't worry, you're not in training for the military by following this recommendation. Standing upright wand sitting straight by avoiding hunching over (or facing down) can reduce the amount of pain in and around your head, neck, and upper back muscles. Pains and aches in these areas often trigger headaches. Work to avoid this by standing tall and sitting straight.

Find A Quiet Space

Use this as a reminder to make time to creating a space to relax to reduce your headache. Constant or loud noises will trigger your headache.

Quick Tips For Menstrual Headaches

Magnesium

Dr. Alexander Mauskop, M.D., director of the New York Headache Center in New York City, reports that about 40-percent of women with migraine headaches during hormonal changes that occur during menstruation, have lowered blood levels of the mineral known as magnesium. 85-percent of women who took a magnesium supplement during this time period during menstruation, reported reduced migraines and immediate relief of headaches. Dr. Mauskop recommends 400 milligrams a day for maximum absorption. You may begin with around 200 milligrams a day and then work up to 400 milligrams a day after about 6-7 days.

*Common Magnesium Sources: avocado, chickpeas, tamarind, basil, dill, ginger, oregano, thyme, any *CBD (cannabidiol) products, nettle leaf, horsetail, red clover, sage, and nopal.*

*CBD oils are almost pure magnesium. To test the purity of CBD oil, send to a lab for testing such as Eurofins Laboratory in Pennsylvania and Texas. To know if it is helpful, you should feel a steady decline in needing to rely upon this substance after this need has been met more often.

Note: You do want to avoid supplemental magnesium due to them promoting and causing diarrhea. You do not want to trade one problem for another one. If you experience some type of diarrhea, it is best to decrease your dosage/intake for a few days until you notice positive changes.

Calcium

Dr. Lawrence Robbins, M.D., director of the Robbins Headache Clinic in Northbrook, Illinois reports that consumption of calcium during menstruation will decrease the frequency of menstruation-caused headaches or migraines. He recommends about 750 milligrams of calcium daily.

Common Calcium sources: sea moss, kale, okra, dandelion greens, turnip greens, lettuce, papaya, and oranges.

Iron

Whenever we bleed, we lose the mineral iron. Iron is the most abundant mineral you will find in the blood. Bleeding a natural part of menstruation. You will want to increase your intake of iron during menstruation to help alleviate symptoms and reduce headaches.

Common Sources of Iron: Wild rice, chickpeas/garbanzo beans, dandelion greens, sarsaparilla, burdock, yellow dock, chapparal, and prunes.

My Personal Remedy:

1 tablespoon of Blue Vervain

2 teaspoons of Valerian

1 teaspoon of Lavender (flowers)

½ teaspoon of African Bird Pepper`1

¼ cup of hemp milk

Mix ingredients together and add to 2-3 cups of boiling water. Let simmer for a few minutes (until hemp milk is mixed in well but not cooked away) and then steep. Drink mixture one to two times a day.

Hearing Loss

Like many health issues, hearing loss can be caused by many issues. Regardless of what may cause your hearing loss, the process is often the same. Over time the nerve cells in the cochlea (organ inside the inner ear that's responsible for hearing) become damaged and destroyed. Similar to many other cells in the body, they can be treated and restored. In this case, when the cells in the inner ear are restored, hearing improves.

Dr. Michael Seidman, M.D., otolaryngologist (ear, nose, and throat specialist) and medical director of the tinnitus center at the Henry Ford Health System in West Bloomfield, Michigan, also works as a researcher. Dr. Seidman's research has involved nutrition and hearing, sponsored by the National Institutes of Health, geared to showing age-related hearing loss that can be slowed and even reversed in rats. Dr. Seidman stated, "In scientific studies, we have treated aging rats with different types of nutrients and improved their hearing by 5 to 10 decibels." In one study, Dr. Seidman tracked the hearing of 18–20-month-old rats until they were 24-26 months old (equivalent of an 80–90-year-old human). During this time period in this study, rats displayed a decline in hearing of 7-10 decibels. When a group of these rats were fed certain nutrients for 6 weeks, their hearing improved by 5-10 decibels, while the rats that weren't fed nutrients, their hearing decrease another 5-10 decibels.

The research Dr. Seidman has highlighted how hearing loss can be improved by focusing on the mitochondria part of the cells. The mitochondria generate the body's fuel. However, as they generate the body's fuel, they also produce pollutants called "free radicals" which damage DNA. The nutrients the rats were given worked to enhance the functioning of the mitochondria. The following nutrients were given to these lab rats:

Acetyl-Carnitine (combination of amino acids)

Alpha-Lipoic Acid (antioxidant0

Coenzyme Q10 (vitamin that carries fatty acids)

Glutathione (enzyme that serves as an antioxidant)

Now, lab rats were used for these research studies. But lab rats are often used prior to human participants in which results must be proven first. The research that Dr. Seidman and his team are conducting are headed towards human participants they have achieved consistent results (they may have already begun). If their human participants achieve similar succeed as these lab rats, their initial hypothesis will carry on. In this scenario, they would have achieved results using chemicals. We then want to recommend natural forms of these substances (ex. promoting regular consumptions of amino acids, antioxidants, and fatty acids).

These items are already widely known to help promote things such as brain health and memory, as well as hearing loss (antioxidants). The challenge (or discovery) is identifying specific amino acids, antioxidants, and fatty acids that are most helpful specifically for hearing loss. This is why Dr. Seidman's studies and research are so crucial for those with this condition.

*Hopefully by the time this book is published, more of Dr. Seidman's research will be promoted and progress has been achieved with these research studies outlined in this section.

Remedies:

Colloidal Silver

In his bestselling book, *The pH Miracle: Balance Your Diet, Reclaim Your Health*, by Dr. Robert O. Young, Ph.D., he states ,"Eye or ear problems, including cataracts, glaucoma, redness, blurred vision, poor eyesight, ringing in the ears, earaches, soreness or swelling of the ears, eardrum damage, hardness of hearing, and (in rare cases) loss of hearing: Use 1 drop of colloidal silver topically (directly in the eye or ear) 3 times a day."

Selective Hearing

We often choose what we hear and give our attention to. People or things we do not want to hear, we essentially muffle our own hearing. Start by asking people close to you, if they feel heard when they speak to you. Their answer can be a key contributing factor towards improving your condition. If no, be more mindful of what they are saying. If yes, try listening closer to help test your hearing. You should find that when you set your intention on listening better, you will hear better as well.

Onion Juice

Use a juicer or blend and strain several medium size or large onions. Take the juice and massage ears with it and/or entire scalp often. Take juice and place into tincture/dropper bottle and put a few drops directly into your ear(s) each day. Do not exceed more than 5 drops per day. Onion juice should be kept in a tight-lid container and will last about 4-5 days in the refrigerator.

Sound Therapy

Do your research around sound therapies that best suit your preferences. You may refer to online resources such as YouTube that have full length videos on combining onion juice and sound therapy together. You can also cut a thin slice of onion and place it in your ear for 20-25 minutes a day and then rinsing your ear (caution on not getting your ear water-logged which can make hearing worse).

Chewing

The jaw muscles that are involved in chewing connect directly to the ears. You will want to chew often when you do eat to create stimulation in this area. Avoid chewing gum which preferences certain teeth. Make sure to chew until t=your food begins to dissolve more often than not.

Iron

In addition to chewing more, you will want blood flow to remain constant and free from obstruction, so getting an adequate amount of iron daily is necessary. Iron transports nutrients. Without enough iron available, necessary nutrients that can be contributing to your hearing loss will continue to not make it to where they are needed.

Common Sources of Iron: Wild rice, chickpeas/garbanzo beans, dandelion greens, sarsaparilla, burdock, yellow dock, chapparal, prunes, raisins, key limes.

*you can eat a few key limes (no more than 3 a day to help increase your iron absorption. Also, you can soak raisins overnight and drink the water for the same purpose.

Heartburn

This condition is actually referred to by doctors as, gastroesophageal reflux. This condition occurs when the valve at the bottom of the esophagus, the tube that leads to the stomach, weakens and results in the stomach acids (reflux) to flow back towards the esophagus, causing a burning sensation to appear near the heart as it pumps, or within the respiratory system near the upper chest or throat. If you experience gastroesophageal reflux disease, you may also experience things such as, a sore throat, coughing, belching, stomach pain, and difficulty swallowing.

Remedies:

Avoid Antacids

"Taking prescription or over-the-counter antacids for months on end for heartburn is crazy" says Richard Leigh, M.D., retired physician in Fort Collins, Colorado. Dr. Leigh notes that "acid indigestion" is actually caused by not generating enough stomach acid to digest food properly. We often run dry of our digestive acids when consuming foods that take longer to digest such as meats, dairy, fried foods, and many processed items made with and assortment of chemicals. Antacids merely tries to mask the root cause of heartburn and eventually add more layers to this condition.

Licorice (herb)

This herb helps to protect the esophagus and help reduce heartburn. This herb can be found in tincture or capsule form or can be used as a tea. There is a specific form of licorice called, "de-glycyrrhizinated licorice" or (DGL) which is a chewable form of this herb. This specific form of licorice has been used as a more effective remedy for treating heartburn without the caution that it can increase blood pressure or lead to developing ulcers as many other remedies can create.

You will want to take DGL (1-2 chewable tablets) three times a day on an empty stomach for best results.

Slippery Elm (herb)

This herb works specifically to reduce acid indigestion while healing the mucous membranes that get damaged or injured from acid reflux. Dr. Pamela Jeanne, N.D., naturopathic doctor in Gresham, Oregon states, slippery elm is a wonderful herb that helps relieve the symptoms of acid indigestion" and recommends taking one capsule of this herb before each meal for best results.

Cayenne Pepper

Take ½ teaspoon of cayenne pepper (powder) and mix it in with a bottle of water. Do not drink excessively but can consume often. Wait at least 30-45 minutes to eat after drinking this to avoid congestion.

Quick Tip: if you feel symptoms of a heart attack coming on, you can consume this same mixture to help reduce some of the symptoms and (hopefully) the heart attack itself.

Sleep (correctly)

Go to sleep on your left side. The left side of your body is where your digestive track rests. If you sleep on your right side, your intestines will "hang" and cause discomfort in addition to slowing down the digestive process, leaving waste materials in the gut which can continue to acid indigestion. This places a strain on your heart also as compared to laying down on your left side in which the heart can rest more easily. It will remain best to sleep on your left side comfortably to help reduce your current symptoms, as well as contribute to improving your sleep where the body naturally works to heal the body.

Common Steps To Avoid Heartburn

No larger than necessary meals. Eating a lot causes the body to produce more acid to breakdown the food. Eat meals necessary for your need. Focus on quality foods that provide adequate nourishment over quantity.

Don't eat soon before bedtime. The body will have difficulty digesting items while also trying to sleep. Laying down after eating will make it easier for stomach acids responsible for digesting food flow towards the esophagus and contribute to your symptoms. Try to eat at least 3-4 hours before you lay down to sleep.

Avoid high fat foods. Consuming fat causes the body to produce a hormone called leptin which weakens the esophageal valve, letting in additional acid into the esophagus.

Avoid coffee. Whether caffeinated or decaffeinated, coffee creates instability within the blood flow in the body. This increases stomach acid production (in addition to other liquid substances).

Cut out chocolate. The amount of fat, sugar, and other ingredients in chocolate ill trigger painful heartburn.

Avoid carbonated beverages. Sodas, beer, and even citrus fruits and items such as tomatoes should be avoided until heartburn is not an issue.

Remain cautious with spicy foods. Although items like cayenne pepper and ginger can be helpful, they can pose an issue when heartburn is present by producing excess acid in the body.

No "nightcaps" or alcohol. Alcohol will increase acid production in the body, but drinking alcohol shortly before going to sleep will almost guarantee a heartburn episode.

Stop Smoking. Smoking weakens the esophageal muscles which allows access for acids to pour into the esophagus.

Avoid specific herbs such as spearmint and peppermint. These herbs typically used to breathe easier, actually loosen the esophageal valve.

Avoid tight-fitting belts and clothing. These can create additional pressure on the body and worsen heartburn symptoms.

Reduce body size. Being 10% - 20% over your ideal body weight places you at a much greater risk for heartburn.

No dairy. Drinking cow's milk is a common remedy promoted to soothe heartburn. Although this substance may feel good, it does not reach the core issue. Cow's milk contains fats, proteins, and calcium which all stimulate the stomach to secrete acid and will prolong your heartburn.

Heart Disease

1 in four people die of heart disease. 2 out of 4 experience symptoms of heart disease. 4 out of 4 most likely know someone who has a heart disease. This is not a small issue or something we are not aware of. The most common formula for creating heart disease is often years of eating high-fat, low-fiber, overprocessed, nutrient-poor foods and beverages, not exercising regularly, and experiencing constant stress. The more these unhealthy habits are present, the less oxygen-carrying blood can get by, leading to heart disease(s).

Remedies:

Exercise (Find What's Needed For You)

Regular exercise helps to control weight, but more importantly exercise helps bring down high blood pressure, lowers blood sugar, and helps to increase the HDL (high-density lipoprotein) cholesterol ("good cholesterol") in the body. According to Dr. Stephen Sinatra, M.D., cardiologist and director of the New England Heart Center in Manchester, Connecticut, all of these factors listed above are the most important factors to preventing and reversing heart disease. This being said, any increased movement will help benefit the heart.

There are many forms of exercise one can do. It is best to identify first any specific recommendations your doctor can make. This is important because your doctor may recommend certain forms of exercise that you do not like that can be the most beneficial to you. We often do not do things we don't like or enjoy, so hearing this from someone else can help give us the kick-start we may need rather than only doing exercises that we enjoy. Next, is identifying exercises you enjoy and incorporating them as much as possible, as long as it does not involve any strenuous activity.

You can also make many minor adjustments that add up over time. Next time you go to the mall or office, don't choose to closest spot to the door and take the stairs instead of the elevator. Walk across the room to change the channel instead of using the remote control and try to go for a walk as often as possible. All of these activities do add up and your heart will be thankful whenever you take the time to do any of these.

Note: maximum heart rate can be at or around 150 beats per minute. When exercising (especially for heart-related issues) you want your heart rate to be around 70%; about 105 beats per minute.

Foods (Only Eat What Comes From The Ground)

Kitty Gurkin Rosat, R.D., registered dietician and nutrition director of the Rice Diet Program at Duke University in Durham, North Carolina has stated, "If we would eat only foods that were just picked, I would need to find a new profession." Foods such as fruits, vegetables, grains, and beans, are al low in saturated fats which are known to cause considerate damage to the heart, in addition to heart-healing fiber, and many essential minerals the heart needs to remain in good health.

Vitamin-E

This is an antioxidant that works to stop free radicals (unstable atoms that can damage cells) from damaging the cells particularly in the heart. Vitamin E helps to process fats and work to avoid damage within the lining of the arteries which contributes to heart disease. Dr. Michael Janson, M.D., consultant physician at Path to Health in Burlington, Massachusetts recommends 400-800 international units of vitamin e daily to protect the arteries.

What we refer to as Vitamin E (tocopherol) is actually a fat-soluble nutrient that is important to vision, reproduction, and the health of your blood, brain, and skin. This nutrient is found in abundance in bell peppers (particularly red bell peppers), walnuts, leafy green vegetables, mangos, and avocados. Working these into your lifestyle more often will allow the body to properly recognize and absorb key nutrients, especially blood and oxygen. "Vitamin-E" helps to increase the body's receptors and help stop the formation of blood clots.

Natural Sources of Vitamin E: red bell peppers, mangoes, walnuts, sunflower seeds (non-processed), avocados, butternut squash, olive oil (for dressings), coconut oil, and avocado oil.

Magnesium

This essential mineral helps to relax the blood vessels, improve circulation, and help lower blood pressure; all critically important to reversing and healing from heart disease.

Natural Sources of Magnesium: avocado, chickpeas, tamarind, basil, dill, ginger, oregano, thyme, any *CBD (cannabidiol) products are helpful. (CBD Oils are almost pure magnesium), nettle leaf, horsetail, red clover, sage, and nopal.

*To test the purity of a CBD Oil, send to a lab for testing or you should feel a steady decline in needing to rely on this substance after your need has been met regularly.

Qigong

Many qigong exercises used in Traditional Chinese Medicine (TCM) help benefit the heart as the body practices, controlled movement with controlled breathing. The practice of Qigong is to provide balance and restoration to the body's life force ("chi") and work to target the blocked chi to help begin restoring balance within the body. the following Qigong exercise specifically targets the heart area:

Place your right palm on the left side of your chest and massage slowly in a clockwise circle. Do this at least once a day for as long as you like. Make sure to match your slowed breath with your hand movement to help calm the heart area.

Yoga

The practice of yoga has far more benefits than can be listed here. There are specific yoga poses and stretches that help focus more on the heart than others. For example, the chest expansion pose helps to promote circulation in and around the heart muscles. For this pose do the following:

Clasp together your hands and slowly stretch your arms upwards.

Keeping your hands clasped, stretch your hands behind you as you gently arch your back.

Hold the stretch for about 5 seconds

Slowly bend forward, dropping your head and stretching your arms downwards for about 10 seconds.

Stand upright, relax your arms on your sides and repeat when ready. Do this a few times daily until you feel completely relaxed. Do not continue if you feel dizzy or lightheaded.

Aromatherapy

Jane Buckle, R.N., nurse and aromatherapist in Albany, New York recommends several essential oils specifically for heart disease. Jane strongly recommends the following essential oils: sweet marjoram, lavender, neroli, or damask rose. Jane believes that damask rose is mostly beneficial for those who have experienced a heart attack.

To use these oils, follow the steps listed below:

Place a few drops of essential oil in a warm bath before soaking for at least 10-15 minutes. Place a few drops onto a cotton ball and place it next to your pillow while you sleep.

Add a few drops to any massage oil prior to receiving a massage.

*Caution: those with heart disease should avoid peppermint oil as it can cause heart palpitations, particularly those who take pharmaceutical prescriptions for heart disease.

Cayenne Pepper (herb)

Cayenne pepper is an herb to mix into your meals as often as possible. In addition to adding to meals, you can take ½ teaspoon of cayenne pepper (powder) and mix it in with a bottle of water. Do not drink excessively but can consume often. Wait at least 30-45 minutes to eat after drinking this to avoid congestion.

Ginger and Clove Tea (herbs)

Take 1tsp of ginger powder (or about ½ fingertip size of fresh ginger) and 1/2 tsp of cloves or clove powder. Mix together with boiling water or mix thoroughly with warm water.

Mugwort Tea (herb)

Take 1.5 teaspoons of this herb and place it in a pot of boiling water (2-3 cups of water). Let steep and drink once a day.

Astragalus Root (herb)

This herb helps improve metabolism and hormonal balances that often interfere with sleep that often contribute to heart disease.

Follow dosage directions on product labels. The recommended dose for a standardized extract is 250 – 500 mg, three to four times a day standardized to 0.4% 4-hydroxy-3-methoxy isoflavone 7-sug. When making tea, boil three to six grams of dried root per 12 ounces of water three times a day. You can get a tincture of astragalus in 30 percent ethanol. The recommended dose is 20 to 60 drops three times a day.

My Personal Remedies:

1 cap of olive oil, 1 cap of key lime (or lime) juice, and spring water.

We want to avoid consuming any oils directly, so it is best to not consume any fried or oily foods and eat mostly raw when doing this. You want to do one step at a time. Consume 1 capful or olive oil, then consume 1 capful of key lime (or lime) juice and wash it down with spring water. Give yourself sometime after drinking this before eating or drinking to allow these ingredients to help clear any congestion or tightness.

Mono-Fasting

Mon-fasting is a fasting routine where one only consumes a limited number of items when they do eat. Spend most or part of the day fasting, and then eating one item every few days. You can eat just apples for a few days, then consume only grapes for a few days, and may want to have just melons for a few days. There's no specific timelines or amounts, but you want to just consume one item at a time. Have as much as you want, but only one every few days.

Food best for mono-fasting (for heartburn): melons, grapes, apples. Try to avoid the very acidic fruits such as citrus fruits for now until you are used to mono-fasting and/or your symptoms significantly decrease.

If you are looking for any specific Fasting routines or recipes, you may reference my book entitled, *Fasting: A Guide To Health and Wellness.*

Heat Exhaustion

When you are becoming low on fluids needed to keep your cool, your body will experience heat exhaustion. Heat exhaustion at its core is when your vital organs are not getting enough blood. The blood transports oxygen and hydrogen together in the form of water (H2O). So, you do not necessarily need cold or cool liquids to remain cool but need enough liquids in the body to help promote proper blood circulation. The body is mostly liquids that come in many forms. We have water, blood, lymphatic fluids (in the form of waste), saliva, semen, sweat, vaginal fluid, and mucus, among others. When the body begins to run low on several of these (or severely low on one) its response is to send receptors in the form of blood cells all around the body on a "wild-goose chase" as they attempt to locate and fill what's become deficient without the proper materials and causes the body's temperature to rise and overheating.

The body overheating and being exhausted from heat are not the same. The body will overheat (meaning above its normal temperature of 98.6°F) from anything involving physical labor to overeating. This involves a short-term process that does not severely hinder the body's ability to function. Heat exhaustion is when the body becomes overheated for an extended period of time where the body begins to lose its ability to function as it normally would with presenting symptoms such as, impaired thinking, slurred speech, headache, dizziness, irritability, and overall weakness in the body.

One thing to take note of is that simply drinking water will not solve the symptoms of heat exhaustion nor the potential long-term effects. Preventing heat exhaustion involves consuming plenty of fluids regularly, make sure you're in a cooler area when exercising inside or outdoors, wearing loose-fitting clothes whenever possible, and incorporating more holistic remedies to supplement the most common steps already listed.

Remedies:

Proper Hydration

Not only drinking about half of your body weight in ounces (ex. if you weigh 100lbs, drink 50oz) but consuming foods that provide water is necessary. Melons, berries, tomatoes, and cucumbers are only a few items that should regularly be in your diet. Consuming items that provide hydration can help wash away and also neutralize the erosive acids that remain in the body from eating things detrimental to our health.

Exercise In A Cooler Area

Whether you're inside or outdoors, you want to avoid the hotter areas when exercising. Not only does this contribute to symptoms of heat exhaustion but can become uncomfortable and even hinder your ability to complete your exercise regimen and help you achieve desired results. You want to move away from any windows or sunnier areas while indoors and work-out in a shaded or partly shaded area when outdoors when you can.

Loose-fitting Clothing

Especially if you will be outside for a considerable amount of time, you want to wear loose-fitting clothing. Allowing your body to feel and absorb any wind or cool air while outdoors can be enough for you to avoid heat exhaustion. Clothing does not necessarily have to feel baggy or extremely loose; the main goal is to avoid any tight-fitted clothes as they can and will block or restrict air flow.

Wearing a shirt can help avoid absorbing as much radiation from the sun when experiencing this issue often. We absorb more when our shirts are off, especially when we do not have a tolerance for increased sun exposure (those from colder climates, or genetically). A shirt can provide protection when needed. However, if you perspire while wearing a shirt, the dried salt from your sweat can impair the breathing quality of your shirt. You want to change and/or wash this shirt as soon as possible if you perspire heavily onto your shirt.

Cotton/Polyester Blend Shirts, Linen, or Hemp Are Best

These types of clothing provide the most "breathability" among shirts as opposed to nylon and other similar materials.

Lemon Balm (herb)

This herb is naturally soothing but can help cool the body more so than many other herbs. Use ¼ cup of dried herb to 1 quart of boiled water. Steep for 30-minutes to 1-hour, strain, and put in the refrigerator until it is cool. Drink this once a day whenever you will be in warmer areas or are feeling hot.

Flower Essence (St. John's Wort)

This herb helps considerably with conditions involving skin sensitivity, as well as many conditions that are related to darkness and light. If you are someone who is sensitive to the sunlight or regularly experience symptoms of heat exhaustion, this herb will be very helpful. Take 4 drops of St. John's Wort flower essence per day for at least a month to test how helpful it is for you. You can take this flower essence for several months until your sensitivity improves.

Avoid Salt Tablets

When we sweat, we also lose electrolytes such as potassium and sodium. To replace sodium, many believe you can take a salt tablet to help offset some of the symptoms. This is not true, and actually makes the condition much worse. The increased salt in the stomach from taking a salt tablet that has to be digested, keeps fluids in the stomach longer from digesting, and interferes with the body being able to send fluids to other areas of the body. Do not take any salt tablets if you are feeling or experiencing any symptoms of heat exhaustion.

You can use a more natural option such as Celtic Salt instead.

Avoid Alcohol

Alcohol fast forwards dehydration. Damages the liver and impact the body's ability to hold onto liquids as the body will respond by wanting to expel liquids due to alcohol making its way to the bloodstream.

Avoid Caffeine and Smoking

Similar to alcohol, caffeine speeds up dehydration where you sweat more than normal. Smoking constricts the blood vessels in the body and impairs your ability to remain in the heat.

Acclimate Yourself

Do not become a person who spends their day relaxing in an air-conditioned space and then go outside for an extended period of time right after. You want to be more in between these two than not. If you use an air-conditioner, you want to acclimate yourself outdoors for smaller amounts of time to help build up your tolerance before staying outside for a long time to help avoid symptoms of heat exhaustion.

Heat Rash

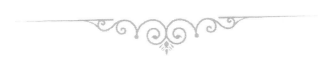

When sweat becomes stuck within the pours and spreads to the surrounding areas and irritating it, you have a rash; when caused solely by the heat, you have a heat rash. A heat rash will appear as small bumps similar to a blister that are itchy and easily irritated. The average heat rash should go away after a few days to a week without doing much, but there are several remedies to apply to reduce the severity of this condition and to make sure it does not last longer than needed.

Remedies:

Herbal Bath

Taking a cool bath with herbs can be very beneficial to healing from a heat rash. Wrap a cup or two of fresh herb leaves (preferably Sandalwood, Comfrey, Coriander, Stinging Nettle, or Neem) in a cheesecloth and fill your tub with cool water. Immerse the herbs wrapped in the cheesecloth in the water for at least 5 minutes. Take the soaked herbs and place onto rash to soak for 5-1 minutes. Repeat as often as necessary until noticeable improvements are achieved.

Calendula (herb)

It is best to find a water-based gel form of this herb. Avoid the ointment or cream as it contains many chemicals that can make the rash worse. Ointments and creams also cover the area and block the air flow which will prolong healing. Take the water-based gel of this herb to apply to the rash. Follow instructions as listed on product package.

Lavender Essential Oil

This essential oil works to regenerate skin cells and skin tissues. apply 1 to 2 drops of lavender oil directly onto the rash and gently rub in. Do these 3 to 4 times a day. You can mis this essential oil with calendula gel as well.

Watermelon (rind)

Using the rind of the watermelon by rubbing it directly onto the skin can help provide necessary moisture and nutrients needed to heal the affected area. You may place it on directly or cut and blend the rind up and make a compress you can keep on the rash.

Myrrh Oil

In test-tube studies, myrrh oil has strong effects against several infectious bacteria, including some drug-resistant ones. Traditional uses of myrrh include treating skin wounds and infections. A test-tube study on 247 different essential oil combinations found that myrrh oil mixed with sandalwood oil was especially effective at killing microbes that infect skin wounds.

Additionally, in one test-tube study, myrrh oil alone inhibited 43–61% of the growth of five fungi that cause skin conditions, including ringworm and athlete's foot.

Myrrh oil contains compounds that interact with opioid receptors and tell your brain you're not in pain. Myrrh also blocks the production of inflammatory chemicals that can lead to swelling and pain.

Sunscreen: One test-tube study found that SPF 15 sunscreen with added myrrh oil was significantly more effective at blocking ultraviolet rays than the sunscreen alone.

Topical Use:

Due to the risk of skin irritation, it's best to dilute myrrh oil in a carrier oil, such as jojoba, grapeseed, or coconut oil. This also helps prevent the myrrh oil from evaporating too quickly.

In general, use 3–6 drops of essential oil per 1 teaspoon (5 ml) of carrier oil for adults. This is considered a 2–4% dilution.

For children, use 1 drop of essential oil per 1 teaspoon (5 ml) of carrier oil, which is a 1% dilution.

You can also add a drop or two of myrrh oil to unscented lotion or moisturizer before you apply it to your skin. Some people add myrrh oil to products used for massage. Avoid applying the oil to sensitive areas, including your eyes and inner ears. Wash your hands with soapy water after handling essential oils to avoid accidental exposure to delicate areas.

Inhaling

You can add 3–4 drops of myrrh oil to a diffuser to distribute the oil as a fine mist into the surrounding air.

If you don't have a diffuser, you can simply place a few drops of the oil on a tissue or cloth and inhale periodically or add a few drops to hot water and inhale the steam.

Quick Tip: apply a few drops of myrrh oil to the cardboard tube inside a roll of toilet paper. When someone uses it, a bit of the aroma will be released.

Heel Pain

Heel pain is caused by constant support and repetitive use when not needed. Sometimes we walk heel to toe with too much pressure paced upon our heels as compared to the rest of our foot. Other

Remedies:

Boswellia (herb)

This herb will help relieve inflammation in the heel and decrease the pain and soreness. Follow instruction on product label for best results as dosage and use can vary. Do not take if pregnant or breastfeeding.

Stretch Your Calf Muscles

Tight calf muscles can be a hidden cause of heel pain. If the calves are tight and cannot absorb the constant pounding of running or frequent walking, the shock goes straight to the heels.

Elevate Your Legs

Although it may feel nice to sit back in a reclining chair or couch, blood flow may rest in your heels and make your heel pain worse. Take 5 minutes a day where you lay down flat on your back with your legs straight up against the wall or flat surface. Your legs do not have to be completely against the wall, but your feet should rest comfortably against the wall. Allow the blood flow in your legs to work away from your heels (and feet altogether) to help reduce the pain and inflammation.

Hemorrhoids

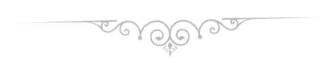

Hemorrhoids are swollen veins in and around the anus. 8 out of 10 adults experience hemorrhoids at one time or another. Similar to varicose veins, hemorrhoids occur when there's additional pressure on the blood vessels. The most common cause of hemorrhoids is a low-fiber diet which creates harder stools in addition to inadequate hydration.

Remedies:

Create Soft Bowel Movements

Straining yourself while on the toilet increases the pressure on the blood vessels located in and around the anus. The veins in the rectum are likely to swell in your rectum. Hard or difficult stools become damaging as they can tear the skin, irritate the area, and add to the pressure. Follow the simple steps listed below to help work past (and avoid) this condition:

Hydration

Drink plenty of liquids while regularly consuming items high in water content such as fresh fruits and vegetables; particularly berries, melons, and leafy green vegetables. If these are already a staple in your lifestyle, increase your intake immediately until relief is achieved.

Fiber

Load up on your fiber. Fiber helps break down your stools and works with the water in your body to soften them as well. You want to fall within the normal range daily at minimum which is between 21-25g per day for women, and between 30-38g a day for men as recommended by the American Dietary Association. This may sound like a lot but, ½ cup of leafy green vegetables can provide about 5g, a small apple is about 3g, and consuming grains like quinoa can provide up to 8g per cup. Just these three items together and you are almost at your daily recommended amount in addition to any other foods you consume that have fiber.

Common sources of Fiber: garbanzo beans, lentils, brussels sprouts, sweet potatoes, avocado, pears, sunflower seeds, flax seeds, hazelnuts, apples and berries (high pectin fruits) and onions.

Soak In The Tub

You will want to soak the area to help clean out (without scrubbing) any bacteria while allowing the area to rest. You want to lay down in the tub while keeping your knees up (feet flat on the tub floor). Warm water is best as it helps reduce the pain while increasing blood flow to the area which works internally to clean out waste materials that create this condition and help shrink the swollen veins.

Don't Scratch

Scratching will make this condition worse by irritating it. When you wash yourself, you want to be as gentle as possible when cleaning this area and avoid using many of your typical cleaning product which may contain many harmful chemicals.

Avoid Heavy Lifting

This does not just refer to exercise and weightlifting. There's not a specific amount of weight to avoid, but whenever we have to strain our bodies to move something, the veins in this area will flare up. It may happen with something that weighs as little as 10lbs. Outside of your typical routine, you want to avoid any heavy lifting that would be difficult to hold or do for more than a few minutes. This may mean making extra trips to your car as you move groceries into your home; unless you have to walk up many stairs in which you should get some assistance and/or plan to make several trips where you take your time. Do not do more than absolutely necessary to complete this step.

Witch Hazel

Using a dab of witch hazel applied to the rectum with a cotton ball can help alleviate external hemorrhoids; if you have internal hemorrhoids, do not attempt to place witch hazel inside your rectum as the side effects can be detrimental to your overall health). Press the cotton ball gently to the area, even if there's minor bleeding. For best results, chill a bottle of witch hazel by placing it in an ice bucket or refrigerator. Soak a cotton ball in the chilled witch hazel and apply to area until the cotton ball is no longer cold.

Stoneroot "Collinsonia" (herb)

This herb helps strengthen the structure and function of the veins in the body by shrinking any swollen veins; particularly helpful to conditions such as hemorrhoids. Take two 375mg capsules twice a day with a 12-ounce glass of water. You also want to drink water in between each meal to help the body properly absorb this herb.

Butcher's Broom (herb)

This herb helps to shrink swollen hemorrhoids. For this herb you want to make an ointment to apply to area. Using a spoon, mix 10-15 drops of butcher's broom tincture (or powder from 5-6 capsules that are 100-200mg in size) into a container of manuka honey (about ¼ cup). Mix well together and apply generously to the area. You may use this as often as necessary, but you do want to gently wash off when you have to begin moving around again. It is also helpful to drink butcher's broom tea during this same time. pour 1 cup of boiling water over ½ teaspoon of the herb and then steeping for about 10 minutes. Strain the herb out and enjoy up to four times a day.

Control Your Salt Intake (and your overall weight)

Excess sodium retains fluids and prevents them from providing relief. A person who is overweight will have more pressure on their lower extremities and in turn, have more complications when dealing with hemorrhoids.

"Donut Pillow"

You've probably seen these pillows on a TV show or given to an older person who has suffered some sort of lower back or hip injury. You will want to get one of these pillows when sitting to provide relief while sitting. Sitting down without it will place an enormous amount of stress and pressure to the area, especially when you move around.

ClenZone

This is an appliance that attaches to your toilet seat and squirts a thin stream of water into your rectum after each bowel movement. Works to serve as a soothing agent while experiencing hemorrhoids.

Herpes Virus

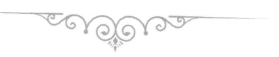

**When it's less than 0.9 they are negative (HSV 1).
HSV2 was measured on a diff scale which is why there's a star next to it.
That's the scale number. HSV1 was what they had and do not have anymore in testing.

Herpes is defined as "a viral disease caused by the herpes simplex virus, affecting the skin (often with blisters) or the nervous system." There are two types of herpes simplex viruses: HSV-1 (Herpes) and HSV-2 (Herpes Type 2). HSV-1 more commonly causes oral infections, while HSV-2 more commonly causes genital infections.

Herpes is generally regarded by the medical establishment as incurable. As such, individuals affected with herpes deal with bouts of recurrences at regular individuals, as medicines or prescriptions given usually suppress the symptoms only for a while. Outbreaks and flareups can involve blisters, irritating skin, fever, scabs, and swollen areas around the genitals and armpits. These flare-ups can last about 7-11 days at a time and vary with severity.

There are however alternate ways of ridding the body of both types of herpes – through the use or herbs, fasting and diet.

To rid the system of herpes, one must take a total approach to heal the body. The quick fix approaches usually don't work. A central nervous system detoxification process is needed for this condition (as identified with remedies listed earlier in this section and in the next section). This process helps to modulate (and turn off) the RNA replication of the virus within our body's system(s). "RNA" refers to what's called "ribonucleic acid" which is present in all living cells. Its role is to become an active messenger that carries instructions from DNA throughout the rest of the body. DNA carries our genetic information. What happens with a virus like herpes is that RNA begins to carry the genetic information, and this keeps the virus alive as the body continues to replicate cells. Turning off this mechanism, allows your body to avoid this and promote a faster recovery when working to reverse this condition.

Remedies (for reducing flare-ups):

Arginine

This is an amino acid that encourages the herpes virus. This amino acid triggers symptoms and can prolong flare-ups. It is best to avoid altogether, but just before or during a flare-up, completely avoid items high in arginine which include, brown rice, whole what products, carob, corn, dairy, oatmeal, chocolate, raisins, nuts, and seeds.

Olive Leaf Extract

James Privitera, M.D., who is an allergy and nutrition specialist in Covina, California, states that, "The (olive leaf) extract gets rid of lesions and helps prevent them from coming back". Olive leaf extract can be taken daily and can work to reduce future flare-ups by working to support the immune system's function. Extract may be available in tincture form or tablet form. If an outbreak-flare-up occurs, it is recommended to take five 500 milligram tablets a day for three weeks. If using a tincture, follow recommendations listed on label.

Water

When the body is not properly hydrated during a flare-up, the body is less likely to flush out toxins that bind with weak immune system cells and can prolong flare-ups and severity of symptoms. Binding with weak immune system cells, essentially allows this virus to re-activate. Drinking the recommended amount of half of your bodyweight in ounces will remain a priority for this condition

Reishi Mushroom

These mushrooms contain an abundant number of antiviral properties that can reduce the frequency and severity of flare-ups and outbreaks. Dr. Janet Zand, O.M.D., licensed acupuncturist and doctor of Oriental medicine, from Austin, Texas, recommends taking 350-500 milligram capsule 1-2 times a day to combat lesions from forming and breakouts from occurring.

Avoid Ointments and Skin Products

Due to having flare-ups, many choose to use ointments and skin care products to alleviate symptoms or just to cover up the area to give the appearance of smooth skin. However, things like petroleum jelly and antibiotic ointments actually block air from flowing in and impairs the healing process.

Note: it is strongly encouraged to NEVER use a cortisone cream as it will inhibit your immune system and help this virus grow stronger.

Wear Loose-fitting Clothing

We need to provide adequate opportunities for the skin to breathe. When a condition involves lesions or blisters, we must allow the skin to breathe even more. This includes wearing minimal clothing when at home and avoiding any tightly stitched or synthetic materials. Cotton is a common source of clothing to wear, from t-shirts to underwear to allow air flow to go to and through areas of the body.

Avoid Touching

This condition can spread to other areas of your body by simply touching an open sore and then touching an area like your mouth or rubbing your eyes, for instance. If you are likely to scratch or itch while sleeping, wearing loose-fitting gloves or covering your sores with gauze will provide additional protection to avoid spreading this virus.

Ask Questions:

Contact the National Herpes Hotline at 919-361-8488 Monday-Friday from 9am-7pm (Eastern Time)

Or STD hotline at 1-800-227-8922 available 24 hours a day, 7 days a week.

You may email ASHA (American Sexual Health Association) at herpesnet.@ashastd.org

How To Treat Herpes Holistically:

These are some herbs used to treat herpes.

Elder Flower, Pau d'Arco, Burdock Root, Contribo (Birthwort/Duck Flower), Olive Leaf, Red Clover, Sarsaparilla, Oregano Oil, Chaparral, Oregon Grape, Dandelion, Yellowdock, Sage

ALL methods to be completed concurrently and continuously. Do not necessarily have to go in order but should be the new foundation for lifestyle until condition is no longer present.

Method 1: Healing The Restrictive Way

Step 1: Cleaning up the system

Detoxifying the system is important to ridding the body of maladies. First, we start by cleaning out the colon (bowels).

Colon cleanse: use the following herbs (Cascara Sagrada, Black Walnut, Rhubarb Root, Prodijiosa, and Pao Pereira)

If you can't buy these u can make your own colon cleanse. Any good colon cleanse recipe should help.

Apple, Onion, Colon cleanse Recipe

1 Apple

1 Large Onion

1 Handful of Pectin (The white part of the citrus. When you peel an orange or lime, that white part you see)

Direction: Blend together with water.

Dosage: Eat about 3 to 4 oz in the morning.

Step 2: Further cleanse to the organs of the body

The Viento (Sapo, Contribo, Chapparal, Valerian, Sea Moss, Hombre Grande) is included in Dr Sebi's small cleansing package because it helps to clean the body at a cellular level. You can make your own Viento formula w/these herbs. One can however go straight to step 3.

Step 3: Clean and nourish the blood

Sarsaprilla, Burdock, Guaco along with Sea Moss and Bladderwrack will help to cleanse the blood, improve circulation to the body and nourish the cells. As noted, you can buy or make your own – it is very easy to do this.

Dosage: Take the herbs as directed.

During this process the diet should be very light, consisting of only alkalizing foods, primarily fruits and vegetables. Follow Dr Sebi's nutritional guide, however, some items on the list should not be consumed when one is trying to reverse serious health conditions.

Things on the list to eat and focus on: Fruits, greens such as lettuce, dandelion greens, mustard greens, amaranth greens and lettuce, mushrooms, vegetables, coconut (water and jelly) herbal teas, green juices and smoothies.

Things on the list to avoid for now: Oils, chickpeas, avocados, nuts (all) and grains (all).

Note: Apart from the teas, everything else you eat should be all raw, i.e. uncooked. Buy organic, if possible, if not, do the best you can, and ensure foods are washed properly before use.

Hydration: Drink plenty of water to flush the system.

Bladderwrack/Seamoss: Add the bladderwrack/seamoss combination to smoothies and have it in teas.

If money is a big factor, in terms of being able to afford the herbs, then go a bit lighter on the herbs.

Start by cleansing the bowel and changing the diet to predominantly fruits and vegetables, preferably 100% raw or as close as possible.

Use the Powder (Seamoss and Bladderwrack) to make shakes and have teas daily.

In addition, add the elder flower, burdock, dandelion, sarsaparilla and ginger to your regimen. Combine them to make teas.

Method 2: Water Fasting

Water fasting can be extremely effective. It is probably one of the easiest ways to rid the body of pathogens and toxins, boost the immune system and allow the body to heal. It is not advisable to begin a water fast with no previous fasting experience.

One however, doesn't need to go to a fasting center in order to fast. If there are no other serious underlining health conditions, one can build up to a fast by preparing the body (so to lessen the effects of detox symptoms). Ensure you have support around you, such as a partner or friend and also, preferably someone with experience of fasting.

Building up to a water fast:

- Start with a 3-day bowel cleanse.

- Consume a total plant-based diet for 7 days.

- Do another 3-day bowel cleanse consuming only raw fruits and vegetables during this period.

- Do a 7-day mono-fast on preferably grapes, mango, melon or apples.

- Follow up with a 3-day juice fast, mainly green juices and the juices of citrus fruits.

- Begin your water fast.

Who should not water fast:

- Pregnant women.

- Anyone coping with anorexia.

- Individuals suffering from debilitating dis-eases and have little strength.

- Advanced stages of dis-eases, such as cancer.

- Individuals suffering from severe mental disorders that require professional treatment. - - If you are suffering from less severe mental disorder, it is necessary to have support around you.

Breaking the fast:

It is important that the fast is broken correctly.

Start with only juices, vegetable juices, non-sweet fruit juices. Have only juices for three consecutive days (assuming a 7 to 10 days water fast. The longer the water fast, the slower and longer the re-feeding period).

Have raw fruits for another 2 days.

Introduce light raw salads.

Slowly introduce other foods.

Note: Eat small meals as needed, chew foods properly, pay attention to the body's signals.

Method 3: Juicing

After the initial bowel cleanse of at least 3 days, have juices and teas only. This includes mainly green or vegetable juices, you will have more of these at the beginning, then add fruit juices (citruses and melons).

Building up to a juice fast

- Do 3 days colon cleanse (as listed above)

- 7 Days all raw fruits and vegetables.

- Start juicing.

- The period varies, aim for a minimum of 21 days. Add herbal teas, such as those noted above, in addition, increase water consumption.

Tip: Swish your juices in the mouth before swallowing.

Method 4: Alternate Water / Juicing

This is where water fasting and juicing are combined.

Building up to the fast

Follow the same method listed in the previous. With this method a deliberate pattern is created consuming a balance of fruit juices and water.

Combined water and juice plan

Juice in the mornings

Water in the days

Juice at nights

Method 5: Mono-meals

21 days, 30 days or 6 weeks minimum of eating only one particular fruit whether for the entire duration of the period or using different fruits for different periods of time.

Fruits to use for mono-meals: Acid and sub acid fruits, avoid sweet fruits as these are high energy foods and less astringent.

The best fruits for mono-meals: Grapes, mangoes, melons, oranges, pears, oranges, lemon/limes. You can however use fruits preferable to you.

Mono-meal medley:

This involves consuming several fruits within the period, for example, days

1 – 7: Apples; days

8 – 14: Mangoes; days

15 – 21: Grapes; days

22 – 28: Melons and so on.

It could also be done in 5- or 3-days period. It is not necessary to juice, just eat the whole fruit. This can be done along with the herbs.

A mono-meal fasting period can be ended with a 2 – 3 days water fasting, followed by 24 hours dry fasting.

Things to note:

Check the urine at regular interval to see if the kidneys are filtering.

Drink plenty of water to help flush the system, however if one notices that urination isn't occurring, despite drinking lots of water, then have some dandelion, hawthorn or horsetail herbal tea; these are diuretics and can be used in instances where the body is holding on to fluids.

Cleansing the colon is important; always start with this first.

Practice deep breathing exercises every day.

Do not use things on the skin you cannot eat.

Do not drink water straight from the tap, filter your water.

Do not shower with regular, store-bought soaps as these will only further irritate the skin.

For blisters and sores

Some things to use for blisters or sores.

Homemade Salve

- Herbal essential oils and salves (e.g.: myrrh, lavender, dandelion, burdock etc)

- Use formation or compresses on affected areas

- Oregano oil

- Olive leaf extract

Even before the end of a cleansing or fasting period one should begin to see positive results.

Adopting a plant-based diet going forward will help you to maintain general health and wellness.

Again, all methods to be completed concurrently and continuously. Do not necessarily have to go in order but should be the new foundation for lifestyle until condition is no longer present.

Hepatitis C

Hepatitis C ("Hep C") is a viral infection that causes damage to one of the main filters in the body (the liver) and increasing the risk of liver malfunction and cancer. The standard protocol for hepatitis c is a drug called *interferon* in addition to many other medications for approximately one year. This treatment leads to fevers, muscle aches, and flulike symptoms and has only been helpful to 60% of clients. The medical model tries to create the natural healing modalities of the body such as flulike symptoms to promote healing this condition, but it is forced upon the body rather than a natural response to the body which is why they have a relatively low success rate of recovery.

You want to instead, consuming liver-protecting herbs while cleansing the body and apply gentle pressure to the areas in the form of acupressure to properly heal from this condition while avoiding additional damage (as the medical model provides). In this section you will learn about natural herbs to consume to make sure your liver is protected while not overworking the body so that it can promote the body's natural healing properties without creating damage.

Remedies:

Milk Thistle (herb)

The herb contains a group of natural chemicals known as silymarin, which work to stimulate the synthesis of protein in the liver which help the liver begin to regenerate itself. Take two 150mg capsules of this herb three times a day. Also available in extract form in which you want to take the recommended dosage listed on bottle. For the extract check the label to make sure it is at least 70 to 80 percent silymarin for best results.

Lemon Balm (herb)

This herb helps to protect the liver by assisting with organizing and breaking down materials being filtered by the liver. Take t teaspoon of fresh or dried herb to 1 cup of boiling water. Steep for 15 minutes, strain, and drink two to three cups a day.

St. John's Wort (herb)

This herb contains some of the benefits mentioned of the other herbs listed above. All you need is one 300mg capsule twice a day.

Avoid Processed Meats Altogether

Processed meats, but particularly red meats are loaded with antibiotics, growth hormones, and steroids. Consuming these items complicates the digestive process, which places additional stress on not only the liver, but the gallbladder, and pancreas, among other organs. Dairy also contains a high amount of fat and sugars which are difficult to digest as well.

Alcohol

Alcohol is notorious for the damage it does to the liver. Sends signals to the organs and reduces the body's alertness and ability to break down harmful substances.

Caffeine

Not only coffee contains caffeine. Sodas, candy, and even over-the-counter medications contain caffeine. This substance places an enormous amount of stress on the liver and will essentially "block" any herbs or lifestyle adjustments that attempt to strengthen or protect the liver.

Tap Water

There are many chemicals that the body just cannot process which are sent straight to the liver. Chemicals such as chlorine and fluoride which contribute to many diseases and illnesses.

Artificial Sweeteners

The liver does not recognize these substances. This disturbs the digestive process, particularly the pancreas and essentially feeds the hepatitis c virus. High-fat and high-sugar foods are the worst for the liver.

Exercise

Exercise stimulates circulation, sends oxygen to the blood, opens up your pours, and filters blood through the liver and kidneys. Exercise is a great fundamental way of opening up the "channels" within the body to promote the removal of toxins in the body. About 30-minutes a day of aerobic exercise daily will be best. Walking, swimming, cycling, and/or jogging are some of the simplest ways to get your 30-minutes a day in.

Acupressure (for smaller episodes)

With most viral conditions, the body will experience minor episodes occasionally. For hepatitis c, the body will feel fatigued, nauseous, and have diarrhea during these minor episodes. Acupressure is a form of therapy that includes pressure on and around the pressure points in the body. Below are specific points to focus on and/or have a professional work on:

PE6 – located on the inside part of the wrist; about three finger-widths above the wrist between the 2 bones of the wrist. This is particularly helpful for nausea.

ST36 – located about four finger-widths below the knee on the outside part of the leg. This is particularly helpful for fatigue.

SP4 – located on the inside part of the foot in the hollow part, behind the bone of the big toe. Also helpful for fatigue.

ST37 – located about four finger-widths below the kneecap on the outside of the shinbone. This is helpful for diarrhea and abdominal cramps.

ST25 – located on the abdomen, about three finger-widths to the right and the left of the navel. Also helpful for diarrhea and abdominal cramps.

Squash, Garbanzo Beans, Mushrooms, and Zucchini

These items will help keep you fulfilled with as you eliminate processed products from your lifestyle as you work through this condition. You can combine these together or make a soup to help feel fulfilled without overworking your digestive system, along with consuming additional fiber that promotes digestion.

Zinc

The body uses Zinc to breakdown bacteria in the body and helps strengthen the immune system. Zinc also helps regulate hormones in the body and balances cholesterol produced by the liver. There have been studies where researchers have found there to be zinc deficiencies associated with hepatitis-C and damaged liver cells which zinc works to replace.

Common Sources of Zinc: chickpeas, mushrooms, zucchini, squash, okra, Brazil nuts, and walnuts.

Dandelion (herb)

Cholesterol being produced by the liver means the liver needs to be taken care of, so the liver's production of cholesterol does not create additional issues within the body. Taking good care of the liver is very important step in regulating the cholesterol levels in your body. Dandelion helps to clean the liver (and pancreas) which affects the way your body metabolizes things like fat (particularly cholesterol derived from fat). Drink 1-2 cups of dandelion tea before each meal for best results. Take 1-2 teaspoons per 10-12 ounces of water to make tea.

Cut The Cholesterol

Our liver organ produces all of the cholesterol that we need. We suppress this from happening when we consume items high in cholesterol, fat, or starch. Cholesterol and other fats are carried in the bloodstream as circular particles called "lipo-proteins". The two most common lipo-proteins are referred to as, low-density lip-proteins ("LDL"), and high-density lipo-proteins ("HDL"). When our liver is overworked, its ability to regularly produce cholesterol needed to fulfill its obligations to provide the body with helping brain and nerve functioning, digestion, breaking down fats, absorbing nutrients, hormone production and balance, and maintaining the integrity of the cells within the body.

You do not want to take something to keep lowering cholesterol levels. Lowering them too much can drastically impair the body. You want to simply avoid consuming additional cholesterol and harmful items that overwork the liver.

High-fat and high-sugar items are the worst for the liver.

High-cholesterol items (**avoid**): processed (deli) meats, red meat, butter, friend foods, palm oil, canola oil, eggs, shellfish, sardines, yogurt (dairy-based).

Items that are damaging and overwork the liver (**avoid**): fried foods, artificial dyes, sodas, white bread, saturated fat (high in fried foods, cookies, pizza, and many baked goods).

Consume more of the following (**add more of these**): cruciferous vegetables (turnips, watercress, maca, arugula, wild mustard greens, broccoli, cauliflower, brussels sprouts, citrus fruits (oranges, lemons, kiwi, berries, grapefruit, pomelo, limes, key limes), olive oil.

Hiccups

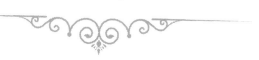

A hiccup is caused by eating too fast and swallowing too much air. We only have about 1 cup of air in our "air pocket", also known as the nasopharynx part of our bronchial tubes that allow us to breathe in air. Whenever we intake food, small bits of air are also consumed as we close open and close our mouths and then swallow the food. As long as we take a moment to breathe after, everything typically adjusts and goes back to normal. However, when we consume bite after bits in small amounts of time, this air pocket tries to hold more air than it can, resulting in pushing the air back up in the form of hiccups.

Note: from a scientific standpoint to "cure" hiccups is to simply increase the carbon dioxide levels in the blood or to disrupt the nerve impulses in the body to temporarily distract the body so the air passageways can re-adjust.

Remedies:

Mac McCallum's Remedy

Richard "Mac" McCallum, M.D., professor of medicine and chief of the gastroenterology and hepatology division at the University of Kansas Medical Center, came across a remedy for hiccups he did for himself and now recommends to patients. McCallum recommends filling a glass full of water, bend over forward, and drink the glass of water upside down. McCallum states, "That always works, and I firmly recommend it for my normally healthy friends."

Blow Out Your Air

Many try to hold their breath as long as possible to prevent hiccups. This simply cannot work as you are simply keeping everything the same. Air has to either go in or out. Since the air is already in, it is important to blow out your air through your mouth in a slow, steady fashion. You may cause or feel uncomfortable for a moment or so, but this will help compress the air passageways and help alleviate your hiccups from reoccurring.

Hold Your Breath (temporarily) While Eating

When you are eating, try eating slowly, one bite at a time. Try to not pick up your next spoonful before swallowing your current bite. While eating, if you feel a hiccup coming on, hold your breath for a few seconds followed by slow, controlled breaths. Then, continue eating. Repeat this while you eat, and you will notice a positive change.

Tickle Remedy

If you want to relive some tension and make this fun, try this remedy. Try holding your breath, then be tickled as you try your hardest not to laugh. This is helpful for children too. This remedy causes you to gasp for air and helps the diaphragm adjust to functioning normally.

Ginger and Mullein Tea

Ginger will help breakdown some of the bacteria that may be sitting around in the body that is obstructing the air pathways. Mullein will help keep the respiratory system to allow the body to breathe much easier. These two herbs together will significantly reduce symptoms and frequency of hiccups. You can take about a fingertip size piece of ginger and 2 teaspoons of mullein and steep them in boiling water for about 12-minutes and then allow to cool off and strain for about 10-minutes. You can drink this as often as you want, just do not exceed 3 cups per day.

High Blood Pressure

High blood pressure is most commonly known as "the silent disease" (hypertension) as there are almost no immediate symptoms for years or even decades. Many people are unaware that they even have this condition. This condition can damage blood vessels, increase risk for stroke, kidney disease, and heart disease, among other conditions. The arteries can only take so much force, so when blood rushes through at a high pressure, the arteries can thicken and harden over time and place additional stress on the heart and the body.

Julian Whitaker, M.D., states that, "Volumes of scientific research show that dietary changes can eliminate high blood pressure…. In spite of that, the routine approach of most doctors is to immediately start a patient on drugs – and usually without any recommendation for dietary change."

Remedies:

Know The Numbers

It is crucial to know what "healthy" numbers are for blood pressure of your age group (and gender). The word "healthy" is in quotes here due to numbers being based on a spectrum of averages where specific numbers don't guarantee overall good health. The only way to know your numbers are to test for it.

Blood pressure is tested by measuring the pressure of the blood within the arteries. It is produced by the contraction of the heart muscle and is recorded by two numbers. The first number (systolic blood pressure - SBP) is measured after the heart contracts and is highest. The second (diastolic blood pressure - DBP) is measured before the heart contracts and is the lowest.

Below are the standard numbers to aim for in order to have *normal* blood pressure for each age range:

Male			Female		
Age Range	SBP	DBP	Age Range	SBD	DBP
21-25	120.5	78.5	21-25	115.5	70.5
26-30	119.5	76.5	26-30	113.5	71.5
31-35	114.5	75.5	31-35	110.5	72.5
36-40	120.5	75.5	36-40	112.5	74.5
41-45	115.5	78.5	41-45	116.5	73.5
46-50	119.5	80.5	46-50	124.0	78.5
51-55	125.5	80.5	51-55	122.55	74.5
56-60	129.5	79.5	56-60	132.5	78.5
61-65	143.5	76.5	61-65	130.5	77.5

Cut Down Extra Weight/Size

If you are overweight, you are two to six times more likely to developing high blood pressure. The first step will be to cut down your overall size to alleviate pressure on the arteries. If you are excessively overweight, the arteries can experience additional pressure by feeling suffocated throughout the day. Any pound you can get rid of will count and be significantly helpful in overcoming this condition. You want to do this in a holistic manner and not rush into anything extreme just to lose weight. Activities such as excessive cardio, you will lose mostly water weight which will be replaced over time. You want to reduce your size while consuming fewer calories and burning any excess fat that you can a little at a time. Even decreasing your overweight by 5%-10% can be enough to lower your blood pressure back into normal range.

Exercise Is Best

Some form of exercise daily is best for reducing high blood pressure. Going for a walk, following a regular routine, targeting certain muscle groups, or even doing things such as gardening will be beneficial for your overall health but increase things such as mobility and strength.

Give Up Cigarettes

Every time your smoke just one cigarette, your blood pressure shoots up high for at least an hour at minimum. Most smokers do not just smoke one cigarette a day. If you are someone who smokes several cigarettes a day, you can constantly be in the danger zone regarding your blood pressure.

Water

Dr. Whitaker states that, "Almost all of the blood pressure medications mimic the effects of increased water intake." These medications work to relax the entire system of the body (particularly the arteries). Water serves this very same purpose for the body and should be used with the same intention. Begin increasing your water intake by making water your primary drink throughout the day and eating more fresh fruits and vegetables.

Reduce Sodium Intake (salt)

Those who are salt-sensitive will have more drastic spikes in blood pressure than those who are not salt-sensitive. However, those who are not salt-sensitive cannot completely avoid high blood pressure; it is just more unnoticeable than those who have more sudden spikes in blood pressure. Everyone can benefit from reducing their sodium intake. Sodium attract water, where consuming too much salt will increase the blood's volume. This raises the blood pressure in the body. No more than 2,400mg of salt should be consumed daily. The important thing is to look where salt (or sodium) is not specifically listed on ingredient labels. Most baked goods, candies, processed foods, and carbonated/flavored beverages contain salt; even condiments such as ketchup and items marketed as whole-grain breakfast foods like cereals have a high sodium content. You will want to avoid adding salt to foods that already contain salt as well. If you can do without, then do so. It may be helpful to use a fine-grained saltshaker which provides fine-grained salt in which you will end up using less salt overall when adding it to specific foods.

Potassium

Potassium and sodium are essentially opposites with how they interact in the body. When potassium levels increase, sodium levels decrease. Not consuming enough potassium can directly contribute to rises in sodium and lead to high blood pressure.

Common sources of potassium: squash, zucchini, bananas, avocado, dried apricots, and herbs such as, guaco (also high in iron), conconsa (has the highest concentration of potassium phosphate), lily of the valley (rich in iron fluorine and Potassium phosphate).

Calcium and Magnesium

These minerals are key contributors of helping the body remain alert and contribute to cleaning the body. With low levels of the minerals, the body's receptors will not work at maximum capacity and can contribute to increased levels of blood pressure.

Common Sources of Calcium: sea moss, kale, okra, dandelion greens, turnip greens, lettuce, papaya, and oranges.

Common Sources of Magnesium: avocado, chickpeas, tamarind, basil, dill, ginger, oregano, thyme, any *CBD (cannabidiol) products are helpful. (CBD Oils are almost pure magnesium.), nettle leaf, horsetail, red clover, sage, and nopal.

To test the purity of a CBD Oil, send to a lab for testing or you should feel a steady decline in needing to rely on this substance after your need has been met regularly.

Omega-3

Omega-3 fatty acids are essential to protecting the brain cells, reducing inflammation in the body, and providing support for the brain and its' receptors. This nutrient can help repair any lingering damage to cells in the body and reduce symptoms of high blood pressure. Consuming these in abundance are a necessary part of the healing process.

Common sources of omega-3 are Walnuts, Brazil Nuts, Avocados, Hemp Seeds, Hemp Milk, Walnut Oil, Olive Oil, and Sea Vegetable such as Nori, Hijiki, Bladderwrack, Kelp, and Dulse.

Hawthorn (herb)

This herb has long been used in Traditional Chinese Medicine (TCM) for reducing blood pressure. Take 1-2 teaspoons of dried or fresh herb and add to cup. Boil water and pour over herb. Let cool, steep, and drink about 12-ounces a day of this tea for best results.

Flor de Manita (herb)

This herb is great for reducing blood pressure and contains a high iron content which helps clean out toxins within the blood. This herb works to clean out anything not needed in the blood to support smoother blood flow, which helps to lower blood pressure. Take 2-3 pieces of this herb and add to a cup. Boil water, add to cup, let cool and strain. Drink two 10-ounce cups a day for best results.

Manage Stress

Stress triggers the heart's impulses. Even if jut temporarily, you want to manage your stress to not experience any symptoms of high blood pressure. Stress can greatly contribute to additional cardiovascular problems that are to be avoided as well. Stress creates salt within the body as well. A nucleus of an atom can only hold 2 electrons in the 1st valance and 8 in the remainder valences (other layers). When we get stressed (heat rises) which causes sodium (Na) molecules in the body to throw electrons off as they lose energy. This makes it unstable and causes it to create a bond with whatever is compatible with it in its current state (this is called "Covalent Bonding"). In this case, the sodium molecule is now compatible with Chloride (Cl) molecule because chloride produces "free" electrons to the body.

A nucleus of an atom can only hold 2 electrons in the 1st valance and 8 in the remainder valances (outer layers). When we get stressed (heat rises) this causes Sodium (Na) molecules in the body to throw electrons off as they lose energy. This makes it unstable and causes it to create a bond with whatever compatible with it in its current state (this is called "Covalent Bonding"). In this case the Sodium molecule is now compatible with Chlorine (Cl) molecule because Chlorine produces "free" electrons to the body.

Now you have Na + Cl which is NaCl which creates Sodium-Chloride which is salt.

If you are cutting out or reducing your salt intake but you are frequently stressed, you are essentially replacing your salt intake, just in another way. Here are some simple, common ways to begin managing ways to reduce your stress.

- When you feel stressed, talk to someone. You do not need to solve whatever has caused your stress. Just simply acknowledging your stress and talking to someone about it can drastically reduce your overall stress in the moment.

- Listen to music that bring up positive emotions within yourself.

- Practice writing down your thoughts and feelings to keep track of how you are down (or how you think you are doing).

- Embrace any emotions that come up when feeling stressed to practice allowing your emotions to pass by. Think of your emotions as "energy in motion" as they remain fluids and are not solid as we are accustomed to thinking. Think of energy in motions rather than an iceberg that has to melt. Allow these emotions to reveal themselves, and simply pass by.

- Connect with a psychotherapist or individual therapist or counselor to help you process your thoughts and work on developing positive coping skills to incorporate into your lifestyle to combat strong feelings of stress.

Clear Up Your Snoring

Regular snoring can be a symptom of sleep apnea, which is a condition where breathing intermittently stops during sleep. Dr. Howard Weitz, M.D., codirector of the Jefferson Heart Institute of Thomas Jefferson University Hospital in Philadelphia, Pennsylvania states, "It (snoring) can definitely raise blood pressure and can also bring about heart irregularities called arrhythmias." Sleep issues can create headaches and tiredness upon awakening which can maintain the need for reducing your blood pressure.

Watch Your Cholesterol

High cholesterol does not specifically result in high blood pressure but can narrow the arteries and cause the blood to push harder to pump through (and around) these narrow arteries and results in higher blood pressure. Having narrowed arteries causes them to be less dilated during activities such as exercise when the heart needs more blood in which this response by the bod contributes to developing additional symptoms of high blood pressure.

High Cholesterol

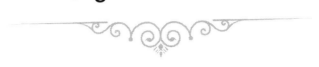

The heart beats about 100,000 times a day. Each heartbeat sends about 2-3 ounces of blood through the vascular system (arteries, veins, and capillaries). The liver produces the cholesterol we need daily when it is clean. However, items in our typical diets and lifestyle contain cholesterol which can alleviate the amount of pressure the liver must produce to help the body maintain positive health. When we consume too much cholesterol or animal fat (which is converted into cholesterol), it clogs the coronary arteries so that blood and oxygen cannot easily get through to the heart, which often causes a heart attack. The lower your cholesterol is away from any high range, the better it will be for your heart and your body.

The problem is not the cholesterol itself that causes these issues; it is when this cholesterol is oxidized (cholesterol that builds up along the arteries).

LDL (low-density lipoprotein), "bad" cholesterol, makes up most of your body's cholesterol. LDL is manufactured and secreted by the liver and is carried to the arteries in the heart. Once it arrives, it will oxidize and create an inflammatory response which harms the area similar to how iron rusts or an apple turns brown after cut and left out. This process makes it harder for blood to pass through. To avoid this inflammatory response the body needs three essential nutrients: vitamin E, vitamin C, and glutathione. These nutrients are most present in fresh fruits and vegetables. Vitamin C can also be oxidized in which vitamin E will come to the rescue by donating some of its own molecules to restore vitamin C. vitamin E bring reduced this way, allows glutathione to replenish it; this is why you need all three to keep your LDL cholesterol at bay.

You may wonder why the liver would intentionally create a substance that inevitably causes some harm to the body? The short answer is, the liver does not intentionally do this, but is a response for when the body is deficient in several essential nutrients. The body works in all aspects to constantly heal itself; even in ways that can cause harm if you are not mindful of its signals it will send to various parts of the body in an effort to help you. You want to keep this level under 100.

HDL (high-density lipoprotein), or "good" cholesterol, absorbs cholesterol and carries it back to the liver to be broken down. You want to keep this level above 40.

Remedies:

Vitamin C, Vitamin E, and Glutathione

These three are essential nutrients that work collaboratively together to protect the bad cholesterol from causing damage to the arteries. Vitamin C and Vitamin E are antioxidants which work to protect cells from eroding, while Glutathione is an amino acid that prepares itself as a building block for protein which are used to promote and coordinate bodily functions.

What we refer to as Vitamin C is a water-soluble nutrient and powerful antioxidant that help form and maintain connective tissues, including the bones, blood vessels, and the skin. This nutrient can help reduce symptoms of allergic reactions and inflammation which will help to avoid any prolonging issues. Vitamin C also is responsible for manufacturing the adrenal hormones which are needed to combat the stress the body goes through when an allergic reaction takes place.

Natural Sources of Vitamin-C: Black Currants, Bell Peppers (red and green), Papaya, Spring Onions, Strawberries, Cantaloupe, Mango, Oranges, Watercress, Raspberries, and Tomatoes.

What we refer to as Vitamin E (tocopherol) is an antioxidant, fat-soluble nutrient that works to stop free radicals (unstable atoms that can damage cells) from damaging the cells particularly in the heart. Vitamin E helps to process fats and work to avoid damage within the lining of the arteries which contributes to heart disease. Dr. Michael Janson, M.D., consultant physician at Path to Health in Burlington, Massachusetts recommends 400-800 international units of vitamin-e daily to protect the arteries.

Natural Sources of Vitamin E: red bell peppers, mangoes, walnuts, sunflower seeds (non-processed), avocados, butternut squash, olive oil (for dressings), coconut oil, and avocado oil.

Glutathione is an amino acid that helps vitamin C and vitamin E perform at their best. The body does not do the best job of absorbing glutathione so increasing your intake is a must. Dr. Philip Lee Miller, M.D., founder and director of the Los Gatos Longevity Institute in California recommends 3,000mg of glutathione a day.

Natural sources of glutathione: okra, leafy green vegetables, strawberries, papaya, bell peppers, oranges, and melons.

Selenium

This trace mineral boosts levels of glutathione. You will want to take 200 micrograms of selenium regularly.

Common Selenium sources: brazil nuts, walnuts, chickpeas/garbanzo beans, kola nuts, dandelion greens, and nettle, and alfalfa. Recommended to consume about 400 micrograms a day.

Zinc and Copper

Both of these minerals work to lower LDL (bad) cholesterol and increase HDL (good) cholesterol. 30 milligrams of zinc and 2 milligrams of copper daily will be a sufficient enough of each of these minerals.

Common Zinc Sources: chickpeas, mushrooms, zucchini, squash, okra, Brazil nuts, and walnuts.

Common Sources of Copper: blackberries, blueberries, guava, apricots, bananas, leafy green vegetables, avocado, sunflower seeds, mushrooms, spring onions, and you can drink sparingly from a copper vessel or bottle.

Guggul (herb)

Use primarily in Ayurvedic medicine practices, this herb is used directly for lowering LDL while increasing HDL cholesterol. Dr. Virander Sodhi, M.D., an Ayurvedic and naturopathic physician and director of the American School of Ayurvedic Sciences in Bellevue, Washington, is quoted as stating, "I have dramatically reduced LDL cholesterol and increased HDL cholesterol with just this one herb." Dr. Sodhi recommends 900 milligrams a day of this herb (taken in 3 doses – 300mg each) until cholesterol levels are normal. Then decrease to 300mg of this herb a day.

Fiber

The recommended amount of fiber is 25-35 grams a day. But the average person only consumes around 12-14 grams of fiber. Fiber is crucial in lowering cholesterol due to fiber absorbing water in the stomach and swells up, causing you to feel full. Fiber when being digested turns into a gel within the intestines and traps cholesterol molecules. As these molecules break down, cholesterol can begin to lower over time. (Helpful Tip: aim to consume at least 5 grams of fiber per eating period during the day to help achieve the recommended daily amount of fiber).

Common sources of Fiber: garbanzo beans, lentils, apples and berries (high pectin fruits) and onions.

Avoid Processed Meats

Processed (deli) meat contains a high amount of saturated fat and cholesterol, which together, can provide a harmful combination to the arteries.

Pectin

Many citrus fruits contain a dietary fiber called pectin which blocks the absorption of cholesterol and other fats into the blood. Apples, berries (particularly blackberries), cherries, bananas, peaches, and apricots are all high in pectin.

Walnuts

Walnuts contain a specific acid known as alpha-linolenic acid which works to lower LDL cholesterol. This same acid is in purslane and olive oil. (Quick Tip: sauté some purslane in a teaspoon of olive oil to easily load up on this acid.

Onions

Add more onions to your meals as onions contain an antioxidant known as quercetin which helps LDL from accumulating in the arteries, while raising levels of HDL. All onions are helpful but focus more on red and yellow onions if you have high cholesterol.

Lecithin

Lecithin granules contain a chemical known as phosphatidylcholine which liquifies cholesterol in the body, so it does not begin to harden or build up along the walls of your arteries. You can take 1 tablespoon of lecithin granules a day. You may also find lecithin (and phosphatidylcholine) in sunflower seeds (and sunflower oil), rapeseeds, and many different beans.

Ginger (herb)

Ginger helps to lower (temporarily) blood pressure while reducing LDL cholesterol levels. You can take a 550mg capsule a day three times a day for best results. Depending ono what your lipid profile looks like after about 8 weeks, then you may take more or less.

Dandelion (herb)

Cholesterol being produced by the liver means the liver needs to be taken care of, so the liver's production of cholesterol does not create additional issues within the body. Taking good care of the liver is very important step in regulating the cholesterol levels in your body. Dandelion helps to clean the liver (and pancreas) which affects the way your body metabolizes things like fat (particularly cholesterol derived from fat). Drink 1-2 cups of dandelion tea before each meal for best results. Take 1-2 teaspoons per 10-12 ounces of water to make tea.

HIV and Aids

HIV (Human Immunodeficiency Virus)
AIDS (acquired immunodeficiency syndrome)

It has been long taught by the medical profession that HIV is the virus that causes AIDS which destroys the immune system and damages the body. Since AIDS is acquired, it is important to remain mindful of the source (immunodeficiency – a deficiency within the immune system). Dr. Jon Kaiser, M.D., director of the Jon Kaiser Wellness Center in San Francisco, California states that, "The progression of HIV disease in my practice is an extremely rare event." What this means, is that HIV can be controlled just like any other virus. Also, like any virus, it can spread and invade the rest of the body; in this case, the virus spreading due to a deficient immune system, and is considered an acquired syndrome. A syndrome is a collection of abnormalities that occur together. We must work to interfere (without interrupting) these abnormalities by building and sustaining the body's immune system and how it functions in order to avoid it from spreading.

Medical doctors have worked on controlling the virus initially, but this can only be one for so long. Once the virus is no longer under control, it spreads and becomes lethal. Dr. Kaiser's holistic methods include whole foods, nutritional supplements, herbs, exercise, stress reduction, and techniques for emotional and spiritual progress, have proven how holistic practices can work to suppress this virus from spreading, while also building/strengthening the immune system. Medical practices simply don't do enough to strengthen the immune system which drastically limits their effectiveness over time.

In this section, we will acknowledge how there is still much more to go with implementing solid, effective holistic remedies for treating this condition naturally, but also identify ways to help strengthen the immune system.

Remedies:

Affirmations

Healing does not come from what we take in, it comes from within. We must start healing by starting with our core beliefs (or creating them) directed towards the healing process. Saying affirmations and creating ones that resonate with you throughout the healing process. Without going into too much detail, it is commonly understood that negative self-talk and being down on yourself will weaken/suppress the immune system. This is the last thing you would want to do for this condition. Here are some affirmations to use while working towards healing: (Feel free to have fun and get creative with making your own).

I am confident and powerful

I am at peace with myself

I am able and calm

I am inspired, disciplined, and energized

I breathe I love and light, and exhale fear and darkness

I will listen to my body's guidance throughout my healing progress.

I am more than I appear to be. All of the world's strength and power rests inside of me

Make sure to write these down in your own handwriting and say them aloud. Take tie to write out your fears. Then create an affirmation in spite of that fear. For example, you may write "I'm afraid I am going to die". You can then write affirmations such as "I am strong and confident" or "I will embrace my challenges as I work through them."

Fatty Acids

Those with HIV often have skin infections and other skin issues. These can be taken care of by making sure there's enough essential fatty acids in the body. Dr. Allen Green, M.D., director of the Center for Optimum Health in Fountain Valley, California recommends between 4,000 to 6,000 milligrams a day of flaxseed oil. However, you do not have to rely completely upon flaxseed oil as there are many items that contain fatty acids.

Common Sources of Fatty Acids: Brazil Nuts, Walnuts, Kola Nuts, Avocados, Bananas, Sea Vegetables (Nori, Wakame, Hijiki, Sea Moss, Bladderwrack), Coconut, Coconut Oil, Olive Oil, Grapeseed Oil, Avocado Oil, Mushrooms, Quinoa, Wild Rice.

"Protein" / "Proteids"

We are taught that protein feeds the immune system so those with an immunodeficiency issue, need as much protein as they can get. However, what must be understood is that before we were taught what proteins were, or that we can only get this substance from animal meats, there were many other terms we would use to describe minerals, nutrients, phytonutrients, and complex bio-available molecules found in plants there were observed to be necessary to maintain life within the human body.

Before the word "protein" was commonly used, the term "proteids" was what we used to describe this item. Since we began using the word protein, it became a label that covers everything from muscle building, to a combination of amino acids, to just about anything referring to repairing the body. This is not an accurate description for what we are referring to when we discuss consuming protein as a part of our dietary regimen.

A proteid, is a complete rich material biomolecule found in all living matter, predominately made of "polypeptides" (large number of amino acids bonded together, along with carbon, hydrogen, and oxygen). When we speak on consuming "protein", it is important to understand that proteids are most abundant in natural fruit and vegetables (living matter). We need proteids, not protein. Gathering living matter is necessary to sustain your own life; not the dead, decaying material found in animal flesh.

Natural Sources of Proteids: seeded grapes, guava, avocado, apricots, blackberries, raisins, cherries, chickpeas/garbanzo beans, squash, brazil nuts, walnuts, hemp seeds, and quinoa.

Recommended amount of proteids (listed as protein) should be about 0.6 grams for every pound of body weight (ex. if someone weighs 150 pounds, at least 90 grams of proteids are needed. 150 x 0.6 = 90).

Quick Tips On Maintaining Proteid/Protein Amounts

Aim for 20 grams per meal

Have snacks around 5-10 grams

Hemp seeds and hemp protein powder (add to smoothies)

Chinese Herbal Remedy For Diarrhea

6 grams of lotus seeds (lian zi)

3 grams of Euryale (qian shi)

3 grams of dried ginger (gan jiiang)

6 grams of dioscorea (shan yao)

9 grams of poria (fu ling)

3 grams of codonopsis (dang shen)

2 red dates (hong zao)

Mix all of these together in a pot and cook with a grain such as quinoa to help deter diarrhea. Chinese practices often recommend this serving to be added to congee (boiled rice pudding), but we are looking to avoid as many starches as possible when trying to holistically treat a condition such as a virus.

Dr. Jon Kaiser's Anti-HIV Nutrient Protocol

Dr. Jon Kaiser has had much success with preventing HIV from spreading and developing into AIDS. Although we are after for official cures as we now have for many other conditions using natural methods, a light should still be shined on this work as it is a strong step in the correct direction.

Note: Dr. Kaiser's protocol involves many things such as "vitamins", artificial supplements that are not often recommended in the holistic realm, however, a similar structure can and should be created or implemented when treating this condition holistically with more natural remedies.

Mineral Support

Vitamin A (beta-carotene): 10,000 – 20,000 international units

B vitamins thiamin, riboflavin, pantothenic acid, and B6): 50 to 100 milligrams

Vitamin B12: 500 to 1,000 micrograms

Vitamin C: 250 to 1,000 milligrams

Vitamin E: 150 to 400 international units

Iron: 9 to 18 milligrams

Zinc: 10 to 25 milligrams

Calcium: 50 to 250 milligrams

Magnesium: 25 to 125 milligrams

Selenium: 100 to 200 micrograms

Multimineral Dosages:

Iron: 9 to 18 milligrams

Zinc: 25 to 50 milligrams

Copper: 1-2 milligrams

Calcium: 1,000 milligrams

Magnesium: 500 milligrams

Selenium: 100 to 200 micrograms

Individual Vitamins:

Vitamin C: 1,000 milligrams twice a day

Vitamin E: 400 international units twice a day

Vitamin B6: 100 milligrams twice a day

Additional Supplementation:

N-acetylcysteine (NAC): 500 milligrams twice a day. This is meant to boost levels of antioxidant glutathione. Studies have shown that those with HIV who have low glutathione levels move more rapidly towards developing AIDS.

Coenzyme Q10: 30 milligrams twice a day. This is meant to provide the cells with additional energy, boost immunity, and help relieve fatigue.

Acidophilus: to be taken daily according to the ingredient label on package that is prescribed to individual. This is meant to avoid digestive problems that often result from taking digestive problems from taking antibiotics and other medications which can destroy the beneficial bacteria in the digestive tract.

Now, after reading Dr. Kaiser's protocol, hopefully you are thinking of the many natural foods and herbs that you may be aware of that could replace some of the items listed above. The important piece of Dr. Kaiser's protocol is the consistency of this daily regimen. This can be difficult to track when consuming whole foods and herbs but is a necessary piece to the healing process. Dr. Kaiser's protocol has helped hundreds continue to prevent their HIV from spreading and developing into AIDS. So, you may see how a diet/lifestyle consistent with whole foods, herbs, and natural practices can achieve the same result and continue to work towards reversal of this condition over time.

Here are some natural sources for the vitamins and minerals identified in this section:

Vitamin-A: mango, papaya, apricots, red bell peppers, winter squash, dark leafy green vegetables, cantaloupe, and lettuce.

B-vitamins (thiamin, riboflavin, pantothenic acid, pyridoxine)

Thiamin ("Vitamin B1"): asparagus, peas, oranges, clementines, lemons, sunflower seeds, sesame seeds, pecans, Brazil nuts, lentils, pecans.

Riboflavin ("vitamin B2"): tomatoes, avocado, sunflower seeds, dandelion greens, swiss chard, kale, quinoa., and edible sea vegetables (Nori, Wakame, Hijiki, Sea Moss, Bladderwrack).

Pantothenic Acid ("Vitamin-B5"): Has been studied to prevent loss of weight in pigeons but that is all known about this so far. No direct link to human need identified at this time.

Pyridoxine ("Vitamin-B6"): avocado, carrots, bananas, peas, lentils, spinach, chickpeas, acorn squash, quinoa, sunflower seeds, brussels sprouts, oranges, pistachios.

Cobalamin ("Vitamin-B12"): You will want to go to local markets and farmer's markets in your area where there is a shorter "farm to table" distance where B12 will remain more present in some capacity. Also growing some of your own plants at home or at a local garden will be best.

Vitamin-C: black currants, red bell peppers, Kakadu plum, camu camu (fruit/berry), gooseberries, papaya, oranges, cantaloupe, raspberry, mango, blackberry, tomato, blueberry, grapes, apricot, and watermelon.

Vitamin-E: red bell peppers, mangoes, walnuts, sunflower seeds (non-processed), avocados, butternut squash, olive oil (for dressings), coconut oil, and avocado oil.

Iron: quinoa, wild rice (not black rice), chickpeas/garbanzo beans, kale, nuts (particularly walnuts), hemp seeds, dates, dried apricots, prunes, watercress, sarsaparilla, burdock (and root), guaco, chainey root, monkey ladder, chickweed, yellowdock.

Zinc: Common Sources of Zinc: chickpeas, mushrooms, zucchini, squash, okra, Brazil nuts, and walnuts.

Calcium: sea moss, kale, okra, dandelion greens, turnip greens, lettuce, papaya, and oranges.

Magnesium: avocado, chickpeas, tamarind, basil, dill, ginger, oregano, thyme, any *CBD (cannabidiol) products are helpful. (CBD Oils are almost pure magnesium.), nettle leaf, horsetail, red clover, sage, and nopal.

Selenium: brazil nuts, walnuts, chickpeas/garbanzo beans, kola nuts, dandelion greens, and nettle, and alfalfa.

Copper: blackberries, blueberries, guava, apricots, bananas, leafy green vegetables, avocado, sunflower seeds, mushrooms, spring onions, and you can also drink sparingly from a copper vessel/bottle.

Hives

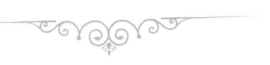

Hives are red bumps on your skin that can become extremely itchy. Most common cause of developing hives is allergens that are triggered. Cells in the body (in the immune system) produce histamine, a chemical produced when blood cells leak fluid into the deepest layers of your skin, causing there to be frequent itching. Aside from allergic reactions, hives can be developed from emotional stress, exposure to cold weather, and/or infrequent exposure to direct sunlight.

Remedies:

Hydrotherapy

When hives are triggered by an allergen, the cells in the immune system release a chemical known as histamine, which leads to developing hives. Taking a warm shower (as warm as you can tolerate) also triggers histamine. When histamine is being released, the itching stops where it will then take a few hours for the body to create more histamine. So, what you want to do is, trigger your own hives by taking a warm shower (at least 10-15 minutes) so that histamine is released while you are washing yourself in which the itching will be relieved shortly afterwards. When itchy you want to apply soothing moisture to it anyway, so during a shower will be your best option. You still want to reduce the cause by getting to the root of the issue, but this remedy can provide temporary relief.

Quercetin

This is a plant pigment found in many plants such as apples, apples, and leafy green vegetables. Works to reduce inflammation and itchiness that comes with hives. Doctors often recommend 500 milligrams of quercetin twice a day, but you can consume the items listed above as a part of your regular lifestyle.

Sandalwood Essential Oil

Sandalwood essential oil offers a cooling (and calming) effect to itchy skin. Add 20 drops of this oil to 1-ounce of a carrier oil such as coconut oil and apply to areas in need every 3-4 hours.

"Rescue Remedy" Flower Essence

Flower essences are prepared for relaxation for the physical body, but also for the mind and emotions. There is a specific flower essence known as "Rescue Remedy" that can help the body work through allergic reactions as well as contribute to reducing the emotional stress of having hives. Typically, you can dd 3-5 drops of oil to a glass of water and drink once a day until symptoms decrease but follow instructions on label for best results.

Cold Compress

Applying a cool compress to your skin can help relieve irritation and swelling. To do this, grab a bag of frozen veggies or fruits, or wrap a handful of ice in a towel and apply it to the affected area for up to 10 minutes. Repeat as needed throughout the day.

Aloe Vera

Is a natural anti-inflammatory. According to the National Center for Complimentary and Integrative Health, applying aloe vera to the skin can help people with acne, herpes simplex, psoriasis, and other conditions affecting the skin. It is typically well-tolerated. But, as with any new remedy, it's important to do a skin patch test before application, especially if you have sensitive skin. Some commercial aloe products may also have added fragrance or other chemicals that can irritate the skin, so be sure to read the label(s).

You can find this plant at most local markets or grocery stores. You want to slice this plant open with a knife, squeeze or scoop out all of the transparent pulp, and then apply directly on the skin covering the affected are(s). You can let this settle in before washing off after about an hour. You can do this as often as you want.

Wear Loose Clothing

All infections or reactions thrive in warm environments. You can avoid this by wearing loose-fitting clothes so that air can keep this area cool. If you exercise or swim, make an effort to change into dry clothes immediately after. It can also be helpful to sleep in the nude also during this time to prevent this area from getting warmer than needed.

Chinese Dittany (dictamus dasycarpus turcz) (herb)

This herb is a flowering herb that has remained helpful for treating hives. A 2021 study published in the *Journal of Pharmacy and Pharmacology, Vol. 73, Issue 12*, examined the phytochemistry of this herb discussed several constituents that have anti-inflammatory, antioxidant, and anti-allergic properties, particularly for the treatment of hives.

Licorice Root (herb)

Licorice root contains the active ingredient *Glycyrrhiza glabra*, had antioxidant, anti-inflammatory, and healing properties that are useful in many applications involving skin inflammation.

Its active compounds are responsible for this healing, and clinical studies in humans and animals have demonstrated licorice as an effective and safe option. Dr. Stengler, N.D., naturopathic physician in San Diego, California, recommends 1,000 – 1,500 milligrams of licorice root in capsule form, or 30 drops of licorice root in a tincture form three times a day on an empty stomach to reduce symptoms.

Hostility

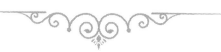

Hostile responses and moments of rage have become very common. Just like any disease or condition, when hostility is left untreated, can sabotage many areas of your life. Those who rationalize getting their anger out in uncontrollable ways are more likely creating more harm for themselves and others than they think. Paul A. Hauck, Ph.D., a psychologist in Moline, Illinois states, "Inappropriately expressed or repressed anger can overshadow all of the great things a person does." Essentially, having explosive anger will take its toll on a person and those around them. There are many research studies that clearly display those who have regular episodes of anger remain at a much higher risk for developing heart disease. Uncontrolled anger has also been linked to other conditions such as asthma, diabetes, anorexia nervosa, and daily pains such as back pain and headaches.

Anger is a part of life that will make its appearance in our lives. How you handle your anger is the key component for what will separate you from those who experience the many issues associated with anger. Ask yourself honestly, are you focused on the problem(s) or the solution(s)? What we focus on becomes more present. We want to identify and practice focusing our awareness on solutions rather than problems to reduce our hostility in ourselves and in others.

Remedies:

Get Moving During The Day

Anger tends to build up during the day, particularly around lunchtime. Pack a lighter lunch and try going for a walk. If you work somewhere and aren't able to leave (or have a regular lunch break) plan ahead time to go for a walk or do something as simple as pushups or squats. This will allow the body to release tension that you cannot see building up and help break apart any lingering thoughts that would have built up if you did not redirect your time and energy. Create your own movement break by finding some form of exercise you can do to alleviate tension and stress in the body to help reduce overall anger and hostility.

Plan Ahead

Avoid the buildup of minor inconveniences that can occur leading up to a planned event or scheduled appearance. Plan and prepare whatever you can to work out the minor details so that you can just focus on the main task.

Prepare For The Crowd

There will always be people that test us or get on our nerves. Many others will trigger certain responses from us; almost as if they thrive off of our uncontrolled responses. We want to prepare for these individuals or groups of people to not give them life which they use to create frustration. Think of ways to ignore or find a humorous response you will have to throw them off balance to help diffuse tense situation (at least within yourself).

Time-out

When you feel anger boiling and know you typically respond out of frustration, tell those around you (don't yell) that you need a moment to yourself and work to compromise a time to speak about the issue later. (Note: if you are not granted a moment to yourself or it can be agreed upon to discuss the issue later on, then those individuals may not want what's best for you and you may want to consider creating distance between yourself and them more often to avoid additional anger from building up).

Think About What's Next

Take a moment to think if what frustrates you will matter to you in a few hours, months, or years. If not, allowing it to go can help avoid potential consequences that will interfere with your future plans.

Keep Tension Elsewhere

When you feel frustrated and want to react, find something to do with your hands, feet, face, or jaw — anything that will help release tension. Grab a towel and squeeze it, have a fidget toy available, bite down a few times, or push your feet downward as hard as you can. These will help redirect your attention but allow you to express your frustrations easier in the moment without it leading to harm for yourself or others.

Yell or Scream

Sometimes the best remedy is to yell or scream. Put you face into a pillow and give it all you got. Or go to a backyard or park and scream at the top of your lungs. Just make sure no large groups or children are around that you may distract or frighten. Sure, if others are around, they may talk about the person they saw outside screaming, but this will only last for a brief moment. It will be worth the investment.

Magnesium

This mineral is a natural muscle relaxer. Many muscle cramps can be attributed to having a magnesium deficiency Dr. Barry L. Beaty, D,O,. orthopedic physician and director of the DFW Pain Treatment Center and Wellness Clinic in Fort Worth, Texas recommends taking 200 milligrams a day spread out throughout the day.

*Common Sources of Magnesium: avocado, chickpeas, tamarind, basil, dill, ginger, oregano, thyme, any *CBD (cannabidiol) products are helpful. (CBD Oils are almost pure magnesium.), nettle leaf, horsetail, red clover, sage, and nopal.*

*To test the purity of a CBD Oil, send to a lab for testing or you should feel a steady decline in needing to rely on this substance after your need has been met regularly.

Exercise

Focusing on an activity such as exercise can help channel your anger around an activity as you work to express yourself. Gradual, controlled movements are best to help a person express themselves while staying grounded. Aerobic exercises such as walking or jogging, are great due to the consistent repetition and ability to simplify while processing what may have caused or triggered your anger.

Breathing

You will want to breathe in slowly and deeply through the nostrils and release through the mouth. This ways of inhaling and exhaling prevents any air from getting "caught" within this process. It is recommended to make some noise (whatever comes most natural to you) when exhaling through the mouth. Release any locked tension and work to release any anger on the surface as you dig a bit deeper with every breath. Breathing is a very crucial piece to the emotional well-being of a person which can be stabilized through deep breathing exercises.

Valerian, Chamomile, and Passionflower (herbs)

These herbs are known for helping relax the body by promoting calmer feelings and lowering stress. Supporting your mood is a great proactive approach for those working to better cope and/or reduce/avoid their anger and contributing factors. Take 2 teaspoons of any of these herbs to drink in tea form twice a day. It can serve you well to make drinking at least one cup of tea once a day to help set your intention for the day or relax the body before you get moving. Any of these teas mentioned can help induce sleep when consumed at night as well which can help to further relax the body and the mind to help balance your emotions.

Reduce The Stimulation

Cut out any noises you can, turn off the phone and/or TV, and move further away from any outside noises. All noises around us get our attention on some level. Reducing or eliminating many of these noises allows us to focus on other things much easier and feel calmer as we are less stimulated and helps to reduce our interactions with other people.

(Also refer to "Anger" section within this text)

Hot Flashes

Hot Flashes are waves of heat that start in the chest area and spread quickly to the head and neck area, resulting in feeling uncomfortable, irritable, hot, and over an extended period of time, sweaty. About 75% of women experience hot flashes that can last for about 3-5 minutes, or longer in some cases. Hot flashes during the evening while sleeping are commonly referred to as "night sweats". These can increase symptoms as they can be more difficult to work through as they are disrupting the sleep cycle.

Hot flashes and night sweats are the result of the drop in estrogen that women experience during menopause (period of time after 12 months of no periods), and perimenopause (2-8 years before menopause). The estrogen deficiency interferes with how the body regulates heat, which can create more hot flashes and/or more inconsistent signals hat hot flashes or night sweats may occur.

Remedies:

Eliminate Processed Sugars

The more processed sugars in your system, the more irritated you will feel and the more you will experience hot flashes. There is not more important step than eliminating processed sugars in all forms from your lifestyle immediately. When we do not eat for a bit of time and then fill our stomach with candy, soda, any processed sugar, your pancreatic enzymes jump in to take care of the increased sugar intake. Then your insulin overshoots and you go into "reactive hypoglycemia" (low blood sugar – even though you just consumed sugar). Your adrenal glands bring adrenaline in to help mobilize the stores of glycogen sugar in your liver to combat the low blood sugar levels. This adrenaline rush stimulates a sudden increase in heart rate (tachycardia). Heart rate increases, body gets warmer due to blood pumping harder, and this contributes to experiencing conditions such as hot flashes. This is why we want to plan regular meals and avoid consuming any processed sugars. The hypothalamus part of the brain relaxes when it knows what to expect. Keep a regular dietary regimen to help the hypothalamus relax and don't send it mixed signals by consuming processed sugars, especially on empty stomach.

No Alcohol

Alcohol consumption is a strong trigger for hot flashes. Alcohol also causes blood vessels to dilate where more blood rushes to the skin, leading to hot flashes.

Wean Off The Caffeine

Caffeine aggravates hot flashes and can make them stronger. The heat from drinks such as coffee or green tea can present a combination of triggers for hot flashes you want to avoid. This does mean drinking sodas are ok. Drinking soda instead will present the same issues; you just won't notice symptoms as quickly.

Exercise

Exercise gives additional strength to the heart and can help drastically reduce the occurrence of hot flashes. Dr. Mary Jane Minkin, M.D., clinical professor at Yale University School of Medicine and obstetrician-gynecologist in New Haven, Connecticut, recommends 30-45 minutes of low to moderate exercise 3-5 times a week at minimum to help reduce menopausal symptoms, improve sleep, keep bones strong, and maintaining good heart health. It is important to find more gently forms of exercise to do more often such as yoga, pilates, or swimming because women experiencing menopause, they will not feel very comfortable sweating.

Know Your Calendar

Keeping track of days, times, and specific times of the month where you notice more severe or more frequent hot flashes is important to prepare for. You want to prepare as much as you can and be mindful to not be caught off guard as often as possible to decrease your symptoms.

Black Cohosh (herb)

This herb is not particularly high in estrogen such as items like soy or flax, but works particularly well with helping to increase the sudden drop in estrogen that can trigger and lead to hot flashes.

Red Clover (herb)

Red clover works to clean waste from the blood and contains blood-thinning properties that help alleviate hot flashes.

Sage

This herb is a common herb used for night sweats. This herb works to decrease the production of sweat. Drinking a cup of this before sleeping will help decrease the amount of frequency you sweat and in turn, reduce your night sweats.

Phytoestrogen Foods

Soy products may increase the estrogen that has dropped but you do not want to trade one issue for another. You may not have hot flashes, but excess or increased soy consumption can disrupt blood flow, create issues with the thyroid, or irritate other areas of the body. You want to consume more natural foods that contain phytoestrogen that can slowly be absorbs within the body. Foods such as apples, strawberries, chickpeas, grapes, plums, pears, onions, leafy green vegetables, and herb such as hops.

Belly Breathing

When experiencing hot flashes, the most common response is to take deep breathes. This can often lead to irritating symptoms if a person begins to breathe too quickly and becomes hot because of this. Doing bely breathing by placing both hands on your abdomen while laying down. As you breath in, you should notice your stomach filling with air and decrease as you breathe out. You want to make your inhale and exhale match as much as possible so that you have slower, controlled breaths to help the body relax and cool off while hot flashes are present. Aim for 6-8 breathes per minute.

Cotton

Wearing cotton will help allow air flow through easier to help keep your cool. Cotton sheets and pillowcases can help keep moisture away from the skin at night and reduce night sweats. Satin, flannel, and polyester trap moisture and does not allow air to flow as freely which can trigger or worsen symptoms.

Load Up On Iron

Iron deficiency alters your thyroid's metabolism which is responsible for regulating your body heat. In a study conducted by the USDA Human Nutrition Research Center in Grand Forks, North Dakota, they measured the effects of iron and its connection to body heat. They found that those who only took 1/3 of the recommended amount of iron for 80 days, lost 29% more body heat than when they were on an iron-rich diet for 114 days.

Common Sources of Iron: Wild rice, chickpeas/garbanzo beans, dandelion greens, sarsaparilla, burdock, yellow dock, chapparal, dates and prunes.

Chasteberry Extract (herb)

Progesterone and estrogen control the menstrual cycle. Dr. Holmes notes that "A deficiency of progesterone, can affect the thyroid gland." Chasteberry extract, commonly known as "vitex" as a name brand supplement, works to stimulate the pituitary gland to increase the production of LH, which results in higher levels of progesterone during the second stage of a woman's cycle known as the luteal phase. Progesterone helps to develop a thick, blood-rich uterine lining into which the fertilized egg can implant. Many women between the ages of 30 and 45 have a sharp drop off in progesterone which leads to shorter cycles and a decreased chance of implanting a fertilized egg. This change can enhance symptoms of hypothyroidism. Make sure to use Chasteberry Extract for several months before attempting to conceive, but generally 14 days before your next cycle. Standard dosage should be about 40 drops of this extract one a day, or one 650-milligram capsule 2-3 times a day. Make sure to follow directions on label instructions.

Hypoglycemia

Hypoglycemia is when low blood sugar is present in the body. The main solution that is often sought out for hypoglycemia is, to consume more sugar. Although this may initially display as not having low blood, this does not identify, locate, or fix the issue long term. Something had to have happened for low blood to remain present in the first place.

For hypoglycemia, the pancreas and the spleen are in need of restoration and repair. The pancreas is responsible for producing hormones that control the sugar levels in the blood stream. The pancreas will stop producing insulin when blood gets too low in order for blood levels to return to their normal levels. The spleen is the organ that harbors stem cells that set forth the ability of the pancreas to create insulin. These two organs working together will either work to heal and self-repair issues regarding blood (and insulin production) or they will signal the body when they are in need for assistance due to blood levels dropping.

Every time we eat, the body is signaled to produce insulin to tell the body to prepare the blood and organs to be ready to use what is consumed for energy. When there is excess fat, artificial, and lack of healthy hormones, the pancreas and/or the spleen will have difficulty functioning properly and increase your risk of low blood sugar.

Remedies:

Astringent Fruits

Persimmons, banana (peels), chokeberries, blackthorn, grapes, kiwi, oranges, starfruit, apples, watermelon, pears, cranberries, cherries, and strawberries, are the most common astringent fruits.

Astringent fruits contain an adequate amount of fiber, minerals, and antioxidant, which together, help to reduce post-meal insulin that is sent to the bloodstream which reduces the body's inability to balance sugar levels. Astringent fruits help enhance insulin sensitivity which contributes to clearing glucose in the bloodstream which allows the kidneys to properly filter fluids within the body.

Acupressure

In Traditional Chinese Medicine (TCM) the energy force within the body (Chi) circulates along the energy tracks in the body referred to as meridians. Apply pressure to areas on these meridians can help send Chi to specific organs. These pressure points can be pressed on each side symmetrically on both sides of the body.

ST36 – about four finger-widths below the lower ridge of your kneecap in front of your shinbone.

SP4 – located at the beginning arch on the inside of the foot, behind the bone of the big toe.

CV6 – this point is two finger-widths below the navel, on an imaginary line running down the middle of the body.

BL20 – located two finger-widths from the spine, level with what doctors refer to as the "11th thoracic vertebra" that is located in between your waist and the middle of your shoulder blades.

Start by searching for images to locate these specific points. Use your thumb or another finger to press each point with steady pressure for about two minutes. For more long-term relief, alternate which points you will focus on each day. Do two points one day and two the next or try alternating points throughout the week. Use these points to mimic the way we have our cars aligned and adjusted as needed.

Reduce The Carbs

Simple carbs such as white s and white flour weaken the pancreas and the spleen by forcing them to overwork themselves trying to filter and process these substances. Simply removing these from your diet and swapping them out for items such as date or coconut, and chickpea or spelt flour, will help to strengthen the pancreas and spleen rather than contributing to weakening these organs.

Snacking On Nuts

Eating nuts (brazil nuts or walnuts) in between meals can help balance your blood levels according to Dr. Michael Janson, M.D., consultant physician at Path to Health in Burlington, Massachusetts.

Mango Leaves

Making tea for mango leaves is an excellent way to balance blood sugar levels, especially for those with diabetes. Mango leaves have the ability to redistribute glucose in the body which helps balance the sugar in the bloodstream.

Minerals

There are many minerals the body is made of. But there are certain minerals to focus on when seeking to support, strengthen, and cleanse the pancreas and spleen. These minerals are:

Magnesium (about 400-500 milligrams/day)

Selenium (100-200 micrograms/day)

Zinc (20-30 milligrams/day)

Chromium (200-400 micrograms/day)

"These levels of nutrients should guarantee that the entire spectrum of vitamins and minerals… is high enough to help remedy hypoglycemia" says Dr. Janson.

Finding these minerals in natural foods is best as they will also contain an assortment of vitamins such as vitamin C and vitamin E that doctors may want to prescribe an artificial supplement for.

Common Sources of Magnesium: avocado, chickpeas, tamarind, basil, dill, ginger, oregano, thyme, any CBD (cannabidiol) products, nettle leaf, horsetail, red clover, sage, and nopal.

Common sources of Selenium: brazil nuts, walnuts, chickpeas/garbanzo beans, kola nuts, dandelion greens, and nettle, and alfalfa. Recommended to consume about 400 micrograms a day.

Common Sources of Zinc: chickpeas, mushrooms, zucchini, squash, okra, Brazil nuts, and walnuts.

Common Sources of Chromium: green beans, orange juice, grape juice, tomato juice, apples, Brazil nuts, dried fruits, broccoli

Impotence

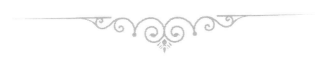

Occasionally, the intended purpose of a drug is not its most effective function. For example, sildenafil citrate (Viagra) was originally developed to treat high blood pressure (hypertension) and chest pain (angina). When Viagra was in its first clinical trial, patients began asking for the drug even though the clinical trials had shown that it was ineffective for treating angina (a condition where there is severe pain in the chest and upper body due to low blood supply to the heart). Another clinical trial was carried out to study Viagra's effects on erectile dysfunction and, ultimately, Viagra became the billion-dollar drug it is today. However, many of the side effects of Viagra include chest pain, dizziness, and can have an impact on blood pressure (ironically). This drug only works to boost blood flow to the penis but does nothing to restore not replenish any damage that has occurred or avoid any blockages that occur that lead to things like erectile dysfunction, otherwise referred to as *impotence*.

About 10-15 million people in America are impacted by impotency.

In this section we will look into the many causes of impotence as well as natural replacements one can take in exchange of items such as Viagra.

Remedies:

Delete The Meat

The penis is a vascular organ, meaning, that the very same things that are well-known to clog arteries (cholesterol and saturated fat) will also clog blood flow to the penis. Slowing blood flow to the penis, creates impotence. You want to refrain from eating animal flesh to reduce clogging blood flow. Dr. Irwin Goldstein, M.D., professor of urology at Boston University School of Medicine states, "High cholesterol is probably one of the leading causes of impotence in this country. It also appears to affect erectile dysfunction."

Arginine

The Viagra pills are designed to block an enzyme called (PDE5) which destroys the nitric acid in the body. Nitric acid is a chemical that is responsible for allowing the penis to fill with blood during an erection. The amino acid known as *arginine*, is the body's main source of nitric acid. 3,000-milligrams a day of arginine should be enough to help show progress. Give it time as it will take a few weeks to take effect. Take at least an hour before intercourse.

Common Sources of Arginine: watermelon, sesame seeds, sunflower seeds, chickpeas, walnuts, butternut squash, watercress, figs (Indian), onion powder, ginger, and coconut kernels.

Ginkgo Biloba (herb)

This herb is most notably known for improving memory and improving blood circulation to the brain. However, this herb also works to improve circulation to other areas in the body, such as the penis.

Say No to Alcohol

Alcohol suppresses the body's nervous system by inhibiting your reflexes, which contributes to impotence. Over time, alcohol will cause hormonal imbalances. Alcohol consumption causes damage to the nerves and the liver. Liver damage prevents the right proportion of testosterone from being produced by the liver, resulting in releasing many other (more feminine) hormones. In men, this leads to not being able to achieve a normal erection. Shakespeare once said that "alcohol provokes desire but takes away performance."

No Nicotine

Dr. Neil Baum, M.D., associate clinical professor of urology at Tulane University School of Medicine in New Orleans, Louisiana, has conducted many studies that show that nicotine can be a blood constrictor. The University of California had researchers summarize 20 years of research showing the connection between smoking and impotence. Approximately 40% of the 3,819 men with impotence studied over these years were smokers, compared to 28% of men who did not smoke.

Skin-To-Skin Arousal

"The skin is the largest sexual organ in the body; not the penis" says Dr. James Goldberg, Ph.D., urologist and professor at the University of Washington in Seattle, Washington. The skin is the first point of contact on the physical body. The skin absorbs and feels touch that stimulates arousal. Alter your focus on skin-to-skin arousal in the form of massage or other activities of intimacy to help relax the body while promoting arousal. Discover (or re-discover) ways to promote arousal and intimacy that aren't centered around getting an erection.

Body Image

When we feel good about our bodies, we perform better. Find some activities that will help you feel good; preferably activities that involve physical movement. Try starting a more specific (short-term) weight-training or exercise plan, practice some martial arts, or commit to working on progress towards sculpting your physique. Find what works for you that does not deplete your energy and makes you feel good while moving.

Relax

When the nerves in the body are not relaxed, the body goes into a more enhanced alert condition known as the "fight or flight" response. Adrenal hormones in the body cause the nerves to send blood to your muscles, away from your digestive tract, and away from your penis. You can turn on this process (no pun intended) just by feeling too anxious or unsettled. You want to do quite the opposite, which is to relax the body as a whole. Even our thoughts

Take Your Time

Working to get a full erection is the easiest way to clog blood flow. Allow yourself to slowly achieve an erection so a slow, steady blood flow is being promoted. It may take longer for older men to get an erection, so it is important to not panic. Use your time to continue activities such as foreplay, massage, or other stimulating activity for your spouse (or for yourself).

Communication

Talk to your partner about what is going on. Chances are, if they are close enough to have intercourse with you, they will be supportive and open to a conversation. Talk to them about what is happening and work together on identifying things that may be helpful. It will serve both of you to work together on decreasing any tension or feelings of inadequacy. This can help strengthen your bond, keep things lively and creative, and also deter those from "cheating" who this may apply to.

Tantric Yoga

This form of yoga is NOT something to do with a family member or friend. It is a form of yoga that teaches techniques for improving sexual performance. Charles Muir, director of the Source School of Tantra Yoga in Wailuku, Hawaii, states that "Most men think that if they don't have an erection, they can't do anything. But these techniques can bring circulation and energy to the penis, causing an erection." Below are the two primary techniques that Charles Muir teaches.

- Holding The Wand – for this technique, either partner grasps the penis with the fingers or hand and manipulates it as if it were a wand, gently rubbing the head across the outside of the vagina, especially over and around the clitoris. Muir says, "The stimulation and contact with your lover's vagina will inspire an erection pretty quickly, but a soft penis can provide a woman great pleasure. A lubricant is necessary in this technique to eliminate friction and enhance enjoyment." Knowing that you and your partner are not about to have sexual intercourse (at least during the yoga class), helps the body relax while focusing attention where it is needed.

- Tapping Into Pleasure – this technique involves tapping the penis against the lips of the vagina and clitoris. Muir states, "Again, either the man or woman can perform this move, holding the penis as if it were a conductor's baton, tapping it to a slow tempo that builds faster and faster, using it to contact the woman with a touch that varies from gentle to firm, then back to gentle." This technique can also be completed were soft or hard.

Aframomum (herb)

Aframomum (also known as Alligator Pepper, Ataare, Grains of Pardise, and Melegueta Pepper) is an African aphrodisiac spice with a similar composition to Ginger. It is a pro-ejaculant herb for men and increases their sperm count. The herb is helpful for all sexual disorders in both genders.

In women, Aframomum boosts libido and make women more sensitive to intimate touch, especially in the lower regions. Additionally, it regulates vaginal lubrication, and increases *sexual* desire in 48-72 hours.

Aframomum promotes circulation making it helpful for erectile dysfunction conditions as well as all other sexual dysfunction plaguing society today.

Bangalala (herb)

Bangalala, native to South Africa and used for centuries by the Zulu tribe, is one of the best herbs for male sexual health. A powerful aphrodisiac and sexual tonic, it boosts and improves libido, counters male erectile dysfunction (improves circulation to the genitalia), increases and improves sexual stamina, increases energy, enhances male potency, and boosts testosterone levels.

The herb enhances sexual performance by increasing blood flow to the penis thus promoting stronger, longer lasting erections. In women, it increases blood flow to the clitoris, heightening sensitivity to the organ and surrounding labia (lips of the vagina).

The herb is also helpful for pregnant women in the last two weeks of pregnancy to help a woman prepare for childbirth. Women suffering from infertility would do well to consume Bangalala religiously.

Mondia Whitei (herb)

Mondia Whitei (also known as Isirigun, White Ginger, Mukombera, and Mulondo), from Nigeria (but also found in Benin), androgenic in nature, is commonly referred to as African Viagra, boosts libido, improves testosterone production and levels in the body, increases size and weight of the testicles, improves male fertility (by improving sperm quality); increases sperm production, boosts strength, energy, and stamina; counters premature ejaculation, helps to heal STDs such as gonorrhea, and improves mental well-being.

Additionally, the herb increases potency by being able to relax the corpus cavernosum muscle thus aiding erection and by improving sperm total motility and progressive motility.

Furthermore, the herb enhances urination, ease birth pains, and increases the quantity and quality of mother's milk.

Fadogia Agrestis (herb)

Fadogia Agrestis (also known as Black Aphrodisiac) from Nigeria, a pro-erectile herb, is one of the most potently effective African erotogens available. It boosts libido, promotes and supports muscle mass, increases energy levels, boosts testosterone levels, strengthens physical/athletic performance, counters impotence/erectile dysfunction, increases stamina, and increases the sex drive. It is a supreme aphrodisiac!

Fadogia Agrestis promotes the production luteinizing hormone which produces testosterone in the male body. Additionally, it helps prevent the accumulation of excess fat in the body and makes one fit by burning fat. It is also loaded with antioxidants and helps keep the immune system fortified.

Fadogia Agrestis is popular herb and ingredient in the Fitness and Supplement World. It is an excellent herb for boosting testosterone levels (which are at all-time lows in the Western world, mostly due to PCBs or Poly-Cholorinated Biphenyls that are literally everywhere in society).

Bulbine Natalensis (herb)

Bulbine Natalensis is a South African herb that boosts testosterone levels by threefold up to six-fold. It is the Number One herb on planet earth for increasing testosterone levels in men, the sad fact which is - today, men in the Western world are experiencing all-time lows in testosterone levels (which mainly due to PCBs [Poly-Chlorinated Biphenyl], Atrazine chemical [in municipal water supplies], and consuming today's female-specific growth hormone [meat and dairy products, derived from farm animals]).

The plant's high testosterone levels greatly boost and repair the male libido.

Additionally, the plant which has anabolic and androgenic properties regulates the hormones (testosterone and androgen), increases testicular size, boosts protein levels in the testes, increases the sex drive, increases intravaginal ejaculatory latency time or EILT

Bulbine Natalensis aids in working out (great for muscle strength). Great for gym-goers and weightlifters (bodybuilders).

While Bulbine Natalensis can increase or boost testosterone levels up to six (6) times, it also lowers estrogen levels three-fold.

Gouro (herb)

Gouro is a natural aphrodisiac from the root of the plant *Turraea Heterophylla* (which is shaped like an erect penis with testicles at the base) which is found especially in Côte d'Ivoire or Ivory Coast in Africa.

It naturally boosts libido and promotes penis enlargement, counters premature ejaculation and sexual weakness. Additionally, it promotes longer lasting erections.

Gouro root highly compliments Yohimbe bark, Mpesu, and Kigelia especially for penis enlargement purposes.

African Pygeum Bark (herb)

African Pygeum Bark, one of the best herbs for adverse prostate conditions, is an anti-inflammatory phytosterol with the ability to normalize male prostate prostaglandins and to help shrink the prostate in males with enlarged prostates. It is very useful for benign prostatic hypertrophy (BPH) to reduce inflammation and pain and normalize the passage of urine.

Pygeum also increases prostatic and seminal fluid secretions. A meta-analysis revealed that men taking pygeum had a 19% reduction in nocturia and a 24% reduction in residual urine volume.

Pygeum bark helps improve semen volume and viscosity via its effect on DHT and through its action on the development and function of the prostate and seminal vesicles. Healthy viscosity of semen allows more sperm to survive for longer.

Mpesu Bark (herb)

Mpesu Bark from South Africa, a pro-erectile, is one of the most potent and effective male-specific aphrodisiac and erotegens on the planet. It counters sexual dysfunction, weak penile erection, premature ejaculation, and boosts libido and sexual stamina.

Mpesu will give a man longer lasting and stronger erections and will help him experience multiple erections and orgasms.

An added benefit of Mpesu Bark is that it is one of a few herbs that actually naturally promotes growth of the male penis. It compliments "Kigelia" and "Akpi" (for promotion of penis growth, length and width).

The herb also naturally and effectively helps to boost testosterone levels.

Yohimbe (herb)

Yohimbe bark, the King of Aphrodisiacs, is a male-specific hormonal stimulant effective in the production of testosterone, and as an aphrodisiac affecting both male impotence and female frigidity.

The bark has a stimulatory effect on the sex organs of both genders. Yohimbe enhances sexual performance and counters erectile dysfunction (ED) in males. In females, the bark increases arousal and sensitivity of the clitoris and counters frigidity.

Yohimbe is also useful in bodybuilding and athletic performance, weight loss, improving body composition, and adverse heart conditions.

Date Palm Pollen

Date Palm Pollen (DPP) from Egypt, Africa is an authentic African substance or product, derived from the male reproductive dust of palm flowers and has traditionally been used to increase libido and improve fertility in both women and men.

It is one of the best substances to counter male testicular and female ovarian dysfunction. A great product for the male and female reproductive systems.

In men, the pollen helps with testosterone (maintaining normal to high levels), libido, and increasing sperm quantity and quality.

In women, the pollen helps to increase female fertility (boosting ovulation) owing to its estrogen-like compounds, sterols, and estrone-like compounds (that do not throw off or counter men's testosterone levels).

Typha Capensis (herb)

Native to South Africa, commonly known as "Love Reed" is an effective African aphrodisiac herb that enhances the production of testosterone thus increasing libido, countering male infertility and aging male problems; enhances male potency, and counters erectile dysfunction (by improving circulation); and enhancing sexual performance.

In women, Typha Capensis is a powerful fertility enhancer. It strongly enhances ovulation. Additionally, it tones the vagina and increases circulation to that orifice, heightening sensitivity in that region during intimacy.

Typha Capensis can be consumed in the last two weeks of pregnancy to prepare for childbirth. It strengthens uterine contractions. Typha Capensis also helps in countering sexually transmitted diseases.

Uziza (herb)

Uziza, an Igbo name (also known as Ashanti Pepper, West African Pepper, Guinea Pepper, and *Ata iyere* in Yoruba) is an African herb, used in Nigeria mainly, that helps improve penile erections, enhances fertility and potency, and improves low sperm counts in men.

In women, Uziza is great for their sexual reproductive health. It improves fertility, enhancing ovulation. During pregnancy, it can be taken throughout pregnancy and especially during the last trimester to prepare for childbirth and to prepare for lactation. It increases uterine wall contraction during childbirth. Additionally, it helps with adverse menstrual issues, especially cramping.

Goran Tula Fruit

Goran Tula fruit (also known as Tree Hibiscus and Snot Apple) increases the libido in both men and women and promotes strong desire for sexual intercourse. It helps couples go multiple rounds *between the sheets.*

The herb is also an effective hormonal balancer, especially for women.

Goran Tula is a reliable fertility enhancer (for both men and women). It also enhances ovulation in women and improves semen concentration and quality while increasing semen volume.

In women, Goran Tula is a vaginal tonic and stimulates the production of vaginal wetness/lubrication and is perfect for keeping the vagina area moist and wet. The herb is one of the best for women who find it difficult to climax or reach orgasm.

Goran Tula is also a vaginal cleanser and deodorizer (helps to eliminate malodors in the vagina) and helps to keep the kitty cat smelling (and tasting) sweet and fresh. Additionally, it helps with adverse menstrual cycle complaints and normalizes the menstrual cycle after childbirth.

Kigelia

Kigelia (also known as Sausage Tree, Worsboom *in Afrikaans*, Modukghulu, *Pidiso in North Sotho,* umVongotsi *in Siswati*; Mpfungurhu *in Tsonga*, and Muvevha *in Venda.*

Because the fruit is shaped in the form of the male penis, pursuant to the herbal doctrine of signatures, its properties are helpful for the male genitalia, especially for naturally increasing the growth and length of the penis (taken consistently or religiously) over time, 3-6 months (to notice significant change).

In men, Kigelia is aphrodisiacal and helps the penis to become larger.

In women, Kigelia counters infertility being naturally rich in phyoestrogens. It is one of the best herbs for the breasts, naturally toning, firming and defining the breasts as well as enhancing their growth (natural breast enhancement or growth factor).

In lactating women, Kigelia stimulates lactation. Additionally, it increases the volume and quality of mother's milk.

Kigelia is exceptional for all gynecological disorders in women. It is useful (in men and women) to counter sexually transmitted diseases (STDs or STIs), especially syphilis and gonorrhea.

Incontinence

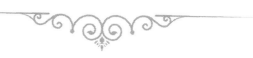

Most doctors only provide three options for incontinence: (1) prescription medications, (2) operation/surgery, or (3) wear a diaper. *Incontinence* involves having a lack of control over your urinary system and bowels where you urinate or defecate. Robert Schlesinger, M.D., urologist at the Faulkner Hospital in Jamaica Plain, Massachusetts, refers to incontinence as a "social disease" because it impacts a person's self-esteem, work life, and social life. More than 13 million Americans experience incontinence.

There are two forms of incontinence: (1) stress induced, and (2) urge induced. If you are someone who leaks small amounts of urine after you sneeze, cough, exercise, or laugh, this is likely *stress incontinence*. If you are someone that loses control of your bladder for no apparent reason which forces you to find a bathroom to urinate, this is *urge incontinence*. Incontinence is not part of getting older that are enhanced due to external triggers. These are internal issues that can be avoided and reversed when addressed properly.

Remedies:

Hydrate Properly

Go easy on hydrating by drinking fluids. Eat fruits and fresh vegetables that have a high-water content so the water can properly absorb into the cells in your body. You can actually become dehydrated by consuming too many liquids as the body will begin storing water in your kidneys in which the body will "leak out" these fluids in the form of regular trips to the bathroom to urinate in which you will lose the opportunity of absorbing the water you are drinking over time and become dehydrated. Melons, berries, and leafy greens are best to consume for proper hydration.

Avoid Caffeine

Caffeine is a diuretic which induces urination. Caffeine irritates the bladder and stimulates muscle contractions more frequently. You want to avoid consuming sodas, coffee, chocolate, and over-the-counter products such as Excedrin, Midol, and Anacin, as they all contain caffeine. The more you make efforts towards decreasing your caffeine intake, the more noticeable improvements you should notice.

Avoid Alcohol

The muscles within the pelvis control the opening of the urethra (tube that urine flows from leaving the bladder). Weak pelvis muscles promote "leakage" in the form of incontinence. Alcohol weakens the muscles within the pelvis. Alcohol is also a strong diuretic which only further promotes conditions like incontinence.

Avoid Grapefruit Juice

This juice is a well-known diuretic which should be avoided when working through this condition. Avoid eating this fruit as well during this time as even a small amount of juice from the fruit itself can trigger symptoms more regularly.

Cranberry Juice

Cranberry juice helps to prevent urinary tract infections (UTI's) which can occur from regularly urinating. This juice can also deodorize the smell of urinating if you have any accidents so that the smell is unnoticeable.

Avoid Nicotine

Nicotine irritates the bladder. This is never a good thing, but when dealing with incontinence, the bladder will believe it has to pass urine when it becomes irritated, and this will lead to more frequent urination. Smoking can also increase stress incontinence due to regular coughing.

Avoid Soft Drinks

The carbon dioxide bubbles in soft drinks make urine more acidic. Not only will this make you urinate more often but will make you more susceptible to contracting an infection (UTI) due to the acidity within your urine. Even "bubbly water" can fall into this same category.

Kegel Exercises

Kegel exercises were further developed in the 1940's by Arnold Kegal, M.D., to help women with stress incontinence and pregnancy. Guidelines from the National Association for Continence include:

- Imagine you are trying to hold a bowel movement (without tightening the abdomen, buttocks, or legs) by tightening the ring of muscles surrounding the anus (sphincter). This step involves the back part of the pelvic muscles.

- While urinating, stop the flow, and then restart. Women may find it helpful to imagine that they are trying to grip a tampon. This step involves the front part of the pelvic muscles.

- As you can now locate these specific areas, you will want to tighten these muscles (back to front). After you tighten these muscles, count to four slowly, then release. Do these for approximately 2-minutes at least three times a day for best results. You should work up to about 100 repetitions a day of these exercises.

Bladder Training

Wait until you are clam to go to the bathroom. We often fear having an accident, so we rush to the bathroom to avoid this from occurring. But all this does is create an unstable feeling about urinating and increase stress. You want to reduce these feelings by controlling the bladder. Simply stopping or holding in your urine won't be enough to prevent this from occurring. A few quick tips on how to control your bladder include:

- When you feel the urge to go, stay put and remain still. This will give you time to notice if you really have to go or if the bladder is just being stimulated.

- Try squeezing your pelvic muscles a few times to inform your body that you are aware of what is happening so that you can remain calm.

- Relax the rest of your body by taking several deep breaths to release additional tension.

- Wait to see if the urge to go changes.

- Walk to a bathroom at a normal pace to not cause the body to feel rushed or anxious.

Do this each time you have to go in order to maintain a better control of your bladder.

Reduce Tension

When the body is unsettled or anxious, any stimulation will appear to be magnified. When dealing with incontinence, you may feel you have to go to the bathroom sooner than necessary which not only creates an additional trip to the bathroom, but also prolongs stress and feelings of uneasiness which will stimulate the bladder and cause you to go again. Do activities to unwind as much as possible. Don't focus too much on setting out to keep busy or occupied, but finding calming and relaxing activities that don't require much effort to help you relax. Maybe go for a walk, visit a museum, or find an area to clean that will help you unwind.

My Personal Remedy:

1 small handful of cornsilk

2 teaspoons of horsetail herb

1 teaspoon of buchu herb

Mix together well and add to cup of boiling water. Drink 2-3 times a day. Take a day or two off from drinking it to track results. Reduce to 1-2 cups a day when results are improving until you do not have to drink this mixture anymore.

Note: You may drink this mixture for several weeks before seeing significant results.

Infertility

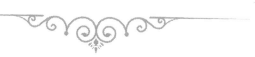

Not everyone develops the capacity to conceive a child. There are many hindrances that get the way that contribute to infertility. Most couples remain on some form of artificial birth control and are unaware of their infertility until they are intentionally trying to conceive a child. Infertility is defined as, "the inability to conceive a child within one year." Conceiving a child involves a process that takes time. being "infertile" does not happen after an initial attempt. A full calendar year (12 months) is given to tract fertility as many factors such as, the time of year, weather, personal fertility cycles, and stress, among other things.

Roger C. Hirsh, O.M.D., doctor of Oriental medicine and specialist in herbal medicine in Beverly Hills, California states that, "Combined conventional and alternative medical approaches are the best ways to treat infertility."

Remedies:
For Women

Birth Control

Whether through natural methods or pill form, if you are a woman over the age of 35, you should avoid birth control if trying to conceive. Fertility and hormonal changes often decrease for women by the age of 35. Around this age, you will want to take advantage of any chances to conceive, which you will further decrease the likelihood of having a child if using birth control. Birth control pills disrupt regular cycles and can actually make it more difficult to conceive in later years.

Finding Your Fertility Weight

Many cases of infertility stem from weighing too much or too little. You want to consult with your doctor about what weight range you should work to maintain.

Exercise

Keeping up with a regular exercise regimen can not only help promote hormonal regulation, but also work to decrease any stress connected to trying to conceive.

Time Your Ovulation

Ovulation is when a woman will release an egg from their ovary. This is about 10-14 days prior to menstruation. Dr. Linda C. Giudice, M.D., Ph.D., director of the division of reproductive endocrinology and fertility at Stanford University recommends using an ovulation detection kit to help track your ovulation. You can purchase one of these kits over the counter and they work by measuring your levels of urinary luteinizing hormone (LH) which is a hormone that stimulates egg maturation and release. It is recommended to use this kit between 8:00am – 10:00am when LH increases. Ovulation detection often will detect about 1 day before you actually ovulate. So, make sure to clear out your schedule that day and the day after so you can increase your chances of conceiving.

No Soy Consumption

Soy can act as a hormone disruptor. Soy will directly interfere with a woman's cycle. Soy contains plant estrogen called, *phytoestrogens*. Phytoestrogens work to compete with a woman's natural estrogen which can throw off a woman's ovulation cycle. Dr. Robert Stillman, M.D., clinical professor of obstetrics and gynecology at Georgetown University School of Medicine in Washington, D.C., and medical director at the Shady Grove Fertility Reproductive Science Center in Rockville, Maryland reports that when woman consume soy products such as soy milk, tofu, or plant-based meats that contain soy, "We've seen women who have stopped ovulating completely."

Chasteberry Extract

Commonly known as "vitex" as a name brand supplement, Chasteberry Extract works to stimulate the pituitary gland to increase the production of LH, which results in higher levels of progesterone during the second stage of a woman's cycle known as the luteal phase.

Progesterone helps to develop a thick, blood-rich uterine lining into which the fertilized egg can implant. Many women between the ages of 30 and 45 have a sharp drop off in progesterone which leads to shorter cycles and a decreased chance of implanting a fertilized egg. Make sure to use Chasteberry Extract for several months before attempting to conceive. Standard dosage should be about 40 drops of this extract one a day, or one 650-milligram capsule 2-3 times a day. Make sure to follow directions on label instructions.

False Unicorn Root (herb)

Yes, that is the actual name of this herb. Although research on this herb to provide scientific data showing more specific proof that this herb helps with fertility, herbalists have named this herb as the primary herb to use to help increase fertility. It is best absorbed in liquid form (tincture) where you use 5-15 drops a day for 3-6 months before trying to conceive.

Vitamin-C

Dr. Jacob Teitelbaum, M.D., a physician in Annapolis, Maryland, cites a study that found women who consume 1,000 milligrams or more increased their chances of infertility. Dr Teitelbaum recommends no more than 500 milligrams of Vitamin C.

Common sources of Vitamin-c: black currants, red bell peppers, Kakadu plum, camu camu (fruit/berry), gooseberries, papaya, oranges, cantaloupe, raspberry, mango, blackberry, tomato, blueberry, grapes, apricot, and watermelon.

Remedies:
For Men

Avoid The Hot Tub

The intense heat from a hot tub can kill the sperm in the testes. Unlike steam rooms where a person sweats, hot tubs leave the testes submerged in hot water which will kill sperm cells over time. It is best to sit in a pool or cool body of water.

No More Tight Underwear

Tight underwear causes more harm than not. It is best to wear loose-fitting underwear so you can allow your testicles to breathe. "Briefs raise the temperature of a man's testicles which can kill sperm or can decrease the ability of sperm to fertilize an egg" says Dr. Linda Giudice, M.D., Ph.D., director of the division of reproductive endocrinology and fertility at Stanford University.

Vitamin-C

Unlike women who can increase their chances of infertility as mentioned in earlier in this section, vitamin c provides benefits for avoiding infertility. Low vitamin c can lead to "sluggish" sperm cells where increasing vitamin c consumption will provide energy and speed to the sperm cells to help improve fertility.

Common sources of Vitamin-c: black currants, red bell peppers, Kakadu plum, camu camu (fruit/berry), gooseberries, papaya, oranges, cantaloupe, raspberry, mango, blackberry, tomato, blueberry, grapes, apricot, and watermelon.

Arginine (amino acid)

Arginine is a semi-essential (not essential or nonessential) amino acid that is necessary in trace amounts to improve fertility. If you have a low sperm count, Dr. Teitelbaum, M.D., recommends 4,000 milligrams a day and up to 8,000milligrams a day if the issue is poor motility. You will want to meet with your doctor to decipher whether you have a low sperm count or poor motility.

Common sources of Arginine: walnuts, brazil nuts, zucchini, sunflower seeds, sesame seeds, pumpkin seeds.

Caution: do not increase arginine intake if you have genital herpes as flare ups can worsen.

Zinc

This mineral helps regulate hormones in the body. When zinc is low in males, they can fail to produce enough hormones that promote fertility. It is recommended to consume about 30 milligrams of zinc daily for a few months to increase fertility.

Common Sources of Zinc: chickpeas, mushrooms, zucchini, squash, okra, Brazil nuts, and walnuts.

Astragalus (herb)

This is a Chinese herb widely used in Traditional Chinese Medicine (TCM) for increasing sperm motility and other conditions such as erectile disfunction. You can use this herb's leaves, root, or in liquid form as a tincture. Follow directions on labeling and recommended dosage(s).

For Women and Men

Condoms & Restraint

Until you are planning to have a child, wearing condoms can be best prior to a relationship. Aside from simply avoiding conceiving a child, wearing a condom will reduce your chances of contracting a sexually transmitted disease that can leave your body infertile (both women and men). Also, practicing restraint where you focus on your partner, and you avoid climaxing together and decrease your chances of conceiving. For men, semen retention can remain key to helping not deplete your body of vital minerals and nutrients where you and your partner may try again later.

Have Self Control

Having sex several times a day can be counterproductive when trying to conceive. A man's sperm count drops immediately after ejaculating which won't help contribute to increasing fertility. It is best to refrain from intercourse temporarily to increase your chances of conceiving.

No Alcohol or Liquor

Estrogen levels rise for men with liver damage which impairs sperm production. Alcohol and liquor damage the liver. Studies have shown that women who drink 5 drinks within a week's span, decrease their fertility over time.

Damiana (herb)

This herb is known for boosting libido and sexual organs but can help increase the body's ability to utilize cells that normally die off during infertility. Drink this herb as a tea twice a day. Take 2 teaspoons and make as a 10-12-ounce tea twice a day for best results.

Acupressure

As stated in other sections throughout this book, acupressure points can be stimulated with the finger or palm to regulate the *chi* ("life energy") within the body along specific pathways called meridians. For men, acupressure point C4 is the best for improving fertility. Located about four finger-widths directly below the navel. This point works to balance and improve the kidneys and also reproductive health in and around the pelvic cavity. To stimulate this area, cover it with the palm of your right hand, then your left palm on top of your right hand, then press down and rub 100 times in a clockwise motion. Apply no more than 10lbs of pressure while doing this to not cause any damage. If you are unsure of how many pounds of pressure you're applying, simply push on your bathroom scale and see if it exceeds 10lbs or if you could apply more.

For women, they can also benefit from this same point but, another point can help enhance fertility even more. The most beneficial point for women is a point known as CV17, which is located in the center of the chest between the nipples. Apply the same technique as mentioned above for best results.

Keep You Abdomen In Good Shape

This does not only refer to exercising your abdomen regularly to promote digestion and strengthening your protection layer of muscles covering your most vital organ, but also the food we eat. You will want to incorporate foods that are more "filling" foods that can be eaten by themselves or with other items. Foods such as grains like quinoa, fonio, kamut, amaranth, and spelt, squash, garbanzo beans, wild rice, and cooked vegetables which take longer to digest than uncooked. All of these items can help warm the uterus by providing protein-rich foods that also provide fiber, so digestion is slowed compared to those one a raw diet or generalized plant-based diet.

Too much heat damages the sperm cells for men. "Cooling" foods are best for sperm count to remain high. Cooling foods can be as simple as eating fruit and leafy green vegetables. These foods will help keep the body cool while providing many essential minerals that can be contributing to infertility. Fruits and fruit nectars are particularly helpful with increasing sperm count and the amount a person can ejaculate.

Relaxation Techniques

Emotions associated with stress that are involved in conditions such as anxiety, depression, and anger can decrease chances of conception. Mind-body techniques are often highly recommended by holistic practitioners because the more tense the body is, the more constricted the body will feel, particularly the reproductive organs.

Dr. Alice Domar, Ph.D., director of the Behavioral Medicine Program for Infertility at Beth Israel Deaconess Medical Center in Boston, MA, reports that mind-body stress release strategies improve chances of conception, and overall quality of life. Dr. Domar advises women to practice for 20 minutes a day some form of meditation, yoga, visualization, or deep breathing to help decrease overall stress. She also recommends breathing from your diaphragm ('belly breathing") where you feel your belly expand as you inhale where you practice breathing in deeply and hen counting down slowly from 10 down to zero with each breath.

Kegel Exercises

Kegel exercises were further developed in the 1940's by Arnold Kegal, M.D., to help women with stress incontinence and pregnancy. Guidelines from the National Association for Continence include:

- Imagine you are trying to hold a bowel movement (without tightening the abdomen, buttocks, or legs) by tightening the ring of muscles surrounding the anus (sphincter). This step involves the back part of the pelvic muscles.

- While urinating, stop the flow, and then restart. Women may find it helpful to imagine that they are trying to grip a tampon. This step involves the front part of the pelvic muscles.

- As you can now locate these specific areas, you will want to tighten these muscles (back to front). After you tighten these muscles, count to four slowly, then release. Do these for approximately 2-minutes at least three times a day for best results. You should work up to about 100 repetitions a day of these exercises.

Doing this can help assist men in toning their prostate which can improve ejaculation power.

Iron

The iron mentioned here is iron-phosphate, which is abundant in plants, not iron-oxide which comes from metallic substances and pharmaceutical medications and prescriptions. While many people may not have low enough iron to be anemic, they can still have an iron deficiency low enough to impact fertility. A standard blood test can be used to test iron levels which measures the *ferritin* (protein in the body that stores iron) to determine if your iron levels are low or not. Dr. Jacob Teitelbaum, M.D., a physician in Annapolis, Maryland, cites how there are many research studies that show that at least half of the women who have low ferritin levels quickly are able to become pregnant once they begin to increase their iron intake. If you do not have access to test your ferritin levels, it is recommended to consume at minimum 50 milligrams of iron a day for several months. It is important to take iron on an empty stomach to maximize absorption. Caution: do not take iron within 6-hours of taking any thyroid medication(s) if applicable.

Common Sources of Iron: quinoa, wild rice (not black rice), chickpeas/garbanzo beans, kale, nuts (particularly walnuts), hemp seeds, dates, dried apricots, prunes, watercress, sarsaparilla, burdock (and root), guaco, chainey root, monkey ladder, chickweed, yellowdock

African Herbs To Assist Men and Women:

Aframomum (herb)

Aframomum (also known as Alligator Pepper, Ataare, Grains of Pardise, and Melegueta Pepper) is an African aphrodisiac spice with a similar composition to Ginger. It is a pro-ejaculant herb for men and increases their sperm count. The herb is helpful for all sexual disorders in both genders.

In women, Aframomum boosts libido and make women more sensitive to intimate touch, especially in the lower regions. Additionally, it regulates vaginal lubrication, and increases *sexual* desire in 48-72 hours.

Aframomum promotes circulation making it helpful for erectile dysfunction conditions as well as all other sexual dysfunction plaguing society today.

Bangalala (herb)

Bangalala, native to South Africa and used for centuries by the Zulu tribe, is one of the best herbs for male sexual health. A powerful aphrodisiac and sexual tonic, it boosts and improves libido, counters male erectile dysfunction (improves circulation to the genitalia), increases and improves sexual stamina, increases energy, enhances male potency, and boosts testosterone levels.

The herb enhances sexual performance by increasing blood flow to the penis thus promoting stronger, longer lasting erections. In women, it increases blood flow to the clitoris, heightening sensitivity to the organ and surrounding labia (lips of the vagina).

The herb is also helpful for pregnant women in the last two weeks of pregnancy to help a woman prepare for childbirth. Women suffering from infertility would do well to consume Bangalala religiously.

Mondia Whitei (herb)

Mondia Whitei (also known as Isirigun, White Ginger, Mukombera, and Mulondo), from Nigeria (but also found in Benin), androgenic in nature, is commonly referred to as African Viagra, boosts libido, improves testosterone production and levels in the body, increases size and weight of the testicles, improves male fertility (by improving sperm quality); increases sperm production, boosts strength, energy, and stamina; counters premature ejaculation, helps to heal STDs such as gonorrhea, and improves mental well-being.

Additionally, the herb increases potency by being able to relax the corpus cavernosum muscle thus aiding erection and by improving sperm total motility and progressive motility.

Furthermore, the herb enhances urination, ease birth pains, and increases the quantity and quality of mother's milk.

Fadogia Agrestis (herb)

Fadogia Agrestis (also known as Black Aphrodisiac) from Nigeria, a pro-erectile herb, is one of the most potently effective African erotogens available. It boosts libido, promotes and supports muscle mass, increases energy levels, boosts testosterone levels, strengthens physical/athletic performance, counters impotence/erectile dysfunction, increases stamina, and increases the sex drive. It is a supreme aphrodisiac!

Fadogia Agrestis promotes the production luteinizing hormone which produces testosterone in the male body. Additionally, it helps prevent the accumulation of excess fat in the body and makes one fit by burning fat. It is also loaded with antioxidants and helps keep the immune system fortified.

Fadogia Agrestis is popular herb and ingredient in the Fitness and Supplement World. It is an excellent herb for boosting testosterone levels (which are at all-time lows in the Western world, mostly due to PCBs or Poly-Cholorinated Biphenyls that are literally everywhere in society).

Bulbine Natalensis (herb)

Bulbine Natalensis is a South African herb that boosts testosterone levels by threefold up to six-fold. It is the Number One herb on planet earth for increasing testosterone levels in men, the sad fact which is - today, men in the Western world are experiencing all-time lows in testosterone levels (which mainly due to PCBs [Poly-Chlorinated Biphenyl], Atrazine chemical [in municipal water supplies], and consuming today's female-specific growth hormone [meat and dairy products, derived from farm animals]).

The plant's high testosterone levels greatly boost and repair the male libido.

Additionally, the plant which has anabolic and androgenic properties regulates the hormones (testosterone and androgen), increases testicular size, boosts protein levels in the testes, increases the sex drive, increases intravaginal ejaculatory latency time or EILT

Bulbine Natalensis aids in working out (great for muscle strength). Great for gym-goers and weightlifters (bodybuilders).

While Bulbine Natalensis can increase or boost testosterone levels up to six (6) times, it also lowers estrogen levels three-fold.

Gouro (herb)

Gouro is a natural aphrodisiac from the root of the plant *Turraea Heterophylla* (which is shaped like an erect penis with testicles at the base) which is found especially in Côte dᴵIvoire or Ivory Coast in Africa.

It naturally boosts libido and promotes penis enlargement, counters premature ejaculation and sexual weakness. Additionally, it promotes longer lasting erections.

Gouro root highly compliments Yohimbe bark, Mpesu, and Kigelia especially for penis enlargement purposes.

African Pygeum Bark (herb)

African Pygeum Bark, one of the best herbs for adverse prostate conditions, is an anti-inflammatory phytosterol with the ability to normalize male prostate prostaglandins and to help shrink the prostate in males with enlarged prostates. It is very useful for benign prostatic hypertrophy (BPH) to reduce inflammation and pain and normalize the passage of urine.

Pygeum also increases prostatic and seminal fluid secretions. A meta-analysis revealed that men taking pygeum had a 19% reduction in nocturia and a 24% reduction in residual urine volume.

Pygeum bark helps improve semen volume and viscosity via its effect on DHT and through its action on the development and function of the prostate and seminal vesicles. Healthy viscosity of semen allows more sperm to survive for longer.

Mpesu Bark (herb)

Mpesu Bark from South Africa, a pro-erectile, is one of the most potent and effective male-specific aphrodisiac and erotegens on the planet. It counters sexual dysfunction, weak penile erection, premature ejaculation, and boosts libido and sexual stamina.

Mpesu will give a man longer lasting and stronger erections and will help him experience multiple erections and orgasms.

An added benefit of Mpesu Bark is that it is one of a few herbs that actually naturally promotes growth of the male penis. It compliments "Kigelia" and "Akpi" (for promotion of penis growth, length and width).

The herb also naturally and effectively helps to boost testosterone levels.

Yohimbe (herb)

Yohimbe bark, the King of Aphrodisiacs, is a male-specific hormonal stimulant effective in the production of testosterone, and as an aphrodisiac affecting both male impotence and female frigidity.

The bark has a stimulatory effect on the sex organs of both genders. Yohimbe enhances sexual performance and counters erectile dysfunction (ED) in males. In females, the bark increases arousal and sensitivity of the clitoris and counters frigidity.

Yohimbe is also useful in bodybuilding and athletic performance, weight loss, improving body composition, and adverse heart conditions.

Date Palm Pollen

Date Palm Pollen (DPP) from Egypt, Africa is an authentic African substance or product, derived from the male reproductive dust of palm flowers and has traditionally been used to increase libido and improve fertility in both women and men.

It is one of the best substances to counter male testicular and female ovarian dysfunction. A great product for the male and female reproductive systems.

In men, the pollen helps with testosterone (maintaining normal to high levels), libido, and increasing sperm quantity and quality.

In women, the pollen helps to increase female fertility (boosting ovulation) owing to its estrogen-like compounds, sterols, and estrone-like compounds (that do not throw off or counter men's testosterone levels).

Typha Capensis (herb)

Native to South Africa, commonly known as "Love Reed" is an effective African aphrodisiac herb that enhances the production of testosterone thus increasing libido, countering male infertility and aging male problems; enhances male potency, and counters erectile dysfunction (by improving circulation); and enhancing sexual performance.

In women, Typha Capensis is a powerful fertility enhancer. It strongly enhances ovulation. Additionally, it tones the vagina and increases circulation to that orifice, heightening sensitivity in that region during intimacy.

Typha Capensis can be consumed in the last two weeks of pregnancy to prepare for childbirth. It strengthens uterine contractions. Typha Capensis also helps in countering sexually transmitted diseases.

Uziza (herb)

Uziza, an Igbo name (also known as Ashanti Pepper, West African Pepper, Guinea Pepper, and *Ata iyere* in Yoruba) is an African herb, used in Nigeria mainly, that helps improve penile erections, enhances fertility and potency, and improves low sperm counts in men.

In women, Uziza is great for their sexual reproductive health. It improves fertility, enhancing ovulation. During pregnancy, it can be taken throughout pregnancy and especially during the last trimester to prepare for childbirth and to prepare for lactation. It increases uterine wall contraction during childbirth. Additionally, it helps with adverse menstrual issues, especially cramping.

Goran Tula Fruit

Goran Tula fruit (also known as Tree Hibiscus and Snot Apple) increases the libido in both men and women and promotes strong desire for sexual intercourse. It helps couples go multiple rounds *between the sheets*.

The herb is also an effective hormonal balancer, especially for women.

Goran Tula is a reliable fertility enhancer (for both men and women). It also enhances ovulation in women and improves semen concentration and quality while increasing semen volume.

In women, Goran Tula is a vaginal tonic and stimulates the production of vaginal wetness/lubrication and is perfect for keeping the vagina area moist and wet. The herb is one of the best for women who find it difficult to climax or reach orgasm.

Goran Tula is also a vaginal cleanser and deodorizer (helps to eliminate malodors in the vagina) and helps to keep the kitty cat smelling (and tasting) sweet and fresh. Additionally, it helps with adverse menstrual cycle complaints and normalizes the menstrual cycle after childbirth.

Kigelia

Kigelia (also known as Sausage Tree, Worsboom *in Afrikaans*, Modukghulu, *Pidiso in North Sotho,* umVongotsi *in Siswati*; Mpfungurhu *in Tsonga*, and Muvevha *in Venda.*

Because the fruit is shaped in the form of the male penis, pursuant to the herbal doctrine of signatures, its properties are helpful for the male genitalia, especially for naturally increasing the growth and length of the penis (taken consistently or religiously) over time, 3-6 months (to notice significant change).

In men, Kigelia is aphrodisiacal and helps the penis to become larger.

In women, Kigelia counters infertility being naturally rich in phyoestrogens. It is one of the best herbs for the breasts, naturally toning, firming and defining the breasts as well as enhancing their growth (natural breast enhancement or growth factor).

In lactating women, Kigelia stimulates lactation. Additionally, it increases the volume and quality of mother's milk.

Kigelia is exceptional for all gynecological disorders in women. It is useful (in men and women) to counter sexually transmitted diseases (STDs or STIs), especially syphilis and gonorrhea.

Inflammatory Bowel Disease (IBS)

A healthy colon has its walls coated with a smooth layer of mucus that serves as protection. When the walls of the colon become inflamed and/or irritated, leading to pains and possibly bleeding, this is when inflammatory bowel disease shows itself. Excess inflammation in the form

of foods we eat and responses to what we consume, begin to apply additional pressure on the colon and cause irritation. We must avoid inflammation, mucus forming foods, while increasing anti-inflammatory foods, in addition to relieving pressure on the colon, are the steps to take for treating (and avoiding) this condition.

Traditional methods of treatment typically involve prescribing drugs that work to prevent the body's immune system from (mistakenly) attacking the intestines in the form of anti-inflammatory drugs. However, these anti-inflammatory drugs do not account for the amount of food or the items that are often difficult to digest. When these drugs and prescriptions are not effective, stronger ones are prescribed with more severe side effects. After stronger drugs are prescribed, if little to no progress is achieved, surgery is recommended to remove the diseased section of the intestines.

The traditional methods in the paragraph before this one will not serve you well long-term. In this section we will review simple ways to incorporate more anti-inflammatory foods while protecting the intestines from further damage to work towards healing this condition.

Remedies:

Glutamine (amino acid)

This amino acid directly feeds the cells' lining in the small intestine. Making sure the small intestine is properly nourished, will help correct the difficulty the small intestine has with absorbing essential nutrients when the bowels are inflamed and irritated with conditions such as inflammatory bowel disease. Increasing intake of this amino acid will help to begin relieving the severity of symptoms to help provide relief.

Common Sources of Glutamine: chickpeas, walnuts, dark leafy green vegetables, parsley, lentils, kidney beans.

Butyrate (fatty acid)

This short-chain fatty acid (SCFA) is produced when the good bacteria in the gut helps to break down dietary fiber in the large intestine (colon). This occurs naturally during digestions. Butyrate specifically supports the gut barrier, which works to keep bacteria and other microbes from entering your bloodstream. The best way to support your gut microbiome to produce Butyrate, is to eat a high-fiber diet that includes sufficient sources of resistant starch and pectin.

Certain foods (particularly those high in fiber) that help promote Butyrate in the gut are: garbanzo beans, lentils, apples and berries (high pectin fruits) and onions.

Boswellia (herb)

This herb provides anti-inflammatory properties without the many side effects that are associated with medications and prescription drugs made for anti-inflammatory or gut health. There are many research studies that show how boswellic acid can prevent the formation of leukotrienes (inflammatory molecules) in the body.

There are four specific acids that are in bowellia resin that contribute to the herb's anti-inflammatory properties. These helps to inhibit an enzyme known as "5-lipoxygenase (5-LO)" which produces leukotriene. The most powerful of the fours acids in Boswellia resin, acetyl-11-keto-β-boswellic acid (AKBA) helps to target the formation and production of leukotrienes.

You can take 300-500mg 2-3 times a day of this herb in tea form. Read directions on ingredient label if bought in various forms (capsules, liquids, etc).

Vitamin-E

Vitamin E helps neutralize free radicals that are released in the bowels for those who have inflammatory bowel disease. Free radicals are unstable oxygen molecules that cause damage to the cells within the intestines. Conditions such as inflammatory bowel disease unleash additional free radicles.

Common Sources of Vitamin E: red bell peppers, mangoes, walnuts, sunflower seeds (non-processed), avocados, butternut squash, olive oil (for dressings), coconut oil, and avocado oil.

Iron

The pressure placed upon the intestines directly impacts iron absorption due to additional blood being pumped to these areas. Prescriptions of artificial iron supplements that are often prescribed to those with bowel issues contain ferrous sulfate which can worsen this condition by slowing or backing up bowel movements. Ferritin, a non-irritating for of iron is better absorbed within the body. If you do not have access to test your ferritin levels, it is recommended to consume at minimum 50 milligrams of iron a day for several months. It is important to take iron on an empty stomach to maximize absorption. Caution: do not take iron within 6-hours of taking any thyroid medication(s) if applicable.

Common Sources of Iron: quinoa, wild rice (not black rice), chickpeas/garbanzo beans, kale, nuts (particularly walnuts), hemp seeds, dates, dried apricots, watercress, sarsaparilla, burdock (and root), guaco, chainey root, monkey ladder, chickweed, yellowdock

Fatty Acids

Due to the instability and frequent discomfort of inflammatory bowel disease, the risk of colon cancer is increased for those with this condition than those who do not have this condition. Essential fatty acids such as omega-3, omega-6, and omega-9 contain two specific acids known to reduce chemical reactions in the body that produce inflammation: (1) eicosapentaenoic acid and (2) docosahexaenoic acid (DHA).

Common Fatty Acid Sources: (Brazil Nuts, Walnuts, Kola Nuts, Avocados, Bananas, Sea Vegetables (Nori, Wakame, Hijiki, Sea Moss, Bladderwrack), Coconut, Coconut Oil, Olive Oil, Grapeseed Oil, Avocado Oil, Mushrooms, Quinoa, Wild Rice.

Liquids

Symptoms of inflammatory bowel disease can be severe and/or unnoticeable (active and/or quiet). To avoid contributing to the severity of the symptoms, it is best to avoid having to digest items that may rub against the intestines. In other words, stick to liquids so that it can slide smoothly through the intestines while being digested, while also providing your body with enough nourishment. Smoothies, juices, herbal tea, and soups (blended) can help you pack together essential minerals to be absorbed into your body, while giving your digestive tract and bowels some relief.

Alfalfa Greens

Contains minerals needed to build intestinal flora for proper digestion, and chlorophyll for healing and cleaning much of the bloodstream. You can take 5-10g of this three times a day in tea form or eat whole after washing.

Ginger (herb)

Aids in improving digestion and relieves upset stomach and gas. Helps reduce various pains and inflammation. Working in herbs to your diet such as Ginger help set daily reminders of your goal to reduce your symptoms while not adding anything that will contribute to or worsen your symptoms. One of Ginger's ingredients (gingerol) helps promote anti-inflammatory propertied you need to break down inflammation within the body.

Take about a fingertip size piece of ginger and add it to tea or break it down and consume with your meals.

Olive Leaf Extract (OLE)

Olive leaf extract (OLE) helps to protect the gut while also boosting the immune system. OLE provides a high amount of natural chemicals that specifically help with breaking down the bad bacteria within the gut. Chemicals such as biophenols (oleuropein and hydroxytyrosol) which improve and maintain the health of the microbiota in the gut. OLE helps to kill and fight off parasites in the gut as well which cause further irritation.

Ingrown Hair

Instead of growing outward like hair is supposed to, an ingrown hair grows inward back into the skin. As the tip of this hair touches the skin (from the inside of the skin) this causes pain and inflammation. The body creates an inflammatory response as a form of protection prevent outside invaders and bacteria from getting inside and making things worse.

Remedies:

Tweezers

The moment you notice a hair growing under the skin, soak the area with a warm, wet compress (small towel soaked in warm water and then wring out the excess water) to help soften the skin on the surface for a few minutes. Then you will want to use tweezers to pull out the ingrown hair. If you can see a hair but cannot reach it, don't try picking at it. This will irritate the skin and area where you may end up in more pain. Allow the hair to grow its way to the surface or grow long enough so that you can reach it. You may be in more frequent pain as this hair grows and pushes against the skin, but once you are able to reach the hair, it will be worth it as you will immediately feel relived without risking an infection.

Grow Your Hair Out (more)

The curlier your hair is, the more you will be at risk for having ingrown hairs. Allow your hair to grow out longer than you usually let it whenever you begin noticing more ingrown hairs. These hairs are more common on our faces so you may want to consider growing out a beard more often than not. At least a week or so you can let hairs on your face grow to avoid going through this, while hair on your arms and legs you don't have to monitor as often. If you shave your legs, allow your hairs to grow a bit more above the surface before shaving again (however long that takes for you).

Batana Oil

This oil as mentioned in other sections in this text helps with any and all issues regarding hair health. If you plan to grow your hair out more or grow more evenly, applying this oil to your hair daily will help. It will also help to smooth out or soften your hair and the skin around it which will help reduce any pain you may have so far.

Soften Your Hair

Not everyone is able to grow a full beard and some ingrown hairs can grow almost by themselves where there's little to almost no hairs. A good remedy to maintain is to apply a hydrating gel or cream and wash your face and hair thoroughly along with water for 2-3 minutes. Rinse off and then pat to dry. This will help soften the hair but also the skin around your hair follicles. This can give time for the hair to correct itself as it grows where you can avoid having an ingrown hair or will help you reach the hair easier to remove it.

Single Razors

Using single track razors will help cut your hairs easier and reduce the risk of ingrown hairs. When you use a double track (or more) razor, the first blade cut the hair but also sharpens it by cutting at an angle, and then the second blade cuts below the skin level. What happens next is, the hair can curl backwards and slip back into the skin and become an ingrown hair. Avoid this by using single razors to provide a closer shave.

Shaving Tips

Our hairs don't often grow straight. Hair on one side of our face may grow one direction while the other side of our face grows in a completely different direction. Rather than shave in various directions, only shave in two directions (1) straight down on your face and (2) up on your neck. Doing this will help to train your hair how to grow straighter and reduce your chances of having ingrown hairs.

Avoid Excess Alcohol On The Skin

Most aftershave gels or lotions contain a ton of chemicals and are mostly made of alcohol. Putting alcohol on your skin immediately after shaving can cause excess bacteria to remain stagnant on the skin. Alcohol can also clog pours on the skin and force hairs to not grow straight, which often results in having an ingrown hair. Reduce or avoid using many lotions.

With The Grain

Most of the time we will shave against the grain to get a closer shave. But all we really need is a good razor and some patience. Try shaving with the grain, not against. People who shave their legs, this goes for your too. Rather than shave ankle to knee, shave downward with the grain to avoid irritating the skin. We know our hair will grow back soon either way, so it's best to not irritate the skin and contribute to having to deal with ingrown hairs.

Inhibited Sexual Desire

When thoughts and feelings aren't shared, intimacy dissolves and sexual desire diminishes. In addition to stress and other barriers in life, communication is the primary reason sexual connection is a challenge for many. We want to work towards identifying ways to increase intimacy that restores the sexual connection.

Remedies:

Yoga

There are many forms of yoga, but doing some form of "couple's yoga" or form that promotes direct intimacy is crucial. These intimacy focused yoga classes essentially help two heartbeats become one where intimacy can become re-connected. If you do not have any classes like those described here, try the following at home with your partner:

Sit in a comfortable position and cross your legs, facing each other. If comfortable, the woman can sit in the man's lap with her legs wrapped around the man. If not comfortable, simply sit on your floor or any flat surface. You may also stand if sitting is difficult.

You and your partner place your left hand over each other's heart.

Lock eyes and work to synchronize your breathing. Feel and locate the energy of one another.

Do this as long as it remains calm and pleasurable.

You may do this with or without clothes on.

If this practice leads to sexual intercourse, don't fight it and be responsible. If not, don't worry about it. Just practice more and identify what section you can improve upon.

Control The Breath

This is an extension of the previous remedy or Yoga when you work to match one another's breath, but without touch. Stare into one another's eyes and synchronize your breathing. As you exhale, you can test out making an "ahh" sound. Paul and Marilena Silbey, of American Tantra in Fairfax, California states that, "This sound feeds the heart just as water feeds a plant." You and your partner want to create and sustain a positive field of energy around you to make way for additional opportunities for intimacy.

Sensitive Touch

For this remedy step, you want to learn (or re-learn) each other's body. take turns touching each part of each other's body with gentle, short strokes. Communicate what areas feel the best for you to your partner in addition to areas you each feel sexually stimulated by. If you only feel sexually stimulated when your partner touches your genitals or sexual organs, this exercise will provide you an opportunity to spread out any stagnant energy in and around your body. communication what is and what is not helpful during sexual intercourse can often lead to frustration and hinder communication. Use this exercise as an opportunity to take a step away from sex and open up the channels for communication and understanding.

Flower Essences

Using flower essences can help stimulate as well as promote sexual intimacy. Below are a few flower essences to boost sexual intimacy and desire.

Hornbean – lacking interest in your partner

Wild rose – more excitement

Olive – lack of sexual desire and fatigue

Note: mix a few drops of any of these flower essences with water and put into a spray bottle. Spray around the room to help set the mood and relax. Make sure to follow instructions on label for best use as some flower essences are safe to apply directly onto the skin, or directly ingested by placing onto the tongue.

African Herbs To Increase Desire and Performance (Men and Women):

Aframomum (herb)

Aframomum (also known as Alligator Pepper, Ataare, Grains of Pardise, and Melegueta Pepper) is an African aphrodisiac spice with a similar composition to Ginger. It is a pro-ejaculant herb for men and increases their sperm count. The herb is helpful for all sexual disorders in both genders.

In women, Aframomum boosts libido and make women more sensitive to intimate touch, especially in the lower regions. Additionally, it regulates vaginal lubrication, and increases sexual desire in 48-72 hours.

Aframomum promotes circulation making it helpful for erectile dysfunction conditions as well as all other sexual dysfunction plaguing society today.

Bangalala (herb)

Bangalala, native to South Africa and used for centuries by the Zulu tribe, is one of the best herbs for male sexual health. A powerful aphrodisiac and sexual tonic, it boosts and improves libido, counters male erectile dysfunction (improves circulation to the genitalia), increases and improves sexual stamina, increases energy, enhances male potency, and boosts testosterone levels.

The herb enhances sexual performance by increasing blood flow to the penis thus promoting stronger, longer lasting erections. In women, it increases blood flow to the clitoris, heightening sensitivity to the organ and surrounding labia (lips of the vagina).

The herb is also helpful for pregnant women in the last two weeks of pregnancy to help a woman prepare for childbirth. Women suffering from infertility would do well to consume Bangalala religiously.

Mondia Whitei (herb)

Mondia Whitei (also known as Isirigun, White Ginger, Mukombera, and Mulondo), from Nigeria (but also found in Benin), androgenic in nature, is commonly referred to as African Viagra, boosts libido, improves testosterone production and levels in the body, increases size and weight of the testicles, improves male fertility (by improving sperm quality); increases sperm production, boosts strength, energy, and stamina; counters premature ejaculation, helps to heal STDs such as gonorrhea, and improves mental well-being.

Additionally, the herb increases potency by being able to relax the corpus cavernosum muscle thus aiding erection and by improving sperm total motility and progressive motility.

Furthermore, the herb enhances urination, ease birth pains, and increases the quantity and quality of mother's milk.

Fadogia Agrestis (herb)

Fadogia Agrestis (also known as Black Aphrodisiac) from Nigeria, a pro-erectile herb, is one of the most potently effective African erotogens available. It boosts libido, promotes and supports muscle mass, increases energy levels, boosts testosterone levels, strengthens physical/

athletic performance, counters impotence/erectile dysfunction, increases stamina, and increases the sex drive. It is a supreme aphrodisiac!

Fadogia Agrestis promotes the production luteinizing hormone which produces testosterone in the male body. Additionally, it helps prevent the accumulation of excess fat in the body and makes one fit by burning fat. It is also loaded with antioxidants and helps keep the immune system fortified.

Fadogia Agrestis is popular herb and ingredient in the Fitness and Supplement World. It is an excellent herb for boosting testosterone levels (which are at all-time lows in the Western world, mostly due to PCBs or Poly-Cholorinated Biphenyls that are literally everywhere in society).

Bulbine Natalensis (herb)

Bulbine Natalensis is a South African herb that boosts testosterone levels by threefold up to six-fold. It is the Number One herb on planet earth for increasing testosterone levels in men, the sad fact which is - today, men in the Western world are experiencing all-time lows in testosterone levels (which mainly due to PCBs [Poly-Chlorinated Biphenyl], Atrazine chemical [in municipal water supplies], and consuming today's female-specific growth hormone [meat and dairy products, derived from farm animals]).

The plant's high testosterone levels greatly boost and repair the male libido. Additionally, the plant which has anabolic and androgenic properties regulates the hormones (testosterone and androgen), increases testicular size, boosts protein levels in the testes, increases the sex drive, increases intravaginal ejaculatory latency time or EILT.

Bulbine Natalensis aids in working out (great for muscle strength). Great for gym-goers and weight-lifters (bodybuilders).

While Bulbine Natalensis can increase or boost testosterone levels up to six (6) times, it also lowers estrogen levels three-fold.

Gouro (herb)

Gouro is a natural aphrodisiac from the root of the plant Turraea Heterophylla (which is shaped like an erect penis with testicles at the base) which is found especially in Côte d'Ivoire or Ivory Coast in Africa.

It naturally boosts libido and promotes penis enlargement, counters premature ejaculation and sexual weakness. Additionally, it promotes longer lasting erections.

Gouro root highly compliments Yohimbe bark, Mpesu, and Kigelia especially for penis enlargement purposes.

African Pygeum Bark (herb)

African Pygeum Bark, one of the best herbs for adverse prostate conditions, is an anti-inflammatory phytosterol with the ability to normalize male prostate prostaglandins and to help shrink the prostate in males with enlarged prostates. It is very useful for benign prostatic hypertrophy (BPH) to reduce inflammation and pain and normalize the passage of urine.

Pygeum also increases prostatic and seminal fluid secretions. A meta-analysis revealed that men taking pygeum had a 19% reduction in nocturia and a 24% reduction in residual urine volume.

Pygeum bark helps improve semen volume and viscosity via its effect on DHT and through its action on the development and function of the prostate and seminal vesicles. Healthy viscosity of semen allows more sperm to survive for longer.

Mpesu Bark (herb)

Mpesu Bark from South Africa, a pro-erectile, is one of the most potent and effective male-specific aphrodisiac and erotegens on the planet. It counters sexual dysfunction, weak penile erection, premature ejaculation, and boosts libido and sexual stamina.

Mpesu will give a man longer-lasting and stronger erections and will help him experience multiple erections and orgasms.

An added benefit of Mpesu Bark is that it is one of a few herbs that actually naturally promotes growth of the male penis. It compliments "Kigelia" and "Akpi" (for promotion of penis growth, length and width).

The herb also naturally and effectively helps to boost testosterone levels.

Yohimbe (herb)

Yohimbe bark, the King of Aphrodisiacs, is a male-specific hormonal stimulant effective in the production of testosterone, and as an aphrodisiac affecting both male impotence and female frigidity.

The bark has a stimulatory effect on the sex organs of both genders. Yohimbe enhances sexual performance and counters erectile dysfunction (ED) in males. In females, the bark increases arousal and sensitivity of the clitoris and counters frigidity. Yohimbe is also useful in bodybuilding and athletic performance, weight loss, improving body composition, and adverse heart conditions.

Date Palm Pollen

Date Palm Pollen (DPP) from Egypt, Africa is an authentic African substance or product, derived from the male reproductive dust of palm flowers and has traditionally been used to increase libido and improve fertility in both women and men.

It is one of the best substances to counter male testicular and female ovarian dysfunction. A great product for the male and female reproductive systems. In men, the pollen helps with testosterone (maintaining normal to high levels), libido, and increasing sperm quantity and quality. In women, the pollen helps to increase female fertility (boosting ovulation) owing to its estrogen-like compounds, sterols, and estrone-like compounds (that do not throw off or counter men's testosterone levels).

Typha Capensis (herb)

Native to South Africa, commonly known as "Love Reed" is an effective African aphrodisiac herb that enhances the production of testosterone thus increasing libido, countering male infertility and aging male problems; enhances male potency, and counters erectile dysfunction (by improving circulation); and enhancing sexual performance.

In women, Typha Capensis is a powerful fertility enhancer. It strongly enhances ovulation. Additionally, it tones the vagina and increases circulation to that orifice, heightening sensitivity in that region during intimacy.

Typha Capensis can be consumed in the last two weeks of pregnancy to prepare for childbirth. It strengthens uterine contractions. Typha Capensis also helps in countering sexually transmitted diseases.

Uziza (herb)

Uziza, an Igbo name (also known as Ashanti Pepper, West African Pepper, Guinea Pepper, and Ata iyere in Yoruba) is an African herb, used in Nigeria mainly, that helps improve penile erections, enhances fertility and potency, and improves low sperm counts in men.

In women, Uziza is great for their sexual reproductive health. It improves fertility, enhancing ovulation. During pregnancy, it can be taken throughout pregnancy and especially during the last trimester to prepare for childbirth and to prepare for lactation. It increases uterine wall contraction during childbirth. Additionally, it helps with adverse menstrual issues, especially cramping.

Goran Tula Fruit

Goran Tula fruit (also known as Tree Hibiscus and Snot Apple) increases the libido in both men and women and promotes strong desire for sexual intercourse. It helps couples go multiple rounds between the sheets.

The herb is also an effective hormonal balancer, especially for women.

Goran Tula is a reliable fertility enhancer (for both men and women). It also enhances ovulation in women and improves semen concentration and quality while increasing semen volume.

In women, Goran Tula is a vaginal tonic and stimulates the production of vaginal wetness/lubrication and is perfect for keeping the vagina area moist and wet. The herb is one of the best for women who find it difficult to climax or reach orgasm.

Goran Tula is also a vaginal cleanser and deodorizer (helps to eliminate malodors in the vagina) and helps to keep the kitty cat smelling (and tasting) sweet and fresh. Additionally, it helps with adverse menstrual cycle complaints and normalizes the menstrual cycle after childbirth.

Kigelia

Kigelia (also known as Sausage Tree, Worsboom in Afrikaans, Modukghulu, Pidiso in North Sotho, umVongotsi in Siswati; Mpfungurhu in Tsonga, and Muvevha in Venda.

Because the fruit is shaped in the form of the male penis, pursuant to the herbal doctrine of signatures, its properties are helpful for the male genitalia, especially for naturally increasing the growth and length of the penis (taken consistently or religiously) over time, 3-6 months (to notice significant change).

In men, Kigelia is aphrodisiacal and helps the penis to become larger.

In women, Kigelia counters infertility being naturally rich in phyoestrogens. It is one of the best herbs for the breasts, naturally toning, firming and defining the breasts as well as enhancing their growth (natural breast enhancement or growth factor).

In lactating women, Kigelia stimulates lactation. Additionally, it increases the volume and quality of mother's milk. Kigelia is exceptional for all gynecological disorders in women. It is useful (in men and women) to counter sexually transmitted diseases (STDs or STIs), especially syphilis and gonorrhea.

Insomnia

Insomnia has become as common as a headache, stomachache, and common cold. Many people believe if they wake up in the middle of the night and have difficulty going back to sleep, that they automatically have *insomnia*. However, it is important to understand the type and severity of you challenges first to know what exactly is going on to best know how to be specific with your treatment. Insomnia is a sleep disorder where you have difficulty falling asleep, and/or staying asleep. This condition can be acute (short-term) or chronic (long-term). Acute insomnia can last for a day or a few weeks, while chronic insomnia can last for at least three nights a week at minimum up to three or more months at a time.

Types of Insomnia:

- Primary Insomnia: sleep problems aren't clearly linked to another health condition or problem.

- Secondary Insomnia: difficulty sleeping directly because of a health condition or substance use issue.

Dr. Gregg Jacobs, Ph.D., an insomnia specialist at the sleep disorders center at Beth Israel Deaconess Medical Center in Boston, MA states, "The majority of physicians consider sleeping pills to be the most effective treatment for insomnia – which they are not – and continue to overprescribe them." These prescriptions can provide short term relief but do not reach the causes directly and a person can adjust quickly to them where they have little to no impact on improving their condition and can also contribute to making their condition worse.

Remedies:

Relax

The harder you try to go to sleep, the more tense your body will remain and the longer you will stay awake. "Stressful life events are the most common precipitators of chronic insomnia" says Dr. Gregg Jacobs, Ph.D. You will want to diffuse these stressful feelings and emotions by practicing and incorporating relaxation techniques into your lifestyle. There are many activities to do to promote relaxation but finds what works best for you that allow you to do the following:

- Be in a space where you will not be disturbed or distracted. Sit down or lie down in a comfortable position.

- Focus your attention on each part of your body. Your body is the container for stress that needs to be released. Notice how each part of your body feels. Certain areas may feel tense, heavy, or nothing. After spending several minutes scanning your body, then take time to notice how the body is relaxing.

- Monitor your breathing by breathing slowly and deeply. Breathe in slowly through your nose until your abdomen expands and then slowly release your breath.

- Practice directing your thoughts away from past events or the typical forever-changing daily circumstances and choose to focus on something neutral such as a word or mantra. This will allow you to be more present and help slow down your thoughts. You may also want to visualize an image that is calming and enjoyable during this time as well.

You can fall asleep while doing any relaxing activity which is fine, but you want to remain awake in order to dissolve what may be blocking your sleep. Also, if you fall asleep, going to sleep later on may be a challenge that you want to avoid.

Avoid Sleeping Pills

People that use sleeping pills take an average of 46 minutes to fall asleep, according to Dr. Jacobs. This is partly due to the body trying to locate what the sleeping pill contains and identify if it meets your bodily needs that are hindering sleep. Sleep pills interfere with brain functioning. This can cause a hangover effect which can hinder your ability to complete daily tasks the following day. Dr. Jacobs states that "After 4 to 6 weeks of nightly use, they're no longer effective. Yet, surprisingly, BZs (benzodiazepines) are routinely prescribed for months or even years." Long term users of sleep pills can develop "rebound insomnia" which can be worse than the insomnia they initially worked on overcoming, in which they remain on sleeping pills or they seek them out. In other words, BZs can become addictive.

In addition to BZs becoming addictive, a person may feel depressed, anxious, or irritable and choose more over-the-counter medication which also come with their own side effects. To wean yourself off of sleep medication(s) you want to start by cutting your dose in half one day per week. This may lead to one restless night a week, but it's to be expected. Eventually you'll adjust better that one night per week and can choose another night to do the same and continue until you can continue to drop your dosage completely as you make room for the remedies covered in this section.

Direct Sunlight

Direct sunlight regulates the chemical in the brain known as *melatonin* that controls and regulates body temperature. Having a normal rhythm with your body temperature, will create more regulated sleep patterns. Think of collecting bits of sunlight as early as possible upon awakening that you can use at night when you go to seep. Keep your window shades open, eat or drink near a sun-exposed window or outside, and/or take an early morning walk to help stimulate the brain producing melatonin that you get to use later on in your quest for a good night's sleep. If you wake too early for work, school, or other obligations, you will need to get out in the sun during the late afternoon or early evening several hours before the sun goes down.

Carbs (carbohydrates)

A small snack that is high in carbohydrates is great for promoting sleep. Carbs increase the brain chemical called *serotonin* which induces sleep. Bananas, apples, mango, dates, goji berries, and quinoa are a few items to eat lightly in the evening at least an hour before bed to help promote serotonin.

Positive Thought Patterns

Negative thoughts will keep you up at night. Every second you are aware that you cannot sleep, these negative thoughts will make it more difficult for you to relax and go to sleep. These negative thoughts about your ability to go to sleep can cause you to feel anxious or depressed. Recognizing and replacing any negative thoughts (about sleep or in general) will help you remain calm enough where the rhythm of your body will promote better sleep. Take time to write down some positive thoughts you want to remember and practice saying to yourself to replace any negative ones. Take your focus away from your inability to sleep. Over time you will gain more control, and this can result in better overall sleep.

Acupressure Points

Traditional Chinese Medicine (TCM) incorporates acupressure in its treatment practices. TCM focuses on where a person's energy (chi) flows along meridians in the body. When *chi* is not flowing, particular meridians are in jeopardy and symptoms begin to come to the surface. Acupressure can be achieved by using needles to apply pressure or through the use of fingers applying pressure (acupressure). When you stimulate nerve points, you can unlock the chi energy for particular conditions. Licensed Acupuncturist Bob Flaws recommends doing the following for 20-30 minutes prior to sleep daily:

(Note: the points described low go from head to toe. They are in no particular order).

- Begin pressing gently with your fingertips the top of your skull. Massage this space gently about 100 times.

- Then, begin to gently massage with your fingertips, the ends of your eyebrows closest to your nose to stimulate the acupressure point BL2. You will want to do this about 20-40 times.

- Using your index finger and thumbs, massage the top part of your eye sockets, followed by the lower edges. Make sure to not touch your eyes directly until these areas feel relaxed.

- Rub your palms together or against your thighs in order to create warmth. Place your warm palms over both of your eyes for about one minute. Then gently rub your closed eyes for another 10-20 seconds.

- Pressure point GB20 is located about halfway behind your ears and the muscles on the side of your spine. This area is more known as the part of the neck most massage when they have a stiff neck or tension headache. Using one hand on each side, press down and massage these areas for a few minutes. Don't massage too long yourself as you may begin to flex your shoulder muscles and create tension in this area.

- There is a pressure point located on the inside part of your forearms between the two tendons known as PE6 (located about 1-2 inches above the wrist). With your thumb, press and gently rub this area. Do this about 40-50 times on each arm; start with your left arm, then do your right arm one time each and then repeat for 40-50 cycles).

- Point HE7 located at the crease of your wrist right below the bottom of your pinky finger helps ease tension in the body. massage this point for about 3-4 minutes.

- Three inches below the outside edge of your kneecap while your leg is bent is point ST36. Massage this point on each leg 30-50 times.

- About three inches above the tip of your inner ankle bone on the back of your lower leg is where point SP6 is located. Press and massage this point on each leg about 40-45 times.

- Point K11 is located just behind the ball of your foot closer to your heel. Rub your palms together and then place the palm of the opposite hand on this spot while it is warm until it no longer feels warm and proceed to repeating for the opposite foot.

Doing all of these points should take about 20-30 minutes but do not feel pressure to complete all of these. Hopefully trying all of these will cause you to feel tired but start by practicing locating each spot and incorporate these practices often. You may work from head to toe, tow to head, or focus on specific areas. The goal is to practice stimulating these points to promote better quantity and quality of sleep.

Create A Sleep Schedule

Regardless of when you begin to feel tired, you want to set a certain schedule you'd like to stick to in order to help your body adjust. If you do not give yourself enough time to rest, you will at minimum wake up feeling drowsy or tired. You want to be able to set and eventually stick to your own personal "body clock". Work to avoid trying to "catch up on sleep" over the weekends or on a day because once you go back to work, school, or other responsibilities, you will feel exhausted after going back into a regular routine.

Aim To Sleep The Moment You Are In Bed

Don't waste your time once you get to bed. Avoid watching TV or videos on your phone. It can help at times, but even avoid reading so you can focus on getting to sleep and not shift your attention elsewhere. As we get older, we essentially need less sleep. Babies need many hours, while there are lower averages for adults ranging from 6-8 hours. If you absolutely cannot sleep, use your time to complete some small tasks so you have less to do the following day to help you begin to feel a need for rest. You want to not feel overly stimulated when trying to go to sleep. The moment you lay down, set your intention on going to sleep.

An hour or so before you intend on going to bed, find a quiet space and just sit. Sit there and reflect upon how your day went. Review and stressors you had and process possible solutions. Work to allow your thoughts to process and pass by in order to clear your mind so you can relax and carry less with you to go to sleep easier.

Avoid Stimulants

Stimulants such as caffeine and nicotine will disrupt sleep patterns and make it difficult to go to bed. Coffee, sodas, chocolate, and cigarettes are the most common items to avoid, especially at nighttime. It is best to not consume these at any time, but especially after 4pm to avoid your body reacting to these stimulants several hours later when you are preparing to go to bed.

Power Down

Visualize your body reducing its activity levels in order to reach the destination of sleep. You cannot sleep while the body is very awake. Insomnia can often be directly linked to stress. Aim to decrease your stress by reducing your activity both, physically and mentally. Work on identifying reasonable ways you can allow your body to "power down" so that you can feel relaxed enough to go to sleep. Redecorate your bedroom to promote calmness if you need to in order to help contribute to you getting to sleep and feeling rested.

Warm Bath

Our body temperatures can decrease at night from where it is for most of the day. Taking a warm bath can help to slightly raise your body temperature so that after you are out of your bath, it will slightly begin to decrease which can help you start to feel tired and go to sleep better.

Ginger Foot Bath

Soak your feet in warm water and add some fresh ground ginger. You can use ginger powder as well. Ginger helps promote relaxation and a steady blood flow throughout the body, helping to promote a more restful sleep. Add about 2-4 tablespoons of ginger or ginger powder to a foot bath and soak your feet for 25-35 minutes.

Valerian Root (herb)

This herb can be used for best results. Taking 150-300 milligrams of this herb can help you fall asleep faster and improve sleep quality.

Kava Kava (herb)

When anxiety is the main cause for your insomnia, this herb can help relax the muscles and calm the brain's receptors. Take one or two 400-500 milligram capsule of this herb about an hour before bed to get to sleep.

Chamomile (herb)

Drink two cups of this herbal tea before bed to help calm the nerves. Take about 2 teaspoons of this herb (dried) or 3-4 pieces of this herb in its natural state and add to a small pot of boiling water for 3-4 minutes. Strain herbs and let steep. Then let cool and drink two 10-12-ounce glasses before bed.

Astragalus Root (herb)

This herb helps improve metabolism and hormonal balances that often interfere with sleep.

Follow dosage directions on product labels. The recommended dose for a standardized extract is 250 – 500 mg, three to four times a day standardized to 0.4% 4-hydroxy-3-methoxy isoflavone 7-sug. When making tea, boil three to six grams of dried root per 12 ounces of water three times a day. You can get a tincture of astragalus in 30 percent ethanol. The recommended dose is 20 to 60 drops three times a day.

Goji Berries

These berries have natural melatonin which helps improve sleep quality. Eat these berries whole or add dried berries to warm water and drink in tea form; and then eat the berries afterwards as they will re-absorb the water and moisture.

Irritable Bowel Syndrome (IBS)

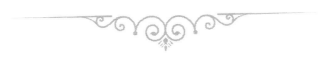

There are smooth, delicate walls on the inside of the intestines that are lined with muscles which contract and release during digestion. Those with irritable bowel syndrome (IBS) have muscles that contract much stronger and take longer to relax afterwards which cause congestion and irritable symptoms in the bowels. As this happens, there is an overgrowth of intestinal bacteria specifically within the small intestine which increases gas and bloating after meals.

IBS will result in any or all of the following: diarrhea, constipation, or abdominal pain. The focus often goes towards worrying about which one of these will make an appearance and working to properly manage these symptoms. It is important to follow the remedies provided in this section to avoid promoting triggers of IBS and effectively improve the overall functioning of the bowels.

The issue is that the *bad* gut bacteria is outweighing the *good* gut bacteria. The goal is to help adjust and change this flow around in the other direction where there's more *good* gut bacteria than *bad* gut bacteria.

Remedies:

Stress Reduction

Douglas A. Drossman, M.D., professor of psychiatry with the division of digestive diseases and co-director of the UNC Center for Functional Gastrointestinal and motility Disorders at the University of North Carolina at Chapel Hill School of Medicine, states that "There's a very good connection between stress and an irritable bowel." He adds that we do not want to become stressed simply *because* we have IBS and create a cycle of symptoms and stress. It is best to recognize early symptoms, acknowledge that this has happened before and will pass, and understand that you will not die because you are having a bowel issue. Anything you do to help relax will help you decrease overall symptoms. Try to become more still, meditation, or even self-hypnosis can help to become calmer.

Stress List

There are certain foods that can trigger you more than others. It is important to list these out to help you avoid them. There are also many people and/or situations that are stressful for you. Could be a conversation with someone or how manage work situations, or how you cope with things such as grocery shopping. You want to personalize what causes you stress and create a list of items you want to remain aware of. Then you can better understand how to manage your day-to-day lifestyle and responsibilities and know what to remain aware of during your day when working to reduce your stressors. Take time to note what you notice happening before, during, and after a stressful event so you know what to focus more on to alleviate your stress. Review this list and keep track of any progress you feel you make over time.

Fiber

Fiber helps promote ease of digestion because it absorbs a lot of water and helps create softer stools, which promote eliminating larger quantities of waste easier. The American Dietetic Association recommends 20-35 grams of fiber daily. This may sound like a lot but, ½ cup of leafy green vegetables can provide about 5g, a small apple is about 3g, and consuming grains like quinoa can provide up to 8g per cup. Just these three items together and you are almost at your daily recommended amount in addition to any other foods you consume that have fiber.

Those with IBS may have diarrhea or small, harder stools due to infrequent and unsteady bowel movements. Increasing fiber will help to regulate bowel movements and directly improve how your body digests items you consume.

Common sources of Fiber: garbanzo beans, lentils, brussels sprouts, sweet potatoes, avocado, pears, sunflower seeds, flax seeds, hazelnuts, apples and berries (high pectin fruits) and onions.

Proper Hydration

The bowels need fluids to help push along thing within the digestive system. Not consuming enough water will slow things down. Be careful to not drink too much water suddenly, but instead, consume more water than you currently are (aim for half of your bodyweight in ounces), and eat more hydrating foods such as fresh fruits and vegetables.

No Dairy

The body has difficulty absorbing lactose which is an enzyme in dairy. The milk this substance is created for (baby cows) only consume this substance for about 6 months, and then they stop and never consume this substance ever again in their lives. Remove dairy from your life to not create an additional workload for your bowels attempting to digest this substance.

Avoid Fattening Foods

We have all heard about good fat vs bad fat and how we want a balance here. However, we do not need the bad fat. The bad fat (white fat) turns into waste, corrodes the systems in the body, and does not provide nourishment. The good fat (brown fat) is essential to organs such as the heart and the brain in which we only need small amounts when we look at our overall diets/lifestyle. Work to eliminate the fried foods, heavy sauces, and oils. These do not join well with water which makes up most of our bodies and cause additional friction within the bowels when working to digest.

Avoid Spicy Foods

Those with IBS are often more sensitive to spicy foods such as peppers and other spices. Switch to eating more "bland" foods if spicy foods are triggering for you. Don't just eliminate the spicier items from your diet because it is often what these foods are eaten with that promote other triggers. Eat more foods that are bland and without many additional spices and see if your symptoms decrease. This will help you avoid overeating which presents additional issue to the bowels as well.

No Coffee, Alcohol, or Cigarettes

These should be avoided regardless of your condition, but they each present issues for the digestive system. They send the body into shock and the body will then take its focus away from digestion or not have enough energy to properly digest things later on if these substances are in your system.

Go For A Jog/Exercise

Dr. James B. Rhodes, M.D., professor of medicine with the division of gastroenterology at the University of Kansas Medical Center in Kansas City, Missouri, notes "Good body tone, good bowel tone." Exercise and cardio where your whole body is moving strengthens and tones the entire body. also helps relieve stress and endorphins which help to control aches and pain better. However, too much cardio or exercise can increase your chances of diarrhea whether you have IBS or not.

Alfalfa Greens

Contains minerals needed to build intestinal flora for proper digestion, and chlorophyll for healing and cleaning much of the bloodstream.

Ginger (herb)

Aids in improving digestion and relieves upset stomach and gas. Helps reduce various pains and inflammation. Working in herbs to your diet such as Ginger help set daily reminders of your goal to reduce your symptoms while not adding anything that will contribute to or worsen your symptoms. One of Ginger's ingredients (gingerol) helps promote anti-inflammatory propertied you need to break down inflammation within the body.

Take about a fingertip size piece of ginger and add it to tea or break it down and consume with your meals.

Olive Leaf Extract (OLE)

Olive leaf extract (OLE) helps to protect the gut while also boosting the immune system. OLE provides a high amount of natural chemicals that specifically help with breaking down the bad bacteria within the gut. Chemicals such as biophenols (oleuropein and hydroxytyrosol) which improve and maintain the health of the microbiota in the gut. OLE helps to kill and fight off parasites in the gut as well which cause further irritation.

My Personal Remedy:

(do not use if pregnant)

Tila (linden), Valerian Root and Ginger Tea

- 1 teaspoon of Tila (linden)
- 1-1.5 teaspoons of Valerian Root
- 1 teaspoon of Ginger
- Add mixture of herbs to empty cup

Boil 3-4 cups of water and add herbs and let steep for about 10-12 minutes. Strain out the herbs and enjoy twice a day.

*Completely avoid anything that takes over 40 minutes to digest to help provide additional relief from the irritation in the bowels while consuming this mixture

Jet Lag

Headache, exhaustion, and sleep deprivation are all symptoms of what we refer to as "jet lag". Our bodies adjust to a different time zone where our body does not believe that the time is correct. You may land and the time is 11:00pm but your body may feel it is 7:35pm or vis versa. This disruption is referred to as our body's "Circadian Rhythm" which regulates our body's sleep-wake cycle, and bodily functions such as bowel movements and hunger. Traveling across two time zones can directly have an impact on our circadian rhythm cycle as we may be ready for bed while it's still early or have trouble staying up until your typical bedtime later in the day.

Remedies:

Direct Sunlight

Allow the sun to reset your internal clock. This internal "clock" in our brains are actually tiny cells that form into a group called the suprachiasmatic nuclei (SCN). This clock is set by being in light. Simplest way to absorb sunlight to help reset our internal clock while moving to avoid any physical symptoms of jet lag is, to take a walk. If you travel east to west, take a walk soon after landing to take advantage of the sunlight that is out. If you are traveling from west to east, find a space to sit or go for a walk around 2am or around this time. you may think going right to sleep will help, but doing so will prolong symptoms and not properly restore the SCN.

Sunlight influences the regulation of melatonin, a hormone that helps synchronize cells throughout the body. Certain cells in the tissue at the back of your eye (retina) transmit the light signals to an area of your brain called the hypothalamus. At night, when the light signal is low, the hypothalamus tells the pineal gland, a small organ situated in the brain, to release melatonin. During daylight hours, the opposite occurs, and the pineal gland releases very little melatonin. Getting direct sunlight properly, can ease your adjustment to your new time zone more than anything else.

Eat Locally

Not just at any store but eating foods that are grown in your area are best with helping adjust to a new climate and region. Telling your body to prepare for a change will put it on notice and the SCN will be prompted to adjust its receptors towards making this adjustment thus, reducing your symptoms of jet lag.

Hydration

Airplanes often have very "dry" air and can cause you to feel dehydrated after your flight lands. It is recommended to drink at least 34 ounces (1 liter) of water for every 6 hours of flying to avoid feeling dehydrated. If you drink any coffee or alcohol before, or during your flight, you will have to drink even more water as coffee and alcohol are harmful diuretics since they flush water out of the body without replacing many essential minerals that can get flushed out also.

Stretching

Stretching your body will help keep it alert to its natural sleep-wake cycle. Make time to do a stretching routine where your body can work to adjust to its new environment and accurately assess your body's needs that you can focus on.

Get Plenty of Rest Before Your Trip

Being well rested upon arriving on your trip will help you adjust better to your environment and avoid feeling generally tired. This starts with getting adequate sleep several days to a week prior to your trip. You will want to sleep on the plane if your flight is during your usual bedtime also to help keep consistent with your rest as you prepare for your new time zone.

Sarsaparilla (herb)

Sitting down for several hours can cause the body to feel stiff and uncomfortable. Sarsaparilla is an herb known for having a very high iron content. Consuming this herb will help to reduce any aches, pains, swelling, or even bruising that can occur after a long flight. This is best in tea form which you can drinking several cups of, but you can get capsules as well where you want to follow instructions listed on the label depending on the size of the capsule.

Blue Vervain (herb)

Increases oxygen delivery to the brain. The body has to be in a stable condition for it to be receptive enough to absorb the increased oxygen intake flowing towards the brain. This herb will essentially help your body wake up or remain awake in order to cope better with symptoms of jet lag.

Kidney Stones

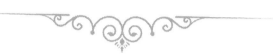

A kidney stone is a dense, collection of tiny sharp-edge crystals that can tear through the delicate tissues of the urinary tract as they leave your body. This is the excruciating pain many go through when dealing with kidney stones. About 70%-80% of all kidney stones are composed of calcium crystals, while another 10% are composed of uric acid crystals. You will need to pass a stone to determine which type you have. Then, you can follow through with specific remedies outlines in this section.

Remedies: for Calcium-Oxalate Stones

"There is no question that a typical high-fat, low-fiber Western diet creates calcium stones" says Dr. Wynne A. Steinsnyder, D.O., osteopathic physician and urologist in North Miami Beach in Florida. This type of diet increases both, the calcium oxalate crystals in the urine and the contributing factors that form a kidney stone.

Low Fats and High(er) Fiber

After reading the quote above, you've probably assumed that this would be the first recommendation. Regular consumption of red meat, processed meats, and white sugars, increase your chances of developing many degenerative diseases such as heart issues, and cancer, as well as kidney stones. Increasing your fiber intake will make passing waste easier and low-fat consumption limits the inflammation present, which contribute to the formation of kidney stones. A general plant-based diet will help steer you in the right direction, but during this time, you will want to avoid things like spinach, swiss chard, and beet roots due to them being high in *oxalates* which are acids that cannot be processed or passed through the urine. Consuming too many of these items can back up the kidneys and begin the process of storing these items, leading to kidney stones.

Common sources of Fiber: garbanzo beans, lentils, brussels sprouts, sweet potatoes, avocado, pears, sunflower seeds, flax seeds, hazelnuts, apples and berries (high pectin fruits) and onions.

Water

Consuming more plants will increase your water intake, but you will still want to hydrate often by placing emphasis on eating fruits and vegetables with a high-water content and drink about half of your body weight in ounces of water. I know it can seem scary to drink water as you may have to urinate and have to pass a stone or several, but as Dr. Steinsnyder states, "Inadequate fluid intake is a major factor in allowing crystals to accumulate in the urine."

Minerals

There are specific minerals to place your focus on when dealing with kidney stones. It is recommended to avoid processed supplements or items with artificial materials. Make sure to do your research around items you can incorporate into your lifestyle that are higher in the following minerals:

Calcium: this is already an essential mineral, but calcium binds to oxalates which can help prevent additional stones from forming as long as you're not consuming more than you need. In a standard diet, about 600-milligrams a day is recommended.

Common Sources of Calcium: sea moss, kale, okra, dandelion greens, turnip greens, lettuce, papaya, and oranges.

Magnesium: the absorption of calcium in addition to the magnesium can help further block stone formation. Most items that contain calcium may contain magnesium. But placing emphasis on consuming these two will also help heal the area after kidney stones are no longer present.

Common Sources of Magnesium: Avocados, Bananas, Chickpeas, Tamarind, Basil, Dill, Ginger, Oregano, Thyme, Butternut Squash, Brazil Nuts, Okra, Leafy Green Vegetables, Nopal, CBD (cannabidiol) products, Nettle leaf, Horsetail, Red Clover, Sage

Gokshura (herb)

An herb to incorporate lightly into your diet during this time is an Ayuvedic herb known as *Gokshura*. This herb can reduce the body's production of calcium oxalates and help prevent these types of stones from being formed. This herb can help clean out bacteria and harmful materials from within the bladder wall and help relieve excess pain associated with kidney stones. Follow label ingredients with this herb and only take minimally if symptoms are more severe.

Low Exercise

It should be difficult to move around a lot while having kidney stones, but you want to avoid sweating more than you may need to. When we sweat excessively, the body has calcium slowly draining out of the bones, and this calcium ends up in your urine (this is why people often have to urinate after working out). The excess calcium that is expelled through the urine, can only add to your kidney stone condition. It is recommended to take a few brisk walks a few times a week rather than exercise or stick to a regular routine or go to the gym. In addition, exercises decrease the amount of available water in the body, even if just for a brief period of time, which can also contribute or trigger symptoms.

Ginger Compress

Fill an 8-quart or larger pot with water and bring it to a boil. Place a piece of fresh ginger the size of your palm in a cheesecloth and tie a string around it to resemble a tea bag. Place the ginger into the boiling water for about 3 minutes. Remove the herb and squeeze the cheese-cloth over the pot so the remains of the softened ginger can go into the pot. Let the water cool off and soak a small towel in the ginger water and wring it out thoroughly. Place a small towel onto your lower back where the kidneys are located. Then, put a piece of plastic over the towel (can use an un-used trash bag as well) followed by a dry towel on top of the plastic.

Repeat this process every 10-15 minutes about 3-4 times a day. Make sure the area stays warm to help the body promote breaking down stones and passing them easier; as well as stimulating the areas such as the bladder and urethra.

Avoid "Vitamin-C" Supplements

These artificial supplements may increase the excretion of oxalates in the urine, as some vitamin-C can be converted into oxalates within the body, according to the Mayo Clinic. In a 2013 research study conducted by the Institute of Environmental Medicine in Sweden, researchers found that vitamin-C supplements doubled the risk of developing kidney stones. Getting Vitamin-C from foods did not post this risk.

Common Sources of Vitamin-C: Black Currants, Bell Peppers (red and green), Papaya, Spring Onions, Strawberries, Cantaloupe, Mango, Oranges, Watercress, Raspberries, and Tomatoes.

Remedies: for Uric Acid Stones

There are typically two ways to prevent and work to reduce symptoms of uric acid stones according to Dr. Steinsnyder; (1) Balance out the pH of the urine, and (2) Reducing your intake of food components that increase uric acid.

pH Balance of Urine

Unlike calcium-oxalate stones, you can drink certain juices that won't irritate your condition. Orange juice, apple juice, and items such as tomato juice can help reduce "purines" (items that increase uric acid) into the urine. You can stick with consuming 2-3 glasses a day of any of the mentioned juices. To reduce purines, you must remove items included but not limited to, anchovies, sardines, gravies, white breads, oysters, ham, asparagus, oatmeal, cauliflower, spinach, mushrooms, and fried foods.

Consuming more than a few ounces of these items builds up uric acid deposits that promote erosion within the body which gets pushed towards the urethra and contributes to your symptoms.

Water

Same as mentioned earlier for calcium-oxalate stones, drink about half your body weight in ounces and seek to include more fresh fruits and vegetables with a higher water content as often as possible.

Corn Silk

Taking the "hair" off of corn and consuming it as a tea (about 1 tablespoon per 10-12 ounces of water) is recommended for breaking down uric acid stones. Corn silk will reduce the friction in the area within the urethra as the stones move along.

Knee Pain

The knee is composed of two bones (1) the femur and (2) the tibia. These two bones are surrounded by connected tissues and muscles. The knee is very specifically designed, but its structure makes it susceptible to various injuries and pains, although it is the strongest of the 187 joints in the body. According to Sharon Butler, a certified practitioner of *Hellerwork* (a structural bodywork and movement therapy) in Paoli, Pennsylvania, she states that, "Proper pain-free function of the knee relies on the balance of all muscles, tendons, and ligaments that wrap the knee joint. When one or more of these elements is tighter or more restricted than the others, knee pain is often the result."

Remedies:

"Tightrope" Exercise

Find an open space at least 6-feet long and place masking tape on the floor in a straight line. Proceed to walk along the tape, one foot in front of the other. Take time to pause at all points; ex. when the toes touch down, the ankle is rotating, foot is completely flat, etc. This exercise helps to align the knee, ankle, and hip bones as they work with one another as you step and shift your weight as you walk.

Reflexology

The foot and knee have many specific pressure points to consider when looking at how to best care and address an issue. Terri Moon, who works as a certified massage technetium and director of Touched by the Moon holistic health center in Santa Rosa, California has steps to properly locate the knee reflect point in your body and ways to care for it.

Step 1: run a finger down the outside edge of the foot. When you come in contact with a bony area midway between your heel and small ("pinky") toe, the spot just below that point on the bottom of that spot is your knee reflex point.

Step 2: for ligament pain, mix one drop of lemongrass oil with 4-5 drops of vegetable oil. For nerve tissues, use geranium oil instead of lemongrass.

Step 3: on the foot of your painful side (knee) put a drop of this mixture and rub it in gently with your fingertips. Gently increase how much pressure you apply to this area.

Step 4: repeat this twice a day until your pain has deceased.

Acupressure

In addition to the knee reflex point on your foot, there are several others to give your attention to. One specific point is called "BL54" which his located in the middle crease in the back of your knee where there's a crease. This point is commonly referred to as the "commanding middle point".

To find this point, bend you knee and place your thumb in the crease behind your knee. Apply firm, steady pressure to this area until you begin to feel stimulation in the area of your knee that is experiencing pain. Use your fingertips to rub gently in small circles for about 30-60 seconds at a time. Repeat several times a day. Make sure to do both knees as a precaution as we may use one side of our body more when having knee issues on the other side.

Rest

Many who experience knee pain are very active. Resting can be difficult but is necessary when experiencing knee pain. For every pound of body weight you have, that's multiplied by about six in terms of stress placed across the knee area. If you are 10lbs overweight, that an additional 60lbs of weight your knee has to carry around according to Dr. James A. Fox, M.D. who specializes in knee surgery at the Southern California Orthopedic Institute in Van Nuys, California. Always seek to modify exercises also as needed. Dr. Fox states, "You don't put a Mack truck on Volkswagen tires" when referring to additional weight on the knees.

Avoid Knee Braces

Unless otherwise determined by a physical trainer and/or if physical therapy will be involved, stay away from knee braces. Knee braces push the kneecap against the joint itself and can lead to more damage.

Exercises Your Hamstrings

This muscle group is often neglected when training legs or exercising. However, this muscle group is located right behind and above the knee joint. When we neglect training this area, we rely more upon our knees to do basic movements. Over time, this will create additional knee pain.

Grapeseed Extract

Use about 50-100 milligrams of grapeseed extract to help reduce inflammation around the joint. Follow instructions on label.

Support Your Ligaments

Muscles provide structure, but the ligaments hold everything together. Some basic exercises you can do to strengthen your knee ligaments are listed below:

Isometric Knee Builder – sit on the floor with your le stretched out in front of you. Slowly tighten your leg until you are able to tighten around the knee for about 30 seconds. Hold for a few seconds and relax as you build up to 30 seconds if needed. Repeat until you feel flexibility in and around the knee.

Sitting Leg Lifts – sit with your back against the wall and place a pillow in the small of your back. Once in position, begin raising one leg and holding it for a few seconds at a time. The pillow against the back is used simply to reduce any back or hip pains. Move closer if needed to complete exercise.

Hamstring Helper – lie on your stomach with your chin to the floor. With an ankle weight or sock full of coins, slowly bring your foot up, bent towards your back and slowly bring towards the floor without touching the floor. Repeats and work slower each time.

Heel Walks – this is a more moderate-to-high strength builder exercise so do so with caution. Lie flat on your back and bring your heels as close to your buttocks as you can. Raise your hips upward and proceed to take steps forward and backward (and side to side) while on your heels. You will want to essentially walk forward until your legs are close to being parallel with the rest of your body and then proceed to walk backwards until you are back in the starting position.

Change Your Running Shoe

Concreate can be one of the hardest surfaces to run on (no pun intended). Run on grass before asphalt, and asphalt before concrete. Running on a flat surface is not always the best if the surface itself is not soft and conducive to your needs. When you run just one mile, your foot hits the ground about 600-800 times. If you are an active runner, try replacing your shoes every three months no matter how much or how little wear and tear is present.

Water Exercises

The buoyancy of training in water helps continue exercises but with less pressure on the knee joint. Water training can allow you to create balance in areas around the knee that typical training in the gym would not reach. Swimming is also a great hobby to strengthen the entire body and help even out your muscle size and strength which will also help reduce direct pressure on your knees.

Pain Relief Remedy (for knees and joints)

2 tablespoons of cayenne pepper powder

½ cup of cold-pressed olive oil

½ inch of grated ginger

Mix all of these items together until they form a paste. Apply directly to affected area. Leave on for a minimum of 20-minutes and then wash off. Do this twice a day.

Lactose Intolerance

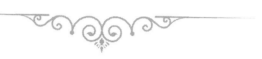

"Ironically, while milk products are the most commonly consumed foods, milk is one of the two or three most common food allergens in the American diet" says James Braly, M.D., an allergy specialist in Boca Raton, Florida.

"Milk is not a perfect food, as is frequently advertised" says Jacqueline Krohn, M.D., physician in New Mexico who also notes how milk can cause allergic symptoms of all kinds, such as diarrhea, asthma, ear infections, rashes, and hives.

Allergic symptoms do not often show up immediately, which is why most do not believe they (or their child(ren)) are experiencing allergic reactions to milk. About 30 million to 50 million Americans fall under the umbrella of being *lactose intolerant*. Lactose intolerance occurs when the small intestine does not produce enough *lactase*, an enzyme required for the digestive tract to digest lactose found in dairy products. "Milk" also contributes to blood loss from gastrointestinal bleeding, and lead to inhibiting iron absorption in the body. Iron deficiency is the most common nutritional problem in the USA. In addition, whole milk contains saturated fat which is very harmful to the heart in which heart disease is the number one leading cause of death in the USA (1 in 10 adults or about 30 million people).

Remedies:

Ditch The Dairy

This is the simplest and most obvious solution to end (and avoid) these issues. However, this is not as easy as it sounds. Most dairy products are filled with additives that create addictions and are often hidden with how ingredients are listed and labeled. One of the main addictive ingredients is *casein*, which releases "casomorphins", which is a substance very similar (chemically) to opioids. These casomorphins can attach themselves to the same receptors in our brains as drugs such as heroin and other narcotics, resulting in a small hit of dopamine (the "feel good" chemical in our brains).

Try setting a goal to go 7-10 days or longer where you can avoid common items such as milk, chocolate, yogurt, and ice cream, while remaining mindful of items such as baked goods, snack foods and others that contain dairy components such as casein, caseinate, lactose, sodium caseinate, or whey. If you're not sure if something contains dairy, do your best to avoid it and do without.

Cook At Home

Cooking at home gives you direct control over what ingredients you use when preparing your food. You want to do your best to avoid processed items with many ingredients when preparing a dish to avoid any hidden dairy ingredients.

Milk Substitute(s)

There are so many other forms of "milk" available today where cow's milk does not even take up the largest section of the milk aisle at most supermarkets. There's coconut milk, hemp milk, coconut milk, walnut milk, cashew milk, and just about every form of "nut milk" you may want to make, or options such as quinoa milk that you can easily make at home.

Calcium Intake

There are many sources of calcium outside of cow's milk (or any animal's milk). Cow's milk is one of the most concentrated due to preservatives, dyes, chemicals, and pus cells that are in it. Because of these other ingredients which do not provide any help to the body, you will not be able to absorb as much as calcium as you may think from reading ingredients labels and how marketing promotes milk for a source of calcium. This is why many people who consume milk believe they are not calcium deficient, until an unfortunate event such as a broken bone or weak joints begin to show themselves. It is best to absorb your calcium intake without creating additional avenues for them to work around.

Note: cow's milk is for infant cows until they are about 6-7 months old. Then they never consume this substance again. They have 3-4 stomachs on average and need a lot of this substance. Us humans, only have one stomach and can be breastfed. We are not breastfed for our entire lives outside of infancy and do not need to consume this as adults.

Calcium is the active mineral that is present in the bones within the body. When a long road or highway is built, cement is poured in and around the cross-linked cables, when bones are being built (and re-built) calcium is the "cement". Dr. Lawrence Robbins, M.D., director of the Robbins Headache Clinic in Northbrook, Illinois recommended about 750 milligrams of calcium daily.

Common Sources of Calcium: sea moss, kale, okra, dandelion greens, turnip greens, lettuce, papaya, and oranges.

Making Your Own Milk

Hemp Milk #1

1 cup of hemp seeds

3 cups of coconut, spring, or distilled water

4 pitted dates (soak in warm water to soften)

1 tablespoon or sea moss gel (or powder)

1 teaspoon of bladderwrack powder

- Blend all ingredients in a high-speed blender.
- Use cheesecloth or cheesecloth bag to strain

Shelf life is about 5 days.

Hemp Milk #2

½ cup of hemp seeds

3-4 cups of water (less water will make thicker milk)

1 pinch of Celtic salt

1 tablespoon of agave

2 teaspoons of cacao powder (to make "chocolate milk")

- Mix all ingredients together in a blender for one minute
- Pour into glass container and refrigerate
- Straining is optional.

Walnut Milk

1 cup of soaked walnuts

2 cups of water

¼ tablespoon or Celtic salt

*Soak walnuts for at least 4-6 hours before. Drain and rinse.

- Blend together all ingredients for one minute.
- Strain with cheesecloth and store in refrigerator until chilled.

Quinoa Milk

1 cup of cooked quinoa

3 cups of water

Blend quinoa with water until it is almost smooth.

Strain in cheesecloth

*Can store in refrigerator for 3-4 days.

Coconut Milk

Scrape out young coconut "meat" from inside of the coconut

2-3 cups of water

Blend together until smooth

"Chocolate Shake"

3 tablespoons of black sesame seeds

¼ cup of dates

¼ cup of walnuts

½ teaspoon of ground ginger

½ teaspoon of cloves

2 cups of coconut milk

6 baby (frozen) bananas

Blend all ingredients together until smooth

Laryngitis

Having a viral infection and/or the common cold are precursors to developing laryngitis. Laryngitis is when there's inflammation of the larynx section of the throat, typically resulting in loss of voice, painful coughs, or harsh breathing.

When we exhale (breathe out) the larynx (voice) box has to vibrate through the vocal cords. This is why when a person's voice sounds different than it usually does, in addition to the many symptoms of laryngitis, it usually means laryngitis is settling in. even a slight change to the larynx can make someone sound completely different. Vocal cords contain several layers of connective tissues. Any alteration or swelling in this area can disrupt the vibration through these tissues. having this area contain excess inflammation is enough to cause pain and prolong many symptoms.

Remedies:

Don't Talk

Even whispering can cause more damage and may feel as if you were yelling. Communicate via the use of technology or writing things down. Any other form of communication outside of using your voice will be best at this time.

Nose Breathing

Breathing through your nose is a natural humidifier. You do not want to expose your vocal cords to any dry or cold air by breathing in through your mouth. During your healing process you may want to read a book entitled, ***Breath: The New Science of a Lost Art*** by award-winning journalist James Nestor which provides many breathing techniques to try and reviews the many health condition attributed to breathing through the mouth.

Avoid Aspirin

Most common aspect of laryngitis is a ruptured capillary (delicate blood vessels) in or around the larynx according to Dr. Laurence Levine, M.D., D.D.S., associate clinical professor of otolaryngology at Washington University School of Medicine in St. Louis, Missouri, and otolaryngology in Creve Coeur in St. Charles, Missouri. Aspirin medication increases blood clotting time which can disrupt the healing process.

Cold Air Humidifier

There's mucous that cover your vocal cords to keep them moist. When they are dry, they become sticky like a piece of wax paper and trap many irritants. Using a cold-air humidifier will help keep your vocal cords moist and help avoid many irritants.

Steam

Steaming can also restore moisture as well. You may stand over a steaming bowl of water for about 5 minutes twice a day. To avoid burning, keep your head about an arm's length away from the bowl and try to not inhale too deep or quickly. Maintain a slow, steady inhale-exhale cycle when breathing.

Gargle Warm Salt Water

You can soothe a sore and irritated throat with warm salt water. Mix 1 teaspoon of salt per 10-12 ounces of warm water, take a sip into your mouth, and gargle it around the back of your throat, then spit it out. Repeat this as often as possible.

Hydration (warm fluids)

Warm liquids will not aggravate this condition like colder liquids can. Use this as an opportunity to drink some herbal tea. I will recommend mullein leaf or mullein flowers (only use the flowers if you have a good strainer to not create an irritant). Take 1 tablespoon of mullein leaf (or 2 teaspoons of mullein flowers) and add to cup. Boil water and add to cup. Let steep and strain after 10 minutes. Drink 2-3 cups a day off this tea.

No Smoking

Smoking in any form can lead to throat dryness. Cigarettes create the most dryness, but even smoking marijuana or other herbs will not be very beneficial to you at this time if you're experiencing any of these symptoms.

Slippery Elm Bark (herb)

This is taken from the bark of the Slipper Elm tree. It has been used primarily for treating upper respiratory tract infections and for reducing inflammation in the air passageways. You can take 2-3 teaspoons a day in tea form. Follow instructions on packaging in capsule or other form.

Ginger (herb)

Ginger's antibacterials properties are helpful for infections of all kinds. Mix together 1-2 teaspoons of ginger (or ¼ inch of raw ginger) to 12 ounces of boiling water to drink twice a day at minimum.

Main Habits to Avoid

While your voice is healing, try to stay away from the following:

- **Singing and shouting:** This will only add unnecessary stress to your vocal cords. This will just lead to more inflammation and a longer healing time.

- **Whispering:** It sounds odd, but whispering actually puts more stress on your vocal cords than speaking normally.

- **Alcohol:** Staying hydrated will help you heal. Avoid any form of alcoholic beverages as they provide a dehydrating effect on the body.

- **Smoking:** Any type of smoking, including e-cigarettes, can irritate your throat, cause coughing, and prolong healing time

Leg Pain

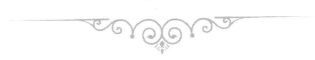

We use our legs more than any other limb on our bodies. Aside from typical aches, most leg pain(s) can be attributed to issues with the arteries or veins (varicose veins, phlebitis, or intermittent claudication). The primary issue with leg pain is that we tend to group all leg pain as "typical wear and tear" from being physically active. What we need to focus more on is not just writing off or ignoring consistent pain(s) because this is when conditions get worse and can even be fatal.

For example, intermittent claudication is a condition where chronic pain is in the calf when walking. We may just attribute this to walking a lot, but it can be a sign of a more serious condition known as, peripheral vascular disease. Similar to how a clogged artery in the heart can start with initial chest pain, intermittent claudication signals a restricted blood flow from the heart to the legs. According to Jess R. Yiung, M.D., former chairman of the department of vascular medicine at the Cleveland Clinic Foundation in Ohio, US, those who have this condition typically have a life expectancy 10 years less than those of the same age that do not experience these symptoms.

In this section, we will review how to take care of typical aches and pain you may already have in your legs, but also ways to remain proactive to avoiding some of the more serious conditions that start out a leg pain.

Remedies:

Stop Smoking Cigarettes

About 75%-90% of those with intermittent claudication are those who smoke cigarettes. Smoking cigarettes essentially substitutes carbon monoxide (from inhaling cigarette smoke) to oxygen, which adds to the legs already being starved of oxygen, which leads to further restricting blood flow and this is what damages the arteries. If this progresses onward, a person could develop this condition known as gangrene, where a limb may have to be amputated.

Start Walking

This is a simple form of exercise that also targets the specific area by promoting a steady blood flow to where it is most needed. Although you may feel some muscle soreness after walking more than usual, it is important to continue to prevent any lingering pains. It is important to work through the first sign of discomfort but once it becomes more moderately painful to walk continuously, take a break for a few minutes and then walk lightly for a few minutes before ending. This is not an overnight remedy as it can take a few months to begin noticing significant progress. Once walking become easier, ride a stationary bike, try jumping rope, stairclimbing, or even go out dancing more to exercise and stimulate the calf muscles.

In a research study that involved walking to help manage symptoms of intermittent claudication led by the Claude D. Peter Older Americans Independence Center at the University of Maryland, patients who participated in this 6-month study, increased the distance they could walk by 134% and blood flow to the calf muscles increased by 30%.

Reduce Your Size/Mass

Obesity is another huge contributor to leg pain(s). Aside from overall health, the weight load and pressure on the legs promotes many symptoms and can create additional pain. This added pressure (and force when exercising) further restricts the blood vessels and contributed to symptoms.

Avoid Heating Pads

Intermittent claudication leads to having colder feet due to the decrease of blood flow to the feet. We may be tempted to warm them up, but the heat will not dissolve symptoms and you may just end up burning your skin instead. You will want to instead, wear loose clothing such as wool socks or stockings to keep some warmth circulating when you are not physically active.

Know Your Numbers

Knowing your blood pressure and cholesterol numbers are very important factors to be aware of at any age. You will want to be aware of any risk factors by controlling these so that ordinary leg pains do not turn into diseases that can result in surgery or can become fatal. A quick internet search of normal blood pressure and cholesterol numbers can be found that will vary based upon your gender, age, height, and weight.

Cut The Cholesterol

Our liver organ produces all of the cholesterol that we need. We suppress this from happening when we consume items high in cholesterol, fat, or starch. Cholesterol and other fats are carried in the bloodstream as circular particles called "lipo-proteins". The two most common lipo-proteins are referred to as, low-density lip-proteins ("LDL"), and high-density lipo-proteins ("HDL"). When our liver is overworked, its ability to regularly produce cholesterol needed to fulfill its obligations to provide the body with helping brain and nerve functioning, digestion, breaking down fats, absorbing nutrients, hormone production and balance, and maintaining the integrity of the cells within the body.

You do not want to take something to keep lowering cholesterol levels. Lowering them too much can drastically impair the body. You want to simply avoid consuming additional cholesterol and harmful items that overwork the liver.

High-cholesterol items (**avoid**): processed (deli) meats, red meat, butter, friend foods, palm oil, canola oil, eggs, shellfish, sardines, yogurt (dairy-based).

Items that are damaging and overwork the liver (**avoid**): fried foods, artificial dyes, sodas, white bread, saturated fat (high in fried foods, cookies, pizza, and many baked goods).

Consume more of the following (**add more of these**): cruciferous vegetables (turnips, watercress, maca, arugula, wild mustard greens, broccoli, cauliflower, brussels sprouts, citrus fruits (oranges, lemons, kiwi, berries, grapefruit, pomelo, limes, key limes), olive oil.

Macular Degeneration

There are cells in the center of your retina part of your eyeballs. This area is called the macula and is responsible for most of your vision. When these cells begin to deteriorate, eyesight becomes blurrier, and you develop a condition known as "macular degeneration". Although most doctors will immediately say there is nothing to do in order to reverse this condition, there are many natural remedies and holistic practitioners that have had clients treated effectively for this condition. Marc Grossman, O.D., an optometrist, licensed acupuncturist, and co-director of the Integral Health Center I Rye and New Paltz, New York, states that "Macular degeneration may be stabilized or reversed with nutritional intervention." In this section we will review some of the more common ways nutritional interventions are applied for macular degeneration.

Remedies:

Lutein

This nutrient is actually a pigment found in leafy green vegetables that can increase the density of the macular pigment which has shown in several studies to prevent and reverse macular degeneration. Dr. Grossman says that lutein is, "By far, it's the number one nutritional treatment for the disease." Most doctors will prescribe a lutein supplement to take, but you can get all of the lutein you need by consuming 5 servings of leafy green vegetables a week (about 2 cups per serving / 16 ounces).

Bilberry (herb)

This helps improve circulation to the retina. You can find lutein-bilberry spray (under-the-tongue) which is easier for older people to take who may have difficulty digesting both of these items. In capsule form, you can take 6-milligrams of lutein and 180-milligrams of bilberry once a day. If you are consuming enough leafy green vegetables for your lutein, you can take bilberry after your meal for best results.

Taurine

Taurine is an amino acid that can help repair and regenerate tissues in the retina. You can take this in liquid form (follow instructions on label). Taurine can be difficult to locate on a plant-based diet, but you can find it in various seaweeds and sea vegetables such as sea moss, and red algae.

Antioxidants

Antioxidants can help stop the formation of free radicals. Free radicles are unstable molecules that cause oxidative damage (internal rust) within the cells. This occurs with conditions such as macular degeneration. You want to consume antioxidants daily. An easy way to work in many antioxidants is to remember to "eat the rainbow" with an assortment of foods that are naturally different colors; not dyes or artificial colorings.

Common Sources of Antioxidants: Berries, leafy green vegetables, spring water, okra, cherries, dates, and raisins, among other items.

Notable Lifestyle Changes To Maintain:

Low-fat, whole-food diet. High cholesterol is linked to macular degeneration, so you want to not overconsume, eat foods high in fat, or items that turn into fat such as processed foods.

Stop smoking. Recommendations are often unnoticeable when a person continues to smoke.

Remove caffeine and alcohol from your diet as it can worsen this condition.

Wear sunglasses often until you begin to notice significant improvements. The retina can become more damaged from ultraviolet radiation (UV rays) produced by the sun.

My Personal Remedy:

1.5 cups of mango

1 ripe burro banana

1 tablespoon of coconut oil

1 cup of amaranth or wild arugula greens

1 cup of walnut milk (preferably homemade)

Blend together and drink daily. If too thick, add some water to thin it out until desired texture is reached.

*this recipe has the primary minerals and nutrients mentioned in this section and has helped me maintain good eyesight after years of wearing glasses.

Male Menopause

The main health change men go through that are most commonly experienced after the age of 45, is a steady decrease of the hormone known as testosterone. In addition to testosterone levels decreasing, other symptoms such as decreased energy, weight gain in their mid-section, memory challenges, less ambition, sore muscles, and many others. Factors such as stress, obesity, diet and lifestyle, and/or disease, over time, alter the signals that the pituitary gland sends to the testes which cause the production of testosterone to decrease or become minimal. The main signal this condition is present is a decreased sex drive or decreased ability to have sex. However, this condition impacts every other system in the body. It takes an accumulation of factors over many years to develop into this condition but, once we reach the ripe age for this condition to settle in, it wastes no time as symptoms can become more severe rapidly depending on how someone's lifestyle has been up to this point. In this section, we will review specific recommendations to focus on in addition to maintaining a healthier lifestyle.

Remedies:

Exercise

Dr. Eugene Shippen, M.D., physician from Shillington, Pennsylvania states that, "All overweight men have lower-than-normal levels of testosterone." As the body accumulates fat, the body produces less testosterone, and converts some of this testosterone into estrogen. The balance of estrogen men has been much different than women. However, as testosterone levels drop, estrogen levels rise, resulting in weaker muscles that aren't able to burn fat as effectively. Exercise, even when not geared towards burning fat helps stop the rise of estrogen and decrease the rate at which testosterone is decreased. Going for a brisk 20-25 minute walk a few times a week can help maintain a lean body mass and prevent the accumulation of fat.

As you lose a few pounds, estrogen levels will drop, testosterone levels will rise, and many symptoms you experience will begin to go away. You do want to also avoid overeating to give your organs a break and reduce your chances of adding any extra pounds.

Zinc

There is an enzyme called aromatase that converts testosterone into estrogen. The mineral Zinc helps to deactivate aromatase and help maintain a steadier balance of testosterone and estrogen. Dr. Shippen recommends 50 milligrams twice a day until you begin to see noticeable improvement, and then maintain around 30-50 milligrams a day going forward. It may take a month or two to begin seeing improvements initially.

Common Zinc Sources: mushrooms, bananas, chickpeas/garbanzo beans, squash, okra, brazil nuts, walnuts, zucchini, and oregano.

Vitamin-C

When the body is low in vitamin-c, levels of aromatase (enzyme that converts testosterone into estradiol hormone) which can decrease levels of testosterone. It is recommended to consume 1,000-3,000 milligrams of vitamin-c daily for 1-2 months. If you do not experience and changes within that time period, reduce your daily amount to 1,000 milligrams a day while you focus more on other remedies outlined in this section.

Common sources of Vitamin-C: black currants, red bell peppers, Kakadu plum, camu camu (fruit/berry), gooseberries, papaya, oranges, cantaloupe, raspberry, mango, blackberry, tomato, blueberry, grapes, apricot, and watermelon.

Antioxidants and Vitamin E

These nutrients help to deactivate free radicals which are responsible for destroying the cells. These both also protect the pituitary gland which controls and regulates the hormones being produced in the body. An issue with the pituitary gland directly decreases testosterone production in the body. Doctors will notify patients of this as the get closer to the age of 75. Most of the time doctors will not mention this due to life expectancy age currently around the age of 78 in the USA and will focus on other areas regarding health.

Common Sources of Antioxidants: blueberries, onions, lettuce, squash, tomatoes, grapeseed extract, and herbs that you can use the flower, root, and leaves for as they contain polyphenolics (compounds that produce antioxidant activity).

Common Sources of Vitamin-E: red bell pepper, mango, avocado, sunflower seeds, brazil nuts, turnip greens, blackberry, black currants, olives, and butternut squash.

Cruciferous Vegetables

Cruciferous vegetables contain a specific compound known as indoles. Which work to break down estrogen, so it does not build up within the body or destroy the available testosterone in the body. it is recommended to eat 3-4 servings (2 ½ cups/day) of cruciferous vegetables a week. We do want to avoid the cruciferous vegetables that are high in oxalates which can decrease vital mineral such as iron in the body. Items such as broccoli, cauliflower, raw kale, brussels sprouts, and cabbage can be avoided altogether or kept to a bare minimum. Items to focus on instead include watercress, arugula, and turnip greens.

Avoiding Alcohol

Alcohol decreases zinc levels in the body and reduces the body's ability to cut down the estrogen levels in the body (specifically the bloodstream).

Avoid Grapefruit

Grapefruit can block the liver's ability to breakdown estrogen. This fruit may not cause many issues while a person is relatively young, but if you are someone who is experiencing male menopause or are over the age of 45, you may want to avoid this fruit.

African Herbs To Boost Libido and Testosterone:

Aframomum (herb)

Aframomum (also known as Alligator Pepper, Ataare, Grains of Pardise, and Melegueta Pepper) is an African aphrodisiac spice with a similar composition to Ginger. It is a pro-ejaculant herb for men and increases their sperm count. The herb is helpful for all sexual disorders in both genders.

In women, Aframomum boosts libido and make women more sensitive to intimate touch, especially in the lower regions. Additionally, it regulates vaginal lubrication, and increases sexual desire in 48-72 hours.

Aframomum promotes circulation making it helpful for erectile dysfunction conditions as well as all other sexual dysfunction plaguing society today.

Bangalala (herb)

Bangalala, native to South Africa and used for centuries by the Zulu tribe, is one of the best herbs for male sexual health. A powerful aphrodisiac and sexual tonic, it boosts and improves libido, counters male erectile dysfunction (improves circulation to the genitalia), increases and improves sexual stamina, increases energy, enhances male potency, and boosts testosterone levels.

The herb enhances sexual performance by increasing blood flow to the penis thus promoting stronger, longer lasting erections. In women, it increases blood flow to the clitoris, heightening sensitivity to the organ and surrounding labia (lips of the vagina).

The herb is also helpful for pregnant women in the last two weeks of pregnancy to help a woman prepare for childbirth. Women suffering from infertility would do well to consume Bangalala religiously.

Mondia Whitei (herb)

Mondia Whitei (also known as Isirigun, White Ginger, Mukombera, and Mulondo), from Nigeria (but also found in Benin), androgenic in nature, is commonly referred to as African Viagra, boosts libido, improves testosterone production and levels in the body, increases size and weight of the testicles, improves male fertility (by improving sperm quality); increases sperm production, boosts strength, energy, and stamina; counters premature ejaculation, helps to heal STDs such as gonorrhea, and improves mental well-being.

Additionally, the herb increases potency by being able to relax the corpus cavernosum muscle thus aiding erection and by improving sperm total motility and progressive motility.

Furthermore, the herb enhances urination, ease birth pains, and increases the quantity and quality of mother's milk.

Fadogia Agrestis (herb)

Fadogia Agrestis (also known as Black Aphrodisiac) from Nigeria, a pro-erectile herb, is one of the most potently effective African erotogens available. It boosts libido, promotes and supports muscle mass, increases energy levels, boosts testosterone levels, strengthens physical/athletic performance, counters impotence/erectile dysfunction, increases stamina, and increases the sex drive. It is a supreme aphrodisiac!

Fadogia Agrestis promotes the production luteinizing hormone which produces testosterone in the male body. Additionally, it helps prevent the accumulation of excess fat in the body and makes one fit by burning fat. It is also loaded with antioxidants and helps keep the immune system fortified.

Fadogia Agrestis is popular herb and ingredient in the Fitness and Supplement World. It is an excellent herb for boosting testosterone levels (which are at all-time lows in the Western world, mostly due to PCBs or Poly-Cholorinated Biphenyls that are literally everywhere in society).

Bulbine Natalensis (herb)

Bulbine Natalensis is a South African herb that boosts testosterone levels by threefold up to six-fold. It is the Number One herb on planet earth for increasing testosterone levels in men, the sad fact which is - today, men in the Western world are experiencing all-time lows in testosterone levels (which mainly due to PCBs [Poly-Chlorinated Biphenyl], Atrazine chemical [in municipal water supplies], and consuming today's female-specific growth hormone [meat and dairy products, derived from farm animals]).

The plant's high testosterone levels greatly boost and repair the male libido.

Additionally, the plant which has anabolic and androgenic properties regulates the hormones (testosterone and androgen), increases testicular size, boosts protein levels in the testes, increases the sex drive, increases intravaginal ejaculatory latency time or EILT

Bulbine Natalensis aids in working out (great for muscle strength). Great for gym-goers and weightlifters (bodybuilders).

While Bulbine Natalensis can increase or boost testosterone levels up to six (6) times, it also lowers estrogen levels three-fold.

Gouro (herb)

Gouro is a natural aphrodisiac from the root of the plant Turraea Heterophylla (which is shaped like an erect penis with testicles at the base) which is found especially in Côte d'Ivoire or Ivory Coast in Africa.

It naturally boosts libido and promotes penis enlargement, counters premature ejaculation and sexual weakness. Additionally, it promotes longer lasting erections.

Gouro root highly compliments Yohimbe bark, Mpesu, and Kigelia especially for penis enlargement purposes.

African Pygeum Bark (herb)

African Pygeum Bark, one of the best herbs for adverse prostate conditions, is an anti-inflammatory phytosterol with the ability to normalize male prostate prostaglandins and to help shrink the prostate in males with enlarged prostates. It is very useful for benign prostatic hypertrophy (BPH) to reduce inflammation and pain and normalize the passage of urine.

Pygeum also increases prostatic and seminal fluid secretions. A meta-analysis revealed that men taking pygeum had a 19% reduction in nocturia and a 24% reduction in residual urine volume.

Pygeum bark helps improve semen volume and viscosity via its effect on DHT and through its action on the development and function of the prostate and seminal vesicles. Healthy viscosity of semen allows more sperm to survive for longer.

Mpesu Bark (herb)

Mpesu Bark from South Africa, a pro-erectile, is one of the most potent and effective male-specific aphrodisiac and erotegens on the planet. It counters sexual dysfunction, weak penile erection, premature ejaculation, and boosts libido and sexual stamina.

Mpesu will give a man longer lasting and stronger erections and will help him experience multiple erections and orgasms.

An added benefit of Mpesu Bark is that it is one of a few herbs that actually naturally promotes growth of the male penis. It compliments "Kigelia" and "Akpi" (for promotion of penis growth, length and width).

The herb also naturally and effectively helps to boost testosterone levels.

Yohimbe (herb)

Yohimbe bark, the King of Aphrodisiacs, is a male-specific hormonal stimulant effective in the production of testosterone, and as an aphrodisiac affecting both male impotence and female frigidity.

The bark has a stimulatory effect on the sex organs of both genders. Yohimbe enhances sexual performance and counters erectile dysfunction (ED) in males. In females, the bark increases arousal and sensitivity of the clitoris and counters frigidity.

Yohimbe is also useful in bodybuilding and athletic performance, weight loss, improving body composition, and adverse heart conditions.

Date Palm Pollen

Date Palm Pollen (DPP) from Egypt, Africa is an authentic African substance or product, derived from the male reproductive dust of palm flowers and has traditionally been used to increase libido and improve fertility in both women and men.

It is one of the best substances to counter male testicular and female ovarian dysfunction. A great product for the male and female reproductive systems.

In men, the pollen helps with testosterone (maintaining normal to high levels), libido, and increasing sperm quantity and quality.

In women, the pollen helps to increase female fertility (boosting ovulation) owing to its estrogen-like compounds, sterols, and estrone-like compounds (that do not throw off or counter men's testosterone levels).

Typha Capensis (herb)

Native to South Africa, commonly known as "Love Reed" is an effective African aphrodisiac herb that enhances the production of testosterone thus increasing libido, countering male infertility and aging male problems; enhances male potency, and counters erectile dysfunction (by improving circulation); and enhancing sexual performance.

In women, Typha Capensis is a powerful fertility enhancer. It strongly enhances ovulation. Additionally, it tones the vagina and increases circulation to that orifice, heightening sensitivity in that region during intimacy.

Typha Capensis can be consumed in the last two weeks of pregnancy to prepare for childbirth. It strengthens uterine contractions. Typha Capensis also helps in countering sexually transmitted diseases.

Uziza (herb)

Uziza, an Igbo name (also known as Ashanti Pepper, West African Pepper, Guinea Pepper, and Ata iyere in Yoruba) is an African herb, used in Nigeria mainly, that helps improve penile erections, enhances fertility and potency, and improves low sperm counts in men.

In women, Uziza is great for their sexual reproductive health. It improves fertility, enhancing ovulation. During pregnancy, it can be taken throughout pregnancy and especially during the last trimester to prepare for childbirth and to prepare for lactation. It increases uterine wall contraction during childbirth. Additionally, it helps with adverse menstrual issues, especially cramping.

Goran Tula Fruit

Goran Tula fruit (also known as Tree Hibiscus and Snot Apple) increases the libido in both men and women and promotes strong desire for sexual intercourse. It helps couples go multiple rounds between the sheets.

The herb is also an effective hormonal balancer, especially for women.

Goran Tula is a reliable fertility enhancer (for both men and women). It also enhances ovulation in women and improves semen concentration and quality while increasing semen volume.

In women, Goran Tula is a vaginal tonic and stimulates the production of vaginal wetness/lubrication and is perfect for keeping the vagina area moist and wet. The herb is one of the best for women who find it difficult to climax or reach orgasm.

Goran Tula is also a vaginal cleanser and deodorizer (helps to eliminate malodors in the vagina) and helps to keep the kitty cat smelling (and tasting) sweet and fresh. Additionally, it helps with adverse menstrual cycle complaints and normalizes the menstrual cycle after childbirth.

Kigelia

Kigelia (also known as Sausage Tree, Worsboom in Afrikaans, Modukghulu, Pidiso in North Sotho, umVongotsi in Siswati; Mpfungurhu in Tsonga, and Muvevha in Venda.

Because the fruit is shaped in the form of the male penis, pursuant to the herbal doctrine of signatures, its properties are helpful for the male genitalia, especially for naturally increasing the growth and length of the penis (taken consistently or religiously) over time, 3-6 months (to notice significant change).

In men, Kigelia is aphrodisiacal and helps the penis to become larger.

In women, Kigelia counters infertility being naturally rich in phyoestrogens. It is one of the best herbs for the breasts, naturally toning, firming and defining the breasts as well as enhancing their growth (natural breast enhancement or growth factor).

In lactating women, Kigelia stimulates lactation. Additionally, it increases the volume and quality of mother's milk.

Kigelia is exceptional for all gynecological disorders in women. It is useful (in men and women) to counter sexually transmitted diseases (STDs or STIs), especially syphilis and gonorrhea.

Marine Bites and Stings

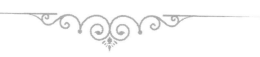

Although jellyfish are by far the most common to sting, there are other fish and sea creatures to be aware of while spending time in the beach. Stingrays, sea urchins, coral, spiny fish, scorpion fish, catfish, and microscopic parasites are always around in some way.

A jellyfish has long, flowing tentacles that are covered with small capsules that sting called, nematocysts. When a tentacle brushes up against our skin, the nematocysts pierce the skin and injected stinging venom which causes the skin to begin burning, throbbing, and itching. The other animals, fish, and sea creatures mentioned in this section also have their own unique ways they sting and bite similar to that of a jellyfish.

Remedies: (Jellyfish Sting)

Vinegar

You can pour this substance over your sting for 30 seconds to help neutralize the nematocysts. Once you have neutralized the nematocysts, you can then pick off the tentacles without spreading the affected area. You do want to wear gloves or use a pair of tweezers when removing the tentacles to avoid being stung again.

Caution: a jellyfish known as "man-of-war" can extend almost 40ft in the water. They can be identified by their blue gas-filled floats. Vinegar can make these stings worse. These stings are already very painful, and vinegar should be avoided if severe pain persists.

50/50 Baking Soda and Salt Water

If you do not have vinegar available, you can mix together 50% baking soda and 50% salt water to form a mixture to prevent the venom from being released. It is best to prepare this ahead of time as a safety precaution and to avoid using freshwater which can stimulate the release of more venom. Note: freshwater essentially the spring water you would drink as opposed to preparing salt-water or using saltwater available while out on a boat. Note: not to be used for man-of-war stings.

Urine

Urinating directly onto your sting can help neutralize the tentacles as well. Urine can help reduce the burning sensation as you incorporate other remedies without concerns of spreading the pain or getting stung again. You will need to be able to urinate (or someone else) in order to do this. Urine is best used warm, so storing in a bag or container may not be helpful if it is not able to be kept very warm.

Saltwater Rinse

If you have absolutely nothing to help neutralize the sting, flush the area with water directly from the ocean. This may appear obvious, but certain bodies of water such as a pond or lake, may have parasites and excess bacteria which will discharge more venom from your sting.

Shaving Cream and Credit Card (or another flat object)

One way to desensitize the nematocysts is to cover the sting with shaving cream which help draw them out. Then get a credit card or other flat object and scrape off the shaving cream. You want to do this only after you've already completed one of the remedies listed previously in this section.

Remedies: (Sea Urchin Sting)

These creatures have sharp, brittle spines that break off and penetrate the skin. Infections can occur if not plucked or removed correctly.

Tweezers

A pair of tweezers is best for these stings. You should be able to see here the skin has been penetrated and you can pluck out any pieces or fragments. You do want to wash the are afterwards with water and slowly wipe clean to locate any smaller fragments or pieces still stuck in the skin. These smaller pieces can remain intact and can lead to an infection if they do not dissolve on their own within three weeks.

Remedies: (Stingray Sting)

These fish like to hide just beneath the sand. At the end of its tail, they have a powerful stinger. Stingrays will often look to retreat when you are close, but they can still sting you as they try to leave and get away.

Note: same protocol can be followed if stung by a catfish or scorpion fish.

Remove, Rinse, and Repeat

Like a bee sting, you want to remove the stinger and rinse with water. Stingrays do leave several stingers at once so you will want to repeat this process a few times to remove any fragments that are leftover. You can rinse with saltwater or freshwater/

Immerse In Hot Water

After removing the stinger(s) and rinsing off the sting, you will want to immerse your sting in hot water for 45-90 minutes. Temperature of water should not be scorching hot; should feel like warmer bathwater for maximum temperature.

Remedy: (Coral Scrapes)

It is common to rub against coral and get a scrape or cut. However, unlike typical scrapes or cuts, there are nematocysts in the coral which can create a fast-acting infection. You want to clean the area well while removing any fragments left in the skin. Then, you want to scrub the area with a gauze pad soaked in freshwater and an antiseptic such as Bactine to avoid triggering nematocysts from flaring up.

Remedy: "Sea Lice" (Jellyfish Larvae)

This type of larvae can get trapped in a t-shirt or bathing suit easily. Once they sit for a while, they can begin to create an itch which feels like an allergic reaction. You want to shower completely, particularly around the waistband (most common area they settle in). then, you can apply any of the remedies mentioned so far in this section.

Memory Problems

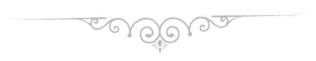

Memory problems can be attributed to many things going on in life such as stress, busy work schedule, to managing several responsibilities. As we age, we tend to forget things as well, but "memory problems" is referring to forgetting things without anything specifically getting in the way. Memory problems are caused by damage to the cells of the brain, called neurons. This damage can be oxidative or inflammatory. Oxidative damage is essentially "cellular rust" from areas of the brain not being used or stimulate enough over time. Inflammatory damage ("cellular burn") is when the cells are eroding due to additional pressure to perform tasks with limited resources, or sources that come in the form of adequate nutrients and proper hydration.

This section will identify natural remedies, memory exercises, and lifestyle adjustments you can make to help improve your memory before a disease or condition is fully developed.

Remedies:

Rosemary (herb)

This herb helps to improve memory. You can just inhale this herb's scent or used as an essential oil. You can place 1-3 drops of rosemary essential oil onto a cotton ball or tissue and keep nearby to inhale its scent. Do not ingest this oil by mouth as it can become toxic and lead to irritations.

Sage (herb)

Holli Ryan, RD, LD/N, has reviewed several research articles around sage helping Alzheimer's patients using sage. Ryan reports that the bioactive compounds in sage help to reduce glucose, cholesterol, triglycerides, inflammation, and help improve mood and cognition. Sage also safety boosts memory in those with and without Alzheimer's.

Sage contains flavonoids such as, apigenin, diosmetin, and luteolin. Apigenin has been shown in clinical studies to stimulate neurogenesis, the generation of neuronal cells in the brain by promoting a process called "neuronal differentiation" which helps to improve memory and slow down the deterioration of brain cells.

You may add sage to soups and stews or sauteed vegetables. This herb can be made as a tea or added to a salad. This herb is also available in extract form where you can take just a few drops a day.

Lion's Mane Mushroom

The lion's mane mushroom also helps to promote the neurogenesis process that sage promotes as mentioned earlier in this section. This mushroom helps to promote the growth of brain cells.

Keep Your Mind Active

We want our brains to remain stimulated, but not too much. Certain areas of our brains have specific tasks they are responsible for, and due to our lifestyles, do not get worked quite enough. We want to do activities to promote stimulation and problem-solving, but not feel overworked. Activities such as crossword puzzles, reading books, playing chess or scrabble, or engaging in martial arts training can all help the brain's capacity to be used in a way that is conducive to using its memory. Anything that does not keep the mind calm, but at ease, will result in memory declining over time.

Create Categories

When we can place certain things into categories, they are easier to remember as there is an increased chance of coming across another item within the same category and help us bridge a connection to what we were trying to remember. Similar to how we structure phone numbers into sections is a helpful way to improve memory. Whether you are studying for a test or going grocery shopping, work to placing all valuable information into specific categories, followed by reviewing each category to help remember better.

Write It Down

When we write things down, we don't have to immediately imprint what we write down into our brains. The ability to wait before we try to memorize something will help us remember easier. Trying to remember something in-the-moment can signal stress which can get in the way of us remembering something. Writing things down can help organize how we remember things as well. We may create lists, bullet-points, or simply thoughts into a few words or phrase(s) which all help support our brains with remembering things better.

Make "Common Spots"

A simple way to make the most of your memory, and to not hinder your memory, is to create some common spots/areas where you leave items or can go to them every day. Items such as car keys, shoes, word badge, etc should have a spot designated for them so you know where they are, and where to put them the moment you get home. This will not only save time, but not use up some of your "memory cells" looking for them the following day or later on. Reducing the number of smaller things, you have to remember is a great way to work towards improving and centering your attention on more important things to remember.

Get Enough Sleep

The brain needs enough sleep in order to properly rest and then function well. How many hours can vary, but you want to feel well rested. You do not want to wake up feeling tired or fatigued. Part of getting enough sleep is preparing to power down before bed and structuring your time around sleep to promote quality sleep. Allan Hobson, M.D., professor of psychiatry at Harvard Medical School and director of the Neurophysiology and Sleep Laboratory at Massachusetts Mental Health Center in Boston, MA, states how "When you're asleep, it works on information you've gathered." Without enough sleep, your cognitive skills can suffer and impair your ability to focus and remember things.

B-vitamins

Dr. Cynthia Green, Ph.D., assistant clinical professor of psychiatry at Mount Sinai School of Medicine of New York University in New York City, reports that, "A vitamin B12 deficiency can cause significant memory loss" and that B-vitamins become harder to absorb as we get older.

Cobalamin ("vitamin B12")

Is naturally created via bacterial synthesis in the gut. Cobalamin is a bacterium that is part of every growing plant that we consume. However, this is often washed off during processing that it is no longer present on these items, and we do not consume this bacterium. Animals will consume foods while they are still in the ground and absorb a larger quantity of cobalamin that goes into their muscle tissue and can be absorbed by anything that eats them. However, eating an animal is a longer route to getting access to this bacterium, and we are unsure if they even have an adequate amount to be absorbed based upon their diets/lifestyle. We can gain consistent access to this bacterium by simply eating more fresh foods that are not processed, and by growing our own foods. The fewer stops from the farm to your table, the better your chances are of gaining access to absorb this healthy bacterium.

We essentially only need about 1 microgram of B12 a day. When we repeatedly do not meet this need, it can become noticeable, but we don't need nearly as much B12 as we do calcium, magnesium, or any other mineral. Since we have worked to kill off any form of bacteria (harmful or helpful) most people remain deficient. If we consume that which is natural and work on eating locally grown produce and growing our own plants (even something small to put in a window at home) we can consume enough B12 and do away with any B12 deficiency (and many others) so that B12 deficiency is no longer a topic of decision.

You will want to go to local markets and farmer's markets in your area where there is a shorter "farm to table" distance where B12 will remain more present in some capacity. Also growing some of your own plants at home or a t a local garden will be best.

Thiamin ("Vitamin B1")

An enzyme that transforms glucose into carbon-dioxide and water. Get destroyed b heating and is most abundant grains.

Common sources of B1: asparagus, peas, oranges, clementines, lemons, sunflower seeds, sesame seeds, pecans, Brazil nuts, lentils, pecans.

Riboflavin ("vitamin B2")

Riboflavin helps the body use nutrients such as carbohydrates, fats, and proteins for energy, and additionally functions as an antioxidant.

Common sources of riboflavin: tomatoes, avocado, sunflower seeds, dandelion greens, swiss chard, kale, quinoa., and edible sea vegetables (Nori, Wakame, Hijiki, Sea Moss, Bladderwrack).

Folic Acid ("vitamin B9")

This is a synthetic man-made vitamin that is added to fortified foods (foods that have vitamins and minerals added to them). It's comprised of several "B-vitamins" but B9 by itself is put together separately to be added to foods. Items that are naturally nutrient-dense should have the combination of "B-vitamins" needed to produce folic acid (vitamin B9).

Common sources of folic acid: avocado, turnip greens, swiss chard, kale, lettuce, dandelion greens, sunflower seeds, oranges, kiwi, quinoa, and wild rice.

*most other B-vitamins are already produced by the body when healthy and can be taken in small amounts.

Niacin ("Vitamin-B3")

Not isolated and its nature is unknown. Believes to boost energy in the body for DNA production and metabolism. Thought to be identical to pantothenic acid found in most whole grains, seeds, and lentils.

Common sources of niacin: mushrooms, peanuts, avocado, peas, chia seeds, broccoli, pumpkin seeds, lentils.

Adenine ("Vitamin-B4")

Is heat destructible and water soluble. Has been studied in rats to prevent a form of paralysis. No human need has been demonstrated at this time.

Common sources of adenine: chickpeas, chili peppers, flaxseeds, pumpkin seeds, sunflower seeds, almonds, mushrooms, hazelnuts, sage, pecans, broccoli, cauliflower, cloves, dandelion greens, peas, lentils, oregano, Brazil nuts.

Pantothenic Acid ("Vitamin-B5")

Has been studied to prevent loss of weight in pigeons but that is all known about this so far. No direct link to human need identified at this time.

Pyridoxine ("Vitamin-B6")

Organic compound composed of hydrogen, oxygen, and nitrogen. It is known for animals to be able to use B6 to utilize the amino acid known as tryptophan which creates melatonin and serotonin to balance hormones, appetite, sleep, mood, and pain. Helps increase the body's utilization from Vitamin-B3 which is needed to energize metabolism and DNA production.

Common sources of pyridoxine: avocado, carrots, bananas, peas, lentils, spinach, chickpeas, acorn squash, quinoa, sunflower seeds, brussels sprouts, oranges, pistachios.

Biotin ("Vitamin B7")

Enzyme that breaks down fats, carbohydrates, and other materials.

Common sources of Biotin: walnuts, pecans, almonds, avocado, sunflower seeds, sesame seeds.

Inositol ("Vitamin-B8")

Is actually a sugar, not a vitamin. Helps regular insulin levels.

Common sources of inositol: oranges, grapefruits, limes, cantaloupe, avocado, lettuce, raisins, cabbage, peas, and most nuts and beans.

Folate ("Vitamin-B9")

Helps with red blood cell production which can promote healthy blood cell function.

Common sources of Folate: asparagus, avocado, oranges, Brussels sprouts, lentils, beets, bananas, leafy greens, hemp, walnuts, chickpeas.

Para Amino Benzoic Acid (PABA) ("Vitamin-B10)

Helps microorganisms in the body. Helps darken grey hairs and protect the skin.

Common sources of PABA: spinach, asparagus, brussels sprouts, dark leafy green vegetables.

Vitamin-B11 (also known as Folic Acid)

Research over time has noticed small differences in structure but orle of B9 and B11 are the same.

Orotic Acid or Orotate ("Vitamin-B13")

Not recognized as a vitamin by health or scientific research but is a molecule that is water soluble and helps with nutrient metabolism and energy production.

Common sources of orotate: carrots, beets, chia seeds, lentils, hemp seeds.

Trimethyl glycine ("Vitamin-B14")

Not yet established as a vitamin but works to increase cell-proliferation in bone marrow.

Common Trimethyl glycine sources: dark leafy greens, avocado, peas, nuts and legume food groups.

Pangamic Acid ("Vitamin-B15")

Not yet recognized as a vitamin. In the1980's was banned due to being an unsafe food additive.

Dimethylglycine (DMG) ("Vitamin-B16")

Combats free radicals, serves as an antioxidant and detoxifying agent.

Common sources of DMG: pumpkin seeds, beans, seeds, grains.

Laetrile ("Vitamin-B17")

Helps control and lower blood pressure. Relieves pain caused by inflammation.

Common sources of laetrile: almonds, apricot kernals, cherry seeds, bitter almonds, lima beans.

Choline ("Vitamin-B18")

Metabolizes fats and cholesterol in the body.

Common sources of choline: sesame seeds, lentils, cauliflower, peanuts.

L-Carnitine ("Vitamin-B20")

Fat burning item often found in many fitness supplements. Transports long-chain fatty acids into the mitochondria so they can get burned off to produce energy.

Common sources of L-carnitine: avocado, asparagus, lentils, potatoes, pumpkin seeds, almonds, chickpeas, cashews.

Vitamin-E

This nutrient is an antioxidant that works to block the harmful effects of free radicles and reduce the buildup of cholesterol and fatty substances that can increase inflammation in the body and the brain which contribute to memory issues.

Common Sources of Vitamin-E: red bell pepper, mango, avocado, sunflower seeds, brazil nuts, turnip greens, blackberry, black currants, olives, and butternut squash.

Gingko Biloba (herb)

This herb can help improve circulation that helps the brain receive all of the nutrients it needs to function well. Alertness, concentration, and overall memory are some of the primary highlights this herb is stated to help with according to many herbalists and holistic practitioner.

Exercise

Increasing and improving blood flow is essential for memory. Dr Green states that "Regular aerobic exercise also protects us from other illnesses such as stroke, diabetes, and high blood pressure, which contribute to memory problems."

Reduce Stress

Those who experience stress often typically have higher levels of the hormone cortisol, which can directly impair the functioning of the hippocampus section of the brain that is responsible for memory. If you remain tense and experience stress frequently, you can also feel very fatigued often which also impairs memory. We cannot avoid stress completely, so it's important to maintain balance through relaxation activities.

Lower Your Cholesterol

High cholesterol diets lead to an increased risk of developing Alzheimer's disease at an earlier age than other animals who get lower cholesterol according to Dr. Gunnar Gouras, M.D., assistant professor of neurology and neuroscience at the Joan and Sanford I. Weill Medical College of Cornell University in New York, New York.

Proper Hydration

Almost 85% of our brains consist of water. Whenever you do not consume enough water, your brain is dehydrated. This is why the majority of the symptoms of dehydration impact the brain, headaches, fatigue, dizziness, confusion, etc. Aim to drink about half of your body-weight in ounces of water daily to remain hydrated. Avoid relying solely on water as the kidneys may retain water and water is void of many minerals that could be consumed easier by consuming fresh fruits and vegetables.

Phospholipids

Phospholipids help the neurons' membranes (outer protection layer) maintain its structure and improves communication between brain cells.

Common Sources of Phospholipids: sunflower oil, kale, seaweeds, walnuts, and brazil nuts.

Fatty Acids (Omega-3, Omeg-6, Omega-9)

Essential fatty acids are essential to the body because of their role in brain and heart health. In the brain, they help protect neuron membranes and promote memory. Dr. Steven Bock, M.D., co-director of the Center for Progression Medicine in Rhinebeck, New York recommends 2 tablespoons of flaxseed oil a day to help get enough fatty acids into your diet.

Common sources of fatty acids are Walnuts, Brazil Nuts, Avocados, Hemp Seeds, Hemp Milk, Walnut Oil, Olive Oil, and Sea Vegetable such as Nori, Hijiki, Bladderwrack, Kelp, and Dulse.

Acetyl-Carnitine ("L-carnitine")

This nutrient helps improves memory, boosts energy in the brain, improves brain receptors, and improve neuron communication, according to Dr. Alan Brauer, M.D., founder, and director of the TotalCare medical Center in Palo Alto, California. 250-2,000 milligrams a day

Common Sources of L-carnitine: avocado, walnuts, garbanzo beans, and seeds (seeds inside fruits and vegetables).

Flower Essences

For Age-Related Memory: rosemary essential oil

For Poor Memory: madia essential oil

For Helping the Brain Find meaning/Connection To Events: shasta dairy essential oil

You may use any of these as needed but you may use all three together for best effects. Take 4 drops of each of these three oils (mixed together in equal parts) 3-4 times a day.

Periwinkle (herb)

This herb helps provide a boost of energy for the brain. Its extract from their seeds help to improve blood flow to the brain. 20-40 milligrams a day is recommended.

Kallawalla (herb)

This iron-rich herb can help regenerate cells and boost oxygen levels within the body, particularly the brain. This herb helps cleanse excess waste in the lymphatic system and can help improve neurological function within the brain that often impacts memory.

Visualization

This may be the primary way to remember things since it's pretty much what we do whenever we're focused on remembering anything. Most of our memory is stored in pictures according to William Cone, Ph.D., a geriatric psychologist in California. He recommends taking anything you want to remember ad making it a picture in your mind. This can act as a connection between two items that help you remember someone's name, a sentence, or anything else you can capture with making it into a picture.

Menopause

Menopause does not categorize as a "disease" but certainly presents itself like one as there's numerous symptoms, and completely alters someone's lifestyle. However, as you will learn in this section, life-altering changes does not have to be met with urgency when we work on preparing ourselves for our aging bodies. Doctors define menopauses as the 366th or 367th day after a woman's last period (about 1 year and 1 day later). This is most common for those in their later 50's and 60's, but can occur much sooner in a woman's 40's where symptoms vary. Ever since puberty, the female body has created and stored about half a million eggs in the ovaries. Typically, by the age of 50, there are only a few eggs left which creates an imbalance that the body has to adjust and account for which often presents as typical menopausal symptoms. The monthly cycle of a woman involves the swelling and bursting of an egg sac, which releases estrogen and progesterone hormones. These hormones being released thicken the uterus with blood that prepares to harbor and nourish a newly fertilized egg. If the egg is not fertilized, there will be shedding of the uterine cells and blood. This process slowly comes to a halt during menopause.

As women age, estrogen levels decrease more rapidly. This triggers many symptoms and also places their body at a greater risk for various diseases, which is why there's often a wide range of symptoms that can be different for every woman. The most common symptoms can include, sudden weight gain, sleep disturbances, emotional changes, vaginal changes (dryness, less elasticity), and hot flashes. The ultimate goal is to not experience any of these symptoms, but also to gradually approach this stage in life so you're aware of what your body specifically needs during this time (just like any other stage or chapter in your life). Many women will opt for hormone-replacement therapy which involves replacing natural hormones which are not being released as often, with synthetic hormones to essential "trick" the body into believing there are no issues. However, this causes the body to then ignore many other issues that can exist, and lead to many other problems over time and inevitably make menopausal symptoms much worse.

Remedies:

Stop Smoking Cigarettes

Mary Jane Minkin, M.D., clinical professor at Yale University School of Medicine and an obstetrician-gynecologist in New Haven, Connecticut, and author of What Every Woman Needs to Know about Menopause, states, "Smokers have a 2-year-earlier menopause on average than nonsmokers." Smoking impacts your reproductive system and overall health. Once you give up this habit you will notice improvements at any age. However, if you don't give up smoking until you're in your 50's, you may not notice as much a change as you would if you would have given up smoking in your 20's or early 30's.

Give Up Alcohol Too...

Drinking alcohol is not helpful to your heart or your bones. Causing lasting damage to these areas will bring upon hot flashes much earlier in your life. If you drink alcohol regularly, you will more than likely experience hot flashes when you are older and will then learn you are going through menopause.

Calcium

Most people do not consume nearly enough calcium a day. Doctors often recommend dairy products as they are higher in calcium than most items, but these also contain a high amount of saturated fats, and calories, which all present their own issues. You want to aim close to 1,000 milligrams a day of calcium.

Common sources of Calcium: sea moss, kale, okra, dandelion greens, turnip greens, lettuce, papaya, and oranges.

Vitamin-E

This nutrient can help properly regulate (and hopefully eliminate) hot flashes. You can start by consuming 200 international units (IU) daily up to five times a day. Start with 400 IU and gradually increase to 1,000 IU a day over the span of about two weeks. Once you begin to feel better you can gradually decrease your dosage back to 400 IU spread out throughout the day. This nutrient can also help reduce vaginal dryness and can also be an "effective substitute for estrogen in the majority of women" says Dr. Susan Lark, M.D., physician in Los Altos, California, USA.

Common Sources of Vitamin-E: sunflower seeds, avocado, brazil nuts, and walnuts.

Vitamin-A

This nutrient becomes deficient for women who bleed often. Dr. Lark cites several studies which show that excessive bleeding leads to lower-than-normal levels in vitamin-A and that fulfilling this deficiency, stops bleeding in almost 90% of women with this issue.

Common Sources of Vitamin-A: mango, papaya, apricots, red bell peppers, winter squash, dark leafy green vegetables, cantaloupe, and lettuce.

Understanding Your Diet/Lifestyle

"Women metabolize foods differently than men," says Larrian Gillespie, M.D., retired assistant clinical professor of urology and urogynecology and president of Health Life Productions, and author of The Menopause Diet and The Goddess Diet. One key difference of how women and men metabolize foods differently is that men use carbs for energy, whereas women use carbs to store as fat in the event women can procreate if there were starvation. Alterations in estrogen levels also have their role in how we process and absorb nutrients. The focus is to identify the "good" carbohydrates such as those in beans, nuts, grains, and most fruits. Not the "bad" carbs in processed foods such as chips, bagels, potatoes, and fried foods which all have a role in boosting your blood sugar levels that often lead to contributing symptoms of menopause such as, nausea, sweating, fatigue, and aches and pains all over your body.

Lubricant (naturally)

Rather than use some chemical-filled lubricant to replace what your body naturally provides during sexual intercourse, it is best to increase more foods that boost the health of the sexual organs in order to avoid side effects from using chemicals that the body cannot absorb or recognize. Dark leafy green vegetables, foods high in omega-3 fatty acids, and fruits help promote vaginal wetness according to researchers from Santa Chiara Regional Hospital in Trento, Italy.

Dark leafy green vegetables (dandelion greens, turnip greens, kale, lettuce)

Omega-3 fatty acids (Brazil Nuts, Walnuts, Kola Nuts, Avocados, Bananas, Sea Vegetables (Nori, Wakame, Hijiki, Sea Moss, Bladderwrack), Coconut, Coconut Oil (do not cook), Olive Oil (do not cook), Grapeseed Oil, Avocado Oil, Walnut Oil, Mushrooms, Quinoa, and Wild Rice).

Fruits (specifically, apples, berries, watermelon, oranges.

Smoothie Recipe (drink 1-2 times a day)

1 cup blueberries

Large handful of chopped watermelon

½ of a small avocado (1/3 of a medium-large avocado)

3-4 dandelion leaves

8 ounces of coconut water

Black Cohosh (herb)

Numerous studies for menopausal women have shown that black cohosh alleviates hot flashes, vaginal dryness, sleep disturbances, night sweats, fatigue, and irritability. Black cohosh extract (remifemin) has been used as an estrogen replacement for many medications over time.

Take up 1-2 40-milligram capsules twice a day or take in extract form ½ teaspoon to 1 teaspoon twice a day.

Milk Thistle (herb)

The majority of the time doctors will prescribe synthetic hormones to decrease the body's initial response to menopause. But excess hormones in the bloodstream essentially clogs the liver as the liver cannot process or breakdown these prescriptions in addition to its other responsibilities. An herb known as Milk Thistle (just the name – no dairy involved in this plant) helps protects the liver from harmful substances and can repair and rejuvenate damaged liver cells. Not only is this herb helpful with repairing already damaged liver cells but can be taken with synthetic hormones without adverse effects as you work to wean yourself off of these prescriptions.

Take 280 milligrams a day of this herb. Typical dosage can be 420 milligrams divided into 23doses a day for about 6 to 8 weeks, then reducing to 280 milligrams a day.

Using Dried Root (milk thistle)

Cut ½ to 1 tablespoon of the root and place into pan with 2 cups of water, cover and simmer for 10 minutes on low heat. Strain tea, let cool until it is room temperature. Drink ½ to 1 cup three times a day.

Motherwort (herb)

Similar to Black Cohosh if Black Cohosh is not available to you in your location. Also use this herb instead if Black Cohosh does not appear to help as effectively within 5 to 6 weeks. Pour 1 pint of boiling water into a pot with 1-ounce oof this herb (leaves). Steep for 10 minutes and let cool. Drink ½ to 1 cup three times a day. In tincture form, you can often take two droppers every 10 to 15 minutes until your symptoms decrease. If this seems to be too much or stressful to do as often, focus on taking two droppers once an hour. The goal is to take frequent doses of this herb but not too frequently.

Sage (herb)

This herb is helpful for hot flashes during the day and those who experience the "night sweats". To prepare this herb for tea, follow the same instructions listed for the Black Cohosh and Motherwort herbs identified in this section.

St. John's Wort (herb)

This herb has been known to be as effective as many antidepressant medications pre-scribed by medical doctors. Depression related to hormonal imbalances during menopause can benefit from using this herb without concern for the side effects that come with antide-pressant medications such as, fatigue, dry mouth, headaches, and loss of sexual interest.

300-milligrams three times a day is recommended. If you get this herb in extract form, follow the dosage recommended on label.

Chasteberry (herb)

This herb is to help symptoms involving hormonal changes and lowered libido. Recommended by Jason Ellis, practitioner of Traditional Chinese Medicine (TCM) in New Paltz, New York, USA. Chasteberry is often found in most retail health stores under the name "Vitex" if you do not have access to a tincture form of this herb. Make sure to use as recommended on product label for at least 3 months before you will begin to have more consistent positive changes.

Hydrotherapy

May sound counterproductive, but intentionally sweating can help release some of the toxins that are often working their way out in small amounts throughout the day which results in regular sweating. Go to a sauna or steam room as often as you can. If neither of these are convenient for you, make sure to take a hot bath for at least 20 minutes as often as possible.

Medical Anthropologists and co-directors of the Institute for the Study of Culturogenic Disease in Hilo, Hawaii tested their hydrotherapy theory by conducting a research study involving 10 women (5 to take a 20-minute sauna or steam bath 6 days a week for one month, while the other 5 do not engage in hydrotherapy). After one month, the 5 who engaged in hydrotherapy experienced "significant or complete relief" while the remaining 5 noted no changes in their symptoms of having hot flashes.

Acupressure

Within acupressure, it is believed that the body's "chi" or energy flows through the body in currents called meridians. Stimulating these spots along the currents in the body can aide and facilitate healing. There are specific spots (acupressure points) that can provide relief to areas impacted by particular conditions.

Stimulating certain points in the feet can help alleviate things like insomnia and anxiety. You want to stimulate each point for at least 3 to 5 minutes for best results.

Point BL62 – use your right hand and press just outside your right ankle, directly below your anklebone. Repeat with your left hand on your left ankle.

Point KI6 – use your left hand and press on the inside of your right ankle directly below the anklebone. Repeat using your right hand on your left ankle.

Exercise / Pilates

"Exercise reduces menopausal symptoms, helps you sleep, helps your bones, and helps your heart" according to Dr. Minkin, M.D. This may seem like common sense to most, but we want to address our main systems in our body regularly to remain in better health and work to reduce symptoms associated with menopause. The most difficult parts of exercising regularly are, staying consistent, and knowing what you are doing to be effective. However, focusing on these two items causes many to overlook what is most important: flexibility. A form of exercise that enhances flexibility without excessive sweating which can trigger symptoms, is Pilates. Pilates is a form of exercise that focuses on strengthening the whole body as a unit without targeting specific areas to promote muscle growth. Pilates is low-impact and a low-sweat alternative as compared to exercises like yoga, running, or swimming.

Kegels

This form of exercise can be completed anywhere. It involves temporarily squeezing the pelvic muscles to help improve vaginal elasticity and increases sexual pleasure. To do this exercise, you want to slowly squeeze and hold for 3 seconds and relax; repeating about 10 times. Next, squeeze the vaginal muscles firmly and relax as rapidly if you can; also repeating 10 times. Complete this cycle 5 times throughout the day.

Yoga ("child's pose")

A common yoga exercise known as child's pose is great for reducing symptoms of anxiety and stress which can help relieve anxiety related to menopause and irritability. Search up this pose as it may sound more difficult to perform simply by reading each step. Find an image that keeps things simple to serve as your reference and hold this pose for as long as you wish, and it is not unbearable.

Affirmations

Affirmations are positive statements that serve the purpose of changing any negative mental or emotional states. You want to sit in a comfortable position and repeat positive statements slowly and clearly, with intention. Find some positive affirmations that you believe will serve you well and write them down.

Menstrual Cramps

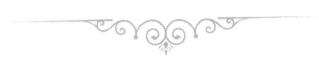

Aside from accepting that it's just a certain "time of the month" for women as a permanent monthly roadblock, there is a biochemical cause for menstrual cramps. There are hormonelike chemicals that we call "series-2 prostaglandins" that trigger contractions in the muscular wall of the uterus. Arachidonic acid stimulates the series-2 prostaglandins. The goal is to cut down the formation of the prostaglandins so the body can adequately process hormonal adjustments without the strong muscular contractions. In this section, we will look at natural remedies to help support both, short-term and long-term relief.

Remedies:

Reduce Specific Fats

Arachidonic acid is a chemical that is in saturated fats., most notably, red meats, dairy products, and palm kernel oil which is found in most processed foods. Consuming these items increase your susceptibility to cramps along with the severity of your cramps. Removing these foods are the most important step. Without doing so, you will normalize a regularly scheduled series of pain each month. It will only be a matter of time before your uterus gets tired of this abuse and will suffer complications such as infertility, or early menopause, among many other issues.

Omega-3 Fatty Acids

While the arachidonic acid in certain fats that triggers the series-2 prostaglandins that causes cramps, omega-3 fatty acids (another type of fat) help keep those series-2 prostaglandins trapped in the cells temporarily so they cannot get into the muscle tissues and trigger spasms and cramps.

532 | **Bryan McAskill's Book of Natural Remedies**

Common Sources of Omega-e Fatty Acids Brazil Nuts, Walnuts, Kola Nuts, Avocados, Bananas, Sea Vegetables (Nori, Wakame, Hijiki, Sea Moss, Bladderwrack), Coconut, Coconut Oil (do not cook), Olive Oil (do not cook), Grapeseed Oil, Avocado Oil, Walnut Oil, Mushrooms, Quinoa, and Wild Rice.

Calcium

This nutrient helps keep the muscles relaxed and evenly tones. This helps prevent all kinds of cramps, but also helps relieve uterine cramps. It is typically recommended to consume about 800-miligrams of calcium a day.

Common sources of Calcium: sea moss, kale, okra, dandelion greens, turnip greens, lettuce, papaya, and oranges.

Magnesium

Magnesium allows the body to absorb calcium and also works to relax the muscles. 400-milligrams is the stand recommendation to consume daily.

Magnesium Sources: avocado, chickpeas, tamarind, basil, dill, ginger, oregano, thyme, any *CBD (cannabidiol) products are helpful. (CBD Oils are almost pure magnesium.), nettle leaf, horsetail, red clover, sage, and nopal.

*To test the purity of a CBD Oil, send to a lab for testing or you should feel a steady decline in needing to rely on this substance after your need has been met regularly.

Vitamin-C

This nutrient helps the body move nutrients to the uterine muscles while also moving waste materials away from the uterus. This nutrient will help reduce the typical fatigue that comes with experiencing menstrual cramps. It is recommended to take 500-3,000-milligrams a day, particularly when experiencing symptoms.

Common Sources of Vitamin-C: Black Currants, Bell Peppers (red and green), Papaya, Spring Onions, Strawberries, Cantaloupe, Mango, Oranges, Watercress, Raspberries, and Tomatoes.

Vitamin-E

This nutrient simply helps to balance the hormones in the body. this is crucial to alleviating severity of cramps, but also helping to avoid symptoms from appearing suddenly.

Common Sources of Vitamin-E: red bell pepper, mango, avocado, sunflower seeds, brazil nuts, turnip greens, blackberry, black currants, olives, and butternut squash.

Niacin

This nutrient works to dilate the blood vessels to bring upon more circulation and oxygen to the uterine wall. 2-200-milligrams of niacin will help to relieve cramps when take 7-10 days before menstruation begins

Common Sources of Niacin: avocado, watermelon, cherries, oranges, nectarines, lettuce, peaches (dried), sesame seeds, walnuts.

Iron

Load up on the right type of iron (Iron Phosphate and Iron-Fluorine) which comes from plants, not (Iron Oxide) which comes from metals which are in many medications and products advertised as containing Iron. Much of the muscle soreness and blood flow is attributed to low iron levels, so many doctors will prescribe "iron-pills", but these do not contain the iron that is needed. And much of the low iron in the body can be traced to poor diets that send blood flow to all areas of the body as it tries to remove toxins and digest unrecognizable materials. Just stopping the consumptions of these items, the body does not recognize is often all that is needed to reduce this issue from continuing, however, the body will need to replace what has been lost, which can be achieved through consuming natural plants that are high in iron (phosphate).

Natural Sources of Iron: Wild rice, chickpeas/garbanzo beans, dandelion greens, soursop, sarsaparilla, burdock, yellow dock, chapparal, dates, prunes, Flor de Manita, Red Clover, Hombre Grande, Blue Vervain, Contribo, Guaco.

Items that rob you of iron:

- chocolate
- cow's milk
- coffee (yes, decaffeinated coffee too and those weight loss coffees as well)
- soda
- yeast
- artificial sugars and food dyes
- foods high in oxalic acids ("oxalates") such as, cauliflower, broccoli, spinach, soy, potatoes, dates, raspberries, navy beans, cashews, and baked potatoes with skin (baked potatoes, French fries, etc). Oxalates deplete and interfere with iron absorption.
- losing blood (this can happen during cycles but not replacing and replenishing your iron when this happens is the issue).

My Personal Remedy:

Combine the following herb tinctures in equal parts:

Black haw – relaxes the uterus

Ginger – moves through positive energy

Valerian – relaxes the uterus

Motherwort – helps restore health for most gynecological imbalances

Dosage: 1 teaspoon of formula twice a day on days that you have cramps.

Motherwort (herb)

This herb in tincture form is powerful enough to help relieve cramps by itself. You can take 5 drops from a tincture, and you do not feel relieve within 10-minutes, you can take another 5 drops. Keep track of the total number of drops it takes to eventually relieve your cramps.

Morning Sickness

Morning sickness is the body's way of adapting to rising estrogen levels. This condition mostly occurs in pregnant women as estrogen levels are more likely to rise during these moments. Morning sickness generally occurs around week 6 of the pregnancy when the placenta of the unborn fetus begins its production of the human chorionic gonadotropin (HCG) which is more commonly known as the pregnancy hormone. Around week 8 or 9, symptoms often peak and then begin to decrease once again after week 13. Having morning sickness is generally a sign that the pregnancy is going well, but there are ways to minimize and reduce the severity of the symptoms associated with morning sickness.

Remedies:

Be Aligned With What Your Baby Consumes

This may sound strange as it is common belief that the baby consumes whatever you eat, but this couldn't be further from the truth. You baby will not seek, digest, or absorb saturated fats, unhealthy oils, or processed sugars. The baby will eventually absorb what's in your bloodstream, but not directly throughout your pregnancy. The baby nourishes itself by searching through your bloodstream for nutrients, particularly glucose. If you do not replenish your glucose supply, your blood sugar levels will drop because your baby is not going to just stop absorbing what it has access to. the best way to keep your glucose supply ready, is by consuming simple sugars from fruit as their glucose supply is already broken down.

Fruits High in Glucose: mangoes, oranges, cherries, watermelon, pears, grapes, and many more you may enjoy.

Avoid Fried Foods

The body takes longer to process and attempt to digest fried foods. Not only does the molecular structure of foods change when they're fried (making them harder to recognize) but they sit in the digestive tract and rot by the time they are digested and reduce the amount of glucose available for storage in the bloodstream.

Keep Small (healthy) Snacks Nearby

Moving around on an empty stomach can trigger or make symptoms worse. So, keep some snacks around to avoid this from happening. You want to avoid any addictive foods like processed foods or junk foods as they will not nourish your or your baby and will deplete your body's energy while triggering symptoms.

Ginger Tea (herb)

This herb can help calm nausea and reduce vomiting. It is best to consume this herb in tea form shortly upon awakening. Take a ¼ piece of a medium sized piece of ginger, place into an empty cup and boil water. Pour the water into your cup and let steep for about 10-12 minutes. Strain out the herb and drink twice a day.

Water and Fruit Juice

Maintaining hydration is key during pregnancy. Drinking enough water will remain helpful to alleviate symptoms and avoid feeling dehydrated. Grape juice is particularly helpful during pregnancy with treating symptoms like nausea and killing any unwanted bacteria which can trigger symptoms. Grape juice will also stimulate your child's immune system and is also high in glucose which your child will seek to nourish itself throughout your pregnancy. Other fruit juices such as orange juice, prune juice, perch juice, guava juice, and strawberry juice, will serve you well during pregnancy as they provide an assortment of vital minerals and nutrients, and all are high in glucose.

Trust Yourself

While pregnant, your body nor your mind will operate how it did before. You will acquire wisdom you were unaware of before and will be guided more naturally. Trust your instincts as long as you know they will not result in harm. Make actions and decisions clear, but allow yourself to be guided, especially in regard to what foods you consume. You may not want to consume certain berries for example. So have something else available on standby. Just make sure to resist temptations for harmful foods.

Remain Calm

This can be challenging as the body is going through many changes you become increasingly more aware of as time goes on. Mindfulness practices and working to find your personal destination of peace and relaxation is crucial to help create balance during this time. find what works best for you that you can do with ease.

Pyridoxine ("Vitamin-B6")

This nutrient has been shown to reduce morning sickness in pregnant women. Vitamin-B6 (pyridoxine) helps our bodies to process certain amino acids (proteins), which may somehow reduce nausea. Some studies show that women who have severe morning sickness have lower levels of vitamin B6 in their blood.

Common sources of pyridoxine: avocado, carrots, bananas, peas, lentils, spinach, chickpeas, acorn squash, quinoa, sunflower seeds, brussels sprouts, oranges, pistachios.

Mint or Spearmint

Chewing mint or spearmint leaves can help reduce a weak or stomach that is in pain. You may drink these in tea form as well if chewing them is too strong for you.

Acupuncture

Some women find that acupressure wristbands ease nausea. Acupuncture, in which hair-thin needles are put into your skin at specific points, might also relieve unnecessary stress and/or tension and promote relaxation.

Aromatherapy

Smelling herbs and fragrances produced by mint, lemon, rosemary, or orange peels may help alleviate nausea. Try placing a cotton ball or tissue infused with scented oil and rub onto the wrist or area you will spend much of your time to help remain relaxed and calm.

Motion Sickness

Motion sickness occurs when the brain receives the wrong information about its environment. When we're at sea, this condition is referred to as "sea sickness". When we're in a car, this condition is referred to as "car sickness". When we're in a roller-coaster, airplane, jet, or any other object, this condition is all the same and is defined as motion sickness.

All of our sensory systems are on alert at all times. They work like computers when everything they notice, organize this information, and it gets sent as a signal to the brain. Once our bodies identify a discrepancy where what we see does not align with the signals being sent, motion sickness settles in. Mixed signals trigger dizziness. Then the body begins to overheat due to the amount of work it is doing to figure out what is occurring which triggers sweating. If things do not improve, feeling of nausea and pale skin settle in and lead to you throwing up. In this section we will review ways to nurse this condition so that the aftereffects can be cut short and remedies to incorporate to hopefully prevent symptoms from settling in.

Remedies:

Shift Your Focus

Much of motion sickness is psychological so when you shift your focus towards something clam and relaxing, the mind and the body won't focus as much on preparing to throw up or feel nauseous. This same method can be applied when you notice others getting sick. It will serve you best to ignore it as they receive help because then your mind will begin to tell you to prepare for the same symptoms and you will get sick. You may have good intentions, but allowing people to follow protocol on their own is best for everyone in volved because it will help another person relax and focus on getting better and prevent you from getting sick by focusing on the sickness.

No Smoking Cigarettes

Many will smoke cigarettes in order to distract themselves, but cigarettes increase your chances of feel nauseous. The moment you begin to feel symptoms coming on, you will want to immediately get to a space where you can breathe easily. If you are on an airplane, train, or bus, and begin to feel symptoms, go to the non-smoking section as soon as possible to not contribute to this process.

Travel At Night

You are less likely to noticing changes in motion at night than you are during the daytime. During the daytime you will notice any change and are more likely to developing symptoms. So, if you can, make sure to travel at night to avoid this from happening.

Alcohol

Drinking alcohol will interfere with the brain's signals which will not only trigger many symptoms but prolong symptoms as well. Alcohol interferes with how the brain processes information and can be multiplied when moving and having more to process. Alcohol can also dissolve into the inner ear which can cause immediate dizziness.

Adequate Sleep

Dr. Roderic W. Gillilan, retired optometrist in Eugene, Oregon, who specializes in motion sickness states, "Your chance of getting motion sickness increases with fatigue." You will want to make sure you get enough sleep each day prior to going on your trip, whether it's on a plane, boat, car, or other mode of transportation. If you have a chance to rest and get a few moments of rest leading up to your trip, take advantage of it by napping.

Be Still

This should go without saying but, it is important to remind yourself to remain still to not create more motion while your head is spinning.

Focus Ahead

In a car we tend to look out the side windows while feeling motion sickness because we're not the ones driving at that point (you don't want a sick driver taking their eyes off the road). It is best to adjust yourself accordingly by sitting in the passenger seat or middle of the back seat(s) and look straight ahead. The view looking to the side can make objects appear to move faster where, looking straight ahead, it can help slow things down for yourself to help you relax. Quick

Tip: If you really want to improve your focus, get off at the next exit and find an empty parking lot or open space and start driving slowly. This will help you become more alert and be able to begin the process of reducing your symptoms.

Read Some Other Time

Reading is a very common way to help pass the time during a long road trip or while traveling. However, the repetitiveness of seeing the words on a page move while riding can trigger symptoms of dizziness and nausea. If you can, try slouching down in your seat and reading at eye level. If this is not an option, you may want to find something else to do to pass the time.

Ginger (herb)

Ginger helps absorb acids in the gastrointestinal tract to help slow down or eve prevent feeling of nausea. In various research studies, two ginger (powder) capsules proved to be more effective than taking a dose of Dramamine (motion sickness pill).

Olives

When experiencing motion sickness, extra saliva is produced by the body. this can increase your chances of feeling nauseous but is the body's response and preparation for throwing up. Olives produce a chemical known as tannins which can make your mouth dry. Upon initially feeling any symptoms of motion sickness, eat a few olives to keep away symptoms from creeping in.

Aromatherapy

Preparing a mist spray in advance to help deter symptoms (particularly nausea). Using a glass bottle is best.

Recipe:

4 ounces of distilled water

70 drops of lavender essential oil

20 drops of dill essential oil

10 drops of cedarwood essential oil

10 drops of spearmint essential oil

The dill and spearmint scents will work to help settle your stomach, while the lavender and cedarwood helps to calm your nervous system. Shake this mixture bottle well after adding drops. When needed, close your eyes and spray above your head about 10 times so the mist will fall in front of you but not directly onto your face. Take deep breaths. Spray periodically throughout you trip as well. You may spray periodically before as a precaution but make sure you have enough leftover if needed.

Note: this spray should have a shelf life of about three years.

Acupressure

(David Filipello, licensed acupuncturist and director of the Acupuncture for health Clinic in San Francisco recommends the following pressure points for motion sickness)

Point #1: there is a pressure point above your upper lip known as GV26. Using your index finger, press down on this point firmly but not to cause any pain for about 30 seconds. Do this every few minutes to prevent and relieve nausea.

Point #2: there is a point on your forearm called PE6 which also relieves nausea. Located on the inside part of your arm (about 3 finger-widths) above the wrist closest to your palm, towards the elbow. The moment you begin to feel nauseous, press n this point firmly for 25-30 seconds every few minutes.

Point #3: there is no specific pressure point but, tugging gently on your earlobes helps increase circulation to your ears which can help prevent and relieve motion sickness. Make sure to do this before and often during your traveling.

Muscle Cramps and Spasms

Muscle cramps are temporarily and sudden constriction of a muscle. A spasm is just a muscle cramp, but one that does not let up. You may feel you've trained a certain muscle group too hard, did not warm up enough, did not have enough minerals or water in your system prior to exercising, or is connected to an older injury that you have aggravated. The truth is, that any or all of these could be what happened and are things you want to consider before your next workout. But once a cramp settles in, recovery is key in making sure it does not happen again or happen often. In this section, we will review recovery methods to incorporate in order to properly heal in addition to the main preventative measure already mentioned in this section.

Remedies:

Pressure

Find the center of your cramp and press on the center firmly. Use the palm of your hand, a closed fist, or your thumb and press firmly so that there's pain but not too much pain. Hold your pressure for about 8-12 seconds and repeat after 30-45 seconds until you notice improvement. Licensed massage therapist Ralph Stevens from Cedar Rapids, Iowa notes that, "The cramp will often vanish by doing nothing more than this exercise."

Stretching (for calves)

Proprioceptive Neuromuscular Facilitation (PNF) stretching is best for the calves according to James Clay, certified clinical massage therapist from Winston-Salem, North Carolina.

Complete the following when doing PNF stretching:

- Sit up in your bed or on a chair/bench.
- Bend your leg and reach down to grasp the sole of your foot.
- Using your fingers to provide resistance, gently press your foot down. Do this to a count of 5.
- Straighten your leg and bend your ankle towards yourself, stretching your calf for a count of 5.
- Return to starting position and repeat.

Stretching (for hamstrings)

If you get a cramp in your hamstring you will want to do this simple stretch. While sitting down, keep the foot of the cramped leg on the floor. Place your other foot on top of that foot and then pull up with the bottom foot with about 10-20% of your strength. Slowly straighten your leg and walk around and your cramp should be relieved.

Tennis Ball

Using a tennis ball to relive your cramp can be your most effective way to address cramps in various parts of your body. We often cannot reach or directly apply a decent amount of firm pressure to every area of our bodies. A tennis ball will come in handy as we can position ourselves onto it in order to help provide relief for things like cramps. To correctly use a tennis ball to address cramps, place the tennis ball onto the ground and cover with a towel. Lie down onto the tennis ball and gently roll into a position where the center of your cramp is making contact with the tennis ball. If you feel comfortable, begin to roll completely over the ball and rest while the tennis ball applied continuous pressure to the area until relief has been reached.

Ice

When you experience a cramp, the nerves in that particular muscle group become very active. Placing ice on the area can slow this down and reduce the severity of the cramp. Wrap an ice pack in a dry washcloth or towel and apply it directly onto the cramped area for about 20 minutes.

Magnesium

This mineral is a natural muscle relaxer. Many muscle cramps can be attributed to having a magnesium deficiency Dr. Barry L. Beaty, D.O., orthopedic physician and director of the DFW Pain Treatment Center and Wellness Clinic in Fort Worth, Texas recommends taking 200 milligrams a day spread out throughout the day. Continue this for a few weeks to notice a change if you have regular muscle cramps

*Common Sources of Magnesium: avocado, chickpeas, tamarind, basil, dill, ginger, oregano, thyme, any *CBD (cannabidiol) products are helpful. (CBD Oils are almost pure magnesium.), nettle leaf, horsetail, red clover, sage, and nopal.*

*To test the purity of a CBD Oil, send to a lab for testing or you should feel a steady decline in needing to rely on this substance after your need has been met regularly.

Potassium

Another mineral that can contribute to cramps when low is, potassium. This mineral transmits nerve signals in the body. Having enough potassium in your body can accurately notify your body that it does not need to cramp so suddenly and also be able to relax itself much faster.

Common Potassium Sources: squash, zucchini, bananas, avocado, dried apricots, and herbs such as, guaco (also high in iron), conconsa (has the highest concentration of potassium phosphate), lily of the valley (rich in iron fluorine and Potassium phosphate).

Chamomile (herb)

Chamomile is to treat a variety of ailments, including muscle spasms. It contains 36 flavonoids, which are compounds that have anti-inflammatory properties. You can drink in tea form or massage chamomile essential oil onto affected muscles to provide relief from spasms. Chamomile tea relaxes sore muscles more so than spasms or cramps but can help be preventative if consumed regularly.

Tart Cherry Juice

People who sign up for marathons train vigorously, often causing a lot of stress on their muscles. In a double blind, controlled study conducted by the Department of Medicine, Oregon Health & Science University, Portland, OR, USA, researchers found that cherry juice helped combat inflammation and muscle pain of runners at baseline, before, and after training. Be mindful that cherries are high in melatonin and can promote sleep.

Antioxidants

Antioxidants are known to help break down inflammation and accelerate recovery from muscle damage. An easy way to work in many antioxidants is to remember to "eat the rainbow" with an assortment of foods that are naturally different colors; not dyes or artificial colorings.

Common Sources of Antioxidants: blueberries, onions, lettuce, squash, tomatoes, grapeseed extract, and herbs that you can use the flower, root, and leaves for as they contain polyphenolics (compounds that produce antioxidant activity).

Vegetable Juice

A glass a day (10 or more ounces) of a vegetable juice provides an assortment of powerful antioxidants, essential nutrients, and helps to break down inflammation in the body. Get creative with making juices with items such as dandelion greens, kale, cucumbers, and adding amount of cilantro. A consistent vegetable juice can provide more than a prescription pill that is given to break down inflammation.

Cayenne Pepper

A substance found in cayenne pepper called, *capsaicin*, is a natural muscle relaxant. Cayenne pepper is often recommended to those who have more serious conditions such as rheumatoid arthritis or fibromyalgia to help reduce their muscle aches and pains. You can add this to meals or find as a cream to rub onto affected area(s).

Vitamin-D

People who have regular muscle pain or spasms might be deficient in vitamin-D. This naturally occurring hormone within the body has to remain presently active in order to help the body. Without vitamin D, the body cannot absorb calcium. It is highly encouraged to sit directly in sunlight for at least 20 minutes a day. Sitting in the sunlight allows the body to produce and absorb its own vitamin-D. 20 minutes of direct sun exposure can provide 200 IU of vitamin-D. this adds up to approximately 40 minutes a day for those under 50 years old, and close to 120 minutes a day for those over 50 years old.

Arnica (herb)

Make your own Arnica Salve to apply to area. If you know an herbalist, you should be able to find Arnica Salve to purchase to use during this time.

My Personal Arnica Salve Recipe:

Step 1: You need to infuse your carrier oil with Arnica and St. John's Wort. Place your dried herbs in a sterile (boil before using) glass jar. I use 1 cup of Arnica and 2 tablespoons of St. John's Wort.

Step 2: Next, add the carrier oils. I use 1 cup of olive oil and 1 cup of coconut oil.

Step 3: Now you will need to infuse the oil. There are several ways to do infuse oils with herbs.

Step 4: Solar Infusion Method: The best method is solar infusion. To solar infuse your oil simply place your jar of oil and herbs in the sun for at least 4 weeks. Swoosh the jar occasionally. This makes the best oil but clearly takes much time to complete.

Step 5: Slow Cooker Method: To use a slow-cooker place a towel in the bottom of your slow cooker and set your jar of oils and herbs on it. Fill the cooker halfway with water and set to warm or low for 8-10 hours. Gently swoosh the jar occasionally.

Step 6: Double Boiler Method: To use the double boiler method place your jar of oil and herbs in a pot filled with water. Warm jar over low heat for at least an hour. The lower the heat and the longer time the better. Gently swoosh the jar every 10 or so minutes.

Step 7: Once your oil is infused with the Arnica and St. John's Wort it is time to strain the herbs out of the oil. I place a metal strainer with unbleached mullein cloths on top of a glass dish, then pour the oil and herbs into it.

Step 8: Allow the oil to drain through the herbs and cloth dripping into the container. Don't be impatient during this step; it takes time. Typically, I end up with about 1 1/2 cups of infused oil. Most will add an essential oil but feel free to skip this step for now. It is now more important to pour the oil into your storage containers. I use glass jars; some prefer plastic or tin. The oil will be hot, so proceed with caution.

Step 9: Allow the jars to cool. It will form into a nice salve rather quickly.

Step 10: Apply cooled salve to affected area and rub in gently. Wash off after a few hours to avoid any contamination.

Peppermint Extract

Often applied to skin in areas to provide pain relief. Peppermint is a hybrid of water mint and spearmint and serves as a cooling agent as well.

Muscle Pain

There are over 600 muscles in the body. whether it is a strain, cramp, or general soreness, they all come from overuse. Either using too much, too often, or too soon in between physical activity. in this section we will review ways to ease your muscle pain anywhere on your body.

Remedies:

Rest

Anytime you exercise, your muscles break down and essentially, become injured. It takes time for the body to recover. Take time to know your body and properly rest as needed. If you are not very active and then go run a marathon, you will need several days of rest with no exercise. However, if you exercise often and run a marathon, you may only need a day of rest, or can tailor your exercise regimen where you engage in low impact activities when training. Set your intention on resting to recover and your body should tell you when it's ok to continue your training.

Ice

Ice helps to constrict your blood vessels which an provide temporary relief. However, it is counterproductive to apply ice for too long as this could kill muscle tissues in the area you're applying ice. You want to wrap ice (or ice pack) in a towel or plastic bag and apply to area no longer than 20 minutes at a time throughout the day.

Use Heat After Ice

Heat helps dilate the blood vessels and can help the body relax. Applying heat after ice is best for strains, sprains, and general soreness. You do want to wait approximately 15 minutes after using ice in order to avoid additional swelling. Heat up a small towel or pad and apply to area shortly after using ice. Apply for 15-20 minutes and then switch back to ice.

Keep Your Feet Up

If you have an injury to the legs or feet, you want to keep this area elevated to reduce blood flow to the area in order to help reduce additional swelling.

Stretching

For cramps and spasms, refer to the Muscle Cramps and Spasms section in this book. Make sure to gradually stretch out your muscles over time. Stretching helps support the healing process by lengthening the muscles that are shortened/constricted during exercise. Unless muscles are able to be lengthened during stretching, you will have re-occurring soreness, tightness, cramps, and injuries.

Neutral Hand Position

Our hands perform a lot of work. From picking things up to typing, writing, scrolling, and texting, our hands perform many tasks. These muscles also need recovery, but we must use them correctly. According to Dr. Scott Donkin, D.C., partner in the Chiropractic Association in Lincoln, Nebraska, "The wrist and hands should be used in what is known as the neutral position. In this position, the wrist is bent neither forward, backward, inward, nor outward." If you are someone who has longer fingers or hands, you may benefit from adjusting your keyboard to a flat surface, so it does not strain any part of your hand. If you have shorter hand and fingers, you may benefit from adjusting devices to be on an incline to make things easier to touch.

Repeat What Made You Sore

If you know what activity caused you to be sore, it can be helpful to repeat it with less intensity. The body will be able to gauge what is needed and also send signals to the area in need of recovery which can promote healing the area faster.

Slow Down

Much of our muscle soreness is caused by torn muscle fiber, according to Dr. Gabe Mirkin, M.D., associate clinical professor of pediatrics at Georgetown University School of Medicine in Washington, D.C. After a hard workout or physical activity, the bloodstream becomes flooded with lactic acid. This acid builds up when there is a lack of oxygen. When these levels reach higher levels, it disrupts the normal chemical reactions in the body and leaves your muscles to temporarily suffer by being sore. To avoid this from happening, we should exercise at a slow, relaxed pace. Now, there are intense forms of exercise and training, but this should be the smaller part of your exercise regimen unless you are a professional athlete and can structure your exercises and dietary needs specifically with trainer and regular monitoring.

New Shoes

A lot of back, foot, leg, and hip pain can come from wearing the wrong shoes. You want to get what is needed for you as opposed to just making your decision off of what feels the most comfortable. For example, when exercising legs or doing things like squats, we want flat shoes so we can have our three points of contact of the foot to press against the floor. If we were to wear running shoes for this exercise, our ankles and other joints are exposed and will probably move more so that the corresponding muscle groups in these areas will become sore quicker, and also increase our risk for injury. Not only do we need the right shoes for certain lifts, but getting the right type of shoe for your style of training is important. Now, don't go out and purchase several pairs of shoes. Get one primary pair, and one secondary pair that you can adjust when needed based on what type of training you will be doing. Then, as they break down over time, you can just replace them.

Hydration

The main cause of cramps and soreness ca be due to dehydration. You want to remain hydrated before, during, and after exercising or any other physical activity. We do want to avoid forcing excess water in our system as it takes time to properly absorb this substance. We want to consume fruits, vegetables, and drink liquids that don't contain artificial sugars, dyes, or chemicals so that we can absorb what is needed. The minerals that are in fresh fruits and vegetables provide us much more to assist us with proper hydration than relying solely upon water. It is best to consume a diet/lifestyle high in fruits and vegetables, while consuming water around training to help maintain proper hydration.

Steps To Avoid Leg Cramps:

Sleep on your side – it is best to sleep on our left side to help support the intestines as compared to sleeping on our right side where our intestines "hang" when we sleep and makes it difficult to sleep. Sleeping on our stomach with legs stretched out and calves flexed invites cramps more regularly.

Loosen the covers – tight covers will increase the tightness of the body. with less room to move around, the body becomes constricted, and cramping is more prone to happen.

Lean against the wall – stand a few feet away from the wall while keeping your heels flat and legs straight. Lean into the wall in front of you while placing your hands on the wall. Begin to lean your upper body downwards, keeping your legs straight to stretch your hamstrings and calves. Do this before going to bed.

Increase calcium intake – Dr. Donkin, M.D., states that a calcium deficiency can cause muscles to be more "trigger-happy" which results in more regular cramping.

Common Sources of Calcium: sea moss, kale, okra, dandelion greens, turnip greens, lettuce, papaya, and oranges.

Antioxidants

Antioxidants are known to help break down inflammation and accelerate recovery from muscle damage. An easy way to work in many antioxidants is to remember to "eat the rainbow" with an assortment of foods that are naturally different colors; not dyes or artificial colorings.

Common Sources of Antioxidants: blueberries, onions, lettuce, squash, tomatoes, grapeseed extract, and herbs that you can use the flower, root, and leaves for as they contain polyphenolics (compounds that produce antioxidant activity).

Nail Brittleness

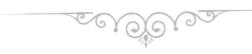

Palm readers would be more effective if they learn to read the other side of our hands, which include our nails. Our nail health can determine our future more than we may believe. Having brittle nails is one of the first signs that something is not right within the body.

Brittle nails come in two forms: hard and sift. Hard nails that will break easily are caused by dehydration. Soft nails that break easily come from too much moisture. Over time our nails become harder as they lose some of their natural moisture (this is more common in the elderly). When we do not replace this moisture, the nails crack easier. If nails are constantly immersed in water, the water causes the nails to expand where they eventually shrink and become brittle.

You want to achieve the right balance between the two of these. Similar to a brick wall that is comprised of the bricks and mortar. The mortar representing the nail bed that helps the nail stick together, and the bricks representing the nail itself. In this section we will review ways to protect and strengthen the nails, so they do not remain brittle.

Remedies:

Avoid Alcohol Ingredients

Many rely upon moisturizers, lotions, and creams for addressing nail brittleness. An important ingredient to avoid is, alcohol. Alcohol presents a drying effect for the nails, making them brittle. You want to avoid any product containing alcohol if you choose to use these types of items.

Keep Them Short

Should go without saying, but longer nails are more likely to break. Now, regardless of their height, our nails should remain strong. But once a nail cracks or breaks, it becomes exposed and is more likely to happen again. So, it is best to keep them short to avoid this from happening.

Proper Hydration

Not only drinking about half of your body weight in ounces (ex. if you weigh 100lbs, drink 50oz) but consuming foods that provide water is necessary. Melons, berries, tomatoes, and cucumbers are only a few items that should regularly be in your diet. Consuming items that provide hydration can help wash away and also neutralize the erosive acids that remain in the body from eating things detrimental to our health.

Gloves

Whenever needed, you will want to wear gloves to protect your nails. Dr. Paul Kechijian, M.D., associate clinical professor of dermatology and chief of the nail section at the New York University Medical Center, recommends getting rubber dishwashing gloves and cotton gloves to wear underneath. The vinyl exterior of the rubber dishwashing gloves keeps water out while the cotton gloves absorb sweat to help maintain this balance and avoid nails from becoming brittle. You can find quality gloves Dr. Kechijan recommends from the George Glove Company online or by calling them at 1-800-631-4292.

Nail Polish Remover

It is recommended to not use nail polish but if you do, you want to seek out nail polish remover that contain a chemical called acetate. It will help remove the nail polish without removing the hydration. Another chemical with similar smelling to acetate which is called "acetone" will remove a lot of moisture from your nails and make them brittle.

Calcium

A lack of calcium in your lifestyle is another cause of brittle nails. If you are under the age of 50, you will want to aim for at least 500-milligrams a day of calcium. If you are over the age of 50, you want to aim closer to 1,000-milligrams a day.

Common sources of Calcium: sea moss, kale, okra, dandelion greens, turnip greens, lettuce, papaya, and oranges.

Horsetail (herb)

This herb is abundant in the mineral silicon. Great for the nails, hair, and skin. For tea, take 2 teaspoons of this dried herb per cup of boiling water. Pour desired amount of water over the herb in a saucepan, boil for about 5 minutes, then let steep for 10-15 minutes. Strain out dried herb and drink when tea is cooled.

Note: do not use horsetail powdered extract as it will dissolve quickly, and you won't absorb this mineral as intended.

Nausea and Vomiting

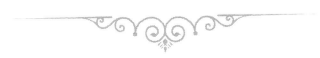

We can feel nauseous from just about anything. Nausea is often well controlled after a few minutes, but the moment it becomes too much, and your stomach begins to turn, you will vomit. In this section we will review ways to decrease feelings of nausea and also learn ways to recover if you do vomit.

Remedies:

Clear Liquids

Even if you feel hungry and want to eat, stick to clear liquids. Allow more time to pass to not trigger symptoms once more. Liquids should remain warm or at room temperature. Any cold liquids will shock your stomach and either you will trigger your symptoms, or you will prolong your recovery. Make sure to sip your liquids slowly (not slurp0 to limit the amount of liquids going to your stomach. Sip 1-2 ounces at a time so your stomach can adjust. You will have a better sense of how much you can consume base upon how your stomach begins to feel. Also make sure to view your urine often too. If it is dark yellow, you're not drinking enough fluids. The paler and lighter your urine gets, the better you're doing at preventing dehydration.

Eat Carbs First

Carbs allow the stomach to settle when consumed in small amounts. Then you want to incorporate other foods, saving any fatty foods for last as they take longer to digest and can prolong symptoms and recovery. Carbs can make you feel tired as they increase the brain chemical serotonin which induces sleep. Bananas, apples, mango, dates, goji berries, and quinoa are a few items to eat lightly while recovering from vomiting or nausea symptoms.

Ginger (herb)

Ginger helps absorb acids in the gastrointestinal tract to help slow down or eve prevent feeling of nausea. In various research studies, two ginger (powder) capsules proved to be more effective than taking a dose of Dramamine (motion sickness pill).

Meadowsweet (herb)

This wildflower can provide soothing properties and relief for the stomach. Mix 1 tablespoon of this dried herb per cup of boiling water and steep for 5-10 minutes. Strain out the herb after it cools off. Sip slowly to not burn yourself and to keep your stomach relaxed. You may add rosemary (herb) to this mixture as well to add to relaxing the body.

Take An Herbal Bath

A caution of drinking herbal tea is that you may vomit out these herbs if your nausea symptoms continue. One way to avoid this from happening is to allow these herbs to soak through your pores. This will allow you to absorb the many benefits these herbs provide without having to drink them. For example, take 1 tablespoon of ginger with a quart of warm water and let it cool. Then soak your hands or feet in a soothing bath until vomiting is no longer an issue. Ginger helps open your pours which helps to sweat and release perspiration and help provide relief for many of your symptoms. Having clogged pours "traps" your sweat and will prolong your symptoms.

Neck and Shoulder Pain

There are 7 vertebrae and 32 muscles that hold up your 10 to 12-pound head. This leaves the neck vulnerable to aches and pains. The shoulders take on some of this load, which also puts additional strain on the neck muscles. Various occupations require more stress on the neck and shoulders than others, but how we use these areas day to day all contribute to creating these issues. Starting from when we wake up in the morning, we often turn out heads in an uncomfortable position, to when we end our nights leaning down to look at our phones or while reading. In this section we will look at ways to help reduce and avoid the typical pains we experience in our necks and shoulders.

Remedies:

Breathing

When we exhale, we reduce the carbon dioxide in our lungs which makes room for more oxygen which will relieve pain and stress. We tend to focus more on inhaling than exhaling due to the body wanting a regular and consistent flow of oxygen. But, when we do not slow down our exhalation, our necks and shoulders can experience more tension which often leads to more stiffness. You can practice this by waiting until you've exhaled, then count for about 5 seconds before inhaling. This can decrease any pains you may have in the neck or shoulder area. It is important to also breathe through our nose, as breathing through our mouths can push more air into the body than is needed and contribute to additional tension.

Laying Down

Many believe that laying down flat on their backs is the best way to support the neck and shoulders. This is not true. When we lie flat on our backs, our neck arches, the chin lifts, and the forehead will either push forward or further back, which all contribute to a constricting position for the neck and shoulders. It is best to keep the chin and forehead in line by putting 2-3 inches of support under your head when you lie down. Place a pillow or folded towel under your knees to reduce any tension in the back while you're at it so pains don't begin to travel throughout the body.

Shoulder Shrugs

Not the exercise you may be thinking of with a barbell or dumbbells. This involves simply to raise your shoulders up and let them drop down on their own. Make sure to not push them down as that can add onto any aches or pains you may have.

Look Down Correctly

When we look down, most will arch the middle of their upper backs. This causes the shoulders to become rounded and places the neck in a compromising position. We want to instead, keep our neck upright while letting the chin drop down so the muscles in the neck can relax. This takes practice to condition yourself to do this so make sure to look down this way whenever possible.

Talking On The Phone

We tend to tilt our heads to the receiver when talking on the phone rather than keep our head straight and bringing the phone to our ears. It is important to focus on bringing your phone to your ear if you are someone who talks on the phone a lot. If your arms begin to get tired, use this as an opportunity to just switch hands or end the conversation.

When Working At A Desk

Many have occupations and home offices where they use a desk. Whether looking down or when working on a computer/laptop, it is important to rest periodically. Rather than stretch and push through or taking a nap, try this method to help rest for a moment so that you can complete your work. Take both of your arms and cross them on top of each other and place them onto your desk. Then, rest your forehead on top of your wrist and sink your head into your arms while relaxing your neck. You should feel relaxed and allow your muscles in your neck and shoulders to get a needed rest. Without falling asleep, focus on your rest these muscles and when you feel better, you can get back to work.

Ice

If there is every any swelling, you want to start applying ice. Wrap ice (or an ice pack) in a cloth to protect your skin and apply your area for 15 minutes. Repeat several times throughout the day every few hours.

Apply Pressure

If you are certain, it is just muscle pain, use your fingertips to apply direct pressure to the area. Constant pressure can force the body to adjust by sending signals to the area to heal and repair. Apply constant pressure with your fingertips and make sure to also massage the area for about 3 minutes at a time.

Ginger (herb)

Ginger is one of many herbs that helps to reduce the production of leukotrienes, which are substances that trigger inflammation and can make any pain worse. Take about 1-2 grams of this herb daily in tea, raw, or capsule form.

Get A Firm Chair

Sitting in a chair without good back support can make neck problems worse and create new problems. To help support your lower back in the meantime, place a rolled towel under the small of your back to help align your spine better.

Don't Sleep On Your Stomach

This places more strain on your lower back and neck. You want to sleep on your side (preferably your left side to help your intestine with additional support). You also want to avoid using a pillow if you do sleep on your stomach as your head will be bending backwards in this position which creates more tension.

Stretch

Allow your head to fall forward with your chin settling into the bottom of your neck. Then bring your head all the way back, letting it hang. Then, lead your head on each side, back and forth. Repeat this while applying pressure to the beck by gently pulling your head to the space it is leaning towards to help stretch the neck muscles. Our necks are often forgotten about when stretching our muscles even though they work nonstop holding out heads up in place. Taking just a few moments to stretch your neck will relieve some pain from your neck and your shoulders.

Nosebleeds

Blood circulates through capillaries in the nose. When blood vessels break, this creates nosebleeds. Whether you've just gotten punched, injured, or are stressed out, the internal pressure applied to this area creates nosebleeds. Nosebleeds can also come from the mucous membranes becoming irritated by cold air. Whatever the cause, all nosebleeds can be treated the same way to stop them.

Remedies:

Blow Out The Clot

You want to blow your nose in order to blow out anything stopping the nose from having a flow of blood. A clot can keep blood vessels open and make it difficult to stop bleeding. Once the clot is out of the way, the blood can begin to slow down from leaking out of your nose. Blood vessels have small elastic fibers around them. Once you clear the nostrils, these elastic fibers can contract around the opening where the nosebleed started, and your nosebleed will slowly start to diminish.

Pinch The Fleshy Part Of Your Nose

We've been told to squeeze the top of our nose to stop bleeding. However, the top part of our nose will not close all of the way, so this won't help. It is best to squeeze the fleshy part of our nose using your thumb and forefinger so it can close more completely. Do this for about 5-7 minutes to allow the blood to start flowing elsewhere in the body and away from your nostrils. If the bleeding does not stop, repeat blowing your nose followed by holding it closed for another 5-7 minutes. After a few cycles at most, you should notice a difference.

Apply Ice

Ice forces the blood vessels to become narrow and can help reduce bleeding. Apply ice to the area by covering some ice or an ice pack in a towel and apply directly to your nose (preferably away from the nostrils to avoid bleeding on your towel) for about 10-12 minutes or until it become uncomfortable. Then, you will want to incorporate other remedies already mentioned dint his section before repeating.

Avoid Picking

It will take about 7-10 days for a ruptured blood vessel to heal. During this time, it can feel irritated, and you will be tempted to pick or rub your nose. If you do this, you run the risk of opening up a scab and will be more likely to having another nosebleed.

Iron

The blood is iron. We will need to replace the lost supply of iron that comes from having a nosebleed.

Natural Sources of Iron: Wild rice, chickpeas/garbanzo beans, dandelion greens, sarsaparilla, burdock, yellow dock, chapparal, and prunes.

Humidify The Air

The air that reaches our lungs must be humidified. This is often why dry air contributes to nosebleeds because the nose has to work harder to remain moist. You can purchase an air humidifier to avoid the air from being dry as you work to recover from your nosebleed.

Control Your Blood Pressure

Those with high blood pressure are more likely to get nosebleeds. You will want to use getting a nosebleed to signify that you will stick to a low-fat and low cholesterol diet. If you do have high blood pressure and a blood vessel breaks as they do in a nosebleed, if it breaks inside rather than outside of the cranial cavity, this can cause a stroke.

(Refer to "High Blood Pressure" section within this text).

Collagen

Collagen, which is a nutrient our body needs to rebuild tissues and cells. Collagen in the tissues of your upper respiratory tract is what helps mucus stick to where it is supposed to, which helps maintain a moist, protective lining within your nose.

Natural Sources of Collagen: Black Currants, Papaya, Spring Onions, Cantaloupe, Mango, Oranges, and Watercress.

Avoiding "Salicylates"

There is an aspirin-like substance known as salicylates, that is present in particular items most people consume that you should avoid until your nosebleed is gone. Items like coffee will irritate your nosebleed, but there are many fruits and vegetables that contain salicylates that you can be sure to avoid. These include, apples, apricots, bell peppers, berries, cherries, cucumbers, cloves, grapes, mint, peaches, pickles, plums, raisins, and tomatoes.

*Note: aspirin can interfere with blood clotting. You should completely avoid aspirin if you are prone to getting nosebleeds.

Oily Hair and Oily Skin

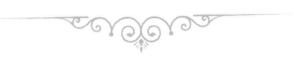

Oily hair is caused by an overly oily scalp, which is caused by a high-fat diet. Just like the bulb of a plant feeds the flower, the hair is fed by the bulbs of the calp. These bulbs are intertwined with the sebaceous glands which produce a substance known as sebum, or what we call, oil. A diet full of fat in the form of fried foods, saturated fats, and other substances such as processed foods that turn into fat when being digested, will create an overproduction of sebum and result in oily hair and oily skin.

Note: men typically have about 311 hairs per square centimeter. Women have about 278 hairs per square centimeter (about a 10%-15% difference). This means that men often are more likely to have oily hair and skin although it appears more noticeable for women.

Remedies:

Low-Fat Diet/Lifestyle

You want to do away with any items you consume that are not helping you. A high-fat diet has never helped anyone do anything but become deceased. I recommend not consuming items marketed as "low-fat" as well because they often contain other harmful ingredients such as chemicals and are only considered to be "low-fat" due to being compared to high-fat items. Many low-fat items would be considered to be high fat if compared to something like a fruit, grain, or vegetable.

We've developed a fascination for consuming healthier fats such as omega-3, omega-6, and omega-9, but often times the body will have to filter these fats from the unhealthy fats which creates additional work for the body. Working on just simply consuming an overall low-fat diet during this time (even from healthy fats) until your hair is no longer oily will be the best thing.

Horsetail (herb)

This herb works to strengthen the hair follicles and cutting the oil production in the hair. Boil.1 cup of distilled water and place 2 tablespoons of this dried herb in the water. Turn off flame after mixing in the herb and let steep for about 10-15 minutes. Let cool and place in a bottle with a sprout. Apply this mixture evenly onto the hair and scalp while massaging it in. leave on scalp for about 5-10 minutes and then rinse out with cool water.

Hemp Seed Oil

Hemp seed oil is suitable for all skin types. It is particularly beneficial for those with dry or mature skin. Make sure to not have on any makeup as it can be runny. But, to remove makeup, wash hands thoroughly before applying a bit of hemp seed oil onto your fingertips and apply to areas you wish to clean. Massage this oil into your scalp and leave in for about 10 minutes before rinsing out with cool water. Hemp seed oil helps to hydrate the skin and regulate the skin's oil production. Skin dryness is actually a sign that the skin may attempts to overproduce oil which in turn, can stimulate acne and other issues you want to avoid. You can use this oil if you have oily hair or skin, but also if you have area of dry hair or skin.

Essential Oils For Hair

These oils can cut the oils in the hair. Add 3-4 drops of rosemary, lavender, and eucalyptus essential oils to 1 ounce of primrose oil. Mix together and apply gently onto your hair and scalp with a cotton ball to prevent this oil from attaching itself to your hands or nails.

Lecithin

Lecithin granules contain a chemical known as *phosphatidylcholine* which liquifies cholesterol and breaks apart fats in the body, preventing it from building up or hardening along the walls of the arteries. This is also helpful with repairing skin and hair cells. You can take 1 tablespoon of lecithin granules a day. You may also find lecithin (and phosphatidylcholine) in sunflower seeds, sunflower oil, rapeseeds, and many different beans.

Essential Oil Remedy #1 (for skin)

Add a drop or two of neroli oil into lavender floral water and spray directly onto your skin wherever there's excess oil. You can spray onto your hair, but the focus is to help clear away the oils on the skin's surface to help provide a healthy remedy for oily hair. Lavender helps tone and cleanse the skin, while the neroli oil works to regulate the production of sebum, according to Barbara Close, an aromatherapist and herbalist from East Hampton, New York.

Essential Oil Remedy #2 (for skin)

Add 5 drops of rosemary, 5 drops of geranium, and 5 drops of juniper essential oils to 1 tablespoon of hazelnut or apricot kernel oil. Mix together well and place 3-4 drops of mixture onto a cotton pad and use gently on the skin. This mixture will help clean the skin and give it a more natural shine than an oily shine. Apply this twice a week.

Cool Water

Warm water activates the oil glands in the body. you want to reduce this as much as possible while working to reduce having oily hair. Gently wash your hair with cool water. Take cooler showers and rinse your hair with cool water often.

Hydrotherapy (for skin)

Steaming helps to provide more of a deep clean to oily hair and skin. Rather than make an appointment at a salon or purchase some expensive self-care products, I recommend the face-over-pot method. Simply boil a pot of water and turn flame off once water is boiling. Stand over the pot so that your face is able to receive a steady steam with consistent warm temperature. Do this for about 8-10 minutes. You can also do this often if cooking something such as a soup or when using a pot to cook. This is more beneficial for the skin, and if you have longer hair you may have to tie it up to avoid burning or damaging your hair (and from making a mess). However, your hair will still benefit from doing this method as it will help slow down the production of oil in the scalp.

Clay and Mud Masks

These are helpful to apply when possible as they both work to cleanse away unwanted oils and bacteria. These masks help absorb many oils in the skin as well to help alleviate washing away oils that have made their way to the surface already.

My Personal Remedy:

Boil 1 cup of water and remove pan from heat. Then add the following:

- 1 tablespoon of yarrow (herb)
- 2 tablespoons of sage

Steep for 30 minutes, strain herbs, and let cool. Use immediately after it has cooled by massaging mixture into scalp and onto hair gently with a cotton ball or by hand. Store any leftover tea in a squeeze bottle which will last for about 3 days in your bathroom, or about 5 days if left in your refrigerator. You may apply this mixture directly onto skin as well.

Osteoporosis

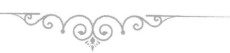

The word *osteoporosis* literally means, "porous bones." The word *porous* means "weak". Healthy bones show up on an x-ray as a lot of white shapes. A person with osteoporosis will display a lot of dark shadows around the bones. Just like out muscles and skin, the entire skeletal system gets worn out by having to constantly rebuild and produce new, healthier cells. Cells known as *teoclasts*, dissolve the bone which leave tiny spaces. Then, cells called *osteoblasts* move into those tiny spaces to build new bone. For osteoporosis to settle in, more bone has to be broken down than what is being produced to replace them.

About 8 million women and 2 million men in the USA have osteoporosis. Millions of others have low bone density which results in bones breaking easily. Osteoporosis takes years to develop, and most won't notice any signs or symptoms until there is pain or an injury. Your best bet is to consume that which helps repair and strengthen the bones in your body without doing anything that contributes to deterioration of your bones. Your bones already constantly create new cells while clearing out older cells. You must capitalize off of this by contributing to the quality of new cells being created through diet and lifestyle.

Remedies:

Leafy Greens

These contain larger quantities of calcium that most single items do and can easily be incorporated into your lifestyle.

Essential Minerals (for the bones):

Most common minerals found in the bones (alphabetical order):

- Boron, calcium, chromium, iron, magnesium, manganese, potassium, phosphorus, selenium, silicon, sulfur, zinc.

Getting these minerals from natural sources will be best. There are apps such as Chronometer which can help you keep track of these levels on a daily basis.

Common sources of Boron: raisins, peaches, prune juice, grape juice, avocadoes, legumes, dried apricots.

Common sources of Calcium: sea moss, kale, okra, dandelion greens, turnip greens, lettuce, papaya, and oranges.

Common Sources of Chromium: green beans, orange juice, grape juice, tomato juice, apples, Brazil nuts, dried fruits, broccoli

Common sources of Iron: Quinoa, Wild Rice (not black rice), Chickpeas/Garbanzo Beans, Kale, Nuts (particularly Walnuts), Hemp Seeds, Dates, Dried Apricots, Watercress, Sarsaparilla, Burdock (and root), Guaco, Chainey Root, Monkey Ladder, Chickweed, Yellowdock.

Common Sources of Magnesium: Avocado, Chickpeas, Tamarind, Basil, Dill, Ginger, Oregano, Thyme, Nettle Leaf, Horsetail (herb), Red Clover, Sage, Nopal, and almost any CBD (cannabidiol) products are helpful. CBD Oils are almost pure magnesium.

To test the purity of a CBD Oil, send to a lab for testing or you should feel a steady decline in needing to rely on this substance after your need has been met regularly.

Common sources of manganese: quinoa, fonio, spelt, walnuts, sunflower seeds, sesame seeds, and hemp seeds.

Common sources of potassium: squash, zucchini, bananas, avocado, dried apricots, and herbs such as, guaco (also high in iron), conconsa (has the highest concentration of potassium phosphate), lily of the valley (rich in iron fluorine and Potassium phosphate).

Common sources of phosphorus: sunflower seeds, pumpkin seeds, Brazil nuts, quinoa, walnuts, pecans, hazelnuts, chickpeas, lentils, amaranth, adzuki (red) beans.

Common sources of Selenium: brazil nuts, walnuts, chickpeas/garbanzo beans, kola nuts, dandelion greens, and nettle, and alfalfa. Recommended to consume about 400 micrograms a day.

Common sources of silicon: horsetail, bananas, almonds, Kenyen beans, red lentils, spinach, dried fruits.

Common Sources of Sulfur: leafy green vegetables, (dried) peaches, onions, watercress, chickpeas, walnuts,

Common Sources of Zinc: chickpeas, mushrooms, zucchini, squash, okra, Brazil nuts, and walnuts.

Calcium

Calcium is the active mineral that is present in the bones within the body. When a long road or highway is built, cement is poured in and around the cross-linked cables. When bones are being build (and re-built) calcium is the "cement."

Magnesium

This mineral works collectively with calcium to constantly build and repair the bones. About half of the magnesium in your body can be found in your bones. Without a consistent calcium-magnesium balance, you will become more likely to develop osteoporosis or some other related bone issue. You want to consume about twice as much calcium than you do magnesium a day for the right calcium-magnesium balance. It is recommended to consume about 2,400 milligrams a day of calcium. So, aiming around 1,000-1,200 milligrams of magnesium is best.

Vitamin-D

This naturally occurring hormone within the body has to remain presently active in order to help the body. Without vitamin-D, the body cannot absorb calcium. It is highly encouraged to sit directly in sunlight for at least 20 minutes a day. Sitting in the sunlight allows the body to produce and absorb its own vitamin-D. 20 minutes of direct sun exposure can provide 200 IU of vitamin-D. this adds up to approximately 40 minutes a day for those under 50 years old, and close to 120 minutes a day for those over 50 years old.

Manganese

This mineral is another foundational nutrient that works to build new bones cells. Can be found in many grains, nuts, and seeds. About 5-20 milligrams a day of manganese is sufficient enough for adults.

Common sources of manganese: quinoa, fonio, spelt, walnuts, sunflower seeds, sesame seeds, and hemp seeds.

Soups

Making soups are probably the simplest way to add minerals such as calcium, and vitamin-D to your diet. You can add an assortment of vegetables, herbs, and spices to increase your intake. Vegetable stock made from scratch can have as much calcium in one cup as an entire carton of cow's milk (is believed to) contain or an entire supplement bottle of calcium.

Reduce Salt Intake

Salt not only dehydrates the body, but it depletes the body's calcium storages. Salt reduces the body's ability to properly absorb calcium, while increasing the amount of salt deposits in the body which gets stored to continue reducing the body's ability to absorb calcium long after you've reduced your salt intake. You will want to make a commitment to reducing your salt intake overall.

Remove Soft Drinks

Soft drinks such as sodas, contain a mineral known as phosphorus which bines with calcium and reduces the calcium's ability to get into the bones. Phosphorus has its role within the body, but when consumed with high amount of sugar, it hinders calcium absorption.

Percussion For Bone Mass

A technique called *tapotement*, is a light tapping form of massage that mimics bone-building stimulation production from exercise. To do this, do the following:

- Bring together the fingers on your right hand.
- Bend your fingers and arch your palm to corm a cup shape.
- Do the same with your left hand.
- Using the tips of your fingers, tap lightly on your hips, ribs, and forearms (these three areas are the most effected by osteoporosis).
- You can have a partner tap other areas of your body also such as your spine or any areas you cannot easily reach.
- Do this twice a day for 5-8 minutes each time.

Exercise:

Regular exercise slows down the rate of bone loss and actually increases bone density. We often view physical exercise as something demanding on our bodies, but this is mostly ties to our joints, ligaments, and connective tissues; not the bones themselves. Finding a form of exercise, you enjoy is the main goal as it will keep you motivated and is what you'll probably do the most of over time. Being able to tone your muscles and keep a steady blood flow in the body will help support bone health as well. Try going for a walk whenever possible and don't avoid those household chores such as vacuuming, going up and down the stairs, squatting up and down, and circular scrubbing motions we use when doing things like dishes or cleaning countertops; all of these greatly contribute to reducing our risks of fractures or sprains.

Coconut Milk

Next to calcium and magnesium, phosphorus is the most abundant mineral you will find in the bones. Without phosphorous being present, the bones do not absorb all of the calcium available. Containing nearly 240 milligrams per cup, coconut milk helps increase bone density.

Note: too much phosphorus will pull calcium out of the bones. So, make sure you are aware of other items that you may consume that has phosphorus in them.

Pain Relief Remedy (for knees and joints)

2 tablespoons of cayenne pepper powder

½ cup of cold-pressed olive oil

½ inch of grated ginger

Mix all of these items together until they form a paste. Apply directly to affected area. Leave on for a minimum of 20-minutes and then wash off. Do this twice a day.

Overweight

This can be a touchy subject as everyone has their own justifications and views on health and nutrition. Many choose to look at body mass index (BMI) while others who exercise regularly may breakdown health into calories, carbohydrates, proteins, and sugars. By definition, everyone who is over the "average" weight is considered to be overweight. Now, there is much more to this than the average weight, as a person's individual health can determine if they are overweight or not.

I recommend viewing "overweight" as an underlying symptom of a fundamental imbalance with the body, emotions, and the mind, while looking at two things to determine if you are overweight: (1) overall size (you'll know if you're larger for your height, age, and weight) that makes it more challenging to perform basic daily tasks, and (2) what you are putting into your body.

When you look at these two things (honestly) you will note specific adjustments that you can make that are clear to you. The challenge then becomes working on the things you cannot see and helping to support the body in restoring its health for optimum longevity. Keep in mind, we can only get rid of waste in the body. We cannot "lose weight" or "drop a few pounds" as there are many other factors in motion at all times.

Having a larger frame for your height, age, or weight will present additional health issues. This being the result of toxins and unhealthy items being stored in the body, will present additional symptoms. Before you know it, you will have to work through a multitude of symptoms and difficulties before you almost anything. The additional stress on the joints and connective tissues begins the breakdown of the structure of the body. Toxins within the body that contribute to creating excess waste will only make symptoms more severe and occur more often. In this section, we will review things to do to help set a solid foundation, and habits to incorporate so that body does not exceed above a more ideal size for your body frame.

Remedies:

Becoming Better Balanced

Address the following:

- Nutritional needs that your body has that are not being provided

- Emotional imbalances where foods are used as a substitute for feeling and emotions.

- Mental imbalances where thoughts predetermine and dwell on past choices (including what you consume) that dictate what you continue to repeat in the present.

- Physical imbalances created by stored toxins that continue to drain your energy and remain stagnant.

"When you in balance, you naturally and easily make food choices that support your overall health, says Shoshanna Katzman, acupuncturist, director of the Red Bank Acupuncture and Wellness Center in New Jersey, and co-founder of the Feeling Light weight-management program.

Positive Self-Talk

You will need an inner force pushing you towards better overall health. Positive self-talk and statements such as affirmation will help you remain on track rather than allow your thoughts, feelings, or emotions, to begin to dictate and determine what you consume once again. Take a few minutes a day and mentally affirm your intentions to become better balanced and it will become more likely to happen. Incorporate some of the following statements listed below to begin with, or create or search up your ones that resonate with you:

- I am in control of myself

- I take personal responsibility for my physical health and wellness

- I eat to nourish my miner, body, and spirit

Rebounding

Rebounding is a term used to describe jumping lightly on a small trampoline. This gets the lymphatic system moving which is responsible for collecting and moving the fluids in the body (particularly waste materials you want to get rid of). The lymphatic system drains these toxins/waste materials easier when doing something such as rebounding. You want to do this for about 20 minutes a few times a week.

Amino Acids

When a person uses food to feel better, the brain releases those natural chemicals in the brain and in turn, causes the body to slowly develop cravings. The chemicals in the brain such as dopamine (energizer), GABA (sedative), endorphin (painkiller), and serotonin (sleep promotor and mood enhancer), are released more often the moment we consume items high in artificial sugars, white flours, and carbohydrates. We begin to crave foods with these in them which are not helpful to us; they turn into waste and create deficiencies which develop into stronger cravings and influence certain emotions that create an unhealthy cycle of consumption.

Amino acids, serve as the building blocks to proteins in our bodies, but also process hormones and neurotransmitters that influence our thoughts, emotions, and thought patterns.

According to Julia Ross, executive director of Recovery Systems in Mill Valley, California, "Scientific studies have confirmed the effectiveness of using just a few targets amino acid precursors to the brain chemicals, thereby eliminating your cravings of food as well as your depression, anxiety, irritability, obsessiveness, and mental dullness." Correcting your brain's chemistry is the most important step in moving towards more long-term health goals. Consuming an adequate number of amino acids will support your brain in correctly filtering and processing neurotransmitters which influence decision-making skill. Over time, where your brain would typically tell you to give in to a certain craving, your brain will step in and disrupt those thoughts and work to set reminders of the healthier lifestyle you are adjusting to.

Natural Sources of amino acids: seeded grapes, guava, avocado, apricots, blackberries, raisins, cherries, chickpeas/garbanzo beans, squash, brazil nuts, walnuts, hemp seeds, and quinoa.

Pyridoxine ("Vitamin-B6")

Vitamin-B6 (pyridoxine) helps our bodies to process certain amino acids.

Common sources of pyridoxine: avocado, carrots, bananas, peas, lentils, spinach, chickpeas, acorn squash, quinoa, sunflower seeds, brussels sprouts, oranges, pistachios.

Healthy Fats

This may sound strange as many people tend to view being overweight as a "fat" problem but, whatever shape you are in, there is a need for healthy fats in the body. Without an adequate amount of healthy fats, the body has more room (and more opportunities) to store waste materials as fat and get in the way of you trying to work close to your ideal weight. These healthy fats appear as "brown fats", while unhealthy fats appear as "white fats". Not to lose weight, but to get rid of unwarranted fats, we must focus on the white fats by not consuming them and making sure to get enough healthy fats in their place. Healthy fats are expressed in the form of omega-e, omega-6, and omega-9 fatty acids. Getting enough of these items regularly helps the body reset its temperature so that you can burn calories and lose some pounds.

Common sources of fatty acids are: Walnuts, Brazil Nuts, Avocados, Hemp Seeds, Hemp Milk, Walnut Oil, Olive Oil, and Sea Vegetable such as Nori, Hijiki, Bladderwrack, Kelp, and Dulse.

Activate Your Brown Fat

Brown fat (good fat) is stored and used for energy. If you do not use this, you will lose it and end up tired and fatigued often. It is best to use this stores energy source to express your energy. This is done through movement activities such as exercising. When you know you have this energy source available, take advantage of it by moving around by going to the gym, walking, yoga, or another form of enjoyable movement activity you can do for a decent period of time. On days you do not feel like being very active, remind yourself that this energy source is stored away (if you've been consuming healthy fats often) and you just need to unlock this through movement. Being able to move your body around will help reduce any limited movements which can cause additional aches and pains.

Colder Showers

When the body experiences colder water, it essentially provides a "shock" to your system as the body will attempt to keep warm. To keep warm, the body will burn white fats as they are disposable material(s). it will only do so for as long util the body adjusts. When showering, before you are ready to turn off the shower, turn the water on cold (not enough that it is freezing) and stand directly under water to provide this shock to your body, allowing the cool water to run down your body. Doing this often will help to burn bits of white fat and inch (pun intended) you closer to your goal of not being overweight.

Evening Primrose Oil

An essential fatty acid known as gamma-linolic acid (GLA) which helps to activate dormant brown fat that is needed to use for energy. Evening primrose oil is rich in GLA. Taking about 2,000 milligrams a day (four 500mg capsules) is best to help your body use your brown fat for energy to get moving rather than turning it into waste.

Parasitic Cleanse

Doing a parasitic cleanse is often the missing link to someone's weight loss journey. This is not a fun experience and can be traumatic to many. But, if you are up for it and want to complete a parasitic cleanse, it is encouraged.

Parasites are in many of the common foods people eat. Foods such as animal flesh, dairy products, and many processed or refined sugars and carbohydrates. These parasites set up shop in the human body and tuck themselves away. They feed off of waste materials. It is best to starve these parasites by not consuming what they feed off of and through developing a fasting regimen. There are many herbal parasite cleanses that should come with a specific protocol available for purchase. Seek out those created and made by an herbalist or holistic health provider as they will have a set intention when putting together herbal compounds made for removing parasites from the body.

Anti-parasite Smoothie

½ large papaya with seeds

4-5 dates

2 bananas

½ key lime (juiced)

1 cup of distilled water

Blend together and enjoy.

Anti-parasite Tea

1 teaspoon of Wormwood

1/2 teaspoon of black walnut hull

½ teaspoon of myrrh

2 thumb-sized pieces of bitter melon

Boil 3 cups of water and add ingredients to a cup. Pour boiling water into cup and let steep for 12-15 minutes. Strain herbs and let cool. Drink twice a day until symptoms decrease.

My Personal Remedy:

Lemon Balm (herb)

Berberine (can be found as a supplement)

Cinnamon

Grapeseed Extract

Start off by making some lemon balm tea. Add in a small amount (you decide) of cinnamon and then recommended amount of grapeseed extract. Mix together well and strain after it cools off. Take recommended berberine dosage and do this around the same time upon awakening. Will help to kick start burning the white fat (bad fat), not the brown fat (good fat) that we need for several vital functions.

Use this to be in addition to more structural changes you will adhere to. Do not use this as a "hack" or anything like that because more than often you will believe you can get away with consuming things not good for your health and will overeat more often than not.

Parkinson's Disease

Connections between the brain and muscles begin to lose their strength, muscles deteriorating, tremors, unstable posture, slow and difficult speech, flat facial expression, and eventually developing the condition known as dementia, where the brain is impaired to where you cannot readily perform many daily tasks occurs. These symptoms and experiences are what we call "Parkinson's Disease".

"There are various nutritional supplements that can help control or delay some of the movement-related and mental symptoms of Parkinson's disease" says Dr. Alan Brauer, M.D., founder and director of the TotalCare Medical Center in Palo Alto, California. Supplements are anything added to the foundation of your diet; not pharmaceutical medications or prescriptions although many will add artificial forms of what will be mentioned later in this section. Upon initially experiencing symptoms, a person should be asking themselves what they can do to significantly slow down the progress of this condition and reducing the symptoms.

Remedies:

Antioxidants

With conditions such as Parkinson's, the free radicals (unstable atoms within molecules that destroy cells) destroy receptive cells in the area of the brain known as the *substania nigra*, essentially a relay station located between the body's muscles and the cerebellum (area in the brain that controls movement). Antioxidants have the ability to block free radical's damage which would slow down the progression of Parkinson's. However, there are several antioxidants that must work together to be effective enough to effectively prevent the damage of free radicals, according to Dr. Phillip Lee Miller, M.D., founder and director of the Los Gatos Longevity Institute in California. The antioxidants that must work together are, (1) vitamin-C, (2) vitamin-E, (3) glutathione (substance made from three amino acids: cystine, glutamate, and glycine). Vitamin-C essentially takes charge of doing its role of transporting nutrients to the muscles and moving waste materials away from the cells until it becomes exhausted. Then vitamin-E fills in with its own special skill set at relaxing the muscles, followed by glutathione stepping in to neutralize the series of events that are taking place.

Vitamin-C – 1,000-4,000-milligrams daily divided into three doses with meals.

Vitamin-E – 600-1,200-international units daily in three divided doses with meals.

Glutathione – 200-milligrams daily.

These are the standard recommendations often made. You will want to compare with intake of items listed that contain these nutrients.

Common Sources of Vitamin-C: Black Currants, Bell Peppers (red), Papaya, Spring Onions, Strawberries, Cantaloupe, Mango, Oranges, Watercress, Raspberries, and Tomatoes.

Common Sources of Vitamin-E: red bell pepper, mango, avocado, sunflower seeds, brazil nuts, turnip greens, blackberry, black currants, olives, and butternut squash.

Common sources of glutathione: okra, leafy green vegetables, strawberries, papaya, bell peppers, oranges, and melons.

Natural Sources of Antioxidants: blueberries, onions, lettuce, squash, tomatoes, grapeseed extract, and herbs that you can use the flower, root, and leaves for as they contain polyphenolics (compounds that produce antioxidant activity).

Thiamin ("Vitamin-B1")

The chemical known as dopamine allows there to be messages sent amongst brain cells. In a condition such as Parkinson's, the availability of dopamine significantly decreases. The nutrient known as "thiamin" works to help the brain produce dopamine. Dr. Brauer recommends 3,000-8,000-milligrams of thiamin daily for those with Parkinson's and those with Parkinson's symptoms.

Common Sources of Thiamin: oranges, bananas, tomato (juice), lettuce, dandelion greens, sunflower seeds, hemp seeds, acorn squash.

Tyrosine (amino acid)

This amino acid also helps the brain produce dopamine. Dr. Miller recommends 00-1,000-milligrams of this early in the day on an empty stomach.

Common Sources of Tyrosine: avocado, bananas, sesame seeds, oranges, peaches, okra, tomato, wild rice.

*note: sticking to recommendation to consume on an empty stomach, it would serve you best to consume some of these items listed in juice form shortly after awakening.

Zinc

Low levels of this mineral will increase a person's chances of developing dementia. You want to remain proactive with making this mineral a staple in your lifestyle. The body uses Zinc to breakdown bacteria in the body and helps strengthen the immune system.

Common Sources of Zinc: chickpeas, mushrooms, zucchini, squash, okra, Brazil nuts, and walnuts.

Muscle Mass

The most visible symptom of Parkinson's is a decreased muscle mass. Medical doctors often prescribe various protein supplements and even some protein powder to help put on size. Many others will recommend a low-protein diet under watchful monitoring where you mostly eat protein at night. However, these products contain chemicals and only stuff the body. The appearance of gaining back size may feel nice and motivating but will weigh a person down even more and although they will believe progress is being made, symptoms often worsen and maintaining these products come to a halt. It is best to add healthy weight without the artificial chemicals that your body will recognize and absorb. There are whole foods that can provide minerals, amino acids and other materials to help feed the muscles and put back on healthier weight.

Here are some common foods that help put back on size:

1. Chickpeas. Also known as "garbanzo beans", are an excellent source of complex carbs, fiber, iron, folate, phosphorus, potassium, manganese, and several beneficial plant compounds, which help decrease cholesterol, regulate blood-sugar levels, lower blood pressure, aid in muscle formation and maintenance, and decrease belly fat.

2. Spelt and Teff. Spelt and teff belong to a category known as "ancient grains". They're both excellent sources of complex carbs, fiber, iron, magnesium, phosphorus, zinc, selenium, and manganese.

3. Hemp Seeds. Hemp seeds are one of the best plant-foods for muscle maintenance, so they are recommended for athletes or very active people. They also contain a good amount of minerals like magnesium, iron, calcium, zinc, and selenium.

4. Amaranth and Quinoa. They both are complete sources of complex carbs, fiber, iron, manganese, phosphorus, and magnesium.

5. Wild Rice. One cooked cup of wild rice provides a good amount of fiber, manganese, magnesium, copper, phosphorus and B vitamins.

6. Mushrooms (all kinds, except shiitake). Due to their "meaty" texture, mushrooms are a common alternative for meat in a plant-based diet. They are filled with minerals such as selenium, potassium, and copper, among many other vital nutrients.

7. Nuts and "Nut Butter". Nuts (walnuts, brazil nuts, kola nuts) are very nutritionally dense foods, as they contain a great amount of healthy fats and other beneficial nutrients.

All of these items provide similar content and even surpass the calorie content in many products doctors will recommend.

NADH

This nutrient is an activated form of the nutrient Niacin which works to produce energy to the brain. This nutrient is often deficient in those with Parkinson's and impairs things like memory and energizing brain cells. Many doctors will prescribe a NADH spray to improve absorption of niacin.

Common Sources of Niacin: avocado, watermelon, cherries, oranges, nectarines, lettuce, peaches (dried), sesame seeds, walnuts.

**boost energy to the brain

Vitamin-D

People with Parkinson disease often have low levels of vitamin-D according to the Icahn School of Medicine at Mount Sinai in New York. Aside from absorbing vitamin-d, (which is an essential fat-soluble nutrient) getting direct sunlight can promote the healthy producing of natural hormones and chemicals within the body and help to reduce triggers that come from being deficient in these key hormones and chemicals. It is generally recommended to get 15-30 minutes of direct sunlight when the sun is at its highest point around noontime. But get in the sun whenever possible, even if you have to take a few minutes in the morning before you start your day, or briefly during a break while at work or school.

Movement Is Medicine

Tai chi, Qigong and yoga can improve balance, flexibility, and range of motion in people with Parkinson disease. They may also boost mood and improve sleep according to the Icahn School of Medicine at Mount Sinai in New York.

Brahmi (bacopa monniera) (herb)

Brahmi is an Ayurvedic herb that is sometimes used to treat people with Parkinson disease. Research studies suggest that it improves circulation to the brain, as well as improving mood, cognitive function, and general neurological function, but it has not been specifically studied for Parkinson disease. If you are interested in brahmi, find a qualified Ayurveda practitioner, and do not take brahmi without informing all your prescribing doctors and practitioners during treatment.

Phlebitis

This condition is presented in two forms: (1) superficial and (2) deep. Deep vein phlebitis (thrombophlebitis) is when there is excess inflammation and clotting in a large vein in your leg where it be very difficult to bend your leg. This form of phlebitis calls for emergency attention as it can at any time generate a blood clot that can break off and become lodged in your heart or lungs and can be deadly. Superficial phlebitis is not as severe as deep vein phlebitis but still very concerning. In this form, a vein near the surface of the sin is visibly inflamed. This occurs when the blood flow slows down, becomes stagnant, and begins to clot (varicose veins are often the first sign of phlebitis). Medical doctors will often prescribe clot-dissolving medications until the condition worsens. However, in this section, we will look at natural ways to strengthen these weaker veins to reverse this condition and wok on restoring your health within the circulatory system in which your blood flows.

Remedies:

Clean The Liver

The weakness in the veins that causes conditions such as phlebitis is, the liver being full of toxins. The job of the veins is to return blood to the heart and then the lungs (where carbon dioxide is dumped, and oxygen is picked up. On the way, the blood stops at the liver where it can be cleaned of toxins. If the liver is full of toxins, the blood cannot be cleaned, cannot flow into the organs, and causes the blood to dilate in the legs where the veins will weaken over time as they never get to feel rejuvenated by being clear of toxins. Once these veins become inflamed, you will have phlebitis. You want to free the liver of congestion. This is where a whole-food, plant-based lifestyle will serve your body the best at directly working to not add toxins to the body.

Herbs To Assist With Cleaning The Liver

My Personal Remedy (for blood, liver, and kidney function):

Yellow Dock (dried: 2-4tsp; powder: 2-3tsp)

Chapparal (dried: 1/2tsp; powder: 1/2tsp)

Nettle (dried: 1tsp; powder: 1/2tsp)

Elderberries (dried: 2-3tbsp; powder: 3-4tsp

Detoxifying organs will begin to expel harmful toxins from the body while cleaning out waste materials in the body.

Liver Detox Tea

Ingredients: Burdock Root, Sarsaparilla, and Yellow Dock. About 750mg/each (about ¼ teaspoon each herb in powder form per 8oz water). Dosage changes for dried herb to about twice this amount at least.

Burdock Root helps promote urinary tract health and healthy liver function. Promotes clear, healthy skin.

Sarsaparilla contains biochemicals called saponins that may promote clear, healthy skin.

Yellow Dock is classified as a bitter herb that helps promote digestion. High in iron.

Liver Cleanse Tea:

The herb called Palo Azul is very helpful for cleaning the liver and breaking down toxins.

(How To Prepare: take 1 large piece or 2-3 medium sized pieces of this herb and place them in a boiling pot of water for approx. 60 minutes. Strain out the herbs and drink 1 cup a day for about 24-30 days).

As mentioned above as a coffee replacement, mixing Roasted Dandelion Root, Black Walnut Hull, and Blessed Thistle, can serve as a natural detoxifier which can help provide some relief for the liver.

(How To Prepare: take 1-2 cups of each herb and mix well together in a bowl or container. Boil water while placing about 1 tablespoon of mixture into a cup and pour boiling water into cup. Let sit for about 10 minutes and then strain out the herbs. You can drink hot or let cool off and add ice for an "Iced coffee". Store herbs in a zip lock bag or container and you can let your drink sit in the fridge overnight as well.

Put Your Feet Up

At least once a day you should put your feet up to take some flow away from your legs; especially if you are in pain or are on your feet much of the day. If you have phlebitis, you should make this mandatory for yourself. For 10 minutes a day, you should lie flat on your back on the floor. Place your lower legs comfortably onto a chair, bed, or other flat surface so that your legs are comfortable and relaxed off of the ground. Doing this will help take some pressure off of your legs and give your body a much-needed rest. This also gives your liver a chance to clean toxins out without feeling overwhelmed. Apply warmth while your legs are up as well to also assist with reducing inflammation.

Bilberry (herb)

This herb works to help strengthen the veins and reduce inflammation. 80-milligrams three times a day of this herb can help prevent flareups as well. You can find this herb in tincture form and follow instructions and dosage on the bottle.

Massage

You can massage your legs a few times a day, applying gently pressure to help improve circulation of the blood. You will want to massage from your ankle to the middle of your thighs on each leg, one leg at a time. this will relieve some of the pressure as you continue to make necessary adjustments.

Avoid Contraceptive Pills

We are 3-4 times more likely to develop phlebitis when taking an oral contraceptive pill. These pills lead to re-occurring vein clotting as compared to non-users according to Dr. Jess R. Young, former chairman of the department of vascular medicine at the Cleveland Clinic Foundation in Ohio, USA.

Go For A Walk

Exercise, primarily walking will help the veins improve circulation and work to clear up stagnation. Minimal activity allows the veins to "pool" which leads to stagnation and clotting. You can avoid this by walking regularly. Plan a daily walk into your schedule and also walk to places nearby rather than driving or getting a ride. If walking around is challenging at the moment, make an effort to stop a few times and walk shorter distances.

Getting Enough Fiber

Fiber helps with bowel movements. Having stagnation in the bowels will cause stagnation in the blood, especially in the legs as we hold up the rest of our bodies with our legs. Reducing feelings of constipation will relieve the pressure placed on your blood cells. Note: make sure to drink more water when increasing your fiber intake as you can feel constipated when hydration is low.

It is recommended for women to aim towards 21-25 grams of fiber a day, while men aim between 30-38 grams of fiber a day.

Common sources of Fiber: garbanzo beans, lentils, brussels sprouts, sweet potatoes, avocado, pears, sunflower seeds, flax seeds, hazelnuts, apples and berries (high pectin fruits) and onions.

Horse Chestnut (herb)

This herb helps to repair damaged blood vessels and work to strengthen the veins. Take 300-milligrams a day twice a day to relieve symptoms. This herb is available in capsule or tincture form.

Vitamin-E

This nutrient contains natural blood-thinning properties which can promote a steadier flow of blood to avoid lotting.

Common Sources of Vitamin-E: Red bell peppers, mangoes, walnuts, sunflower seeds (non-processed), avocados, butternut squash, olive oil (for dressings), coconut oil, and avocado oil.

Stop Smoking

Smoking damages the blood cells by depriving them of oxygen. The body will pull oxygen from other parts of the body as a response which can lead to clotting.

Plantar Warts

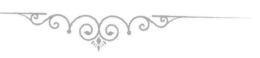

A plantar wart is a wart located on the bottom of your foot. A wart is a virus that takes over genes (DNA) and forces them to produce more viruses as well as forces your body to send blood to the area with blood vessels and nerves. A plantar wart then becomes covered with calluses. Many podiatrists will remove a wart, but this does not guarantee they won't return.

Due to warts being a virus, we want to gear our focus towards strengthening the immune system first. In this section we will review things to apply directly to the area, and ways to naturally strengthen then immune system.

Remedies:

Tea Tree Essential Oil

This essential oil is antiviral and is very effective at treating plantar warts. Apply drops as recommended on product label ad stop after 3-4 months.

Fatty Acids

The reason oils are very helpful are that they often contain the fatty acids that we are deficient in when experiencing symptoms of Arthritis or any joint or bone pains. Four specific fatty acids are to be focused on when a person has Arthritis. They are:

Alpha-linolenic Acid (LNA) Acid

Eicosatetraenoic Acid (EPA)

Docosahexaenoic Acid (DHA)

Gamma-linolenic Acid (GLA)

These four fatty acids not only help reduce inflammation, but they also help repair a weakened immune system that has been battling a disease and toxic environment for an extended period of time.

Common Sources of Fatty Acids: Brazil Nuts, Walnuts, Kola Nuts, Avocados, Bananas, Sea Vegetables (Nori, Wakame, Hijiki, Sea Moss, Bladderwrack), Coconut, Coconut Oil, Olive Oil, Grapeseed Oil, Avocado Oil, Mushrooms, Quinoa, Wild Rice.

Zinc

The body uses Zinc to breakdown bacteria in the body and helps strengthen the immune system.

Common Sources of Zinc: chickpeas, mushrooms, zucchini, squash, okra, Brazil nuts, and walnuts.

Vitamin-C

Steven Subotnick, D.P.M., podiatrist in Berkeley and San Leandro, California recommends 1,000-milligrams of vitamin-c daily to help strengthen and kick start the immune system. What we refer to as Vitamin C is a water-soluble nutrient and powerful antioxidant that help form and maintain connective tissues, including the bones, blood vessels, and the skin. This nutrient can help reduce symptoms of allergic reactions and inflammation which will help to avoid any prolonging issues. Vitamin C also is responsible for manufacturing the adrenal hormones which are needed to combat the stress the body goes through when an allergic reaction takes place.

Common Sources of Vitamin-C: Black Currants, Bell Peppers (red and green), Papaya, Spring Onions, Strawberries, Cantaloupe, Mango, Oranges, Watercress, Raspberries, and Tomatoes.

Astragalus (herb)

This herb helps to boost the immune system and kill off viruses (pretty convenient for cold sores). This herb is most potent in capsule or tincture form. A typical dosage can span from 9-30g a day in tincture form and two 80mg capsules a day in capsule form for no more than 6 weeks at a time.

Selenium

This mineral is very crucial when it comes to our body's immune system. Selenium combines with several other substances in the body to form a compound known as "glutathione peroxidase", which allow your immune system to sample organisms that are inhabiting (but not yet overgrowing) on the outer layer of the skin. This not only reduces any overgrowth, but also allows the immune system to respond accordingly and destroy any organisms that may be harmful to the body.

Common sources of Selenium: brazil nuts, walnuts, chickpeas/garbanzo beans, kola nuts, dandelion greens, and nettle, and alfalfa. Recommended to consume about 400 micrograms a day.

No More Gluten

Gluten provides no essential nutrients. It is a protein found in wheat, oats, barley, certain breads, cakes, soy products, white pastas, and various vegetarian or vegan "meats". Although gluten is more associated with celiac disease, the immune system establishing the norm of attacking an organ in the body will make the immune system become more easily compromised and easier to be persuaded to attack other organs such as the pancreas which is the norm for type-1 diabetes. We want to avoid gluten items as they cause unnecessary damage to our bodies with no essential nutrients in them. Gluten will create additional work for our immune systems that we can do without so that we can ward off other potential illnesses and symptoms of disease.

Cut Out Refined Carbs

"Sugar and white flour weaken the immune system and rob the body of energy" says Dr. Metzger, M.D., Ph.D., medical director of Helena Women's Health in San Francisco, California, and Palo Alto, California. When excess sugars and white flour are consumed, this creates an enormous workload on the digestive system and due to their toxicity, the immune system t-cells respond by treating this as a foreign invader. The body can do without the additional immune response which can be better served focusing on other areas of the body and avoid accumulating waste within the body.

Freeze It Off

Going to see your doctor, they can apply ways to freeze your wart off. Freezing the wart can reduce stimulation to the area and also help the wart come off of the skin. There are many products that can be purchased at a local pharmacy or drug store but be cautious to not damage the skin around your wart as this can come with complications.

Olive Leaf

The olive tree contains powerful compounds that break down infections. The active ingredient in olive leaves (oleuropin) should be found on the product label for best effects. Olive leaf can come in dried form, tinctures, or capsules. Make sure to follow instructions on label depending on which form of this plant you decide to use.

Oregano Oil

Oregano oil contains *carvacrol*, the main active compound in oregano oil and a type of antioxidant called a phenol. Also contains *thymol*, which may help protect against toxins and fight fungal infections.

These antioxidant and anti-fungal properties help to break down a wart/infection from the inside out. One way of using oil of oregano is to add 2–3 drops to water or juice and drink the mixture. However, people should be careful to use oil of oregano and not oregano essential oil. The latter is much stronger and is not safe to consume. Follow direction on label as not all oils are made for the same usage but look for those you can apply directly onto the skin to help breakdown this infection that's located in a specific area before it spreads.

Pneumonia

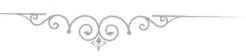

Pneumonia is an infection of your lungs. It is not simply a "bad cold". The body work to expel this mucus ore muscles, difficulty breathing, headaches, and symptoms of fever, chills, and by you coughing out rust-colored or green mucus, chest pain, and excessive sweating. You want to target the respiratory system and the blood for this condition. Many will try and even many doctors will recommend strengthening your immune system as the focus for this condition but, only doing this forces your body to fight, hoping that you survive the battle. This is why many people die from this condition. Not because strengthening the immune system is not helpful, but because the immune system can run out of "fighters" and if the battle goes on longer than initially anticipated, the body may not survive or be able to fully recover without complications. In this section, we will review what to do in addition to strengthening the immune system, to help thin the mucus, help make it easier to expel toxins, clean the lungs, and clean the blood cells in order to recover fully from this condition.

Remedies:

Bromelain

This digestive enzyme helps to thin mucus and help boost the killing of bacteria that eventually turns into additional mucus.

Common Sources of Bromelain: watermelon, bananas, papaya, pineapple.

Vitamin-A

This nutrient helps to strengthen what we call the epithelium, what is the tissue that lines the lungs. Protecting this layer of the lungs helps to keep harmful bacteria out and will help promote recovery by allowing the lungs to focus on breaking down and removing mucus.

Common Sources of Vitamin-A: mango, papaya, apricots, red bell peppers, winter squash, dark leafy green vegetables, cantaloupe, and lettuce.

Vitamin-C and Vitamin-E

Whenever the body fights an infection, it produces free radicals (unstable molecules that damage cells, making them more susceptible to being invaded by bacteria. Vitamin-C works to stop free radicals, according to Dr. Peter Holyk, M.D., director of the Contemporary Health Clinic in Sebastian, Florida. As vitamin-C works to prevent free radicals, vitamin-E help support vitamin-C, helping to make them more effective.

Common Sources of Vitamin-C: Black Currants, Bell Peppers (red and green), Papaya, Spring Onions, Strawberries, Cantaloupe, Mango, Oranges, Watercress, Raspberries, and Tomatoes.

Common Sources of Vitamin-E: red bell pepper, mango, avocado, sunflower seeds, brazil nuts, turnip greens, blackberry, black currants, olives, and butternut squash.

My Personal Remedy For Pneumonia

Step 1: Commit to remove dairy products (milk, cheese, yogurt, etc.) for 14 days straight. (will help much more if all meats are removed as well).

Step 2: Drink Mullein Leaf, Guaco, Red Willow Bark, Elderberry, and Dandelion Root.

Dosage for each herb:

Ages 2 to 4 years = 2 teaspoons (once/day)

Ages 4 to 7 years = 1 tablespoon (once/day)

Ages 7 to 11 years = 2 tablespoons (once/day)

Ages 12+ = 2 tablespoons (can drink more regularly per day; or more than 8oz cup).

<u>*Refer to the following sections in this book for additional recommendation to apply: Colds and Flu, Coughing, Emphysema, and Fever.</u>

Pregnancy Discomfort

There are serious concerns when pregnant such as, potential for miscarriage, toxemia (from high blood pressure), and gestational diabetes from elevated blood sugar levels. Pregnancy discomfort is what may appear to be the inevitable discomfort that goes along with being pregnant that don't require immediate help. For example, back pain from the baby's weight on your muscles, heartburn from the swelling of the uterus pushing your stomach upwards, the varicose veins from the constant pressure applied to the blood flow, and many more.

In this section we will visit and review remedies for some of the primary discomforts associated with pregnancy an identify ways to provide relief.

Remedies:

Morning Sickness

visit the "Morning Sickness" section in this book.

Heartburn and Indigestion

During pregnancy, the sudden increase of hormones such as estrogen and progesterone, can slow down digestion and relax the valve that keeps acid in the stomach. Aside from eating a clean diet void of meats, dairy, and processed foods filled with chemicals, there's an herb that can serve as your primary remedy for heartburn and indigestion called Meadowsweet.

Meadowsweet (herb)

A woman can take 15-45 drops of this herb in tincture form diluted in water 1-4 times a day. Monitor your dosage and determine if you need more or less. You may also drink this herb in tea form by taking 1-tablspoon of this herb, placing it into a cup, and pouring 1 cup of boiling water over it. Let steep for 15-20 minutes, strain, and sip slowly. Do this once a day.

Insomnia

Your baby's movements in the middle of the night can wake you up and can make it difficult to get to sleep most nights.

visit "Insomnia" section in this book.

Calcium and Magnesium

We cannot properly absorb calcium without magnesium so it's important to have both of these minerals around the same time, particularly before going to bed. Both of these minerals will help calm the muscles and nerves in the body and help promote sleep. It is important at times to eat right before going to sleep. Ordinarily this would keep you up as the food will be digesting and will prevent you from sleeping. But eating a small snack right before going to bed will help keep your baby occupied with absorbing minerals and processing materials that they remain calmer. It is recommended these snacks consist of the items listed below which are high in calcium and magnesium.

Common sources of calcium: sea moss, kale, okra, dandelion greens, turnip greens, lettuce, papaya, and oranges.

*Common Sources of Magnesium: avocado, chickpeas, tamarind, basil, dill, ginger, oregano, thyme, any *CBD (cannabidiol) products are helpful. (CBD Oils are almost pure magnesium.), nettle leaf, horsetail, red clover, sage, and nopal.*

To test the purity of a CBD Oil, send to a lab for testing or you should feel a steady decline in needing to rely on this substance after your need has been met regularly.

Varicose Veins

A growing child places additional pressure on the circulatory system. So, the blood going through the body will often pool (remain stagnant) in the legs and leads to varicose veins.

visit "Varicose Veins" section in this book.

Horse Chestnut (herb)

After the first trimester, use this herb for relieve and for promoting circulation. Take -15 drops of this herb diluted in water (about ¼ cup) 2-3 times a day.

Exercise

Doing "pelvic tilts" is a great daily exercise to help with circulation. A lot of movement in the pelvic area becomes stagnant while pregnant due to the baby growing in this area and more demand for sitting. To bring back more flow to this area, stand with your feet about shoulder-width apart. place your hands on your hips and slowly push your pelvis forward, then backwards. Gradually increase your speed until you can do so vigorously. Then try rolling your hips to make a figure-8, or side to side where you can feel a nice stretch. Light cardio in the form of walking is also highly recommended to keep your hips aligned and maintain flow within the circulatory system while pregnant.

Back Pain

*visit the "Back Pain" section in this book and apply what is helpful (not harmful) for pregnant women.

Premature Ejaculation

Premature ejaculation is defined as ejaculating in 4-minutes or less. However, premature ejaculation is most commonly referred to as, ejaculating earlier than your partner is able to orgasm. This condition was not referred to as a condition until it was proven that women need more time to reach an orgasm than men. The goal is to simply learn to delay your natural ejaculation reflexes to prolong having intercourse with your partner to help them reach an orgasm. In this section, you will learn ways to prolong your erection to avoiding premature ejaculation.

Remedies:

Kegel Exercises

These exercises involving squeezing the muscles in the anus as if you were trying to stop the flow of urine. This allows you to strengthen the muscle known as the "pubococcygeus (PC) muscle", which serves as a sling for the sexual organs. Dr. Alan Brauer, M/D., psychiatrist. Sex therapist, and co-author of the book entitled, Extended Sexual Orgasm, which aimed towards teaching men how to have orgasms that last for a half-hour or longer, states that, "The more awareness and control you have over the PC and sexual muscles, the more control you'll have over ejaculation." Dr. Brauer recommends that instead of only tightening the muscles in the anus, that it is important to push down as if you're forcing out urine or bowel movement (make sure you do not have to go when doing this). This pushing down movement can help stop ejaculation during sexual intercourse. As you take deep, slowed breaths, you will want to practice both, squeezing and pushing the muscles in the anus. When doing either, count from one to five, then as you exhale slowly, count from five back down to one. Make sure your partner is aware of you doing this in order to practice and take breaks as needed. Don't feel embarrassed.

Your partner will more likely appreciate your efforts more than anything and offer support and guidance as you make progress.

Note: during the day when not having sex, practice both of these exercises about 50 times throughout the day.

Self-Stimulation

Athletes practice specific moves to build muscle memory. You can do the same here. The more practice a man can get close to ejaculating but not completing, the more familiar they will be and the less urgency they will have to ejaculating too early. Dr. Brauer recommends masturbating gently to help the muscle fibers and blood flow become more even and slowed down in order to decrease the urgency and prolonging your erection.

Scrotal Pull

This technique involves pulling down the scrotal sac (area that "hugs" your body when you're sexually aroused). During sex, you can gently pull down on this area pr ask your partner to do it. This will help regulate blood flow and contribute to lasting longer.

External Prostate Spot

There's a specific area called the perineum, which is the space between the anus ad the back of the scrotum that stimulates the prostate (the gland that supplies the fluid for semen during ejaculation). Pressing gently but firmly on this spot when you are aroused can help prevent ejaculation. You may press this spot periodically during sex at any point after you've achieved a full erection. If you are not fully erect, pressing on this point can cause pain throughout your sexual experience.

Breathing

Making sure to take slow, deep breaths is vital to maintaining the body's to prolonging an erection. You do not want to visualize and ending and bring that thought closer, so focus on your breath to keep circulation going throughout your body and not just towards your sexual organs. Breathing will help to decrease the urgency of the body wanting to ejaculate.

African Herbs That Support Sexual Organs (Men and Women)

Aframomum (herb)

Aframomum (also known as Alligator Pepper, Ataare, Grains of Pardise, and Melegueta Pepper) is an African aphrodisiac spice with a similar composition to Ginger. It is a pro-ejaculant herb for men and increases their sperm count. The herb is helpful for all sexual disorders in both genders.

In women, Aframomum boosts libido and make women more sensitive to intimate touch, especially in the lower regions. Additionally, it regulates vaginal lubrication, and increases sexual desire in 48-72 hours.

Aframomum promotes circulation making it helpful for erectile dysfunction conditions as well as all other sexual dysfunction plaguing society today.

Bangalala (herb)

Bangalala, native to South Africa and used for centuries by the Zulu tribe, is one of the best herbs for male sexual health. A powerful aphrodisiac and sexual tonic, it boosts and improves libido, counters male erectile dysfunction (improves circulation to the genitalia), increases and improves sexual stamina, increases energy, enhances male potency, and boosts testosterone levels.

The herb enhances sexual performance by increasing blood flow to the penis thus promoting stronger, longer lasting erections. In women, it increases blood flow to the clitoris, heightening sensitivity to the organ and surrounding labia (lips of the vagina).

The herb is also helpful for pregnant women in the last two weeks of pregnancy to help a woman prepare for childbirth. Women suffering from infertility would do well to consume Bangalala religiously.

Mondia Whitei (herb)

Mondia Whitei (also known as Isirigun, White Ginger, Mukombera, and Mulondo), from Nigeria (but also found in Benin), androgenic in nature, is commonly referred to as African Viagra, boosts libido, improves testosterone production and levels in the body, increases size and weight of the testicles, improves male fertility (by improving sperm quality); increases sperm production, boosts strength, energy, and stamina; counters premature ejaculation, helps to heal STDs such as gonorrhea, and improves mental well-being.

Additionally, the herb increases potency by being able to relax the corpus cavernosum muscle thus aiding erection and by improving sperm total motility and progressive motility.

Furthermore, the herb enhances urination, ease birth pains, and increases the quantity and quality of mother's milk.

Fadogia Agrestis (herb)

Fadogia Agrestis (also known as Black Aphrodisiac) from Nigeria, a pro-erectile herb, is one of the most potently effective African erotogens available. It boosts libido, promotes and supports muscle mass, increases energy levels, boosts testosterone levels, strengthens physical/

athletic performance, counters impotence/erectile dysfunction, increases stamina, and increases the sex drive. It is a supreme aphrodisiac!

Fadogia Agrestis promotes the production luteinizing hormone which produces testosterone in the male body. Additionally, it helps prevent the accumulation of excess fat in the body and makes one fit by burning fat. It is also loaded with antioxidants and helps keep the immune system fortified.

Fadogia Agrestis is popular herb and ingredient in the Fitness and Supplement World. It is an excellent herb for boosting testosterone levels (which are at all-time lows in the Western world, mostly due to PCBs or Poly-Cholorinated Biphenyls that are literally everywhere in society).

Bulbine Natalensis (herb)

Bulbine Natalensis is a South African herb that boosts testosterone levels by threefold up to six-fold. It is the Number One herb on planet earth for increasing testosterone levels in men, the sad fact which is - today, men in the Western world are experiencing all-time lows in testosterone levels (which mainly due to PCBs [Poly-Chlorinated Biphenyl], Atrazine chemical [in municipal water supplies], and consuming today's female-specific growth hormone [meat and dairy products, derived from farm animals]).

The plant's high testosterone levels greatly boost and repair the male libido.

Additionally, the plant which has anabolic and androgenic properties regulates the hormones (testosterone and androgen), increases testicular size, boosts protein levels in the testes, increases the sex drive, increases intravaginal ejaculatory latency time or EILT.

Bulbine Natalensis aids in working out (great for muscle strength). Great for gym-goers and weightlifters (bodybuilders).

While Bulbine Natalensis can increase or boost testosterone levels up to six (6) times, it also lowers estrogen levels three-fold.

Gouro (herb)

Gouro is a natural aphrodisiac from the root of the plant Turraea Heterophylla (which is shaped like an erect penis with testicles at the base) which is found especially in Côte d'Ivoire or Ivory Coast in Africa.

It naturally boosts libido and promotes penis enlargement, counters premature ejaculation and sexual weakness. Additionally, it promotes longer lasting erections.

Gouro root highly compliments Yohimbe bark, Mpesu, and Kigelia especially for penis enlargement purposes.

African Pygeum Bark (herb)

African Pygeum Bark, one of the best herbs for adverse prostate conditions, is an anti-inflammatory phytosterol with the ability to normalize male prostate prostaglandins and to help shrink the prostate in males with enlarged prostates. It is very useful for benign prostatic hypertrophy (BPH) to reduce inflammation and pain and normalize the passage of urine.

Pygeum also increases prostatic and seminal fluid secretions. A meta-analysis revealed that men taking pygeum had a 19% reduction in nocturia and a 24% reduction in residual urine volume.

Pygeum bark helps improve semen volume and viscosity via its effect on DHT and through its action on the development and function of the prostate and seminal vesicles. Healthy viscosity of semen allows more sperm to survive for longer.

Mpesu Bark (herb)

Mpesu Bark from South Africa, a pro-erectile, is one of the most potent and effective male-specific aphrodisiac and erotegens on the planet. It counters sexual dysfunction, weak penile erection, premature ejaculation, and boosts libido and sexual stamina.

Mpesu will give a man longer lasting and stronger erections and will help him experience multiple erections and orgasms.

An added benefit of Mpesu Bark is that it is one of a few herbs that actually naturally promotes growth of the male penis. It compliments "Kigelia" and "Akpi" (for promotion of penis growth, length and width).

The herb also naturally and effectively helps to boost testosterone levels.

Yohimbe (herb)

Yohimbe bark, the King of Aphrodisiacs, is a male-specific hormonal stimulant effective in the production of testosterone, and as an aphrodisiac affecting both male impotence and female frigidity.

The bark has a stimulatory effect on the sex organs of both genders. Yohimbe enhances sexual performance and counters erectile dysfunction (ED) in males. In females, the bark increases arousal and sensitivity of the clitoris and counters frigidity.

Yohimbe is also useful in bodybuilding and athletic performance, weight loss, improving body composition, and adverse heart conditions.

Date Palm Pollen

Date Palm Pollen (DPP) from Egypt, Africa is an authentic African substance or product, derived from the male reproductive dust of palm flowers and has traditionally been used to increase libido and improve fertility in both women and men.

It is one of the best substances to counter male testicular and female ovarian dysfunction. A great product for the male and female reproductive systems.

In men, the pollen helps with testosterone (maintaining normal to high levels), libido, and increasing sperm quantity and quality.

In women, the pollen helps to increase female fertility (boosting ovulation) owing to its estrogen-like compounds, sterols, and estrone-like compounds (that do not throw off or counter men's testosterone levels).

Typha Capensis (herb)

Native to South Africa, commonly known as "Love Reed" is an effective African aphrodisiac herb that enhances the production of testosterone thus increasing libido, countering male infertility and aging male problems; enhances male potency, and counters erectile dysfunction (by improving circulation); and enhancing sexual performance.

In women, Typha Capensis is a powerful fertility enhancer. It strongly enhances ovulation. Additionally, it tones the vagina and increases circulation to that orifice, heightening sensitivity in that region during intimacy.

Typha Capensis can be consumed in the last two weeks of pregnancy to prepare for childbirth. It strengthens uterine contractions. Typha Capensis also helps in countering sexually transmitted diseases.

Uziza (herb)

Uziza, an Igbo name (also known as Ashanti Pepper, West African Pepper, Guinea Pepper, and Ata iyere in Yoruba) is an African herb, used in Nigeria mainly, that helps improve penile erections, enhances fertility and potency, and improves low sperm counts in men. In women, Uziza is great for their sexual reproductive health. It improves fertility, enhancing ovulation. During pregnancy, it can be taken throughout pregnancy and especially during the last trimester to prepare for childbirth and to prepare for lactation. It increases uterine wall contraction during childbirth. Additionally, it helps with adverse menstrual issues, especially cramping.

Goran Tula Fruit

Goran Tula fruit (also known as Tree Hibiscus and Snot Apple) increases the libido in both men and women and promotes strong desire for sexual intercourse. It helps couples go multiple rounds between the sheets.

The herb is also an effective hormonal balancer, especially for women.

Goran Tula is a reliable fertility enhancer (for both men and women). It also enhances ovulation in women and improves semen concentration and quality while increasing semen volume.

In women, Goran Tula is a vaginal tonic and stimulates the production of vaginal wetness/lubrication and is perfect for keeping the vagina area moist and wet. The herb is one of the best for women who find it difficult to climax or reach orgasm.

Goran Tula is also a vaginal cleanser and deodorizer (helps to eliminate malodors in the vagina) and helps to keep the kitty cat smelling (and tasting) sweet and fresh. Additionally, it helps with adverse menstrual cycle complaints and normalizes the menstrual cycle after childbirth.

Kigelia

Kigelia (also known as Sausage Tree, Worsboom in Afrikaans, Modukghulu, Pidiso in North Sotho, umVongotsi in Siswati; Mpfungurhu in Tsonga, and Muvevha in Venda.

Because the fruit is shaped in the form of the male penis, pursuant to the herbal doctrine of signatures, its properties are helpful for the male genitalia, especially for naturally increasing the growth and length of the penis (taken consistently or religiously) over time, 3-6 months (to notice significant change).

In men, Kigelia is aphrodisiacal and helps the penis to become larger.

In women, Kigelia counters infertility being naturally rich in phyoestrogens. It is one of the best herbs for the breasts, naturally toning, firming and defining the breasts as well as enhancing their growth (natural breast enhancement or growth factor).

In lactating women, Kigelia stimulates lactation. Additionally, it increases the volume and quality of mother's milk.

Kigelia is exceptional for all gynecological disorders in women. It is useful (in men and women) to counter sexually transmitted diseases (STDs or STIs), especially syphilis and gonorrhea.

Premenstrual Syndrome (PMS)

Once a month, approximately 2 weeks before a woman begins to menstruate, the hormones (estrogen and progesterone) begin to build. These hormones regulate the menstrual cycle and affect the central nervous system as they work in tandem by contrasting one another. If one of these hormones begins to outwork or overshadow the other, this is when issues arise, and we have what's referred to as "premenstrual syndrome". Think of these two hormones as opposing armies that battle. Each month they go back and forth, but it's not until one arm begins to destroy the other, that the balance they provide by opposing one another, that there's any issues. These issues can turn into strong symptoms that last days.

PMS impacts about 1/3 – ½ of all women ages 20-50 years old. Having several children, stress, and existing health issues all increase the risk of PMS.

Remedies:

Exercise

Consistent, moderate exercise increases and improves the blood flow in the body, relaxes the muscles, and helps to fight fluid retention which all impact PMS. According to Dr. Edward Portman, M.D. a PMS consultant and researcher and former director of the Portman Clinic in Madison, Wisconsin, "exercise increases your brain's production of endorphins, natural opiates that make you feel better all over." Find an exercise you enjoy that you believe you can gradually improve upon so that you push yourself week after week.

Destress Your Immediate Environment

An imbalance of hormonal changes can cause a person to become more sensitive to environmental stressors. Try surrounding yourself with soothing colors, soft music, and removing any clutter in your space to decrease the sensitivity ad help remain calm.

Mineral Bath

Help your muscles relax all over your body. add 1 cup of sea salt, 1 cup of baking soda to warm bathwater. Add some essential oils and even some herbs you may enjoy, providing a relaxing effect.

Chasteberry

Progesterone and estrogen control the menstrual cycle. Dr. Holmes notes that "A deficiency of progesterone, can affect the thyroid gland." Chasteberry extract, commonly known as "vitex" as a name brand supplement, works to stimulate the pituitary gland to increase the production of LH, which results in higher levels of progesterone during the second stage of a woman's cycle known as the luteal phase. Progesterone helps to develop a thick, blood-rich uterine lining into which the fertilized egg can implant. Many women between the ages of 30 and 45 have a sharp drop off in progesterone which leads to shorter cycles and a decreased chance of implanting a fertilized egg. This change can enhance symptoms of hypothyroidism. Make sure to use Chasteberry Extract for several months before attempting to conceive, but generally 14 days before your next cycle. Standard dosage should be about 40 drops of this extract one a day, or one 650-milligram capsule 2-3 times a day. Make sure to follow directions on label instructions.

Invest In Sleep

If you are lacking sleep due to insomnia from PMS symptoms, work on going to bed several hours before your usual bedtime. It may take longer for you to go to sleep, so laying down in your bed earlier will help increase your chances of getting rest. At the least, you may get brief moments of rest that ad up over time to the point you feel rested upon awakening.

Avoiding Empty Calories

This step is true for every condition but is very important to avoid for those with PMS. Digesting, processing materials, and sending blood to the digestive tract, all without gaining any necessary nutrients will waste any energy you may have left. You are already running low on energy and feel fatigued. The last thing you need is to spend some time and energy performing another task without receiving anything from it. Low-nutrient foods like junk items and processed foods, soft drinks, and items containing refined sugars are to be avoided completely.

Avoiding Dairy

Not only is dairy full of hormones, but it also contains lactic acid which creates muscle soreness. Lactic acid forms in the body whenever oxygen is absent. Consuming that which is deprived of oxygen is like adding interest to already sore and fatigued muscles in the body. The lactose sugar in dairy also block's your body's ability to absorb magnesium which works to reduce muscle soreness, regulate estrogen levels, and increase energy.

Decrease Sodium Intake

Sodium creates water retention. You do not want to retain fluids while dealing with PMS due to further disrupting your period during your monthly cycle. Besides avoiding items with moderate to high sodium, you want to view the ingredient lists of items such as commercial soap, salad dressings, and other items you do not think has a high sodium content.

Fiber

Fiber helps clear out excess estrogen through digestion. Being able to contribute to breaking down the estrogen for its removal, help significantly decrease the workload the body has to do by itself. High-fiber foods contain a natural chemical known as "indole-3-carbinol" which helps estrogen from binding with breast tissue.

Fiber helps promote ease of digestion because it absorbs a lot of water and helps create softer stools, which promote eliminating larger quantities of waste easier. The American Dietetic Association recommends 20-35 grams of fiber daily. This may sound like a lot but, ½ cup of leafy green vegetables can provide about 5g, a small apple is about 3g, and consuming grains like quinoa can provide up to 8g per cup. Just these three items together and you are almost at your daily recommended amount in addition to any other foods you consume that have fiber.

Common sources of Fiber: garbanzo beans, lentils, brussels sprouts, sweet potatoes, avocado, pears, sunflower seeds, flax seeds, hazelnuts, apples and berries (high pectin fruits) and onions.

Cut Your Caffeine

Caffeine is a hormone disruptor. This substance contributes to bodily aches and pains, anxiety, and irritability. Caffeine also decreases oxygen delivery to the brain which further promotes and onslaught of moderate to severe symptoms of PMS.

Avoid Diuretics

Diuretics work to flush items out of the body. usually this is not a bad thing, but you may lose many vital minerals and nutrients currently in your body that are helping you avoid many symptoms. You do not want to contribute to worsening your symptoms or condition.

Cut Your Sugar Cravings

Dr. Susan Lark, M.D., physician in Los Altos, California states that, "In my experience, getting women of sugar is the secret of curing many cases of PMS. Here are some tips on how to begin cutting your sugar cravings.

Sea Salt

Place about ¼ teaspoon if sea salt into a cup of warm water and drink it. This will help an immediate sugar craving. You want to monitor and not overconsume salt in general but use this method sparingly only once a day at most and during your strongest cravings.

Ginger (herb)

This herb helps relieve many symptoms PMS. Ginger also provides a similar "mod lift" that we get from items such as chocolate, and caffeinated drinks such as coffee or soda.

Eat Foods to Stabilize Blood Sugar

When the body's blood sugars levels are not stable, the body responds by craving sugar. Consuming carbs in the form of fruit, vegetables, and grains are best as they are light on the digestive system and consume natural sugars our bodies thrive off of while having carbs to break down in the meantime to provide glucose to the body to enhance your ability to performing tasks and alleviating many symptoms of PMS.

Avoid Aspartame

This toxin is an artificial sweetener found in many processed items. Contains addictive qualities that contribute to things such as depression, anxiety, poor sleep patterns, headaches, and fatigue. These are many of the very same symptoms many experience with PMS, so consuming this substance will increase the frequency and severity of symptoms.

Sunlight

The hormones melatonin and serotonin can decrease naturally during ovulation. If melatonin is low, we do not sleep well. If serotonin is low, we feel tense and experience symptoms of depression. Exposure to direct sunlight boosts the body's levels of both of these hormones. You want to spend at least 20-30 minutes a day in direct sunlight to help stimulate and boost these hormones. This may sound like a lot of time, but you can sit outside somewhere, get up when the sun is rising, or go for a walk in an open area outside. Every minute spent in the sun is an investment into helping regulate and balance these hormones in your body.

Calcium

This mineral helps work on reducing the fluctuation of calcium-reducing hormones that are stimulated by estrogen (and progesterone) during the latter half of the woman's menstrual cycle. Dr. Susan Thys-Jacobs, M.D., an endocrinologist at St. Luke's-Roosevelt Hospital in New York City cites several research studies that compared women who took 1,20-miligrams of calcium to women who did not, and the end result was, "twice as many on calcium stated they felt les moody and depressed than those not on calcium."

Common Sources of Calcium: sea moss, kale, okra, dandelion greens, turnip greens, lettuce, papaya, and oranges.

Pycnogenol

This nutrient can be found in the seeds inside of grapes and from pine bark. Pycnogenol helps reduce bloating, fluid retention, and even things like breast tenderness that can occur during a woman's cycle. Dr. Lark recommends 50-miligrams of this nutrient 1-2 times a day.

Evening Primrose Oil

This oil is a great source of omega-3 fatty acids which work to reduce fluid retention and mood disturbances. It is recommended to take 2,000-3,000 milligrams a day for as long as you need to not experience these symptoms.

My Personal Herbal Remedy:

Add the following to an empty cup:

1 tablespoon of dried sage (to relieve headaches)

1.5 teaspoons of dandelion leaf (to decrease bloating)

1 teaspoon of St. John's Wort (to decrease irritability and depression symptoms)

1 teaspoon of cleavers (for breast tenderness)

Boil water and pour over herbs. Let steep for 20-minutes, strain and enjoy 1-2 times a day. When you feel symptoms coming on, begin preparing this tea, or make it a plan to make the following day until symptoms decrease.

Prostate Cancer

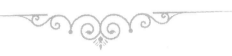

Each year, about 185,000 men are diagnosed with prostate cancer. The prostate is a small nut-sized gland located below the bladder that supplied the fluid that caries sperm during ejaculation. Al forms of cancer essentially include the same treatments (surgery, chemotherapy, radiation, and anti-hormone therapies). While these treatments have the intention of getting rid of the cancer that is visible, it is more important to strengthen the body's defenses to control the spread of these cells. In this section you will learn about helpful steps to take in order to control the spread of this condition and how reliving the body of many other ailments will help to begin reversing this condition completely.

Remedies:

Bathroom Stool

Get a small stool to place your feet onto when using the toilet to defecate. The position it will place your digestive tract and more importantly, your prostate, will allow you to pass stools much easier. When we sit at an almost 90-degree angle, our anal muscles squeeze and contract closer together which places an enormous amount of pressure on the prostate. Sometimes frequent straining can damage the prostate long-term and create other health issues.

Selenium

This mineral helps control free radicals in the body that damage cells and DNA which triggers the formation of cancer and many other conditions. In a research study, researchers found that hundreds of men who took 20-miligrams of selenium cut the incidence of prostate cancer by 60%. Dr. Michael Schachter, M.D., director of the Schachter Center for

Complementary Medicine in Sufern, New York treats his patients for prostate cancer with 400-600 micrograms of selenium daily.

Common sources of Selenium: brazil nuts, walnuts, chickpeas/garbanzo beans, kola nuts, dandelion greens, and nettle, and alfalfa. Recommended to consume about 400 micrograms a day. You may also plan to purchase a tasteless, odorless, liquid form of selenium by the brand Aqua Sel where you take 1-2 drops per day (or no more than 190mg daily).

Zinc

The prostate gland has the highest concentration of zinc in the body. having additional amount of zinc in the body will either, address a deficiency contributing to the growth of cancerous cells, or help this organ battle cancer cells as the body works towards healing.

The body uses Zinc to breakdown bacteria in the body and helps strengthen the immune system. This mineral helps regulate hormones in the body. When zinc is low in males, they can fail to produce enough hormones that promote fertility. It is recommended to consume about 30 milligrams of zinc daily for a few months to increase fertility.

Common Sources of Zinc: chickpeas, mushrooms, zucchini, squash, okra, Brazil nuts, and walnuts.

Soursop

According to the National Institute of Health (NIH), soursop fruit, leaves, and extract inhibits the proliferation of PC-3 human prostate cancer cells. Traditional uses of soursop have been used to treat bacterial and fungal infections, as it possesses anthelmintic, antihypertensive, anti-inflammatory, and anticancer activities. In the NIH study, they found that soursop seeds induce apoptosis, helping to inhibit colorectal cancer cells and breast cancer cells. Also, that soursop leaves inhibited prostate cancer cells and colon cancer cells.

You can find soursop extract to take topically, and soursop leaves which you can make into a tea. The soursop fruit can be found at. Local markets but prices can vary where it is expensive in some areas.

Jaboticaba Fruit or extract ("Brazilian Berry")

Jaboticaba is a fruit that resembles a small plum but tastes similar to "blueberry yogurt". This plant grows in abundance in southeastern Brazil. A study carried out by the University of Campinas in Brazil through the School of Food Engineering, and their Instituted of Biology, researchers found that jaboticaba extract prevents prostatic damage associated with again and high-fat diet intake. The peel of the jaboticaba plant is rich in fibers and bioactive compounds such as, anthocyanins, delphinidin, and cyanidin 3-glucoside, which show high antioxidant capacity and antiproliferative action against leukemia and prostate cancer cells.

Saw Palmetto (herb)

This herb is known to shrink the tissues of the prostate. This is often the main caution of taking this herb, but when dealing with prostate cancer, the male hormone known as testosterone, helps feed the cancerous cells in the prostate. Saw Palmetto helps block testosterone. Typically, we would not want to block testosterone, but we do want to shut of the source of anything helping feed cancerous cells during the healing process of a condition such as prostate cancer. Dr. James Forsythe, M.D., medical director of the Cancer Care Center in Reno, Colorado recommends 80-miligrams of saw palmetto herb twice a day as a part of the treatment protocol for treating prostate cancer.

Fatty Acids

Fatty acids contain an abundance of nutrients that work to control the development of cells. All forms of cancer are conditions in which cell growth and development out of control. Essential fatty acids (omega-3, omega-6, omega-9) help repair the cellular damage that has taken place over the years from consuming too many artificial sugars.

Common Sources of Fatty Acids: (Brazil Nuts, Walnuts, Kola Nuts, Avocados, Bananas, Sea Vegetables (Nori, Wakame, Hijiki, Sea Moss, Bladderwrack), Coconut, Coconut Oil, Olive Oil, Grapeseed Oil, Avocado Oil, Mushrooms, Quinoa, Wild Rice.

Items To Cut

Items listed in this section are geared towards avoiding the development of prostate cancer in the first place. However, removing these items will help to reduce the chances of this condition form spreading as well.

Saturated fats – these weaken the immune system and increase your risk of prostate cancer. Red meat, dairy products, and processed foods are the main items with these types of fat.

Coffee and alcohol irritate the prostate and hinder its strength and function.

Lycopene

A pigment called lycopene works to block free radicals that damage cells and help stimulate the immune system. Both of these benefits provide what someone needs who is battling prostate cancer. Dr. Robert Roundtree, M.D., co-founder of the Helios Health Center in Boulder, Colorado prescribes 1 teaspoon a day of tomato paste for his patients with prostate cancer. The reason he does this is because the pigment lycopene is abundant in tomatoes. Dr.

Roundtree notes that, "Lycopene has more potent antioxidant properties than beta-carotene, and it has anti-cancer properties." Oxidative stress (imbalance of free radicals) remains the primary cause of depleting lycopene from the body.

Common Sources of Lycopene: tomatoes, watermelon, papaya, pink guava, and pink grapefruit.

Isoflavones

Isoflavones are anti-cancer phytochemicals that inhibit a biochemical response that can cause cancerous cells to dissolve. It is recommended to consume two 70-milligrams tablets with each meal for those with prostate cancer ranging from about 300-400 milligrams a day of isoflavones.

Common Sources of Isoflavones: currants, raisins, chickpeas-garbanzo beans, and herbs such as alfalfa, hops, thyme, and the verbena species.

Damiana (herb)

This herb is known for boosting libido and sexual organs but can help increase the body's ability to utilize testosterone and strengthen the prostate. Drink this herb as a tea twice a day. Take 2 teaspoons and make as a 10-12-ounce tea twice a day for best results.

Rattlesnake

The rattlesnake (dried) and meat has been used in some cultures to treat various cancers; primarily the Asian Sand Viper and the South American Rattlesnake (RDB) according to researchers at the Jinnah University for Women in Pakistan, and the Red Diamondback Rattlesnake in Arizona, USA, according to researchers at Wright State University in Ohio, USA, who've researched snake venom being a treatment for various illness including cancer.

Researchers at the Jinnah University for Women in Pakistan have researched proteins such as, "eristostatin" and "contortrostatin" that have been found in the venoms of Asian sand viper and South American rattlesnake respectively have the ability to fight against cancers. "Mambalgins" (from the venom of black mamba) are believed to have analgesic and anti-inflammatory effects as well which can prevent cancer from spreading.

Prostate Problems

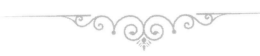

One of the more common problems for men involving the prostate is, frequent need for urination (particularly at nighttime). Frequent urination is often an early sign of diabetes, but this is usually throughout the day along with several other signs and symptoms involving blood sugar. The prostate gland is located directly beneath the bladder and is responsible for producing most of the fluids that are in semen. The prostate begins as the size of a pea until it begins to grow during puberty when testosterone levels rise. When a man reaches his middle 40's the prostate may begin growing once again due to hormonal changes and can lead to a condition called "benign prostatic hyperplasia" (BPH) or more commonly known as, an enlarged prostate. Those with an enlarged prostate are at risk for additional prostate-related issues as they get older. Most men don't experience any additional problems, but with many others, the prostate begins to press against the urethra (the tube that urine passes through). This leads to feeling stimulated to urinate, along with many other urinary-related issues.

Many other men will develop a condition known as prostatitis when the prostate gland becomes inflamed. This condition impact nearly 50% of men which can range from symptoms such as, pain after ejaculation, frequent burning, to severe back pain, and blood in the semen. Regardless of the severity of symptoms, there are steps outlined in this section to help begin the process of alleviating many of these symptoms as you work towards healing any issues impacting the prostate.

Remedies:

Saw Palmetto

The berry extract of this palm tree is widely used to treat BPH. Compounds in this plant helps to lower the DHT (dihydrotestosterone) a metabolite of the hormone testosterone. "High levels of DHT as associated with an enlarged prostate" says Dr. Winston Craig, R.D.,

Ph.D., professor of nutrition at Andrews University in Berien Spring, Michigan. Dr. Craig recommends two to three 50-milligram capsules a day f saw palmetto extract.

African Pygeum

Several European studies have found this fruit of the African evergreen tree effective for diminishing inflammation in the prostate. Dr. Craig states that, "The active extract seems to reduce symptoms of frequent nighttime urination and difficulty urinating." Standard dosage is usually 10-20 milligrams a day in capsule form.

Nettle Root (herb)

This plant in extract form also has anti-inflammatory properties that befit men with BPH according to Dr. Craig. You may take no more than six 30-miligram capsules a day and can take in combination with saw palmetto.

Zinc and Copper

Zinc is essential to the production of semen. A deficiency of this mineral can set the stage for prostate problems. It is recommended to take about 30-milligrams a day of zinc. However, it is important to note that copper and zinc together can create an imbalance, even when taking zinc for a long period of time. it is recommended to consume zinc, but also 2-milligrams of copper regularly as well to avoid any imbalances.

Common Sources of Zinc: chickpeas, mushrooms, zucchini, squash, okra, Brazil nuts, and walnuts.

Common Sources of Copper: blackberries, blueberries, guava, apricots, bananas, leafy green vegetables, avocado, sunflower seeds, mushrooms, spring onions, and you can also drink sparingly from a copper vessel/bottle.

Lycopene

This pigment, which is very abundant in tomatoes (responsible for their red color) can relieve symptoms of prostate issues and prevent the progression of prostate cancer. When cooked in some sort of oil, lycopene is essentially multiplied which helps increase the protection of the prostate.

Common Sources of Lycopene: tomatoes, watermelon, papaya, pink guava, and pink grapefruit.

Stand Up During Breaks

Men who have jobs and careers where they sit a lot, they are at an increased risk of BPH and prostate problem due to the constant pressure forced upon the prostate by sitting. Making time to stand up more often will increase circulation in the body, particularly the abdomen and legs. Whenever you are on break, spend a few minutes standing up, or make time to go for a brisk walk after working all day.

Exercise

Elizabeth Platz, Sc.D., assistant professor in the department of epidemiology at Johns Hopkins University Bloomberg School of Public Health in Baltimore, Maryland has studied more than 30,000 participants in various studies and states that, "Men who exercise more are less likely to have symptoms of BPH." She found that men were almost 41% less likely to developing BPH symptoms by exercising more as compared those who did not exercise, in which they were 42% more likely to develop BPH and more severe symptoms. Walking was the most common form of exercise used in these research studies and Dr. Platz recommends a minimum of 2-hours a week dedicated to light to moderate exercise.

Stop Smoking Cigarettes

Men who smoke cigarettes are 35% more likely to developing BPH symptoms than those who do not smoke, according to Dr. Platz.

Wear Looser Briefs

You want to wear briefs that are not tight and restrictive to not disrupt blood flow to the area. Many times, our undergarments trap sweat and does not allow the skin to breathe. Accumulation of toxins on the skin in an area just above the prostate can negatively impact this gland.

Bathroom Stool

Get a small stool to place your feet onto when using the toilet to defecate. The position it will place your digestive tract and more importantly, your prostate, will allow you to pass stools much easier. When we sit at an almost 90-degree angle, our anal muscles squeeze and contract closer together which places an enormous amount of pressure on the prostate. Sometimes frequent straining can damage the prostate long-term and create other health issues.

Damiana (herb)

This herb is known for boosting libido and sexual organs but can help increase the body's ability to utilize testosterone and strengthen the prostate. Drink this herb as a tea twice a day. Take 2 teaspoons and make as a 10-12-ounce tea twice a day for best results.

Psoriasis

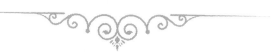

Typically, skin cells renew themselves every 30 days or so. When these skin cells renew themselves after just a few days (the time it takes for a new skin cell to make its way to the surface), the skin becomes irritated, itchy, and develop raised area in the skin. This sequence of events is known as psoriasis. Skin cells usually die off like any other group of cells in the body but, because there are so many cells in the skin, these raised areas in the skin (plaques) turn white as they have dead cells flaking off. This condition goes through cycle of flare ups where the skin can turn red and become itchier, particularly during colder weather. Medical doctors often treat this condition with topical skin creams and lotion and prescription medications, but all of these only cover up the visible sign of psoriasis. These items more often make this condition worse as they interact with the bloodstream once they are in contact with the body and essentially add interest to this condition by disrupting the normal sequence of skin cells renewing themselves.

Psoriasis originates within the intestinal tract. It directly coincides with intestinal permeability ("leaky gut syndrome"). The walls of the small intestine become thin and permeable which allow toxins such as fats, bacteria, acids, and developing yeast) to enter the bloodstream which ordinarily would have been removed by the digestive tract. The body tries to eliminate these toxins via the sweat glands, but as they come into contact with the skin, they turn into legions and irritable skin until a psoriasis diagnosis is made.

In this section we will review ways to cope and work to prevent this condition from occurring and/or re-occurring.

Remedies:

"Stewed" Fruits

Stewed fruit is when fruit is slightly cooked in liquid until it begins to gel together. Ordinarily fruit does not need to be cooked as it is best in its natural form but, for a condition like psoriasis, we want to help clean the gut without losing vital nutrients. Slowly cooking fruits (sparingly) can help create a laxative effect that will help clean the bowels while providing adequate fiber so that vital nutrients are lost in the process. You will want to eat a serving or two a day every few days then take 2-3 days off, then repeat.

Fruits To Use: apples, figs, raisins, pears, peaches, apricots, and prunes.

Water

Immediately upon awakening drink some water. Moisten up your organs and prepare your body to be prepared for cleansing activity. Drink two 8-ounce glasses of water.

Exercise

Exercise stimulates circulation, sends oxygen to the blood, opens up your pours, and filters blood through the liver and kidneys. Exercise is a great fundamental way of opening up the "channels" within the body to promote the removal of toxins in the body. About 30-minutes a day of aerobic exercise daily will be best. Walking, swimming, cycling, and/or jogging are some of the simplest ways to get your 30-minutes a day in.

Olive Oil

Rub some olive oil onto any legions you see to help moisturize the skin without irritating it. Don't be concerned if the legions do not appear to change much after adding olive oil this step is just geared towards hydrating the skin while the real work is to be completed internally.

Avoid Deodorants

Aside from the high aluminum content, deodorants block (and even clog up) the sweat glands and pours and prevent the normal elimination of toxins through the skin. For those with psoriasis, blocking elimination creates accumulation, which will turn into and make already existing lesions worse.

Hydrotherapy

Taking a bath will help soothe the nerve ending and help clean off any debris that may be on your skin that you did not clean off thoroughly when showering in fear of tearing the skin or causing more irritation.

Avoiding Saturated and Hydrogenated Fats

Saturated and hydrogenated fats cause excess inflammation. These fats are in red meats, processed foods, and items such as butter and margarine.

No Nightshade Vegetables

A plant-based lifestyle is recommended for any condition as it provides many necessary minerals and nutrients without the harmful items such as fats, artificial sugars, and other things detrimental to our health. However, nightshade vegetables for those with psoriasis, nightshade vegetables contain alkaloid compounds (cause physiological changes in the body) that can be harmful and increase irritation. We essentially, are trying to create a "new self" by reversing this condition, but due to the fact that the skin cells are already replicating much faster than what is typical, we do not want to add to this and want to instead, gear our focus on cleaning out what's already there.

*Common Nightshade Vegetables (**To Avoid**): tomatoes (are the worst), eggplant, peppers, paprika, white potatoes.*

No Junk

Not that junk food items are technically "food", these should be avoided as they will add interest to the irritation due to be made primarily of toxins and chemicals. Soda, chips, candies, pies and pastries should be avoided. Remove shellfish, alcohol, and processed foods that cook coconut oil or palm oil as these irritants will make symptoms worse and get in the way of your healing journey.

Slippery Elm (herb)

This herb helps to coat the inner lining of the digestive tract to protect it during the healing process. Take ½ teaspoon of powder (dried herb can deteriorate quickly after picked) into a cup of war, water. Let cool for 15 minutes then stir together. After drinking this do not eat for at least 30-minutes to 1-hour to allow this herb to make contact with your intestines uninterrupted. Do this every other day.

Yellow Saffron (flower)

This flower when consumed in tea form helps to heal the intestines while also flushing the liver and kidneys. Take ¼ teaspoon of saffron into a cup, add boiling water, and let cool for 15 minutes. If you begin urinating excessively or experience symptoms of a bladder infection, stop use and drink warm water instead.

Oregon Grape Root (herb)

This herb helps to fight bacteria to reduce lesions and skin issues. Look for the extract of this plant so it can better assimilate into the body as compared to capsules or tea which must be digested first. Follow instructions on label.

Sunlight

In studies tracking how sunlight impact those with psoriasis, results show that 95% of people show improvement regarding a decrease in symptoms. Psoriasis patients tend to experience more difficult challenges in the winter or in colder climates. Spend at least 30-minutes in direct sunlight daily. Just remain cautious of avoiding a sunburn so you do not have additional skin issue.

Stress

Stress triggers psoriasis. Any absence from daily stress will remain helpful. Find a consistent, healthy way you can relieve stress and make it a priority to do daily or whenever possible. You may want to meditate, read a book, stretch, or sleep if possible. Anything that you can commit to doing regularly will add up over time and your body will thank you.

Rashes

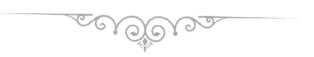

Everyday our bodies come into contact with many materials that can irritate the skin. Other times, we may consume or rub our skin against materials that create a rash or develop a rash due to allergens. Regardless of how we get a rash, the skin is sending a message to you stating that it is not happy with something and that it will remain until something is fixed.

Most common allergens for rashes:

Urushiol – an oil that is in poisonous plants such as poison ivy, oak, and sumac.

Rubber – found in products such as latex gloves, shoes, elastic waistbands, and rubber bands.

Nickle – metal found in costume jewelry, cookware, or mixed with other metals we come in contact with such as coins, belt buckles, and zippers.

Chromate – chemical that is in home products such as paint, and cleaning materials.

Preservatives and fragrances found in hand creams and lotions.

Dairy – animal's milk but often components such as casein, caseinate, lactose, sodium caseinate, and whey that can create a rash by irritating the body and eventually the skin itself.

Neomycin – ingredient in many over-the-counter medications, prescription creams, ointments, lotions, ear drops, and eyedrops.

Ethylenediamine – preservative added to creams.

Sodium silicate, sodium phosphate, sodium carbonate – often found in many laundry detergents and fabric softeners.

Remedies:

Change Your Jewelry

If you are having a rash around the areas you notice a rash, you may have a reaction to nickel. Change your jewelry to alleviate this issue and/or find out if your jewelry is the cause of your rash. Make sure to not sweat while wearing jewelry to avoid irritating your skin (even if there's no rash). If it is within your budget and price range, getting gold can be best as there are no concerns about gold irritating the skin. Dr. Larry Millikan, M.D., chairman of the department of dermatology at Tulane University Medical Center in New Orleans, Louisiana states, "I've never heard of anyone who's allergic to pure gold."

Wear Gloves (and wash your hands)

Chromate, a chemical found in household products, paint, and other items are very common ways to attract a rash. Since we use our hands the most when cleaning or using any specific products or painting, it is best to wear gloves to avoid any direct contact or irritating the skin. Washing your hands will further ensure that nothing was left in your skin.

Use Lighters

Some matches contain chromate where touching the match can irritate the skin. Matches are often placed on a countertop or in your pockets which can add to your risk the next time you reach into your pockets for something or leave something on the countertop. Use a lighter instead if you are someone who smokes.

Read Labels

If you see any of the ingredients listed in the introduction part of this section, put it back on the shelf and do without. You want to avoid anything that contains a lot of chemicals. As you notice improvements while avoiding specific ingredients, remain consistent with these changes.

Gloves

If you notice regular rashes on your hands or arms, try changing out you rubber gloves for vinyl gloves as a substitute. Powderless rubber gloves can be less allergenic but work to avoid rubber gloves if they appear to be giving you issues.

Check Your Shoes

Besides probably containing rubber, there are many other materials used in shoes that interact with the rubber that may cause issues. Items like leather, adhesives, and dyes can cause a reaction that results in a rash. Hypoallergenic shoes can be difficult to find but may be a suitable option for you if your shoes are giving you problems.

Echinacea (herb)

Mix 1-part echinacea tincture with 3 parts of distilled water and rinse your infected area(s) several times a day to soothe itching and reduce inflammation.

Chickweed (herb)

Get 1 cup of fresh chickweed herb (8 ounces)

Wrap herb in cheesecloth and crush it with a rolling pin until you have finely grained everything

Fill jar with crushed herb. Add sunflower oil to cover the chickweed with at least ½ inch of oil at the top of the jar.

Label jar with ingredients and date, and place in a cool, dark place for 2 weeks.

After 2 weeks, use a paper coffee filter and strain the oil.

Pour oil into a glass bottle and store in refrigerator. Should last about 6 weeks

Saturate oil onto a compress and place cloth over the injured area for 15-20 minutes once a day (make sure injured area is no longer open).

My Personal Remedy:

1 small scoop of bentonite clay (mix with water until it forms a thick goo.

Add 1/4 - 1/2 teaspoon of powdered Oregon grape root to mixture and 1 drop of lavender essential oil

Spread this mixture over the infected area to dry up blisters and control the itch. Remove when it begins to wear off or gets itchy once again.

Poison Plant Rashes

About 85% of people are susceptible to becoming allergic and getting a rash from coming in direct contact with poison ivy, oak, or sumac.

First step is being able to properly identify each of these items:

Poison Ivy – contain clusters of three shiny leaves together ("leaves of three, let it be"). Poison Ivy most often grows as a vine or shrub, but always has hairs on its trunk/base.

Poison Oak – this also can be a high-climbing vine or shrub. It has notches in its leaves and grows berries in clusters. This plant is green in the summer and white in the winter, poison oak also mostly grows in the western or southeastern states in the USA.

Poison Sumac – this plant contains stems that have 7 to 13 leaflets. Sprouts green berries in the summertime that turn yellow-white in the winter. Mostly found in the northern states in the USA and deep southern states. Even during the winter, when this plant has no leaves, the plant's bark and roots remain poisonous.

Wash Off Well

Water is your best remedy when noticing a rash, especially a poisonous one. Rinse and wash the entire area well. Soap and other products are unnecessary as water is what inactivates urushiol (poisonous compound in poisonous plants). "Alcohol followed by water is the best treatment" says Dr. William L. Epstein, professor emeritus of dermatology at the University of California, San Francisco, School of Medicine. Make sure to not use any washcloths as you will just spread the poisonous chemicals. If you do not have any alcohol to use, then use whatever you have that's close to it such as baby wipes. It is also a good idea to clean everything you can such as your clothes after you've been in contact with a poisonous plant.

Baking Soda (or Zinc Oxide)

May not feel as soothing as calamine lotion but can be just as effective.

Cover With A Compress

Place a cotton cloth soaked in cool water over the entire rash and let a fan or cool air blow over it. The cooling effect can provide similar relief to most lotions.

Colloidal Oatmeal

This substance works to dry up oozing blisters. Apply this onto area with a cloth or use it in a bath. Products have step-by-step instructions to follow as well.

Jewelweed (herb)

You cut a slit in the stem of this herb and put the juice from it onto the rash. Botanist James A. Duke, Ph.D., taught herbal healing at the Tai Sophia Institute in Columbia, Maryland, and use to work for the Agricultural Research Service of the USDA, states, "I ball up this whole plant and make sort of a washrag out of it and wipe the poison sap off." This plant may be difficult to find in a health food or local herbal store. However, it is simple to locate if you know what you're looking for. This orange species blooms from June to September in moist, shaded areas. If you cannot find this plant close to you, you can order a 4 ounce bottle of this by sending a written letter to Rainbow's End Herbals, 514 Gidsville Road, Amherst, VA, 24521 or find their product online at http://www.greenpeople.org/listing/Rainbow-s-End-Herbals-24412.cfm?lckeyword=jewelweed

Raynaud's Phenomenon

This condition involves a decreased blood flow to the fingers (also the hands, toes, nose, and ears). The result is constant coldness and pain. What occurs in this condition, is that blood vessels constrict blood flow to the extremities and a spasm occurs. Over time, the condition can impair the ability to touch and have weakened fingers and hands.

Note: About 5%-10% of those with Raynaud's Phenomenon are those who put forth damage to the blood vessels through vibration from power tools such as chain saws or drills. Many others are a result of various medications.

Remedies:

U.S. Army Remedy

This technique helps to train your hands to heat up in the cold. Place yourself in a room with temperature that's comfortable for you and place your hands into a container of warm water for 3-5 minutes. Then dry off your hands and go into a cold rom and dip your hands again in the container of warm water, but for 10 minutes this time. The colder environment typically causes our blood vessels to constrict, but the warm water forces the blood vessels to open.

Arm Movements

Donald McIntyre, M.D., retired dermatologist in Rutland, Vermont would have clients pretend to be a baseball pitcher by swinging their arm behind their back (downwards), and then upward in front of your body. do this for about 80 twirls a minute. This windmill effect, according to Dr. McIntyre, forces blood to the fingers through both, gravitational and centrifugal force.

Load Up On Iron

Iron deficiency alters your thyroid's metabolism which is responsible for regulating your body heat. In a study conducted by the USDA Human Nutrition Research Center in Grand Forks, North Dakota, they measured the effects of iron and its connection to body heat. They found that those who only took 1/3 of the recommended amount of iron for 80 days, lost 29% more body heat than when they were on an iron-rich diet for 114 days.

Common Sources of Iron: Wild rice, chickpeas/garbanzo beans, dandelion greens, sarsaparilla, burdock, yellow dock, chapparal, and prunes.

Eating Filling Meals

The act of eating sets forth a rise in body temperature as items are being digested and sent in all directions to be either absorbed or filtered out of the body. this process is known as thermogenesis. Eat something before you get moving to help the body remain relatively warm to combat some of the symptoms you may experience with Raynaud's Phenomenon.

Hydration

If you are even relatively dehydrated, this can aggravate chills by reducing the blood's volume. You want to hydrate by eating fresh fruits every day, and consuming about ½ your bodyweight in ounces on days you don't eat as much fruit.

Avoid Caffeine

Caffeine restricts the blood vessels. This is never helpful. You do not want to interfere with your blood circulation if you have this condition.

Avoid Alcohol

Drinking alcohol increases blood flow to the skin, giving the temporary appearance that your body is getting warm. But what actually happens is that the body feels warmer when blood is sent to the skin, but this causes the warmth to evaporate and inevitably makes you colder. If you drank an excess amount of alcohol and was suddenly placed in the cold, severe issues such as hypothermia or frostbite can settle in.

Dress Appropriately

We often attempt to dress warmer than we need to when it's cold out. This causes us to sweat, where the heat evaporates and leaves the body. It is important to choose correct fabrics when out in the cold. Polypropylene, a synthetic fabric can be used instead of wool for items such as socks for example. The key is to remain warm without sweating. Making sure your clothing is somewhat loose allowing for air to pass through, but also trap the warmth (air pockets) that is produced by the body for a longer period of time.

Wear A Good Hat

This is often a missing piece to keeping warm. Much of our warmth is stored in our heads. The blood vessels in our head will not appear to restrict like the blood vessels in our hands and feet will and can go completely unnoticed.

Wear Mittens

These are a better option of keeping hands warm as opposed to gloves which only attempt to keep one finger warm at a time. Mittens work to keep the whole hand warm at the same time.

Foot Powder

Using a foot powder can be a helpful way to keeping your feet dry. Many powders are often used for conditions like athlete's foot because they prevent moisture. The same concept is helpful here with this condition.

Avoid Cigarettes

Cigarette smoke forms plaque around your heart arteries. Nicotine (the addictive ingredient0 causes spasms that narrow the blood vessels and restrict the amount of blood available to keep your hands and feet warm. Dr. Frederick A. Reichle, M.D., former chief of vascular surgery at Presbyterian University of Pennsylvania Medical Center in Philadelphia, Pennsylvania notes that "Raynaud's patients are sensitive even to other people's smoke."

Calm Yourself

Being stressed, nervous, or unsettled can create the traditional "fight or fight" response where blood is pulled from the hands and feet to the brain and internal organs to enable you to think and react quickly. This can produce the same effects as the body remaining in the cold. To avoid this, you want to remain calm. Relaxation techniques such as deep breathing or forcing tension in the form of "progressive relaxation" that involves you creating tension for the muscles and the release. You clench or tighten certain muscles such as the muscles in your head, jaw, hands, and/or toes, followed by a release to allow these areas to relax.

Repetitive Strain Injury (RSI)

Repetitive strain injury (RSI) is a condition where inflammation and injury in some part of the upper extremities, fingers, hands, wrists, forearms, shoulders, or elbows. This condition is caused by repetitive action using these specific body parts. RSI is referred to as a "cumulative microtrauma" as it can be the result of a combination of many activities such as, typing on a keyboard, clicking buttons on your phone, cutting your hair or items with scissors – over and over again, frequently.

Remedies:

Modifications

Identify ways to make specific things in your life easier. Use voice-command options on things like your cell phone where you can talk-to-text, type notes, or make things like your grocery list. Save certain websites on your home page or desktop so you can just click to save time and energy typing. And make sure to ask for help whenever it's needed.

Posture

Keeping correct posture can help reduce many symptoms such as chronic aches and pains. Make sure to not strain yourself too much trying to force yourself to keeping a good posture. Visit a local chiropractor and get an adjustment/alignment or target specific areas that are most in need.

Stretching

Keep a standard of taking a break every 30 minutes or so to stretch your fingers, wrists, or any area in need. Always make time to stretch your neck side to side, and up and down to avoid any leaning in one direction which can influence the rest of your body to lean on these areas of weakness or cause more stress to them.

Wear Gloves

When the hands are warmer, they are able to function well and work better without hindrance. Get a pair of wool gloves that leave the fingers open to use. During your day, take a moment every so often and placed your hand on your cheek to see if any part of your hand is cold. If so, put your glove on and continue working.

Gingko Biloba (herb)

This herb helps to improve circulation in the body, particularly the extremities such as the hands and fingers. Dr. Robert E. Markison, M.D., a hand surgeon in San Francisco, California, recommends 60mg once a day with 16 ounces of water so this herb is properly absorbed into the body.

Water

Proper hydration is key as you want liquids in your system. We often don't drink nearly enough water that we need. Aiming towards drinking about half of your body weight in ounces will help steer you in the right direction. Consuming foods with high water content is highly recommend as well. A well hydrated body promotes a stronger circulation it the body and makes it easier to send vital nutrients into areas in need, according to Dr. Markison.

Cut The Caffeine

Caffeine is a diuretic which drains water from your body. less water equals a poorer blood circulation which leads to more frequent and severe symptoms of RSI.

Nicotine and Alcohol

Nicotine is necessary to remove for those with RSI. Dr. Markison states that, "A single puff of nicotine (from cigarettes) can shut down blood flow to the hands by as much as 60 percent." Alcohol increases inflammation which worsens areas of RSI.

Vegetable Juice

A glass a day (10 or more ounces) of a vegetable juice provides an assortment of powerful antioxidants, essential nutrients, and helps to break down inflammation in the body. Get creative with making juices with items such as dandelion greens, kale, cucumbers, and adding amount of cilantro. A consistent vegetable juice can provide more than a prescription pill that is given to break down inflammation.

Weight

Anyone who is 20-30 pounds above relatively ideal weight can quadruple their chances of developing RSI and/or RSI symptoms. Any additional crowding of fat in the body will create excess inflammation. Refer to the "Overweight" section in this book for suggestions on how to begin decreasing overall size and weight.

Stress Reduction

Stress reduces blood flow to the extremities. This worsens conditions such as RSI. Try visualization techniques and even guided meditations to help reduce any built-up stress that has remained present in your life.

Restless Legs Syndrome

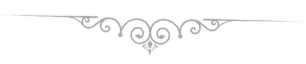

This condition feels like an electrical current flowing through the legs, according to members of the Restless Leg Syndrome Foundation. Restless leg syndrome (also known as "Ekbom syndrome") tends to be a chronic annoyance rather than a symptom to a larger developing issue. It is most common for the entire lower body to be affected, but one leg/limb can experience this condition by itself as well.

Restless Leg Syndrome essentially comes down to an imbalance in the brain's chemistry, instability with the body's iron metabolism, and genetics can play a role.

Remedies:

Iron Deficiency

"Iron deficiency may be the cause of restless leg syndrome" says Dr. Ronald F. Pfeiffer, M.D., professor, vice chairperson, and director in the department of neurology at the University of Tennessee Health Science Center in Memphis. Dr. Pfeiffer sites many research studies pointing to a strong connection between iron deficiency and restless leg syndrome.

Common Sources of Iron: Wild rice, chickpeas/garbanzo beans, dandelion greens, sarsaparilla, burdock, yellow dock, chapparal, dates, and prunes.

Items that rob you of iron:

- chocolate
- cow's milk
- coffee (yes, decaffeinated coffee too and those weight loss coffees as well)
- soda
- yeast

- artificial sugars and food dyes
- foods high in oxalic acids ("oxalates") such as, cauliflower, broccoli, spinach, soy, potatoes, dates, raspberries, navy beans, cashews, and baked potatoes with skin (baked potatoes, French fries, etc). Oxalates deplete and interfere with iron absorption.
- losing blood (this can happen during cycles but not replacing and replenishing your iron when this happens is the issue).

If you choose to implement Iron supplements into your lifestyle, understand that Ferrous Sulfate will not properly provide you with what you need. *Ferrous Gluconate, Iron Gluconate,* and *Iron Picolinate* digest and absorb much easier into the body as compared to Ferrous Sulfate and should be sought out within the ingredient labels on products. It is strongly recommended to incorporate more natural items such as those listed above, however, everyone can be at different stages in their journey.

Stop Eating After 8pm

This is more of a headline to catch your attention. 8pm is not the specific time to stop as there's nothing too special about this time aside from this being a few hours before most will go to bed. You want to avoid digesting things later at night as this can interfere with your sleep. According to Dr. Lawrence Z. Stern, M.D., professor of neurology at the University of Arizona College of Medicine in Tucson, "It may be the activity of digesting a big meal that triggers something that causes symptoms."

Avoid Sleep Meds

Sleeping meds make it easier to relying on them and you build up a tolerance quickly to them over time. These medications contain chemicals that mimic what actually goes on inside of your brain when you are going to sleep which add (and creates) the chemical imbalances that occur in the brain which contribute to the symptoms of restless legs syndrome.

Cut The Caffeine

Dr. Pfeiffer states, "Some studies have shown an association between relief of restless legs syndrome and stopping caffeine." Caffeine decreases oxygen delivery to the brain and add onto the imbalances of the brain's chemistry and disrupts blood flow needed to avoid symptoms of restless legs syndrome.

Avoid Cold and Sinus Meds

"These have been reported to increase the symptoms" according to the Restless Legs Syndrome Foundation.

Give Up Smoking

In a study at the University of Kentucky College of Medicine involving more than 1,800 participants, smokers were significantly more likely to develop restless legs syndrome than those who did not smoke. Many participants experienced relief of symptoms after one month of not smoking and remained symptom free after several months of not smoking.

Massage Your Legs

Keeping your legs stimulated can relieve symptoms and work to preventing you from experiencing this condition. Before bed make time to massage your legs and do some light stretching.

Walk Before Bed

"Exercise changes chemical balances in the brain – endorphins are released – and may promote more restful sleep" says Dr. Stern. Even if it's close to your bedtime and you feel the urge to move, satisfy this urge as it will help alleviate symptoms from settling in.

Reduce Stress

Stress creates instability and irritableness within the body. These feelings support triggering symptoms of restless legs syndrome. Make some time for yourself, practice some deep breathing techniques, and work on ways of reducing stress before you go to sleep.

Soak Your Feet In Water

Try to immerse your feet in cold (not freezing or frigid) for about 8-10 minutes then dry your feet off. If this is helpful, make it a part of your bedtime routine. Note: if it's helpful do not try to do more by immersing your feet in ice or anything colder than what is helpful as this could lead to other issues. If cold water does not work, try this same method with warm water. Some people prefer cold water, while others may feel better after using warm water. Find what works better for you and make it a habit.

Road Rage

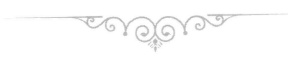

This condition may not seem like an issue in need for treatment or remedy, but it is an everyday issue that evokes stress, anger, and frustration that we can do without. Road rage can be described as, the deliberate, criminal attempt to hurt someone, or have an intent to follow through (or respond to) a threat with acts of violence. Road rage is responsible for 28,000 deaths in the USA each year. While most may not specifically identify with committing acts of road rage, many are aggressive drivers.

In a survey covering most states in the USA, results showed that 80% of drivers considered others to be aggressive drivers, while only 30% admitted they drive aggressively. This shows that about 50% of drivers don't even realize they're aggressive drivers. Most often only view their driving as "aggressive" based upon their own preferred levels of risk upon others. For example, those who tailgate or honk their horn the second a green light is shown at a traffic stop may feel that others are too slow.

We tend to dehumanize one another once we get behind the wheel. We see the car and know a person is driving, but do not view them as an equal person and remove any feelings of concern or compassion. We even look to process who's to blame first when there's an accident. In this section, we will review ways to work towards eliminating these added frustrations by focusing on ourselves and keeping things in the proper perspective while on the road.

Remedies:

Help Someone Out

We can often tell who's in a rush or may be new to driving while we are on the road. Try making some space for them to change lanes, get ahead of you, or take a turn first. When you take time to help support another driver, your stress decreases and your mind is able to not focus on your developing frustration(s). To know we helped contribute to avoiding an accident or allowed someone to become the victim of road rage is a relief as well.

Try The Right Lane

Most avoid driving in the right lane as they feel they will arrive at their destination much slower. Research show that driving in one of the fast lanes will get you to your location about 3-4 minutes sooner. Spending about 3-4 more additional minutes driving at a steady pace while avoiding any interactions with aggressive drivers may be worth it to help decrease your stress and deter your own aggressiveness if you are an aggressive driver.

Don't Give Others Fuel

When frustrated while driving you'll likely want to respond, but this will only escalate the situation. Getting called a name or having someone get close to harming your vehicle is no light issue, but once you notice what the other driver(s) are trying to do, this will remind you to relax and remain calm until they pass by.

Listen

We tend to ignore any complaints other people such as passengers may have about our driving. Maybe we pass it off as personal preferences, or we just don't want to hear any critiques. But it may be more beneficial to listen to some statements or points made by others as their concerns may be valid and can make you a better, safer driver.

Respect Your Passengers

Many drivers feels as if their passengers have to adhere to their personal rules and adjust to their driving. This can create issues when dealing with things such as road rage because the driver may feel a need to be "in charge" where they display this through driving aggressively. However, when you think of your passengers and their preferences, your anger and thought of acting on your frustrations can dissolve much easier during those moments of anger. You will be more prone to let things go and even distract yourself in the moment with conversation or sharing observations about aggressive drivers with your passengers, so that you do not act on your frustrations.

Avoid Honking When Not Needed

Honking has turned into a form of disrespect rather than an alert or sign of caution to other drivers. Make sure to only honk (lightly) when absolutely needed to avoid triggering other drivers and to avoid using as a tool to display your own frustration.

Teach The Children

Babies and toddlers learn a lot while in their car seat. It is of no surprise why many children play aggressively with toy cars from a very young age. Children may witness certain actions while in a car, but most often learn to use a car as a tool for themselves rather than understanding that they are sharing the road with many others. Also ask your children for help while in your car as they may remind you to do things such as put on your seatbelt, or even remind you of behaviors you've displays while driving. Sometimes the embarrassment and guilt you may feel from a child reminder you of unnecessary behaviors you displayed while driving can be enough to deter you from any aggressive driving.

Refreshing Scents

Tie some herbs to your dashboard or get some air fresheners that evoke calmness such as lavender, rosemary, or eucalyptus. You may also keep these fresh herbs in your car so as you drive, you are inhaling herbs that help you relax. Find the right scent that keeps you calm and add it to your car. You may also find a scent you enjoy that calms you that you can smell before you get into your car and drive.

*(Also refer to "Anger" section in this book)

Rosacea

Rosacea (pronounced "rose-AY-shah") is an inflammatory skin condition that often results I redness of the skin on the nose, cheeks, forehead, and chin. This skin condition impacts almost 14 million Americans and is most common with those who have a lighter skin complexion. The average doctor may assume it is an allergy or an acne issue. When this condition is left untreated or just treated as an allergy or an acne issue, the tiny blood vessels become more visible (redness), pimples develop more often, the nose may swell, and the eyes can remain watery or bloodshot. What is needed besides a correct diagnosis is to identify what things are triggering these flare-ups. In this section we will review what some common contributors that create flare-ups, while identifying simple ways to manage these flare-ups before they become worse.

Remedies:

Pick Your Time In The Sun

Heat can trigger symptoms, so you want to remain aware of when the heat begins to feel uncomfortable for you. Limit your time in direct sunlight until symptoms are more under control and stay in the shade whenever possible when outdoors. You want to make sure your cover your head the most as symptoms impact this area of your body the most.

Remove Alcohol From Your Lifestyle

Alcohol can bring upon some of the more severe symptoms and reactions. Flare-ups will occur quicker an often get worse over time as long as you consume alcohol.

Avoid Warm or Hot Beverages

Hot or warm beverages cause the face to flush more often as the heat can promote dehydration, even though it's a liquid. If you drink something like hot coffee, switch to a colder form. If symptoms and flare-ups continue, work to remove coffee altogether as caffeine may be your trigger ad not the warmth.

Keep Track Of Your Foods

Hot, spicy foods such as cayenne pepper can cause you to sweat internally (from heat), and this can immediately trigger flare-ups. Other foods such as avocados, chocolate, cheeses, beans, citrus fruits, eggplant, vinegar, yeast, spinach, cauliflower, and vanilla are common triggering foods as well. Dairy and foods that contain oxalates appear to be the foods that provide stronger triggers. Oxalates are acids that cannot be processed or passed through the urine. Consuming too many of these items can back up the kidneys and begin the process of storing these items, often leading to kidney stones. Many items that involve gene-splicing and combing two plants such as broccoli, eggplant, spinach, and cauliflower contain higher amounts of oxalates that interfere with how the body functions ad in turn, creates flare-ups.

Low-intensity Workouts

Exercise is always recommended, but pushing yourself very hard will exert your body closer to its physical limitations. Too much exertion can send the blood pumping quicker to the upper body and triggers symptoms that impact the face, neck, and head areas. Try to not strain yourself by doing any very difficult exercises or lifting too much weight.

Keep Cool

When exercising drink liquids regularly to not get too warm. You may also use a spray bottle to spray your face when working out or while at home to remain cool.

Completely Remove or Considerably Reduce Wearing Make-Up

While dealing with acne and skin blemishes many will try to offset these by wearing a contrasting color or foundation to reduce the appearance of any redness or scars from pimples. We don't want to try and cover up this issue as bad as we want to hide it until symptoms are better. Be prepared to make some necessary changes and lifestyle adjustments in order to achieve greater results than adding make-up which can aggravate flare-ups and prolong this condition.

Wear The Right Tones

As stated above, we don't want to hide these flare-ups by covering them up but, we can make adjustments that can support flare-ups not being so visible. If you were to wear a red, black, or white shirt, flare-ups would be very noticeable. Try wearing softer shades of blue, green, and yellow instead.

Work To Cleaning The Blood

Anytime you have a skin issue, there's an underlying blood issue. The blood goes everywhere in the body; it is sent closer towards the skin when flare-ups occur. You will want to incorporate many herbs that are high in iron-phosphate (from plants) and work to eliminate items such as white sugars, dyes, unhealthy fats, and starches from your diet to help promote a clean, steady blood flow.

Common Sources of Iron: Wild rice, chickpeas/garbanzo beans, dandelion greens, sarsaparilla, burdock, yellow dock, chapparal, and prunes.

Items that rob you of iron:

- chocolate
- cow's milk
- coffee (yes, decaffeinated coffee too and those weight loss coffees as well)
- soda
- yeast
- artificial sugars and food dyes
- foods high in oxalic acids ("oxalates") such as, cauliflower, broccoli, spinach, soy, potatoes, dates, raspberries, navy beans, cashews, and baked potatoes with skin (baked potatoes, French fries, etc). Oxalates deplete and interfere with iron absorption.
- losing blood (this can happen during cycles but not replacing and replenishing your iron when this happens is the issue).

If you choose to implement Iron supplements into your lifestyle, understand that Ferrous Sulfate will not properly provide you with what you need. Ferrous Gluconate, Iron Gluconate, and Iron Picolinate digest and absorb much easier into the body as compared to Ferrous Sulfate and should be sought out within the ingredient labels on products. It is strongly recommended to incorporate more natural items such as those listed above, however, everyone can be at different stages in their journey.

Shea Butter

Shea butter is great for evening out and moisturizing the skin. In various parts of Africa, a child will be scrubbed with shea butter daily (their entire body) for the first few months of their life to serve as a protection for the skin to help reduce chances of various illnesses. Shea butter can be found in stores, but you want to get it without the added chemicals and artificial ingredients for best results.

My Personal Remedy:

(You can increase the amount of shea butter, nopales, and batana oil to your desired texture. All other ingredients remain the same).

Shave off thorns or nopales and peel off skin. You can use one large or 2 medium sized nopales pads. Large should be considered larger than the size of your opened hand. Blend together or place into food processor.

Add 2oz of burdock root to boiling water. Cook for 8-10 minutes, then let steep until cooled off.

Add nopales, burdock (tea), ½ cup shea butter, 8 drops of chamomile oil, and add a small scoop or batana oil and mix together thoroughly. Apply as much as you feel is needed directly onto skin twice a day.

Scarring

Scar tissue(s) are the skin's new connective tissue that have been formed after there has been damage afflicted to the skin. This could be from a cut, a wound, or from some form of surgery. Every time the skin gets cut a scar will form. Scar tissue works to repair and regenerate the skin cells and surrounding parts, but they can present additional issues during the healing process. Scars that are not properly cared for, can create keloids which are large, hard growths on the surface of the skin. Keloids can be essentially harmless, but can become itchy, sensitive to touch, and become unsightly. Scars from surgery can form an adhesion where the tissue binds with other tissues which can create pain and limit movement. In this section we will review ways to properly care for any scars to promote fully recovery.

Remedies:

Don't Pick Your Scabs

This not only prolongs your healing but increases the size and severity of your scar.

Lavender Essential Oil

Immediately flowing an injury, place a few drops of (undiluted) lavender essential oil onto the skin. This will prevent excess scarring. For best results, clean area by washing first, then pat to dry before adding essential oil and then cover area with a sterile pad.

Massage

Particularly after stitches have been removed, more damaged cells will be in need of repair. Once stitches have been removed and incision is closed, begin gently massaging this area to help stimulate blood flow and repair to the area. Massages will help to prevent adhesions. Use your fingers (not fingertips, but where your fingerprints are) and gently massage he skin tissue around your scar. Normal skin tissue will move easily in all directions, but where there's an adhesion, the skin tissues will provide resistance where you do not want to pull hard against; just continue to press gently around the area to help decrease tension and resistance again. You should be able to notice slight improvements over the course of a few weeks when massaging the area and later on notice even more significant improvements as you continue your massages.

Chickweed (herb)

When a wound begins to heal, it will create a crust (or scab) that covers the incision to protect it from outside bacteria and other materials. Chickweed helps to soften the area that will scab over to keep the scarring to a minimum. If you have a scab and scratch or accidentally rub against something, it can tear the skin more and add to a deeper scar. To use this herb, you will need to do the following:

- Get 1 cup of fresh chickweed herb (8 ounces)
- Wrap herb in cheesecloth and crush it with a rolling pin until you have finely grained everything.
- Fill jar with crushed herb.
- Add sunflower oil to cover the chickweed with at least ½ inch of oil at the top of the jar.
- Label jar with ingredients and date, and place in a cool, dark place for 2 weeks,
- After 2 weeks, use a paper coffee filter and strain the oil.
- Pour oil into a glass bottle and store in refrigerator. Should last about 6 weeks
- Saturate oil onto a compress and place cloth over the injured area for 15-20 minutes once a day (make sure injured area is no longer open).

You may also use this remedy for rashes, boils, and eczema.

St. John's Wort (herb)

Keloids can become an uncomfortable nuisance. To reduce this discomfort, you can use St. John's Wort oil. This herb is an antiseptic and an analgesic; meaning it prevents growth and relieves pain. Follow instructions on label but you can use this 1-2 times day and use as long as you like.

Zinc

The body uses Zinc to breakdown bacteria in the body and helps strengthen the immune system. Wounds heal faster when there's adequate zinc in the body according to Beverly Yates, N.D., physician and director of the Natural Health Care Group located in Seattle,

Washington. Loading up on this necessary mineral will help relieve you of your potential scarring.

Common Sources of Zinc: chickpeas, mushrooms, zucchini, squash, okra, Brazil nuts, and walnuts.

*Zinc: 15 milligrams a day within diet is recommended

Shower Gently

Sweat glands, oil glands, and hair glands are all destroyed by scarring. A larger scar can take up many of the nutrients and oils the skin has available which can take it away from other areas of your skin, leaving it susceptible to abrasions or other skin-related issues such as dryness, acne, sunburn, or rosacea, among other conditions. When we shower, we wash away many of these natural oils and clean the skin from head to toe. We want to avoid pulling off any scabs or brushing the skin too harshly in other areas as the skin where there is no scarring may become more sensitive at this time. Be particularly careful using any washcloths or brushes.

Frankincense Oil

This oil can help fade scars that you have. Follow directions on label. Most labels will state no more than 4 drops a day of this oil to apply and gently rub into skin a day.

Hemp Cream

There are many CBD oil and creams out there that can provide adequate results. To simplify, you can get some hemp-based cream to apply to affected area and use as instructed. Participants in a research study published in the La Clinica Terapeutica Journal, tracked 20 participants who applied CBD-enriched ointment to scarred areas of skin twice a day for three months. After three months, researchers found that the CBD ointment significantly improved the skin's appearance in categories such as, elasticity, hydrations, and helping to fade scarred areas.

My Personal Remedy #1:

Mix together the following: 2 drops of clary sage oil, 8 drops of roman chamomile oil, 4 drops of frankincense oil, and 30ml of rosehip seed oil. Apply 4 drops a day onto scar and gently rub in.

My Personal Remedy #2:

(You can increase the amount of shea butter, nopales, and batana oil to your desired texture. All other ingredients remain the same).

Shave off thorns or nopales and peel off skin. You can use one large or 2 medium sized nopales pads. Large should be considered larger than the size of your opened hand. Blend together or place into food processor.

Add 2oz of burdock root to boiling water. Cook for 8-10 minutes, then let steep until cooled off.

Add nopales, burdock (tea), ½ cup shea butter, 8 drops of chamomile oil, and add a small scoop or batana oil and mix together thoroughly. Apply as much as you feel is needed directly onto scar twice a day.

Sciatica

The sciatic nerve stretches down the lower back, down the back of the legs, all the way to the ankles. Anything that puts pressure on this specific nerve will result in a sharp pain down your leg. Common injuries such as a herniated spinal disk, a bone spur, or a spinal misalignment can result in sciatica. These injuries can be long-lasting, especially as our bodies go through constant changes as we age, along with many other contributing factors such as stress, weight-fluctuation, exercise, and posture. Over time, simple things such as bending over, sneezing, or having a bowel movement can trigger sciatic pain depending on the damage to the nerve. In this section we will review ways to manage sciatic pain and gear your efforts towards healing and repairing this condition completely.

Remedies:

Ice

Once you notice a symptom, apply a cold compress (small bag of ice cubes wrapped in a thin cloth, or icepack) to your lower back for 15-20 minutes every 2-3 hours. "The cold helps reduce the inflammation and will prevent painful muscle spasms", says Andrew J. Cole, M.D., at the Spine Center at Overlake Hospital Medical Center in Washington State. A gel pack can be very helpful as well since the gel pack will adjust to the area in need and stay cold for a while.

Heated Pad

After applying a cold compress for a day or two, it is recommended to use heat, as advised by John, J., Triano, D.C., Ph.D., director of the chiropractic division of the Texas Back Institute in Plano, Texas. Use a heating pad or hot water bottle to apply to your lower back for at least 15 minutes at a time once an hour throughout the day. The heat works to relax the muscle around the sciatic nerve to (hopefully) prevent painful muscle spasms and increases circulation to the area.

Swimming

Unlike going for a run or a jog (or even brisk walking) is that water supports the lower back and joints much easier so that the muscles are able to relax and relieve pressure on the sciatic nerve. Swimming and spending time in water can be one of the greatest rehabilitation tools a person can use. You do want to initially rest after experiencing sciatic pain as straining these muscles can cause the pain to worsen. Make sure to always rest a while before getting into the water for a swim or just walking in the water at least waist deep to cover you lower back.

Go For A Walk

Walking regularly is a way to keep the muscles well-toned and improve circulation in the body; particularly around the sciatic nerve. If you are in pain or walking with a limp, try one of the other remedies covered in this section first before going for a walk to not aggravate the condition.

Strengthen Your Core

When we hear the word "core" we often picture only our abdominal muscles. But our core involves so much more. The hips, buttocks, muscles that surround the spine, all the way up to our shoulders are involved in our core. Basic compound exercises such as squats and deadlifts help immensely with these core muscles when performed correctly. Other exercises such as "bridges" where you lay ono you back, feet flat on the floor placed close to your buttocks, and you press your feet down while raising your hips all the way up, can be a great movement to loosen your lower back. Other movement activities such as yoga can relieve any tension while sculpting and shaping (while also aligning) your core muscles.

Massages

Find a local setting where you can get a full body massage. A massage will help improve circulation in the body and help the muscles become more flexible over time which in turn can reduce the severity of symptoms and any pains you may experience.

Lift With Your Legs

The worst possible movement you can if you have sciatica is bend over at the waist. This will not only create a painful stretch but put an immense amount of pressure directly upon your sciatic nerve. Always make sure to lift with your legs whether something is light or heavy. Even when you do something like drop your keys or a pencil, make sure to squat down and use your leg muscle to not strain your sciatic nerve. After picking something up or holding something, make sure to always hold it close to your body to avoid any added tension to your lower back.

Cut The Sodium

Sodium (mineral most commonly found in salt) in the body can provide an additional spark of energy, but too much creates chaos. Although this substance is necessary in the body, once it gets into the bloodstream and creates tension within the body, it begins to interrupt anything it may come into contact with. Removing items that are high in sodium (processed meats, junk items, cookies and cakes, sodas, etc.) help reduce additional and unnecessary activity in the body.

Magnesium

Magnesium is responsible for regulating the nerves in the body (among other responsibilities). Whenever you are low on magnesium, the response your body will give will mimic many of the symptoms attributed to sciatica. Too little magnesium in the body does not allow the system to charge the muscles and nerves for optimum performance. Magnesium also helps stimulate digestion within the body, so the cells know what to absorb and what to not absorb. Reducing this workload on the body will tremendously help reduce many of the symptoms associated with sciatica.

Common Sources of Magnesium: Avocado, Chickpeas, Tamarind, Basil, Dill, Ginger, Oregano, Thyme, Nettle Leaf, Horsetail (herb), Red Clover, Sage, Nopal, and almost any CBD (cannabidiol) products are helpful. CBD Oils are almost pure magnesium.

*To test the purity of a CBD Oil, send to a lab for testing or you should feel a steady decline in needing to rely on this substance after your need has been met regularly.

Frequent Breaks

Dr. Triano states that, "If you have sciatica, your enemy is a prolonged, static posture." This can happen whether you are active or not. If you are very active during the day, try scheduling in breaks periodically to give yourself time to relax. If you are sitting most of the day at home or at work, take a break from that as well by scheduling in frequent breaks throughout the day. Sitting can actually put twice as much pressure on the spine as standing.

Deep Breathing

How fast your heart beats depend on the sympathetic nerves and parasympathetic nerves (vagal nerves) contracting. When the heart beats, the sympathetic nerves are dominant. You want to help the parasympathetic nerves to be in control as this network of nerves are the "brakes" for the heart to begin slowing down as these nerves become more dominant. The parasympathetic nerve system become stimulated when we take deep breaths. You want to incorporate deep breathing exercises daily, as often as you make time for them to help stabilize your heart rate.

Put Your Foot Up

The spine has a natural curve. When standing, this curve is accentuated. This can aggravate the sciatic nerve. If you have one leg that is often triggered more often or more severely, it will benefit you to elevate your foot and then the other while standing. While sitting, it can help to place one leg up higher to help relax the steady pressure that is placed on the sciatic nerve during the day. Whenever possible, put your foot on a stool or something that is higher than the ground to help alleviate this pressure.

Maintain Healthier Weight

Every pound you may have of unwanted weight will place more pressure on your sciatic nerve. Particularly if your stomach is larger for your size, this will lead to lower back problems and trigger your sciatic pain more often. You want to shed any unnecessary weight you may be carrying and maintain a weight where your sciatic pain is not triggered easily or often.

Reduce Your Car Time

The way car seats are designed, they place a lot of pressure on the lower back. Not only is this uncomfortable, but cars vibrate as they move which can create pain for someone with sciatica, but cam lead to muscle inflammation, muscle spasms, and can even damage disks in your back. You want to not have any extended stays in your car. Avoid traffic whenever possible, work to limit how much you drive daily, and stretch immediately after going for a drive.

Find Your Favorite Position

Anyone who experiences sciatic pain has at least one position when they lay down that cause little to no pain. You want to find your most comfortable position and maintain it whenever there is pain. However, the position must be functional to help long term. If your most comfortable position is when your back or neck re twisted around, this will just create additional issues later on and will not properly cope with this pain in the moment.

Avoid Cigarettes

Dr. Cole states that, "Some surgeons won't perform surgery unless patients quit smoking." This is because cigarette smoke weakens the spinal disks and slows recovery when in pain. Operations will then be a much higher risk; a risk surgeons may not want to take.

Sit Down (Don't Lean Back)

One of the main reasons we have back, leg, and neck pain, is leaning backwards while sitting. When you lean back while sitting it flattens the lower area of the back which deprives it of its natural curve. This adds an additional amount of stress on not only the spine, but the ligaments, and disks. Sitting like this, puts added weight on the buttocks which can pull and apply unnecessary pressure to the sciatic nerve where you can develop sciatica and shooting pains down each your legs.

Tips For Improving Posture:

- Sit while lifting your breastbone.
    - o Will help relieve tension from the pelvis and hips. You want to "lengthen" the space between your belly button and upper chest. You simply raise your chest upwards while also tilting the hips towards your back to help promote the natural curvature of the spine.

- Align your head, first
    - o The rest of your body will follow the motion of your head. This extra weight will drive your spine either forward or backward. You want to position the head in a neutral position to avoid the spine leaning towards one way. Doing this will help alleviate some of the muscles in the back that are getting overused and want to relax.

- Driving
    - o If you drive a lot, you most likely have back pain. The way car seats are designed to have your knees higher than your hips places an incredible amount of pressure onto your back. To minimize this from happening, you want to adjust your car seat so that your knees and hips are at least at the same level. You essentially want to drive in the same position that you sit (when sitting correctly). If your seat does not adjust much, consider sitting on a folded towel or small pillow. The last adjustment to make is making sure your steering wheel is not too far forward that you have to reach for it. This can cause you to round your back which does not promote healthy posture.

Acupressure

Exercise #1: Spine

The spine is the primary crossroad of all the meridians (pathways of energy in the body). when you increase the flow/energy within the spine, ease of pain can travel throughout the body.

Start by rolling a towel into a tube shape (preferably the length of your spine) and lay down on your bed, wooden board, or comfortable surface while the towel is underneath the right side of your spine. As you lay there, take slow, controlled breaths, and press down on a specific point on your hand ("S13") located right underneath the knuckle on your smallest finger. From this point, press upwards at a slight angle toward your ring (4th) finger. Press firm enough and repeat until you experience relief. Start with your right hand and then repeat with your left hand.

Note: Only lay down with towel under your back if you can lay down comfortably. If not, remove towel.

Exercise #2: Spine and Hips

Start by sitting upright in a chair. Then, let your head drop forward and bend until your shoulders meet with your knees or thighs. If you can only bend slightly forward do not go past discomfort. Also, if you feel dizzy, stop this exercise, hydrate and go back to sitting upright until your dizziness goes away. Breath deep into your navel while down (similar to the Hara Breathing mentioned earlier in this text) and work to release tension in the body in the spine and hips. Continue this exercise and work to stretch deeper until you can place your arms inside of your thighs and touch your ankles.

While down touching your ankles, take your thumb (or any finger that can reach) and press on point "K16") which is located about an inch below the peak of the anklebone on the inside part of each foot. Press down steadily for 4-5 breaths or as long as you feel comfortable. Then proceed to press down on the same location but pressure point located on the outside of the foot (point "BL62").

If you can, try reaching down and applying pressure to all four pressuring e points at the same time while also massaging around each area to provide relief.

Exercise #3: Fingers, Wrists, and Arms

Pressure point "TW5" can provide much relief to the areas surrounding the hands and arms. This pressure point is on the outside of the upper arm, about two inches from the wrist, and right in the middle of your arm between the two bones. Press firmly on this spot for about one to minutes.

Exercise #4: Feet and Toes

For relief in the feet and toes, you want to locate pressure point "GB41"). This is located between the fourth and fifth toe (your big toe is your first toe). Beginning at the web between these toes, press firmly between the toes directly on the bone towards the ankle. Press for about 1-2 minutes each side, one foot at a time, and repeat as needed until you notice relief.

Exercise #5: Large Joints In The Body

The large joints in the body are typically, the shoulders, knees, elbows, and hips; essentially any joint connecting two main bones/areas of the body are considered "large joints". There are two main points to focus on for large joints which are, "TW5" and "GB41". You should already know where TW5 is as listed earlier in this text. GB41 is located towards the top part of the bone in your 4th toe (away from the toe). If you cannot reach GB41, you may use a soft tool or cane-like object to press down on this area. You do want to be careful to not press down much harder on any point more than the others; they are all equally necessary and damage to these areas can worsen your symptoms.

Exercise #6: Lay Down

A lot of the aches and pains we have is just tension or areas of the body that have remained stagnant for lack of relaxation and/or movement. Start by lying flat on your back (preferably on a flat surface) and bend your knees so that your feet are flat on the surface about 12 inches from the rest of your body. elevate your head slightly off of the surface with a pillow or small stack of books and rest your hands on your stomach alongside your ribs while your elbows remain at your side.

Remain in this position until you feel your shoulders, neck, lower back, and various parts of your back relax. Allow these areas to become softer and softer for about 12-15 minutes. Do this daily as a part of your morning or evening routine to help alleviate any tightness or pressure in these areas.

Seasonal Affect Disorder (SAD)

During the autumn season, the days become shorter due to daylight savings time where many people begin to develop symptoms of "feeling down" as we move towards the winter months. As time goes on these people experience mild to severe symptoms of depression, fatigue, desire to sleep and decrease activity, and often have cravings for things like refined carbs and artificial sugars which stimulate the brain's chemicals without movement. Then, as we get closer to the spring months, these symptoms decrease and people begin to feel more energized, social, and genuinely happier and motivated. This series of events and symptoms as referred to as, Seasonal Affect Disorder (SAD).

Remedies:

Get Outside!

Go outdoors on a bright sunny day and soak up all of the sun that you can. Even if it's a cloudy day, you can still get more sunlight than you can while inside. Natural sunlight affects the hormone known as melatonin which peaks in the brain at night and helps to regulate your internal body clock. Light also helps stimulate the neurotransmitter in the body known as serotonin which regulates your mood.

Bring In More Light

Open your window blinds and open your drapes to let more light in to flow throughout your home. You want to do this while you're home of course as much as possible.

Awaken To Light

Set a timer and get up before the sun has fully risen. Sit comfortably outside or stand as the sun slowly rises. The eyes are more sensitive upon awakening but are more absorbent to light.

Exercise

You will want to combat many symptoms of SAD by staying physically active. Find a simple exercise activity you can do often and continue in the winter months such as walking, jogging, or cycling on a stationary bike. Slowly add other exercises for variety and set reasonable goals you may want to work towards. Daily exercise should be looked at as a requirement for those who experience SAD. Not that this is an additional task but viewed as more of being an activity to avoid being stagnant. It's not necessary to develop a body-building schedule or spend all of your free time at the gym. Simply going for a walk for 20-30 minutes a day can be very beneficial to alleviating symptoms of depression. Keith W. Johnsgard, Ph.D., professor emeritus of psychology at San Jose State University in California, USA states that, "the changes in brain chemistry provoked by exercise appear to parallel those of the major antidepressant drugs".

Music

We have all most likely listened to music when feeling down or upset. Music has the ability to not only provide connection and understanding but help improve our mood and feelings of well-being.

Prepare For The Winter

Anticipate the winter as being a time where your energy may feel that it has decreased. Complete tasks during the warmer months to give you more time to do enjoyable activities during the winter.

Get Comfortable With The Right Foods

Don't begin searching for or buying comfort foods that are high in carbohydrates such as cookies, candy, cakes, potatoes, breads, and pasta. Aim to cook more soups and stews instead where you can provide yourself a load of minerals and nutrients while taking up your time to do something relaxing such as cooking. You can cook these items to remain warm and store away for a few days that you can reheat.

St. John's Wort (herb)

This herb has shown to have positive effects in studies for decreasing symptoms of depression. 300-milligrams of this extract daily is recommended. Note: this herb can make you more sensitive to light. If this occurs, simply stop its use and continue with your light therapy when exposed to natural sunlight.

Avoid Self-Diagnosis

Our minds are not in the healthiest space when we are experiencing SAD. Yes, we can simply refer to the diagnosis listed in this section and confirm what we feel is accurate, but it is important to meet with a professional as there are many assessments that can provide more clarity to our current situation. We may agree with all parts of the criteria listed for SAD when we are alone. Seek out a mental health provider and work to provide more clarity to what is going on and connect with helpful services.

Go To Therapy!

A therapeutic relationship can at times be the only remedy needed. Having a therapeutic relationship with someone who can provide structure and support on treating your signs and symptoms is vital. Being able to peel back the layers of your life and examine without judgment will help dissolve your symptoms as you work to create, establish, and fine-tune healthy coping skills. Regular assessments can be reviewed as perspective-taking can take place in this therapeutic setting as you work towards exploring all areas of self-identified growth. You will also be able to learn more about your diagnosis and have access to more valid information that you can remain mindful of.

Socialize

You do not necessarily need to go out with friends to socialize. Simply acknowledging other people as you encounter them is a great way to work away from your typical symptoms due to you placing yourself outside of your normal comfort zone and bringing your awareness to something else that will keep you stimulated, even for brief moment of time. Go to a local restaurant, sporting game, park, or just go for a walk and make it a point for you to increase socializing. Maybe start off with setting a small goal of saying "hi" to one or more people, or even planning to have a small conversation with someone. These regular encounters we can create will remain helpful towards working away from that negative perception we may have of ourselves if SAD is present.

You can perhaps keep a frequent schedule of being out more by going to the gym, walking around your neighborhood, or meet this need through some other job/volunteer service in your community such as coaching a sport, helping organize various food pantries or soup kitchens, or attending local youth or performance-related activities.

Create A Regular Schedule

When your inner world appears chaotic and difficult to manage, having a regular schedule can help regain some control and maintain order in your life. You don't want to be too strict on your schedule or develop a regular routine that does not allow much time for yourself or flexibility.

Forgive Yourself

Knowing you have an internal battle that challenges you, try to not hold any grudge towards yourself and work on laughing at the smaller accidents or inconveniences that would normally disrupt your day. We will always feel just about anything throughout the day, so work on making more room for letting go of the feelings you don't want to remain present when you can. Don't immediately blame yourself when something does not go as planned.

Shingles

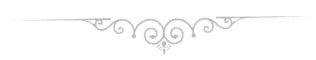

Shingles appears after the condition known as herpes zoster ("chickenpox") reawakens in the nerve cells which makes its way to the skin, resulting in burning pain, tingling, painful rashes, blisters, and numbness. Stress, frequent illness, and maintaining a vulnerable immune system contribute to this condition.

Remedies:

St. John's Wort (herb)

This herb works as an antiviral which can reduce symptoms of this virus that looks to spread around the body. Take 200-300 milligrams of this herb 2-3 times a day until you notice your pain being gone.

Olive Leaf (extract)

This herb helps to serve as an antiviral while also boosting the immune system. Take 500-milligrams three times a day until your symptoms are gone.

Lysine

This substance is an amino acid. When a virus looks to spread, it reproduces itself by combing with the amino acid arginine. However, when a cell is already occupied by another amino acid (Lysine), the virus does not have a place to call home and can die off if the conditions are right. Many doctors will provide an artificial form of Lysine to take but there are natural forms if it as well. The important part when taking a natural approach is consuming what's helpful, while avoiding what's not (in the moment). So, in the case of herpes zoster (chickenpox and later on, shingles) you will want to load up on your Lysine while avoiding your Arginine consumption.

Common Lysine Sources (consume): quinoa, olives, wild blueberries, grapes.

Apply A Cool Washcloth

Take a washcloth and wet it in cool water (the cooler, the better) and then rinse out any excess water. Apply to affected area to help calm flareups you may experience.

Remain In A Cool Setting

Avoid going out into the heat and being in humid settings. These both will irritate the skin and prolong recovery.

Hydrogen Peroxide For Infections

If you have any blisters that burst and become infected, apply hydrogen peroxide. You don't have to dilute this in water and can use straight from the bottle.

Cayenne Pepper

Cayenne pepper contains an extract known as capsaicin which is in main pain-relieving creams. Use some as often as possible when you are eating meals. Tailor some meals to make that would benefit from adding cayenne pepper to it.

Ice Bag

If your blisters have healed but pain persists, fill up a plastic bag with ice and stroke the skin. Although this may initially feel uncomfortable, doing this will help confuse the nerves so they don't remain stagnant and contribute to symptoms as the nerve cells replicate.

Shin Splints

Shin splints are tiny sections are torn muscles of the tendon or muscle on the shin bone located on the front of your leg between the knee and ankle. They are the beginning of a stress fracture. Aerobic exercises are often the cause of shin splints. Athletes who run track or jog/run regularly are more prone to getting shin splints. The average person can get shin splints by going from a sedentary lifestyle to suddenly being very active in a short time period. Within this section, we will review simple strategies for overcoming shin splints without simply stopping or halting all physical activity.

Remedies:

Rest

Make additional time to rest. Put your feet up and relax whenever possible to reduce blood flow to the area to help reduce inflammation. The more activity and stress you put on your legs, the longer it will take to properly heal. Once you can get moving again, prioritize grass and dirt spaces over asphalt. Perform activities in a soft gym floor or on a wooden floor.

Having The Correct Shoes

You want to wear shoes appropriate for what you're doing. If you wear heavier shoes while running, you will be more likely to having shin splints. It would be best to wear lightweight running shoes instead for jogging or running longer distances often. If you weightlift and do any heavy lifting, you will want to have shoes with harder soles on them to take the pressure off of your legs (or go barefoot to allow the body to adjust better for these lifts if applicable to the gym you go to).

Rub Out The "Bumps"

Whenever you feel any soreness or prior to going for a run or physical activity, rub in between where the muscle and bone meets in the leg where your shin is located. Don't press enough to cause any pain but press firm on this area up and down your shin.

Go Bike Riding

Looking for a great exercise that also works your legs and keeps you active? Go bike riding. This will alleviate pressure from your legs but still allow you to maintain your physical fitness routines. You may use a stationary bike as well if you are not interested in riding a bike outdoors.

Arnica (herb)

Make your own Arnica Salve to apply to area. If you know an herbalist, you should be able to find Arnica Salve to purchase to use during this time.

My Personal Arnica Salve Recipe:

Step 1: You need to infuse your carrier oil with Arnica and St. John's Wort. Place your dried herbs in a sterile (boil before using) glass jar. I use 1 cup of Arnica and 2 tablespoons of St. John's Wort.

Step 2: Next, add the carrier oils. I use 1 cup of olive oil and 1 cup of coconut oil.

Step 3: Now you will need to infuse the oil. There are several ways to do infuse oils with herbs.

Step 4: Solar Infusion Method: The best method is solar-infusion. To solar infuse your oil simply place your jar of oil and herbs in the sun for at least 4 weeks. Swoosh the jar occasionally. This makes the best oil but clearly takes much time to complete.

Step 5: Slow Cooker Method: To use a slow-cooker place a towel in the bottom of your slow cooker and set your jar of oils and herbs on it. Fill the cooker halfway with water and set to warm or low for 8-10 hours. Gently swoosh the jar occasionally.

Step 6: Double Boiler Method: To use the double boiler method place your jar of oil and herbs in a pot filled with water. Warm jar over low heat for at least an hour. The lower the heat and the longer time the better. Gently swoosh the jar every 10 or so minutes.

Step 7: Once your oil is infused with the Arnica and St. John's Wort it is time to strain the herbs out of the oil. I place a metal strainer with unbleached mullein cloths on top of a glass dish, then pour the oil and herbs into it.

Step 8: Allow the oil to drain through the herbs and cloth dripping into the container. Don't be impatient during this step; it takes time. Typically, I end up with about 1 1/2 cups of infused oil. Most will add an essential oil but feel free to skip this step for now. It is now more important to pour the oil into your storage containers. I use glass jars, some prefer plastic or tin. The oil will be hot, so proceed with caution.

Step 9: Allow the jars to cool. It will form into a nice salve rather quickly.

Step 10: Apply cooled salve to affected area and rub in gently. Wash off after a few hours to avoid any contamination.

Sulfur (MSM)

The mineral sulfur helps reduce muscle soreness and inflammation. There is a supplement often prescribed by doctors called methylsulfonylmethane ("MSM") which was developed specifically to relieve athletes of muscle soreness. 1-gram a day for a few weeks has been able to speed up muscle recovery and soreness according to Dr. Stanley W. Jacob, M.D., professor of surgery at Oregon Health Sciences University in Portland, Oregon.

Common Sources of Sulfur: leafy green vegetables, (dried) peaches, onions, watercress, chickpeas, walnuts.

Massage

Gently but firmly press your thumbs down both sides of your calf or along the shin bone (starting from your knee, going down to your ankle). Use your left thumb on the left side and right thumb on the right side. Repeat several times on each leg 2-3 times a day.

Visualization

We must rest in order to recover from shin splints, but we must also rest our mind. Visualizing healing the body helps to direct our thoughts towards something more specific and allows our mind to rest from all of the concerns we may have. It can help to visualize you performing the task(s) that contribute to your shin splints but performing them completely healed with no pain. Examine and assess how this feels (literally). This exercise (pun intended) will serve as a measuring tool towards tracking your recovery when you are more active again. You can enhance your ability of knowing when to stop and what surfaces suit you better to walk, jog, or run on while recovering. Take time to imagine positive flow back in your legs and shift your energy towards healing. Set your intention on healing and then preserving your body. you do not want to heal and then immediately be in pain once again.

Ice

Pour water into a dixie (paper) cup, and slowly roll up and down on your shins. Do not press hard to avoid more pain or soreness. Just gently rub up and down on your shins equally until it begins to melt. Use a towel to avoid any freezer burn on your fingers.

Sinusitis

Facial pain, tooth pain, headache, cough, and clogged nose are the combination of symptoms that represent a bacterial infection in the sinuses around the nose. This condition is called Sinusitis. Sinusitis can be acute, lasting only a few days, or become chronic, lasting several weeks and then re-occurring often. Sinuses are tiny air-filled pockets that serve as air-quality control operators just under your cheekbones, above your eyes, above your nose, and behind your eye sockets. Their primary duties include: maintaining warmth, moisten, purify, and clean up the air that you breathe before it goes into your lungs. When bacteria attempt to enter, it is caught and filtered out and trapped by mucus and tiny nostril hairs. When the sinus openings become clogged, the mucus becomes stagnant, pressure builds, and this bacteria can breed and spread amongst your sinuses. Once an infection settles in, inflammation settles in, and you now have sinusitis.

Remedies:

Avoid Antibiotics

Antibiotics destroy the good bacteria in the gut that keeps digestion normal. Destroying this bacteria often leads to diarrhea, inflammation, and digestion issues. This can trigger additional health issues. The more antibiotics you take, the harder it will be for the body to create the good bacteria within the gut, meaning your next battle with sinusitis will be more unbearable. "Recurrent doses of antibiotics for sinusitis usually make things worse" says Guillermo Asis, M.D., director of Path to Health in Burlington, Massachusetts.

Check Your Allergies

Chronic sinusitis can be an aggressive response by the body to combat allergies such as pollen, dander, dust mites, or foods. You will want to review the Allergies section within this book for more specific recommendations.

Salt Water

Saltwater kills bacteria. You can relieve many of your symptoms by spraying this under your nose. You will want to get a nasal douche ("neti pot") which is a small glass or hard plastic pipe with a hole in the side. Make a solution with ½ teaspoon of sea salt per cup of distilled water. Taste a small amount to make sure it tastes salty and that you haven't diluted it too much. Fill the neti pot full of this mixture, hold one finger over the hole, then snort and immediately move your finger away from the hole. This will send a rush of this mixture into your nose to help clean out the area. You may blow your nose and notice excess mucus coming out. This is what you want to see until you have no more mucus and can breathe easily. You want to do this twice a day.

Let Your Head Hang

Lie down fat on your back on your bed or the side of your couch. Allow you head to hang slightly over the edge. Remain in this position while controlling your breath for 5-8 minutes. You should feel your sinuses begin to drain into your pharynx and eventually into your digestive system to be expelled out of the body. this technique will help you drain your sinuses to help relieve pressure and symptoms in the affected area.

Hydrotherapy

Put a warm, wet washcloth or small towel over the painful area for 30 seconds. Then switch to a cold, wet washcloth for 30 seconds. Alternating warm and cold applications can help improve circulation to the affected area where it can move out congestion. You can repeat this remedy as often as you want during the day.

Eucalyptus Essential Oil

Boil water in a large pot and add a few drops of eucalyptus essential oil to it. Place the pot onto the counter or leave on stove with flame turned off. Cover your head with a towel and lean over the pot and breathe in deeply. Do this a few times a day. Eucalyptus not only will help you relax, but will help relieve your headache and reduce the pain you are experiencing.

Cayenne Pepper

Cayenne pepper contains an extract known as capsaicin which is in main pain-relieving creams. Capsaicin works to stimulate nerve fibers that can promote the breakdown of mucus within the sinuses. Use some as often as possible when you are eating meals. Tailor some meals to make that would benefit from adding cayenne pepper to it.

Flush Your Sinuses

There are many store-bought products and devices available to help flush the sinuses. Sinus infections will make symptoms worse over time. try to look at flushing your sinuses as "mucous drainage" because that's what you are doing. A simple remedy goes as followed:

Mix ½ teaspoon of fine-grained sea salt in 1 cup of warm water. Pour solution into your cupped palm and inhale it through one nostril while holding your other nostril closed (temporarily). You want to repeatedly blow out of the nostril you just inhaled through to help discharge any mucous that is trapped. Then repeat with your other nostril. Do this as often as possible, not just when you get a cold or feel sick to remain proactive with this condition.

Load Up On Flavonoids

Flavonoids are items that look like tiny crystals located in foods that fight inflammation. Common foods such as onions, apples, berries, and prickly pears, flavonoids give these items their color. Flavonoids not only strengthen the capillary walls which can make breathing easier, they are antioxidants, so they also work to protect the airways from pollution.

Go For A Walk

With all of the congestion taking place, you may feel irritated, or angry/frustrated. Walking helps to release adrenaline which constricts the blood vessels in the body, increasing the swelling in the sinuses. Reduce this constant pressure by taking a walk.

Snoring

Snoring impact about 45% of all adults. Because it is so common, it does not always appear to be anything other than a nuisance or that it can be effectively managed.

Remedies:

Control Your Weight

This does not mean you have to be lean or thin. You just have to work more towards a size suitable for your body to not respond by snoring. Dr. Earl V. Dunn, M.D., professor in the department of family medicine at the United Arab Emirates University in Al-Ain, and professor emeritus at the University of Toronto in Canada states, "We've found that if a moderate snorer loses weight, the snoring becomes less loud, and in some people it actually disappears." You will want to make necessary adjustments to diet and physical activity in order to begin losing some excess weight as you work towards decreasing your snoring.

Avoid Alcohol

Besides the health risks that are covered in other section in this book, alcohol relaxes all of the muscles in the throat that vibrate. The more you drink alcohol, the louder your snore will be.

Avoiding Sedatives (sleeping pills)

Anything that relax the tissues around your head and neck will not decrease snoring. The worst part is that it will be more difficult for you to notice as it will be harder for you to wake up after being sedated. Sleeping pills make help you sleep but they won't decrease snoring or help your partner sleep.

Stop Smoking Cigarettes

Smoking cigarettes increase swelling and inflammation within the throat tissues, leaving them more likely to vibrate and increase snoring.

Remove Your Pillow

Anything that keeps your neck in a compromised position, will increase your snoring. Get use to sleeping without your pillow to relive your neck.

Addressing Your Allergies

You will want to take some time and review the Allergies section in this book and apply each step. Many people who snore, developed this condition after years of allergies.

Ginger (herb)

This herb helps soothe the throat. Start adding it to meals and practice drinking as a tea in the evening a few hours before you go to sleep.

Peppermint and Spearmint

Both of these forms of mint are *mentholated*, meaning they help open the airways which can contribute to decreasing snoring. You can make these together or by themselves as a tea or you can chew them. Chewing them, may be very strong for many but you want to wash the leaves first and make sure to avoid chewing any stems. Chew a few at a time any time of the day that you want to help provided relief when sleeping.

*peppermint oil can also help clear congestion in the chest which can decrease or eliminate symptoms.

Nasal Strips

Sometimes all you need is a consistent open airway. Putting on a nasal strip can help reduce snoring. You do want to take notice if your snoring decreases overall, and/or if you continue to snore when you do not use them.

Sore Throat

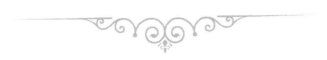

A sore throat can be caused by many things. The focus is to remain on recovery while you reflect upon what you noticed as being the cause. You could have been exposed to low humidity, been talking or yelling more than usual for you, were exposed to a bacterial infection, or could be an early warning sign of contracting a condition such as the flu. Note: if your sore throat is caused by a viral infection, antibiotics won't help.

Remedies:

Phenol

This is a mild anesthetic that numbs raw nerve endings to help reduce the soreness by killing bacteria and allowing the body to build up its resistance during recovery. Typical lozenges ("cough drops") are soothing but don't contain phenol so they don't contribute to healing. There re sprays and cough drops that contain phenol that will serve you best as you work to recover quickly.

Oil of Oregano

Oil of Oregano contains: carvacrol, the main active compound in oregano oil, and a type of antioxidant called a *phenol*. Also, oregano oil contains *thymol*, which helps protect against toxins and fight fungal infections.

One way to use oil of oregano is to add 2-3 drops to water or juice and drink the mixture. However, people should be careful to use oil of oregano and not oregano essential oil. The latter is much stronger and not generally safe to consume.

Argan Oil

Is rich in natural phenols (organic compound) that are primarily used to benefit the hair follicles. This oil can contribute to hair growth, as well as thicker hair. Massaging this oil into your hair is another way of consuming this oil that can contribute to reducing symptoms.

Zinc Lozenges

Zinc can help sore throats that are linked to a cold or flu. There are zinc lozenges available to help increase your zinc consumption during this time.

Common Zinc Sources: chickpeas, mushrooms, zucchini, squash, okra, Brazil nuts, and walnuts.

Gargle Frequently

You will want to gargle often to help soothe your sore throat. Swallowing food and liquids may hurt at this time. You can gargle often to help track your progress with how sore your throat is.

Salt Water – mix 1 teaspoon of sea salt in 2 cups of room temperature water. You can gargle this mixture once an hour.

Chamomile – steep 1 teaspoon of dried chamomile in 1 cup of hot water, strain, and let cool until room temperate. Start by gargling a few sips for about 20 seconds each time. then drink the remaining tea slowly to help reduce the irritated membranes.

Humidify Your Space

We are more likely to breathe through our mouths when the air is not humid enough. Mouth-breathing will only contribute to the dryness and irritation we have in our throats. Find out if cool-mist or warm-mist is best for you. You can purchase a bedside humidifier online or at most retail stores.

Breathe in Steam

In your home, fill up a pot of water and bring to a boil. Reduce heat to low. While the water is being boiled, wrap your head in a towel so you can lean over the pot and inhale the warm, moist air. Keep about 10-inches away to avoid burning. You can do this several times a day for 5-10 minutes each time, taking small breaks as needed.

Walk By The Sea

If you can, head on over to a local beach and breathe in the air. The mist produced by the sea is great to breathe in to help soothe your sore throat.

Drink The Right Fluids

Room temperature water will help keep your throat moist. You want to avoid a few liquids during this time.

Orange Juice – this may add to a burning sensation you may already feel.

Cow's Milk – this is a mucus-producing substance that can make it more difficult to breathe.

Caffeine Drinks – and counteract remedies that are applied and stimulate hormonal changes which can trigger a response that overworks the thyroid glands and create more congestion in the throat.

Chamomile Wrap

Take 1 tablespoon of dried chamomile flowers to 2 cups of boiling water. Allow to steep for 5-7 minutes before straining. Soak a cloth or towel in this tea, wring out excess liquids, and apply to the infected area. Leave on until the cloth or towel is cool. Repeat up to three times a day until you find relief.

Get A New Toothbrush

Using the same toothbrush while having a sore throat can prolong your recovery. Your current toothbrush may also be the cause of your sore throat as bacteria can collect on the bristles. The moment you are feeling ill, get a new toothbrush. Then get another one once you feel you have recovered.

Manuka Honey

Manuka honey is produced by bees that pollinate the flowers found on a manuka bush; a kind of tea tree. The form of honey originates from parts of Australia, New Zealand, and Honduras. Traditionally used to heal wounds, sore throats, and to prevent tooth decay. However, this honey has become more commonly known to treat acne, prevent ulcers, and treat eye deficits. This form of honey is much different from traditional honey as it comes from a different source and provides additional benefits. Manuka honey is an antioxidant, and antibacterial substance.

Mix two tablespoons of manuka honey with a warm glass of water. You may boil water first to make a tea. This honey will work to reduce inflammation and fight against bacteria that can cause pain in the throat. Researchers at The Hebrew University, Hadassah School of Dental Medicine in Jerusalem, Israel found that manuka honey helps specifically decrease the type of bacteria most present in sore throats, streptococcus mutans.

Note: like any other honey, manuka honey does contain a high amount of sugar made from fructose and glucose. So, you will want to remain mindful of this if you have diabetes, liver disease, heart disease, or want to avoid consuming excess calories.

Homemade Cough Syrup

To avoid the many chemicals which can trigger additional reactions within the respiratory system, making your own cough syrup will help soothe the areas that are triggered and can help decrease symptoms as well.

Recipe:

1 cup of elderberries

2 tablespoons of ginger root powder

3.5 cups of distilled water

¾ cup of agave (for taste)

Add elderberries and ginger root powder to boiling water. Let simmer for about an hour, until about half of the water has evaporated. Then let sit and cool for about 15-minutes. Store in a mason jar or container and mix in agave. Have 1-2 tablespoons daily.

Mullein, Red Clover, and Ley Lime Tea

For this recipe, take 2 teaspoons of mullein leaf (or mullein flowers), 2 teaspoons of red clover, and 1 key lime to juice. Add mixture to boiling water and let steep for about 15-minutes or until cooled off. Drink 1-2 times a day to provide relief and help keep the respiratory system clean.

My Personal Remedy:

2 teaspoons of mullein

2 teaspoons of burdock root

1 teaspoon of nettle

1 teaspoon of tila

1-2 pieces of star anise

Boil 4 cups of water and add herbs. Simmer on low for about 15-20 minutes. Strain herbs and let cool off. Drink 2-3 times a day.

Sprains and Strains

A sprain involves an injury (overstretching) to the ligaments that connects the bone to other bones. You've essentially asked your muscles to do more work than they could handle in which the ligaments then are stretched which results in the area becoming swollen, warm, painful, and even bruised.

A strain involves a similar process of a sprain but involves an injury to the tendons (tissues connecting muscles to the bone).

Both injuries can benefit from the same treatment however, recovery may just vary depending on severity and past history of either injury you may have endured. In both cases, you will tear some tissues or microfibers of tissues. where there is some tearing, there will be internal bleeding where dead cells can bind together and promote things like deeper bruising and swelling. Not until the swelling goes down will healing be completely attainable.

Remedies:

RICE Method

R = rest

I= ice

C= compression

E=elevation

Rest is imperative to any healing protocol because whenever you use an injured area, this will cause further damage to it. Ice helps to control any internal bleeding. Wrap ice or an ice pack in a towel. Keep on injury for 20-minutes, then take off for 40-minutes. Repeat this as often as possible during the day as long as there's swelling. Compression is when you place an elastic compression bandage ("Ace bandage") around the area to help stop internal bleeding. You want this bandage to fit well without being too tight to allow for normal circulation. Elevation is to help drain any fluids or waste materials away from the area to reduce swelling.

Get Comfortable

You want to find the most comfortable position in order for your sprain or strain to heal. You want to rest in a position that take the tension and pressure off of your injury. Control your breathing while in this comfortable position as it will be your main resting position while you heal and recover from your injury.

Apply Pressure

Once you have found your comfortable position, you can now begin to apply direct pressure to the area. Using your thumb or index finger to locate spots that hurt and begin to gently press on them. Hold your pressure for a few seconds and then relax your pressure to allow the pain to ease. Ligaments and muscles tighten when they are injured as a defense mechanism to avoid further injury. Pressing on these tender spots will allow for maximum contraction which in return, allow the muscle, ligament, or tendon to relax.

Plantain (Weed not the fruit)

This plant is a weed that is loaded with tannins (natural chemicals that help tighten the skin and surrounding tissues) that help reduce inflammation and itchiness around the affected area. The weed grows all over but is abundant in areas that are damp and shady. Grows about 6-18 inches tall and has deep purple veins from top to bottom. From the summertime until the fall, this plant sprouts green, pipe cleaner-like flower spikes.

You can chew this plant if you get bitten by a bee or mosquito. But for sprains and strains, take the leaves, and rinse them off as you place a handful of the leaves directly on the affected area to instant relief. You may also rub the leaves together after you rinse them off until they create a "juice" which you can apply to the infected area.

You may make tea and let sit for about 10-15 minutes in a cooled area. To make tea, take ¼ cup of dried plantain leaves to a quart of boiled water and let steep for 20-30 minutes. Place a small towel in the water and apply directly to affected area to help reduce inflammation and pain.

Urine Wrap and Soak

A helpful remedy to help alleviate swelling, but not sending the white blood cells away, is a form of Urine Therapy. Filling up a plastic bag (same bag you would ordinarily use for ice) with your own urine and wrapping it around your ankle will help apply heat and pressure but contain many minerals where the body can detect them and know how many white blood cells are needed. Our urine is intelligent. It contains many vital minerals and parts of our DNA which can communicate more with our injury than a bag of ice or a heated towel can.

After the warmth of the urine wears off, you can choose to soak the affected area in your urine as well. You can start by pouring some onto a small towel and allowing to soak while elevated. You want to place a small collection pan or tray for any liquid that may run off just as you would when soaking a towel with water. As your swelling decreases and you become active again, it is recommended to continue to soak your previously injured area(s) in your urine after training or any strenuous exercise.

Arnica Salve

Make your own Arnica Salve to apply to area. If you know an herbalist, you should be able to find Arnica Salve to purchase to use during this time.

My Personal Arnica Salve Recipe:

Step 1: You need to infuse your carrier oil with Arnica and St. John's Wort. Place your dried herbs in a sterile (boil before using) glass jar. I use 1 cup of Arnica and 2 tablespoons of St. John's Wort.

Step 2: Next, add the carrier oils. I use 1 cup of olive oil and 1 cup of coconut oil.

Step 3: Now you will need to infuse the oil. There are several ways to do infuse oils with herbs.

Step 4: Solar Infusion Method: The best method is solar-infusion. To solar infuse your oil simply place your jar of oil and herbs in the sun for at least 4 weeks. Swoosh the jar occasionally. This makes the best oil but clearly takes much time to complete.

Step 5: Slow Cooker Method: To use a slow-cooker place a towel in the bottom of your slow cooker and set your jar of oils and herbs on it. Fill the cooker halfway with water and set to warm or low for 8-10 hours. Gently swoosh the jar occasionally.

Step 6: Double Boiler Method: To use the double boiler method place your jar of oil and herbs in a pot filled with water. Warm jar over low heat for at least an hour. The lower the heat and the longer time the better. Gently swoosh the jar every 10 or so minutes.

Step 7: Once your oil is infused with the Arnica and St. John's Wort it is time to strain the herbs out of the oil. I place a metal strainer with unbleached mullein cloths on top of a glass dish, then pour the oil and herbs into it.

Step 8: Allow the oil to drain through the herbs and cloth dripping into the container. Don't be impatient during this step; it takes time. Typically, I end up with about 1 1/2 cups of infused oil. Most will add an essential oil but feel free to skip this step for now. It is now more important to pour the oil into your storage containers. I use glass jars, some prefer plastic or tin. The oil will be hot, so proceed with caution.

Step 9: Allow the jars to cool. It will form into a nice salve rather quickly.

Step 10: Apply cooled salve to affected area and rub in gently. Wash off after a few hours to avoid any contamination.

Massage

Massaging the area stimulates blood flow and circulation. We want circulation and blood flow to go away from any areas of swelling, but once there's little to no swelling, you will want to massage the area. Massage with your fingers and/or palm of your hand in a circular motion. Use this to see which areas are still tender and gently massage for about 5-10 minutes a few times a day.

Foot Spelling (for ankle injuries)

This exercise involves writing each letter in the alphabet, with your foot. You will want swelling to be gone so that you have your mobility to move around. Sit comfortably in a chair or stand upright. While moving the foot from the ankle (not the knee), pretend to trace each letter of the alphabet as if your big toe is the tip of your pen or pencil. You may pretend you are using lowercase or uppercase letters (or both). Take your time and then take note of which letter were difficult to identify which motions were more challenging for you so that you can practice and also mark your progress.

Toe Pickups

Place a towel on the ground. Standing upright or sitting down, place your toes on top of the towel and then use your toes to pick up the towel. This is a great exercise to test not only your mobility but strengthen some of the muscle tissues that need to get stronger to avoid future injuries.

Newspaper Squeeze (thumb or toe injuries)

If you are dealing with a thumb or toe injury, get yourself a newspaper and place one sheet down onto a table or floor. To restore strength, use your toe or thumb to crumble up the sheet of newspaper. Squeeze slowly to not aggravate the injury. Do this twice a day to test your strength and also mark your progress.

Wear Correct Shoes

As a general rule, you want to wear shoes for activities you do the most. You wouldn't want to wear lightweight running shoe for when you play basketball. They have the ankle support you will need to avoid these types of injuries. After an injury, you want the proper support to be in place. Try to avoid wearing ankle shoes, crocs, or slides if you just had an ankle injury. It won't take much to lean to one side and aggravate your injury.

Stretch

After achieving mobility without pain, you want to stretch the area impacted by injury. When we have a sprain or strain, our muscles, tendons, and ligaments become constricted and tight. Over time, they become more relaxed and don't hurt. However, small areas can remain tight weeks after you feel better. You will want to stretch this are daily to help regain strength and also loosen out the impacted area so that blood flow can go in and out as needed without interference.

Stress

Stress is something we all experience as it is difficult to avoid. We do want to manage our stress so that it is not too much for ourselves individually. Everyone can manage a different amount of stress, but understanding your personal threshold and tolerance is key. Often, stress can be a great motivator to reach a deadline, complete a test, or compete in a sport. However, when we experience stress that becomes unbearable for us, this is when stress becomes toxic. In this section, we will review preventative measures and ways to remain proactive with relieving stress when it is present and ways to work on minimizing stress in your daily lifestyle.

Remedies:

Cut The Sodium

Sodium (mineral most commonly found in salt) in the body can provide an additional spark of energy, but too much creates chaos. Although this substance is necessary in the body, once it gets into the bloodstream and creates tension within the body, it begins to interrupt anything it may come into contact with. Removing items that are high in sodium (processed meats, junk items, cookies and cakes, sodas, etc.) help reduce additional and unnecessary activity in the body.

Excess stress also creates salt in the body. A nucleus of an atom can only hold 2 electrons in the 1st valance (outer layer) and 8 in the remainder valences. When we get upset or frustrated (heat rises) this causes the sodium (Na) molecule to throw electrons off. This makes it unstable and causes it to create a bond with whatever is compatible with it in its' current state (this is called "Covalent Bonding"). In this case, the sodium (Na) molecule is now compatible with chloride (Cl) because chloride produces "free" electrons to the body which the sodium molecule is looking to replace. Chloride maintains metabolism and energizes the cells.

Now you have Na + Cl which is NaCl, which creates Sodium Chloride aka "salt".

We can eat right but if we're around people who get us upset or situations that make us upset, we'll continue to accumulate salt within the body. These people and situations will create the same thing we're looking to escape from. Salt is a crystal. All crystals serve as conduits for healing (good energy in, bad energy out). Salt however, especially coupled with an unhealthy environment (the body), will cause the body to remain negative and only be capable of projecting negatives words, feelings, or behaviors. In a more positively functioning environment/body, stress turns into motivation and positive movement expression. This is why eating right (in my opinion) helps support further positivity and improvement.

Understand How You Respond To Stress

Almost anything in life can and has happened to someone and life still goes on. Outside of the event of someone dying by suicide, it's most often less important what happens, but how you respond to these events that determines your stress. Next time you notice someone else experiencing stress, take a moment too observe them and learn. Some will yell and scream, others will clench their jaw, then hands and feet begin to show movement, sweat may make an appearance, and many other things that signify a stressful response. Use this as a learning tool to help you become more mindful of what you do when you are stressed so that you can change it.

The Chinese word for "crisis' is, *wuji*, where it is represented by two characters that separately mean "danger" and "opportunity". Stress incites a crisis within the body, but if we can use it as a response to identify other outcomes (hopefully the outcome we want) then we can make the most out of these natural opportunities in which stress not only dissolves, but it no longer represents a roadblock in our lives or our daily routines.

Work to challenge your current beliefs about certain situations as you work to changing a lifestyle of stress and discomfort, into a life of challenge and excitement.

Anti-stress Affirmations

You can imagine gently thoughts in your spare time to remain calm, but this is practice for using these in the moment during times of stress. It is necessary to think certain thoughts to help begin changing how you receive messages that create stress. Below are a few affirmations to say to yourself to help decrease your stress.

- "There is nothing I have to do at this moment."
- "This moment is here, and it shall pass soon enough."
- "There are no problems I have to solve at this time."
- "There's no place I have to go right now."

Counting Up or Down

Something to do when experiencing stress is to start counting. You may count up or down. Counting down from 10 to 1 is helpful for some, but others may want to continue counting in order to provide themselves more time to calm themselves. Doing this will provide you with some sense of control and help shift some of your attention away from whatever may be triggering stress inside of you.

Look Somewhere Else

Our eyes often focus on the stressor. Look somewhere else to divert your attention, and your body will be inclined to do the same. Spot certain colors, shapes, or designs that catch your attention and count them to help shift your focus away.

Deep Breathing

When stress is present, our pulse begins to race which triggers faster breathing. We must work on slowing down our breath to tell the body that you are working to become calm. Practicing deep breathing (slow, controlled breaths) teaches the body to control our responses via the nervous system. Forcing yourself to breathe deeply, you also slow your heart rate, send oxygen to the brain allowing it to take in other data besides the stressor, and ease tension in the body, allowing you to shift your awareness towards allowing the stress to pass.

Meditation

You may picture someone sitting with their legs crossed, eyes closed, blocking out all noise, with a slight grin on their face whenever you hear the word "meditation", right? Although many of these things can be a goal, they are the result of regular practice of calming and relaxing the body. meditation is used to help induce a relaxation response within the body. our responses and awareness can vary depending on the situation. However, we can go towards a desired, internal destination that is void of these stressful events through the practice of meditation.

Do not be concerned about if you are meditating "correctly". Just explore different forms of meditation that you feel you can add to your lifestyle and focus on the relaxation. Accept the challenge that there will still be distractions and stressful events, but that you are doing something about it, and that you are the one who will absorb the many benefits to be acquired through this practice or re-wiring your mindset.

Stretching

Stress creates tension. Stretch to help relieve them of tension in order to channel its release from your body. this can include activities such as yoga but can be applied daily at any time to help the body feel less constricted as it does when we are stress. Implement a morning and/or bedtime stretching routine to do and be mindful of simple stretches you can do while sitting or during certain moments throughout the day.

Soak Yourself

Whenever we are stressed, blood flow that is sent to our extremities is reduced. This causes disruption with our circulation, causing adrenaline to build and often leads to muscle tension. Soak certain parts (if not your whole body) in warm to hot water. Placing warm water on certain areas like the forehead, hands, and feet, can help the body return blood flow to these areas and relax. You may also try letting warm water run over your hands in a sink to help restore blood flow and promote relaxation. Note: cold water will do the opposite as it will mimic many of the symptoms we experience during moments of stress.

Music

The vibrations and sounds in music we enjoy can shift our awareness and help reduce stress. Music can be used to relax, or to inspire. We can use stress in many ways, but we want to control it. Put on some music you enjoy and just zone out. After feeling better, take some time to reflect and examine ways you can void whatever was causing a stressful response.

Stroke

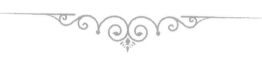

A stroke is like a heart attack, but specifically towards the brain. When a stroke occurs, an artery to the brain is obstructed where tiny blood vessels burst. Many who survive a stroke will still have speech challenges, paralysis, and poor memory from the oxygen-deprived brain tissue that died during a stroke. The number one risk factor for decreasing your risk of a stroke is, high blood pressure. If you've already experienced a stroke, decreasing your risk factors so another stroke does not occur will be your focus.

Remedies:

Ways To Reduce Blood Pressure

Below are the standard numbers to aim for in order to have normal blood pressure for each age range:

Male			Female		
Age Range	SBP	DBP	Age Range	SBD	DBP
21-25	120.5	78.5	21-25	115.5	70.5
26-30	119.5	76.5	26-30	113.5	71.5
31-35	114.5	75.5	31-35	110.5	72.5
36-40	120.5	75.5	36-40	112.5	74.5
41-45	115.5	78.5	41-45	116.5	73.5
46-50	119.5	80.5	46-50	124.0	78.5
51-55	125.5	80.5	51-55	122.55	74.5
56-60	129.5	79.5	56-60	132.5	78.5
61-65	143.5	76.5	61-65	130.5	77.5

Note: keep note of the numbers on this chart and review the High Blood Pressure section in this text to learn more about ways to reduce and avoid high blood pressure.

Bromelain

This digestive enzyme can dissolve unhealthy bacteria which is crucial in preventing a second stroke.

Common Sources of Bromelain: watermelon, bananas, papaya, pineapple.

Fatty Acids

Fatty acids (omega-3, omega-6, and omega-9) are a form of *polysaturated fat* which work to help provide the body build healthy cell membranes. These help with maintaining hydration and absorbing nutrients. These fats bind to cell membranes increasing fluidity, which is important for the functioning of each brain cell. The benefit of membrane fluidity is that it helps the brain change and adapt to new information.

Common Sources of Fatty Acids: Brazil Nuts, Walnuts, Kola Nuts, Avocados, Bananas, Sea Vegetables (Nori, Wakame, Hijiki, Sea Moss, Bladderwrack), Coconut, Coconut Oil, Olive Oil, Grapeseed Oil, Avocado Oil, Mushrooms, Quinoa, Wild Rice.

Antioxidants

According to the National Institutes of Health (NIH), antioxidant therapy seems to be an effective treatment in the management of oxidative stress relevant to inflammatory disorders like stroke.

Natural Sources of Antioxidants: blueberries, onions, lettuce, squash, tomatoes, grapeseed extract, and herbs that you can use the flower, root, and leaves for as they contain polyphenolics (compounds that produce antioxidant activity).

Scalp Acupuncture

This is the number one treatment for reducing risk for stroke in China. This treatment works by increasing blood flow into small blood vessels of the brain. A hyperbaric oxygen chamber, where the atmospheric pressure is raised, you can breathe oxygen easier which helps with recovering from a stroke. After a stroke occurs, certain areas of the brain go into hibernation. Hyperbaric oxygen absorbed through breathing allows these areas of the brain to thrive again. Opening the channels to supply oxygen to these areas of the brain allows the cells in these areas to recover and new blood vessels can grow into areas previously deprived of blood. Scalp acupuncture has a long history or relieving stress but has maintained a positive impact on preventing and assisting with the recovery from those who have suffered a stroke.

Yoga and Mindfulness Activities

Practicing Yoga, Meditation, and Mindfulness will help to reduce the stressors in the body. when the body experiences stress, many of the muscles will tighten up which can trigger symptoms. These exercises also help to open the airways in the body as well. Basic movements will help regenerate, re-build, and restore many of the physical symptoms of a stroke.

Acetyl-Carnitine ("L-carnitine")

This nutrient works to energize the brain cells. The brain cells that have not died off or are severely damaged can essentially be revived from this nutrient. This nutrient helps improves memory, boosts energy in the brain, improves brain receptors, and improve neuron communication, according to Dr. Alan Brauer, M.D., founder, and director of the TotalCare medical Center in Palo Alto, California. 250-2,000 milligrams a day.

Common Sources of L-carnitine: avocado, walnuts, garbanzo beans, and seeds (seeds inside fruits and vegetables).

Breathing

Sit as comfortably as possible. Take time to tone your body down to relax. Begin taking slow, controlled breaths until you go into a deeper state of awareness where you are thinking of the future or the past. Only awareness on the present. Getting to this space take practice. Once you are able to reach this space, send your awareness to your lungs to keep the air flowing to and through your body. Keeping the body relaxed can help reduce blood pressure and maintain healthy cells within the brain.

Affirmations

During your breathing or meditation time, use this space to also affirm your intentions and visualize to activate healing. You are telling your nervous system what direction to go in when you do these activities. You can affirm that your muscles will get stronger, you will speak more clearly, and continued to feel motivated, among many other things you want to affirm. Create personalized affirmation that resonates with you and what you need. Make sure to not only speak what you want to achieve, but what you wish to avoid along the way as well.

Visualization

Visualizing can help you picture the types of actions you wish to perform better. Set your intentions when visualizing on what you want to improve upon, and away from processing the negative aspects that are challenging for you at the moment. Visualize all movements you want to step closer towards and then put your visualizations to practice as you are able to make progress. You also want to visualize how you want to feel during your progress so your body can detect these emotions and be prepared for them so that you are attracting what you most desire.

Whether you're recovering forma stroke, r trying to prevent one, you will want to incorporative more of the following:

Vitamin B-12, B-6, and B-9

Cobalamin ("vitamin B12")

Is naturally created via bacterial synthesis in the gut. Cobalamin is a bacterium that is part of every growing plant that we consume. However, this is often washed off during processing that it is no longer present on these items, and we do not consume this bacterium. Animals will consume foods while they are still in the ground and absorb a larger quantity of cobalamin that goes into their muscle tissue and can be absorbed by anything that eats them. However, eating an animal is a longer route to getting access to this bacterium, and we are unsure if they even have an adequate amount to be absorbed based upon their diets/lifestyle. We can gain consistent access to this bacterium by simply eating more fresh foods that are not processed, and by growing our own foods. The fewer stops from the farm to your table, the better your chances are of gaining access to absorb this healthy bacterium.

We essentially only need about 1 microgram of B12 a day. When we repeatedly do not meet this need, it can become noticeable, but we don't need nearly as much B12 as we do calcium, magnesium, or many other minerals. Since we have worked to kill off any form of bacteria (harmful or helpful) most people remain deficient. If we consume that which is natural and work on eating locally grown produce and growing our own plants (even something small to put in a window at home) we can consume enough B12 and do away with any B12 deficiency (and many others) so that B12 deficiency is no longer a topic of decision.

B12 helps to regenerate the neurons in the brain that help with communication. These neurons typically die off during and after a stroke. Repairing them and providing rejuvenation to this area is very crucial in avoiding and recovering from a stroke.

You will want to go to local markets and farmer's markets in your area where there is a shorter "farm to table" distance where B12 will remain more present in some capacity. Also growing some of your own plants at home or a t a local garden will be best.

Pyridoxine ("Vitamin-B6")

Organic compound composed of hydrogen, oxygen, and nitrogen. It is known for animals to be able to use B6 to utilize the amino acid known as tryptophan which creates melatonin and serotonin to balance hormones, appetite, sleep, mood, and pain. Helps increase the body's utilization from Vitamin-B3 which is needed to energize metabolism and DNA production. B6 helps promote circulation in the body which helps stroke patients improve utilizing any areas that may be paralyzed or temporarily paralyzed.

Common sources of pyridoxine: avocado, carrots, bananas, peas, lentils, spinach, chickpeas, acorn squash, quinoa, sunflower seeds, brussels sprouts, oranges, pistachios.

Folate ("Vitamin-B9")

Helps with red blood cell production which can promote healthy blood cell function. This is particularly helpful in avoiding a stroke as folate helps to reduce the reoccurrence of plaque that build up and contributes to a stroke or prolongs the recovery process.

Common sources of Folate: asparagus, avocado, oranges, Brussels sprouts, lentils, beets, bananas, leafy greens, hemp, walnuts, chickpeas.

Sunburn

Asunburn is due to overexposure of the sun while not being prepared. If you are not properly hydrated for example, then overexposure can mean being outside for a few minutes. There are many contributing factors to developing a sunburn that we will review in this section as well as ways of working to prevent getting a sunburn.

Remedies:

Proper Hydration

Not only drinking about half of your body weight in ounces (ex. if you weigh 100lbs, drink 50oz) but consuming foods that provide water is necessary. Melons, berries, tomatoes, and cucumbers are only a few items that should regularly be in your diet. Consuming items that provide hydration can help wash away and also neutralize the erosive acids that remain in the body from eating things detrimental to our health which work their way through the bloodstream and into the skin that is in direct contact with the sun and causes a sunburn.

Lavender Essential Oil

Add a few drops of lavender essential oil directly onto the skin. You can add with water to spread to other areas of the body as well.

Zinc

Zinc can help sun burns heal more effectively, according to Dr. Bradley Bongiovanni, N.D., naturopathic physician in Cambridge, Massachusetts.

Common sources of Zinc: chickpeas, mushrooms, zucchini, squash, okra, Brazil nuts, and walnuts.

Antioxidants

The sun causes damage to the skin cells. Antioxidants help to rebuild skin cells. Antioxidants can help stop the formation of free radicals. Free radicles are unstable molecules that cause oxidative damage (internal rust) within the cells, contributing to sunburns You want to consume antioxidants daily. Ann easy way to work in many antioxidants is to remember to "eat the rainbow" with an assortment of foods that are naturally different colors; not dyes or artificial colorings.

Common Sources of Antioxidants: Berries, leafy green vegetables, spring water, okra, cherries, dates, and raisins, and herbs that you can use the flower, root, and leaves for as they contain polyphenolics (compounds that produce antioxidant activity).

Apply A Cool Compress

Dip your towel into cool water, rinse out excess water and carefully lay it over your burn. Repeat each time after the towel warms up from your body heat. Do this for a minimum of 15-20 minutes a day.

Lettuce

Boil lettuce leaves in water, strain, and then let the liquid cool off for a few hours in the refrigerator. Dip cotton balls into the liquid and gently apply to the affected area.

Don't Wash With Soap Or Bodywash

You do not want your burn to come in contact with soap or bodywash as they will irritate the burned skin. Avoid using these items.

Aloe Vera

Is a natural anti-inflammatory. According to the National Center for Complimentary and Integrative Health, applying aloe vera to the skin can help people with acne, herpes simplex, psoriasis, and other conditions affecting the skin, including sunburns. It is typically well-tolerated. But, as with any new remedy, it's important to do a skin patch test before application, especially if you have sensitive skin. Some commercial aloe products may also have added fragrance or other chemicals that can irritate the skin, so be sure to read the label(s).

You can find this plant at most local markets or grocery stores. You want to slice this plant open with a knife, squeeze or scoop out all of the transparent pulp, and then apply directly on the skin covering the affected are(s). You can let this settle in before washing off after about an hour. You can do this as often as you want.

Drain Larger Blisters

If you have blisters, they can come in all different shapes and sizes. You don't want to accidentally tear one and it get infected. To drain the fluid, first sterilize a needle by holding it over a flame. Then puncture the edge of the blister and press gently to allow the fluid to come out. Then leave these blisters alone after gently washing dry. Note: you may use a safety pin in place of a needle if you have any concerns about needles.

Tachycardia

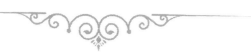

Rapid heartbeat can appear suddenly. What is considered "rapid" is when your heart is beating faster than 100 beats per minute. Average heartbeat can range from 60 to 85 beats per minute, where more elite athletes can average 40 beats per minute. Tachycardia occurs when your atria (chamber in the heart that receives blood from the veins and pumps it into the ventricles to be sent back out throughout the rest of the body, the atria keep a steady rhythm, but when tachycardia is present, the rhythm can be three times faster than normal.

Remedies:

Rest

Tachycardia occurs to signal the body to stop what it's doing and rest. Choose any way you can minimize movement to help relax.

Deep Breathing

How fast your heart beats depend on the sympathetic nerves and parasympathetic nerves (vagal nerves) contracting. When the heart beats, the sympathetic nerves are dominant. You want to help the parasympathetic nerves to be in control as this network of nerves are the "brakes" for the heart to begin slowing down as these nerves become more dominant. The parasympathetic nerve system become stimulated when we take deep breaths. You want to incorporate deep breathing exercises daily, as often as you make time for them to help stabilize your heart rate.

Massaging The Right Carotid Artery

Massaging the right carotid artery that connects in the neck underneath the jaw is another way to stimulate the parasympathetic nerves.

Avoid Stimulants

Stimulants such as coffee, soda, chocolate, and processed foods put you more at risk for tachycardia. These items also can be more difficult to process and digest, causing more blood flow to be sent to the digestive tract and increasing your heart rate.

Protect Your Hypothalamus

Your hypothalamus section of your brain is to keep the body in a stable state (homeostasis). This section of the brain sends signals to the heart where the body responds to maintaining stability and control over your nerves and nervous system. When we consume unhealthy foods, avoid exercising, and do not maintain a positive mental state, we experience "sympathetic overload" where pollutants cause the hypothalamus to go into overdrive.

When we do not eat for a bit of time and then fill our stomach with candy, soda, any processed sugar, your pancreatic enzymes jump in to take care of the increased sugar intake. Then your insulin overshoots and you go into "reactive hypoglycemia" (low blood sugar – even though you just consumed sugar). Your adrenal glands bring adrenaline in to help mobilize the stores of glycogen sugar in your liver to combat the low blood sugar levels. This adrenaline rush stimulates a sudden increase in heart rate (tachycardia).

This is why we want to plan regular meals and avoid consuming any processed sugars. The hypothalamus part of the brain relaxes when it knows what to expect. Keep a regular dietary regimen to help the hypothalamus relax and don't send it mixed signals by consuming processed sugars, especially on empty stomach.

Magnesium

Magnesium helps balance the effects of calcium in the body which stimulates muscular contractions with the cells in the heart. Magnesium can promote more regular rhythmic contractions and relaxation, making the heart less irritable.

*Common Sources of Magnesium: avocado, chickpeas, tamarind, basil, dill, ginger, oregano, thyme, any *CBD (cannabidiol) products are helpful. (CBD Oils are almost pure magnesium), nettle leaf, horsetail, red clover, sage, and nopal.*

*To test the purity of a CBD Oil, send to a lab for testing or you should feel a steady decline in needing to rely on this substance after your need has been met regularly.

Potassium

Potassium is a mineral that relaxes the heart and reduces irritability of the muscle fibers. Note: you can deplete your body of potassium if you consume a high amount of sodium.

Common sources of Potassium: squash, zucchini, bananas, avocado, dried apricots, and herbs such as, guaco (also high in iron), conconsa (has the highest concentration of potassium phosphate), lily of the valley (rich in iron fluorine and Potassium phosphate).

Copper

This mineral works to lower LDL (bad) cholesterol and increase HDL (good) cholesterol, helps balance iron metabolism and absorption, produces red blood cells, supports the immune system, and turns sugar into energy for the cells, among many other tasks. Lowering the "bad: cholesterol will help reduce the excess work on the heart which can reduce palpitations and other issues. 2 milligrams of copper daily will be a sufficient enough for the body to perform its daily tasks and responsibilities.

Common Sources of Copper: blackberries, blueberries, guava, apricots, bananas, leafy green vegetables, avocado, sunflower seeds, mushrooms, spring onions, and you can drink sparingly from a copper vessel or bottle.

Fiber

Fiber helps digestion which is needed to help the body continue to clear out toxins and unnecessary waste. Dr. Stengler, N.D., a naturopathic physician in San Diego, California notes that the indigestible portions of many whole-food plant-based foods help to remove excess cholesterol from the body also which promotes heart health. We do not necessarily absorb every bit of every nutrient provided by what we consume, but unlike many processed food items, plant-based foods help cleanse out additional waste even the indigestible parts. It should be a goal to consume about 5 portions of plant-based foods daily, regardless of any specific dietary regimen you may follow. It is recommended for women to aim towards 21-25 grams of fiber a day, while men aim between 30-38 grams of fiber a day.

Common sources of Fiber: garbanzo beans, lentils, brussels sprouts, sweet potatoes, avocado, pears, sunflower seeds, flax seeds, hazelnuts, apples and berries (high pectin fruits) and onions.

Exercise

When we perform exercises that raise the heart rate, the heart tends to reset at a lower level. Those who don't exercise often have a heart rate around 80 beats per minute. Doing some light running or cardio, the heart's rate may go up to 150-170 but then rest at 60-65 beats per minute. Regular exercise helps you become more resistant to excess adrenaline release which decreases your risk of tachycardia.

Vagus Nerve Stimulation

The vagus nerve in the body has many functions, but most importantly it connects the communication between the brain and the heart. The vagus nerve is directly involved with communicating to the heart to beat faster. We want to help this connection become calmer so that the heart doesn't beat faster unless it is reasonable.

Take a cold shower: splashing cold (not freezing) water onto your face helps stimulate this nerve. Helps to increase awareness and help the brain communicate that there's not an immediate threat for the heart to beat faster and relaxes the nerves. You can do this in the shower or apply a cold towel or ice pack (covered) for 20-30 seconds.

Chant "om" or cough: this also helps stimulate the vagus nerve, telling the body to make space for relaxation. If you cough, do so under control to not invoke unwarranted stress.

Hawthorn Berry (extract)

This extract is great for digestive issues and high blood pressure. Recent studies have shown positive impacts of reducing heart palpitations. In a study conducted by the National Institute of Health (NIH) they conducted a 2-year study with 952 participants who were experiencing heart failure. One group received hawthorn berry extract in addition to treatment and therapy, and the other group did not receive any hawthorn berry extract but received the same treatment and therapy. The study found that the group who received hawthorn berry extract saw a steady decrease in heart palpitations compared to the group who did not receive the hawthorn berry extract.

Clean The Liver

The liver sends out the good cholesterol our body needs. When the body is overworked, the liver becomes backed up and cannot send out toxins. Most toxins are filled with chemicals which end up in the bloodstream and can immediately trigger symptoms and impact neurotransmitters in the brain (i.e. "send mixed signals). The liver is one of the primary detoxifying organs in the body. Keeping this organ clean will help to remove many of the chemicals and excess waste we do not need in our body.

Tips on how to clean the liver:

Herbal Teas:

The herb called Palo Azul is very helpful for cleaning the liver and breaking down toxins.

(How To Prepare: take 1 large piece or 2-3 medium sized pieces of this herb and place them in a boiling pot of water for approx. 60 minutes. Strain out the herbs and drink 1 cup a day for about 24-30 days).

As mentioned above as a coffee replacement, mixing Roasted Dandelion Root, Black Walnut Hull, and Blessed Thistle, can serve as a natural detoxifier which can help provide some relief for the liver.

(How To Prepare: take 1-2 cups of each herb and mix well together in a bowl or container. Boil water while placing about 1 tablespoon of mixture into a cup and pour boiling water into cup. Let sit for about 10 minutes and then strain out the herbs. You can drink hot or let cool off and add ice for an "Iced coffee". Store herbs in a zip lock bag or container and you can let your drink sit in the fridge overnight as well.

Liver Detox Tea

Ingredients: Burdock Root, Sarsaparilla, and Yellow Dock. About 750mg/each (about ¼ teaspoon each herb in powder form per 8oz water). Dosage changes for dried herb to about twice this amount at least.

- Burdock Root helps promote urinary tract health and healthy liver function. Promotes clear, healthy skin.

- Sarsaparilla contains biochemicals called saponins that may promote clear, healthy skin.

- Yellow Dock is classified as a bitter herb that helps promote digestion. High in iron.

Teething

An infant's teeth actually begin developing several months before birth (around the 7th week of pregnancy). The teeth just do not show themselves or work completely through the gums until a few months after birth. All 20 primary teeth should sprout over their first 2 ½ years. It is common for their teeth (around 4-8 months) to push through quickly which results in the baby's gums becoming swollen and causes the baby to become irritable and restless. This is when "teething" has occurred. In this section we will review some tips on how to make this process less painful and challenging for the infant and everyone involved.

Remedies:

Cooling The Teeth

Chewing on something cool can help soothe the child's gums. If you have your child using a teething ring, place it in the refrigerator to keep cold before giving it to your child. For children 6 months or older, they can use a cold washcloth to chew on.

Caution: Avoid teething rings with anything besides water inside. They can break and the liquid can be toxic for your child to consume.

Clean The Drool (avoid wiping)

Teething will cause the baby to drool more than usual. Use a warm washcloth to pat to dry and gently wipe drool to prevent a rash from developing.

Massage The Gums

Use a slightly moist gauze pad to massage the baby gums with your forefinger. Doing this helps to remove bacteria buildup which can cause additional discomfort. You can start this a few days after being born; you don't necessarily have to wait until teething begins. Daily massaging gums helps develop healthier gum tissue and can help make teething less painful.

Baby Safe Feeder

Instead of a teething ring, you can use a product called Baby Safe Feeder where you can give your baby frozen grapes or other items they can suck on. This product works to eliminate choking while holding the food easier for them to suck or chew. You can use this product to help introduce healthier foods and developing their taste buds so they can maintain a healthier diet as they get older.

Chamomile Compress (ages 8 months or older)

Any water under the age of 6 months can present a choking hazard. A child can drink chamomile tea but making tea to let cool then soak a small towel in to chew on will be most helpful. Chewing on chamomile tea will help reduce the irritableness a child experiences when teething. Chamomile will provide a soothing effect.

Clove Oil

You want to start by diluting clove oil as it can be very strong. Mix one drop of clove oil with one teaspoon of coconut oil and apply it directly to the child's gums. You may also add a few drops of clove oil to water and soak a towel in for a child to chew on.

make sure to use clove oil sparingly. Too much or too often can resulting vomiting and nausea.

Amber Teething Necklace

You want to get an Amber necklace made from Baltic amber beads. These beads are believed to release natural oils containing succinic acid. The child's body heat releases succinic acid from the amber which is absorbed into the skin and helps them remain calm. These beads can help reduce inflammation and provide pain relief. You do want to give you child this necklace with caution as the small beads or necklace may break which can present a choking hazard. Remove necklace whenever they are asleep.

Weleda Tooth Powder

Weleda is a natural and organic personal care company. Ingredients include several herbs such as chamomile and calendula which help soothe the gums and alleviate pain. Follow directions and use a small amount of this powder per use. Massage gently onto their gums or add a small amount to a clean spoon to have your child swallow.

You can purchase Weleda's teething relief powder here; https://www.weleda.com.au/product/b/baby-teething-powder-oral-powder

Temporomandibular Discomfort

In this condition, the joint that connect the lower and upper halves of the jaw is either damaged, or not aligned properly. This results in headaches, pain in the skull, dizziness, tingling in the hands, or the jaw remaining (painfully) locked in one position. Temporomandibular discomfort (TMD) is not just a dental issue as it may appear to be; it is a whole-body issue that should be addressed correctly. In this section we will review whole-body healing methods to effectively treat this condition.

Remedies:

Ice and Stretch

Tense neck muscles are often the source of head and jaw pain. Ice helps slow down the blood flow and sends signals to the nervous system to override the pain, making it a bit easier to stretch. You will want to wrap a single ice cube in a small towel and rub it against the side of your neck from just above your shoulder all the way up to behind your ear. Apply gentle but steady pressure to this area on each side of your neck for about 1 minute each side. After doing one side, gently stretch your neck to the side for about 10-15 seconds. Then switch to the other side. After each exercise, make sure to warm up the area with your hand to improve circulation back to the area.

"Fishhook" Stretch

The facial muscles on the side of the jaw are often in pain from TMD. Stretching this area will help reduce some pain. Take your index finger on each hand and "hook" the inside corners of your mouth. Gently pull on these areas by stretching them apart for a few seconds and then release. Repeat a few times until you feel these areas are loosened up.

Acupressure Points

Tradition Chinese Medicine (TCM) incorporates the use of pressure points to stimulate areas where there is blocked energy (chi) that needs to be released. For TMD, there's a specific spot located on each forearm known as the "M" spot. For pain on the left side of your face, lay your left forearm down with your palm facing up. Put your finger from your right hand on your left forearm so that your index finger is in the fold of your elbow and the rest of your fingers are next to one another. By gently moving your middle finger, you should feel a ligament in your arm at the edge of your right index fingertip. This is the point you need to press on. Press with your finger firmly for 15-seconds and then release. Do this 3-4 times, pausing for 29-seconds in between. Switch sides to relieve pain on the right side of your face. This will be sensitive at first, but you will build up your tolerance as you continue to practice.

Acupressure For Eye Pain

It is common for there to be a sharp pain behind the eyes at times for those with TMD. If you are experiencing pain behind either of your eyes, follow these steps. If you're having pain behind your left eye for example, you will take your left pinky finger and place it in your mouth all the way back until your fingertip is behind the last molar tooth in your mouth. Then, press up against the gum behind the tooth and hold for a few seconds. Repeat on the other side with your other pinky finger. Apply steady but firm pressure to these areas to help reduce the amount of pain you have behind your eye(s).

Unclench Your jaw

Those with TMD may believe it is normal for everyone to clench their jaw or be unaware of when they are doing this. When the jaw is clenched, the muscles will tighten. Tight muscles on add more tension to the areas most impacted by this condition. To help practice unclenching your jaw, keep your tongue on the roof of your mouth, lips together, and teeth apart. it can help if you repeat these steps to yourself throughout the day. Then, begin practicing putting the tip of your tongue on the roof of your mouth but behind your front teeth. This minor adjustment will help to center the jaw and help relieve tension created by not being aligned and favoring one side of the jaw over the other.

Support Your Posture

Whenever we lean forward, this creates additional tension on the jaw, neck, shoulders, and head. This is the last thing anyone with TMD wants to happen. Make sure your back is supported whenever you are sitting. When standing, make sure your cheek bone is slightly over your clavicle ("collar bone"), while your ears are never far in front of your shoulders.

Keep these points stabilized and your posture will improve and not only avoid causing pain but relieve much of the pain you may consider to be normal with this condition.

Adjust Your Pillow

Our pillows can apply additional (and unnecessary) pressure to our heads, neck, shoulders, and jaw. Taking your pillow and placing it between your knees instead, will be much more beneficial. Placing your pillow between your knees will help mobilize and straighten your spine, helping to improve posture. This will take pressure off of your back which in turn, relieves pressure from all areas impacted by this condition.

Stop Chewing Gum

This probably feel redundant by now, but additional chewing during the day, sometime for hours will place a great deal of strain on your jaw and add to the tension you may feel. Too out your gum completely.

Avoid Hard or Crunchy Foods

Biting down hard has no way of helping you. These items present additional issues and are also unpredictable on how they will break and what teeth you will need to use to chew them with. Chose softer foods and liquids whenever possible.

Tendonitis

Tendonitis is inflammation in and around the tendon that connects the muscle to the bone. This condition is painful. Unlike muscle soreness, which is often temporary, tendonitis can be persistent and more long-term. In this section we will review ways of reducing the impact tendonitis has on the body.

The main cause is sudden overuse. We often have a regular schedule that our body adjusts to. When we suddenly use an area of the body more than usual, this contributes to the development of one, or both of these conditions.

Tendinitis often has 3 stages:

- A dull ache following activity, which improves with rest
- Pain with minor movements (such as dressing)
- Constant pain

Remedies:

Rest

This can be difficult, especially for athletes but, you cannot realistically get better or improve if you're in constant pain. You may have to take a day or two off of work or avoid all activities after work or school in order to get better. You will have to make room of rest before anything else. You do want to be reasonable about your rest as you don't want to rest for too long and develop "atrophy" which us where the muscles will begin to decline and waste away from non-use. This is much more common in athletes, so you will want to maintain low-level activity at most while recovering.

Take A Warm Bath

Many take ice baths to reduce inflammation which can be beneficial, but a warm bath will help improve circulation and help avoid stagnation in the blood cells so that you can at least move around enough to do low-level exercises. Warming up the tendon before putting it through a stressful activity is best as well.

Wrap It Up

Place a warm, moist towel over the tendon. Then place a plastic bag over that, then a heating pad, and then wrap loose elastic wrap over everything to keep things in place. Keep it on for 2-6 hours. Make sure to keep the heat pad on low to avoid burning yourself. Make sure each layer has some space so it is not too tight where it will decrease or cut off your circulation. Keep your injured area elevated higher than your heart as well to slow down blood flow and activity to the affected area.

Don't Stretch Cold Muscles

You always want to warm up your muscles before stretching. And you should always stretch before exercising at full speed. Stretching after warming up (you should break a sweat before stretching) will help prevent the muscles from "shortening" where the muscles feel constricted and push together where blood flow is hindered, and tendonitis symptoms can spread or begin to re-appear.

Take Frequent Breaks

Tendonitis does not only appear when exercising. It can appear from handling items at work or typing for too long on a computer or laptop. Tendonitis can appear almost anywhere in the body, not just the main areas like our arms and legs. We want to take breaks often to avoid inflammation from building up. Avoiding the buildup is more than half the battle when dealing with tendonitis.

Ice

Using ice to soothe these inflamed areas is best practice for the first 24-hours. An ice massage can help reduce the inflammation and help prevent some of the irritableness of these conditions. Using a bag of frozen fruit or vegetables to help as their shapes can feel like smaller ice cubes but do not shrink in size like ice cubes do. You can plan to regularly massage the area with ice for about 5-10 minutes and then remove for 5-10 minutes. You don't want to leave this on too long so that the area become numb because then it can be hard to determine if any of the symptoms are going away.

Fatty Acids

Omega-3 is the fatty acid to focus on if you have tendonitis or bursitis. Dr. Edwards, M.D. a physician from Fresno, California states that, "A person who gets omega-3 fatty acids in adequate amounts will not get bursitis or tendonitis as readily".

Common Sources of Fatty Acids: Brazil Nuts, Walnuts, Kola Nuts, Avocados, Bananas, Sea Vegetables (Nori, Wakame, Hijiki, Sea Moss, Bladderwrack), Coconut, Coconut Oil, Olive Oil, Grapeseed Oil, Avocado Oil, Mushrooms, Quinoa, Wild Rice.

Gently Move The Area

Eventually you will want to move the area that is in pain to detect when recovery is achieved. Start by gently moving the area by stretching, moving slowly around in a pool or hot tub.

White Willow Bark

A natural chemical known as "Salicin" serves as an anti-inflammatory which reduces pain within the nerves in the body and do away with much of the lingering pains from tendonitis.

Boswellia (extract)

Boswelic acid produced from this extract has anti-inflammatory properties that can help reduce swelling and pains associate with tendonitis.

Say No To Artificial Sugars

These sugars in most processed items decrease immune function which slows down healing by increasing inflammation and often contributes to unwanted extra weight that can worsen symptoms of tendonitis.

Reduce Sodium Intake

Too much sodium counteracts potassium, which helps reduce inflammation. This also contributes to the loss of important nutrients from your body that are needed to facilitate the healing process.

Shockwave Therapy

A relatively new concept but Shockwave therapy works to reduce pain in the body by increasing blood flow. In studies conducted on animals, researchers have discovered that this form of therapy increases the number of stem cells by signaling and activating stem cell mitochondria, promoting a faster recovery time for conditions such as tendonitis.

RICE Method

R = rest

I= ice

C= compression

E=elevation

Rest is imperative to any healing protocol because whenever you use an injured area, this will cause further damage to it. Ice helps to control any continued swelling. Wrap ice or an ice pack in a towel. Keep on injury for 20-minutes, then take off for 40-minutes. Repeat this as often as possible during the day as long as there's swelling. Compression is when you place an elastic compression bandage ("Ace bandage") around the area to help prevent frequent swelling. You want this bandage to fit well without being too tight to allow for normal circulation. Elevation is to help drain any fluids or waste materials away from the area to reduce swelling.

Thyroid Issues

The hormones pumped out by the thyroid gland work to regulate your body's temperature. When these hormones are low, so is your temperature, and in result, many of the body's energy-producing enzymes not being able to do their job, inevitably leading to your body feeling fatigued, sore, trouble concentrating, and experiencing consistent symptoms of depression and anxiety.

For best results regarding thyroid health, you want a selenium-rich, processed sugar-free, gluten-free, Vitamin-B complex diet.

Remedies:

Selenium

This mineral works to prevent cell deterioration and Zinc helps the immune system detect and remove weaker cells from the body which can happen when we have issue with the thyroid. Selenium is very crucial when it comes to our body's immune system. Selenium combines with several other substances in the body to form a compound known as "glutathione peroxidase", which allow your immune system to sample organisms that are inhabiting (but not yet overgrowing) on the outer layer of the skin. This not only reduces any overgrowth, but also allows the immune system to respond accordingly and destroy any organisms that may be harmful to the body.

Common sources of Selenium: brazil nuts, walnuts, chickpeas/garbanzo beans, kola nuts, dandelion greens, and nettle, and alfalfa. Recommended to consume about 400 micrograms a day.

No More Gluten

Gluten provides no essential nutrients. It is a protein found in wheat, oats, barley, certain breads, cakes, soy products, white pastas, and various vegetarian or vegan "meats". Although gluten is more associated with celiac disease, the immune system establishing the norm of attacking an organ in the body will make the immune system become more easily compromised and easier to be persuaded to attack other organs such as the pancreas which is the norm for type-1 diabetes or hormonal imbalances which take place when there are thyroid issues. We want to avoid gluten items as they cause unnecessary damage to our bodies with no essential nutrients in them. Gluten will create additional work for our immune systems that we can do without so that we can ward off other potential illnesses and symptoms of disease.

Energy Level Exercise

The thyroid gland is one of seven organs in the endocrine system (system that generates hormones). Located under the throat just below the larynx ("voice box"). Dr. Claire Holmes, N.D., naturopathic physician and clinical hypnotherapist in Kuli, Hawaii recommends incorporating the throat chakra into treatment. she states, "To really bring the thyroid back into balance, a person must be willing to balance the energies associated with the throat chakra, which are the energies of expression."

To do Dr. Holmes' recommended exercise, do the following steps:

- Lie flat on your back on a comfortable surface.
- Gently massage your upper abdomen for a minute or so to help warm up your diaphragm (the source of your breath and your voice).
- Take slow, controlled breaths.
- Place one and over your throat as you exhale.
- Start making a sound (any sound) while you exhale.
- Imagine this sound coming directly from your thyroid.
- Do this for 5-10 minutes a day.

Sunlight

Direct sunlight stimulates the pineal gland (endocrine gland in the middle of your brain). This stimulation helps to positive stimulate (not overwork) the rest of your endocrine glands, most notably, the thyroid. Go outside within the first hour of sunrise or watch the sunrise. Make sure to stare in the direction of the sun and not directly at it if you have never done this activity before. Remove any eyeglasses, sunglasses, or looking through any windows for best effects.

Avoid Hormonal Foods

If your hormones are not stable, don't consume additional hormones as they will only add more to your challenges. Meat, dairy, processed foods, and eggs (have synthetic hormones) will throw off the balance and over functioning of the thyroid.

Damiana (herb)

This herb is known for boosting libido and sexual organs but can help increase the body's ability to utilize hormones needed for proper thyroid function. Drink this herb as a tea twice a day. Take 2 teaspoons and make as a 10-12-ounce tea twice a day for best results.

Chasteberry Extract

Progesterone and estrogen control the menstrual cycle. Dr. Holmes notes that "A deficiency of progesterone, can affect the thyroid gland." Chasteberry extract, commonly known as "vitex" as a name brand supplement, works to stimulate the pituitary gland to increase the production of LH, which results in higher levels of progesterone during the second stage of a woman's cycle known as the luteal phase. Progesterone helps to develop a thick, blood-rich uterine lining into which the fertilized egg can implant. Many women between the ages of 30 and 45 have a sharp drop off in progesterone which leads to shorter cycles and a decreased chance of implanting a fertilized egg. This change can enhance symptoms of hypothyroidism. Make sure to use Chasteberry Extract for several months before attempting to conceive, but generally 14 days before your next cycle. Standard dosage should be about 40 drops of this extract one a day, or one 650-milligram capsule 2-3 times a day. Make sure to follow directions on label instructions.

Tyrosine

The amino acid combines with iodine to make thyroxine, a thyroid hormone.

Common Sources of Tyrosine: avocado, bananas, sesame seeds, oranges, peaches, okra, tomato, wild rice.

*note: sticking to recommendation to consume on an empty stomach, it would serve you best to consume some of these items listed in juice form shortly after awakening.

Fatty Acids

These components of fat are involved in the production of thyroid hormones. In cold weather we should aim to consume more fatty acids to help offset hormonal imbalances and changes due to weather.

Common sources of Fatty Acids: Brazil Nuts, Walnuts, Kola Nuts, Avocados, Bananas, Sea Vegetables (Nori, Wakame, Hijiki, Sea Moss, Bladderwrack), Coconut, Coconut Oil, Olive Oil, Grapeseed Oil, Avocado Oil, Mushrooms, Quinoa, Wild Rice

Ginger (herb)

This herb is rich in minerals such as potassium and magnesium which help combat inflammation which is one of the primary causes of thyroid issues. You can take about one fingertip-sized piece of ginger and make tea with about 10-12 ounces of water. You can also utilize ginger when cooking meals.

Iodine (addressing the thyroid)

Common conditions that impact the Thyroid are Hypothyroidism (underactive thyroid – doesn't produce enough hormones) and Hyperthyroidism (overactive thyroid – produces too many hormones). The thyroid functions off of Iodine just like the bones thrive when having enough calcium. You will want to include many items such as Sea Moss and Elderberries as well as many sea plants such as Hijiki, Dulse, Nori, and Bladderwrack.

Note: If you have Hypothyroidism, you will want to incorporate more Bladderwrack into your diet. This plant is often found in products that contain Sea Moss but can be consumed in capsule or powder form. If you have Hyperthyroidism, you will want to consume as herb named, Bugleweed often in tea form.

Hypothyroid Smoothie:

- Large handful of watercress

- 2 apples

- 1 key lime (juiced)

Hyperthyroid Smoothie:

- 2-3 green apples

- 4-5 large dandelion leaves

- 1 handful of cilantro

- 1 key lime (juiced)

**Both of these smoothies are not a "cure" but a way to help deter many of the symptoms associated with each form of Thyroidism. They help the body begin to function well in preparation of additional dietary adjustments that can and should be implemented in a timely manner.

Drink This Tea (daily): Tamarind Juice, Ginger, and Key Lime (juice).

This tea can help cleanse out unnecessary waste materials while promoting a natural way of balancing hormones within the body.

Vitamin-B Complex

Below is a brief list and sources of where to find each "B-vitamin"

Thiamin ("Vitamin B1")

An enzyme that transforms glucose into carbon-dioxide and water. Get destroyed b heating and is most abundant grains.

Common sources of B1: asparagus, peas, oranges, clementines, lemons, sunflower seeds, sesame seeds, pecans, Brazil nuts, lentils, pecans.

Riboflavin ("vitamin B2")

Riboflavin helps the body use nutrients such as carbohydrates, fats, and proteins for energy, and additionally functions as an antioxidant.

Common sources of riboflavin: tomatoes, avocado, sunflower seeds, dandelion greens, swiss chard, kale, quinoa., and edible sea vegetables (Nori, Wakame, Hijiki, Sea Moss, Bladderwrack).

Niacin ("Vitamin-B3")

Not isolated and its nature is unknown. Believes to boost energy in the body for DNA production and metabolism. Thought to be identical to pantothenic acid found in most whole grains, seeds, and lentils.

Common sources of niacin: mushrooms, peanuts, avocado, peas, chia seeds, broccoli, pumpkin seeds, lentils.

Adenine ("Vitamin-B4")

Is heat destructible and water soluble. Has been studied in rats to prevent a form of paralysis. No human need has been demonstrated at this time.

Common sources of adenine: chickpeas, chili peppers, flaxseeds, pumpkin seeds, sunflower seeds, almonds, mushrooms, hazelnuts, sage, pecans, broccoli, cauliflower, cloves, dandelion greens, peas, lentils, oregano, Brazil nuts.

Pantothenic Acid ("Vitamin-B5")

Has been studied to prevent loss of weight in pigeons but that is all known about this so far. No direct link to human need identified at this time.

Pyridoxine ("Vitamin-B6")

Organic compound composed of hydrogen, oxygen, and nitrogen. It is known for animals to be able to use B6 to utilize the amino acid known as tryptophan which creates melatonin and serotonin to balance hormones, appetite, sleep, mood, and pain. Helps increase the body's utilization from Vitamin-B3 which is needed to energize metabolism and DNA production.

Common sources of pyridoxine: avocado, carrots, bananas, peas, lentils, spinach, chickpeas, acorn squash, quinoa, sunflower seeds, brussels sprouts, oranges, pistachios.

Biotin ("Vitamin B7")

Enzyme that breaks down fats, carbohydrates, and other materials.

Common sources of Biotin: walnuts, pecans, almonds, avocado, sunflower seeds, sesame seeds.

Inositol ("Vitamin-B8")

Is actually a sugar, not a vitamin. Helps regular insulin levels.

Common sources of inositol: oranges, grapefruits, limes, cantaloupe, avocado, lettuce, raisins, cabbage, peas, and most nuts and beans.

Folate ("Vitamin-B9")

Helps with red blood cell production which can promote healthy blood cell function.

Common sources of Folate: asparagus, avocado, oranges, Brussels sprouts, lentils, beets, bananas, leafy greens, hemp, walnuts, chickpeas.

Para Amino Benzoic Acid (PABA) ("Vitamin-B10)

Helps microorganisms in the body. Helps darken grey hairs and protect the skin.

Common sources of PABA: spinach, asparagus, brussels sprouts, dark leafy green vegetables.

Vitamin-B11 (also known as Folic Acid)

Research over time has noticed small differences in structure but orle of B9 and B11 are the same.

Cobalamin ("vitamin B12")

Is naturally created via bacterial synthesis in the gut. Cobalamin is a bacterium that is part of every growing plant that we consume. However, this is often washed off during processing that it is no longer present on these items, and we do not consume this bacterium. Animals will consume foods while they are still in the ground and absorb a larger quantity of cobalamin that goes into their muscle tissue and can be absorbed by anything that eats them. However, eating an animal is a longer route to getting access to this bacterium, and we are unsure if they even have an adequate amount to be absorbed based upon their diets/lifestyle. We can gain consistent access to this bacterium by simply eating more fresh foods that are not processed, and by growing our own foods. The fewer stops from the farm to your table, the better your chances are of gaining access to absorb this healthy bacterium.

We essentially only need about 1 microgram of B12 a day. When we repeatedly do not meet this need, it can become noticeable, but we don't need nearly as much B12 as we do calcium, magnesium, or any other mineral. Since we have worked to kill off any form of bacteria (harmful or helpful) most people remain deficient. If we consume that which is natural and work on eating locally grown produce and growing our own plants (even something small to put in a window at home) we can consume enough B12 and do away with any B12 deficiency (and many others) so that B12 deficiency is no longer a topic of decision.

You will want to go to local markets and farmer's markets in your area where there is a shorter "farm to table" distance where B12 will remain more present in some capacity. Also growing some of your own plants at home or a t a local garden will be best.

Orotic Acid or Orotate ("Vitamin-B13")

Not recognized as a vitamin by health or scientific research but is a molecule that is water soluble and helps with nutrient metabolism and energy production.

Common sources of orotate: carrots, beets, chia seeds, lentils, hemp seeds.

Trimethyl glycine ("Vitamin-B14")

Not yet established as a vitamin, but works to increase cell-proliferation in bone marrow.

Common Trimethyl glycine sources: dark leafy greens, avocado, peas, nuts and legume food groups.

Pangamic Acid ("Vitamin-B15")

Not yet recognized as a vitamin. In the1980's was banned due to being an unsafe food additive.

Dimethylglycine (DMG) ("Vitamin-B16")

Combats free radicals, serves as an antioxidant and detoxifying agent.

Common sources of DMG: pumpkin seeds, beans, seeds, grains.

Laetrile ("Vitamin-B17")

Helps control and lower blood pressure. Relieves pain caused by inflammation.

Common sources of laetrile: almonds, apricot kernals, cherry seeds, bitter almonds, lima beans.

Choline ("Vitamin-B18")

Metabolizes fats and cholesterol in the body.

Common sources of choline: sesame seeds, lentils, cauliflower, peanuts.

L-Carnitine ("Vitamin-B20")

Fat burning item often found in many fitness supplements. Transports long-chain fatty acids into the mitochondria so they can get burned off to produce energy.

Common sources of L-carnitine: avocado, asparagus, lentils, potatoes, pumpkin seeds, almonds, chickpeas, cashews.

Tinnitus

This condition can be irritating as it causes people to hear clicking, ringing, and/or buzzing sounds inside of their head. The cause is often damage to the tiny hairs located on the auditory cells within in the inner ear, which causes portions of the brain to generate these sounds internally. Constant exposure to loud music or other sounds can be a main cause in addition to many contributing factors. Tinnitus is often accompanied with another condition known as hyperacusis, which is a sensitivity to sounds.

Remedies:

Avoid Loud Noise

Don't listen to music on maximum volume, loud cars, power tools, even using loud vacuums when cleaning your home. Make necessary adjustment needed to avoid persistent loud noises. Note: if you are at least 8-10 feet away from someone and one of you needs to raise your voice to hear the other, the environmental noise is too loud for you to remain there much longer.

Earplugs

To make sure to avoid loud noises, or if you know you will be in a setting that will produce loud noises, get a pair of earplugs to block out the sound. Headphone can work as well, but you will want to test them out first which you may not be able to do at most stores. If you already have a decent pair of headphones, make sure to wear them, or get a pair of wireless ones so you can block out the sound without risking the wire getting caught on something or in your way during an activity.

Earmuffs

These are not ideal and can make you sweat, but are great at blocking out noise and can be something to wear at home while trying to relax or when doing things like going to for a walk.

Humming

Humming activates a muscle in the inner ear which helps prevent some sound waves from getting in which can reduce the impact loud noises have on you. A good example to keep in mind is that humming is something drummers are taught to do right before the louder parts of songs to help drown out some of the sound. You can use this same technique during your daily life.

Let Your Ear Hairs Grow A Bit Longer

This may not be desirable or attractive, but many will often trim or pluck some hairs from their ears. Allowing your hair in your ears to grow a bit will provide a few decibels (unit of measuring sound) of protection that you may need at this time. Trimming these hairs can expose you to more sound and can lead to longer-lasting damage.

Rest

If you are around loud noises, you want to immediately take time to rest and relax afterwards. Having additional noise (even if it's quieter) following loud noises can prolong your recovery and can worsen your condition.

Distract Yourself

It is often hard to ignore noises, but it can become easier to do when we distract ourselves with other activities and shifting our awareness to other things. You will want to keep your auditory system busy when distracting yourself. Playing low music in the background, listening to birds far away make noises, or leaving your television on for background noise, can all help contribute to keeping your auditory system stimulated but not overworked.

Wearable Sound Generator

Audiologists provide sound generators that are similar to wearing a hearing-aid, but they play soft white noise to help drown out louder noises.

Avoiding Sulfides

Certain items contain a chemical known as sulfides which contribute to developing tinnitus. Red wine, chocolate, pickles, and processed foods containing artificial sugar are to be avoided.

Bryan McAskill's Book of Natural Remedies

Salt

Meniere's disease isa condition that results in excessive amounts of fluid in the ears. Tinnitus often comes after developing this condition unknowingly. Consuming a high sodium intake (more than 2,000-milligrams) a day contributes to fluids accumulating within parts of the body such as the ears. You will want to reduce your sodium intake at this time to no more than 2,000-milligrams a day mostly by cutting the use of table salt and processed foods.

Caffeine

Caffeine constricts blood vessels and temporarily raises blood pressure which can make the sounds of Tinnitus, much louder. Avoiding coffee, sodas, chocolate, soft drinks, and junk items are necessary.

Cigarettes

Smoking cigarettes also constricts the blood vessels like caffeine does and should be avoided. If you do not smoke, you will want to avoid any second-hand smoke you may come in contact with.

Baby Oil

Earwax may build up from the ears constantly working hard to tune out and adjust to a variety of noises all of the time. This may block out some noise but will impair hearing more than anything else. Apply a few drops of baby oil with an eyedropper 1-2 times a day. As the earwax softens, gently flush the ear canal with warm water using a bulb syringe. Repeat several times in order to remove excessive wax from the ears.

Reduce Stress

Stress will impact the weakest parts of your body. if you have tinnitus, higher levels of stress will likely make ordinary sounds seem louder than they actually are, according to Dr. Dhyan Cassie, Au.D., doctor of audiology and coordinator of the Tinnitus/Hyperacusis Management Clinic for Speech and Hearing Associates at the College of New Jersey in Ewing, New Jersey.

"Sweet Oil"

This oil is easy to find and is often made from olive oil and almond oil. Follow instructions on label but you can either drop in a few drops directly into your ear, or massage into the skin in and around the ear daily until there's less earwax buildup and/or until any pain decreases.

Therapy

Tinnitus is associated with a high level of emotional stress where depression, anxiety, and insomnia are present as well, Cognitive Behavioral Therapy (CBT) can help assist with identifying healthier ways to cope and manage this emotional stress and accepting this condition where it is in your life. The goal is to improve your overall quality of life so that tinnitus is not the main focus.

Individual or group therapy is strongly encouraged for having an outlet for verbally expressing yourself in a controlled setting with a professional who often has the therapeutic tools that can remain supportive as you work through these challenges.

CBT is a therapeutic approach where clients learn to do the following:

- Cope better with difficult life situations
- Positively resolve conflicts in relationships
- Deal with grief more effectively
- Mentally handle emotional stress caused by illness, abuse or physical trauma
- Overcome chronic pain, fatigue and other physical symptoms

The specific steps in Cognitive Behavioral Therapy include:

- Identification of situations or circumstances in your life that lead to trouble
- Awareness of your thoughts and emotions surrounding anger triggers
- Acknowledgement of inaccurate, negative thought patterns
- Relearning of healthier, positive thought patterns

Very few risks are associated with cognitive behavioral therapy, and you will likely explore painful feelings and emotions, but you will do it in a safe, guided manner. Cognitive Behavioral Therapy (CBT) is considered a short-term approach and generally lasts about 10 to 20 sessions depending upon your specific disorder, the severity of your symptoms, the amount of time you've been dealing with symptoms, your rate of progress, your current stress levels, and the amount of support you receive from friends and family. Engaging in CBT will help work to take an assessment of the root of your challenges to help it dissolve and re-wire your responses to typical triggers, resulting in an improved quality of life.

Mindfulness-based Stress Reduction (MBSR)

Mindfulness is an awareness approach to help develop skills to control attention and draw focus away from uncomfortable feelings. One study led by Jennifer Gans, PsyD, mindfulness teacher and clinical psychologist who has a private practice in San Francisco, California, found that people who participated in an 8-week program designed specifically for tinnitus, reported a significant improvement in their symptoms.

Colloidal Silver

In his bestselling book, *The pH Miracle: Balance Your Diet, Reclaim Your Health*, by Dr. Robert O. Young, Ph.D., he states ,"Eye or ear problems, including cataracts, glaucoma, redness, blurred vision, poor eyesight, ringing in the ears, earaches, soreness or swelling of the ears, eardrum damage, hardness of hearing, and (in rare cases) loss of hearing: Use 1 drop of colloidal silver topically (directly in the eye or ear) 3 times a day."

Toothache

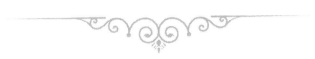

Toothaches can be almost anything. You could have an infection in your gums somewhere, a crack in your tooth, or a cavity. Whatever the cause is, you will want the pain to stop. In this section you will learn about remedies to incorporate to help relieve your toothache so that it hopefully goes away for good, or help you at least manage it on your own before getting an official diagnosis from a dentist.

Remedies:

Chamomile or Calendula (herbs)

Using either of these herbs helps to draw out toxins in an infected tooth. Once a day, moisten a small amount of either herb (or in an herbal tea bag) and place it in the painful area for 15 minutes. Repeat this for three days. If pain decreases, you can continue monitoring your toothache. If no changes occur after 3 days, go make plans to visit a dentist.

Clove Oil (herb) – cavities or hole in tooth

Cloves are often recommended for oral health as this herb can help kill and reduce harmful bacteria. For a general toothache with a visible hole in the tooth or cavity, getting this herb in oil form, is best. Take a small piece of a cotton ball or gauze pad and put 2-3 small drops of clove oil onto it. Place it right inside the hole with a small amount sticking out to help remove later on. Leave in for as long as you notice relief and remove no later than 60 minutes. Use a new ball or gauze pad each time you apply.

Coconut Oil Pulling

Take 2- teaspoons of coconut oil and swish it around in your mouth for about 20 minutes. This is commonly referred to as "oil pulling" or "heavy metal pulling", but this will help provide some relief with underlying issues. You want to closely monitor any additional pain you may feel afterwards, and you can mix in some clove oil or clove powder as well.

Myrrh Powder (herb)

Follow suggested dosage on label and mix in with warm water until dissolved. Swish this around your mouth until toothache pain goes away.

Arnica (herb) - tincture

This herb can work to reduce swelling in the affected area. Swelling mostly appears in the gums which can then prolong recovery. Take a small piece of a cotton ball and apply a few drops of arnica oil onto it. Place next to swollen area on gums. Use this anytime you need relief.

Avoid White Flour and White Sugar

These toxins are highly acidic and can quickly cause cavities and gum damage. Once a tooth issue begins, consuming these items will irritate the nerve in the tooth and cause more severe and frequent toothaches. These items can be very addicting and should be avoided completely.

Hydrogen Peroxide (use with caution)

You will want to floss first and then swish a mouthful of 3-percent solution of hydrogen peroxide for about 5 seconds. Spit it all out and rinse your mouth thoroughly with water. Do this once a day for 3 days at the most.

Caution: make sure to not swallow any as it can damage your esophagus and cause severe stomach cramps. Don't try this more than 3 days as it can begin damaging your gums.

Avoid The Heat

If you are dealing with an infection, you want to remain in a cool, dry area. If you are in a warm or hot area, the heat will draw the infection to the outside of your jaw and make your infection worse. Stay indoors and away from the heat when you have a toothache or tooth infection.

Ice Massage

Rather than placing ice onto your cheek and risking temporary damage and irritation to the skin, try an ice massage instead. Wrap an ice cube in a thin cloth and gently place directly onto area that is affected. Take the ice cube and slowly (and gently0 move it around the area to duplicate a massaging motion. Hold for a few minutes on each section temporarily while massage area. Moving, rather than holding ice around the impacted area will help stimulate more impulses along the nerve pathways and promote recovery. Massaging the area will help outweigh the pain as the area is stimulated and circulation is improved steadily.

Tooth Decay

When we eat sugary foods, bacteria in our mouths eat the leftovers. This issue with this is that the bacteria eats whatever is left over, but also holds onto them, forming a sticky substance called plaque which ends up on your teeth. This plaque coats your teeth with acid that begins to rob minerals from the tooth's outer surface (enamel) while also preventing the teeth from absorbing many minerals consumed through diet/lifestyle. To prevent your teeth from decaying, you will need to avoid sugary foods (not sugars from fruit), and brush and floss regularly. In this section we will review items to avoid and preventative measures we can take to avoid tooth decay.

Remedies:

Avoiding Artificial Sugar

Our teeth are not just small, tiny bones as they may appear to be. They are complex units of living tissue within our bodies that are comprised of many minerals and small, microscopic tubes (tubules) that go from the nerves inside each tooth, to the enamel on the outside of each tooth. These tubules contain a nourishing and cleansing fluid that flows from the inside of the tooth to the enamel (similar to sweating). When we consume artificial sugars, they are not absorbed into the body and get sent back into the bloodstream, in which this flow from the inside of the tooth to the outside of the tooth, becomes reversed, deepening the bacteria in the teeth and leading to tooth decay. Good dental hygiene cannot prevent tooth decay in those who consume diets loaded with artificial sugars located in processed foods, candy, junk items, and things like sports/energy drinks.

Mercury Fillings

Mercury is a poison. Somehow, we've been led to believing that the silver/mercury fillings we have in our mouth are safe, all because we do not die immediately. The silver fillings (dental amalgam) contain about 50% mercury, with additional metals such as copper, silver, and tin.

Experimental trials conducted on lab rats showed that when these rats inhaled the same level of mercury that's in our mouths, they developed legions similar to those with Alzheimer's disease. Chewing gum and sucking candies causes mercury vapor in your mouth to rise. Mercury fillings have been banned in many countries such as Germany, Sweden, England, and Austria due to their danger to the body, particularly harm within pregnant women. Symptoms of mercury poisoning include, fatigue, headaches, insomnia, high blood pressure, irregular heartbeat, allergies, and symptoms of depression.

If applicable, you can choose composite resin, porcelain, or zirconium as replacements for silver-mercury fillings. These fillings are made from a form of plastic that is reinforced with powdered glass. Composite resin has become more popular based on their appearance blending in with the color and texture of teeth, their durability, and lower cost.

Selenium

This mineral helps to displace mercury and help work it out of your system. Dr. David Kennedy, D.D.S., dentist in San Diego, California recommends 200-micrograms of selenium a day.

Common sources of Selenium: brazil nuts, walnuts, chickpeas/garbanzo beans, kola nuts, dandelion greens, nettle, horsetail, and alfalfa. Recommended to consume about 400 micrograms a day.

Cilantro (herb)

Dr. James Hardy, D.M.D., holistic dentist from Winter Park, Florida cites that cilantro is "the best herb for removing heavy metals such as mercury" from the body. he recommends adding ½ ounce of cilantro to salads daily or whenever we're consuming leafy green vegetables.

Cut The Soda

Soft drinks, most notably sodas contain phosphoric acid which eats away at tooth enamel and decreases the protection your teeth have against harmful bacteria and other materials.

Rinse Often

You will want to begin rinsing your mouth with water every time you eat if you are experiencing tooth decay in order to reduce the potentially harmful bacteria from building up.

Tooth Grinding

Teeth grinding or frequent clenching of your teeth often has an emotional cause. Dr. William Payne, D.D.S., dentist in McPherson, Kansas cites that over the several decades he has in practice, those who are emotionally and spiritually aware have better control over avoiding tooth grinding than those who aren't as aware. He concludes that we will grind our teeth rather than deal with the issue in our lives that should be addressed and worked on. When avoiding dealing with stress or concerns effectively, our mind essentially "chews" over these issues and we will begin clenching our jaw or grinding our teeth as a replacement response. In this section we will review calming ad awareness strategies to help gain better control of this unhealthy habit of grinding our teeth.

Remedies:

Designated Time To Rest Before Sleep

To help prevent grinding your teeth while asleep, designate time (20-30 minutes) where you do not do anything stressful before going to sleep. We must not go to sleep irritated. Try taking a warm bath, listen to calming music,

Herbal Tea

Drinking herbal tea can be calming and something soothing to do in the evening, or other part of the day you may have time to relax. Herbs such as chamomile, hops, valerian, blue vervain, lavender, and skullcap are herbs that promote relaxation and deeper sleep. Have fun experimenting with trying different herbs and see which ones you prefer and enjoy the most so you can select them and make drinking herbal tea a habit.

Practice Enunciation

Saying each vowel (A, E, I, O, U) while exaggerating each sound, can help stretch, but also relax the muscles in the face. You will want to do this several times a day to stimulate the muscles in and around the mouth to help deter you away from grinding your teeth. You may also benefit from trying to learn a new language and practicing the pronunciation or new words and phrases as well.

Don't Eat Late

You want as much time between your last meal or snack and the time you lie down to rest. You want your body to feel as relaxed as possible before sleep and have a long gap between chewing your teeth while eating and when going to sleep. Finish eating at least 2-3 hours before going to bed to increase digestion and stimulate metabolism so you're less likely to grind your teeth.

Note: you will also want to avoid carbs and caffeine at night because they will keep the body very active and will disturb your sleep.

Night Guard

Not all cases of teeth grinding are caused by stress and emotional instability. Sometimes people may have a jaw alignment that is not level, or a misaligned bite which results in frequent teeth grinding. A night guard is a mouthpiece made of hard acrylic that prevents you from grinding your teeth. The grinding movements may still persist, but without frequent damage to the teeth which can over time, work to reduce how often the body responses by grinding your teeth. These guards are something you should speak with a dentist about getting as they should be able to provide a custom fit just for your needs.

Tooth Sensitivity

Tooth sensitivity is when the tooth enamel has been worn away. They can't help but be sensitive. Enamel can be worn away from brushing your teeth too hard, chewing on hard objects, and chewing too much on things like gum and candy, among others. Medications and prescribed/recommended mouth rinse to minimize the pain don't solve the issue, which is to re-build and strengthen the enamel. All these products do is allow your body to ignore the continued damage being inflicted on your teeth. In this section we will review ways to naturally work on strengthening and re-build enamel.

Remedies:

Cloves (herb)

This herb is often recommended for sore teeth where you can just suck on this herb. However, for tooth sensitivity, it is best to make a salve to ensure that it stays but can soothe the area(s) in need. Mix ¼ teaspoon of clove powder with a few drops of water. After every meal you eat, gently wipe your teeth clean and apply just enough to cover the sensitive area. Note: don't put this on a tooth that is cracked or has a hole in it to avoid infection.

Calcium Hydroxyapatite

This form of calcium helps to regenerate enamel according to Dr. Edward M. Arana, D.D.S., retired dentist and former President of the American Academy of Biological Dentistry in Carmel Valley, California.

Avoid Cold Items

Eating things with ice or are cold can trigger your teeth sensitivity. Even healthier versions of things like ice cream can worsen this issue. It is best to avoid cold items until your condition improves.

My Personal Remedy:

(mix together in equal parts – liquid extracts)

White oak bark – contains tannins which tighten and clean gum tissue.

Horsetail – rich in selenium to decrease bleeding.

Fennel – high in potassium, sulfur, and sodium which "quiet" the nerves in the teeth.

Option 1:

Take 8 drops of mixture and apply directly onto each tooth that is sensitive.

Option 2:

Dilute 8 drops of this mixture into a cup of water and use as a rinse.

Tooth Stains

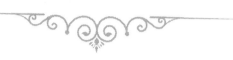

Items such as soda, coffee, cigarettes, acidic juices, medications, and highly processed foods can caused stains on your teeth. Our teeth are naturally light yellow like the rest of our bones, but often darken as we get older. Over time, if we consume some of the items listed above, surface enamel begins to crack and erode, causing more permanent stains. Yellow stains are often initial plaque buildup and can be easily removed, while brown stains are often deeper damage on the tooth and can be difficult to remove. In this section we will review simple wats to address tooth stains and ways to prevent future damage.

Remedies:

Brush and Rinse After Every Meal

You want to completely avoid the items listed at the beginning of this section, but even if you eat healthy, you will want to brush and rinse after every meal to avoid any bacteria or plaque buildup. You will have a decreased chance of developing stains.

Baking Soda and Hydrogen Peroxide Mix

Mix 1 teaspoon with a few drops of hydrogen peroxide and put onto your toothbrush, or brushing stick, and gently brush your teeth. Do this daily and monitor your hydrogen peroxide use as too much can burn your teeth and gums if you use too much.

Plaque Quotient

Go visit a dentist that will provide you with an opportunity to be able to see how much plaque remains after brushing. This is the plaque we cannot often see with our eyes after brushing or rinsing. Locating specific spots that signify plaque can help you focus on these areas and avoid things such as cracking, plaque buildup, cavities, etc.

Miswak

Brushing your teeth with a miswak stick can help reduce bacteria in the mouth. No toothpaste is needed, only water. You can chew or lightly brush your teeth directly.

Ulcers

Ulcers are very common conditions that are often ignored. About 350,000 new cases are diagnosed each year. The stomach pain, sudden weight loss, bloating, burping, and nausea, are often considered to be a part of "normal life" by those who experience these symptoms, and the development of an ulcer(s) gets ignored. Every time that we each anything, our stomachs bathe the food in acids that begin the digestion process. There are proactive tissues in and around the digestive system to help prevent damage to these areas when digesting foods. Sometimes these tissues do break down and bacteria gets inside which creates sores that are knows as, *ulcers*.

Many small ulcers can go away on their own, but most can be attributed to extensive rest. The reoccurrence of these ulcers is the goal in providing more permanent relief to these areas of the body, reversing this condition, and to restore the body.

Remedies:

Reduce Acid Production

Acidic foods mixed with acidic digestive acids, creates excess acidity in the body. Not only acidic foods such as those that taste sour, but items that have a low pH (potential Hydrogen) level. Anyone can review a pH chart and focus heavily on avoiding anything with a pH below a 7.0 which signifies somethings that is acidic or neutral; anything above a 7.0 is alkaline. In addition to this general rule, avoid consuming things such as orange juice, tomatoes, or things like grapefruits or lemons which can taste sour and bitter. These substances when broken down can contribute to irritating these ulcers and can make this condition worse by prolonging symptoms.

Remove Dairy

Cow's milk in all forms stimulates an increase in acid production in the digestive tract which will cause you to feel worse. The texture of milk itself may appear soothing initially, but the damage will come later. Milk ferments quickly in the gut and contains many of the same forms of bacteria that creates ulcers.

Licorice Root (herb)

Glycyrrhizic acid is the chemical found in this plant that helps reduce the symptoms of an ulcer. Dr. Stengler, N.D., naturopathic physician in San Diego, California, recommends 1,000 – 1,500 milligrams of licorice root in capsule form, or 30 drops of licorice root in a tincture form three times a day on an empty stomach to reduce symptoms of an ulcer.

Glutamine

Glutamine (also known as I-glutamine) is an amino acid. It's the most abundant amino acid in the human body. It works to help nourish and repair the digestive tract which is an essential part of the healing process of an ulcer.

Common Sources of Glutamine: chickpeas, walnuts, dark leafy green vegetables, parsley, lentils, kidney beans.

Eat Smaller Meals Several Times A Day

Although every time we eat our stomachs produce acids and our pancreas produces insulin, having foods present in our bodies help to provide a "buffer" so that ulcers do not corrode so quickly. Besides stimulating acids to help break down and digest foods, blood flow is also sent to the stomach when we eat which also helps protect ulcers from being surrounded by digestive acids. Besides committing to 2-3 medium to larger meals a day, work on eating smaller meals and snacks about 5-6 times a day instead.

Reduce Stressors

It has been difficult for doctors and researchers to determine if stress specifically creates ulcers by themselves. However, stress contributes to the brain's perception of pain and can directly contribute to the many symptoms connected to ulcers. Everyone works to regulate and have control of stressors in different ways. The goal is to not control, but to prevent stress from playing a larger role in our lives during this time.

Water

Drinking about half of your body weight in ounces is recommended daily regardless of having a condition or an illness. Water will help dilute the acids in the stomach and provide the same soothing feeling the cow's milk appears to provide, just without the aftereffects and discomfort.

No Smoking or Caffeine

Dr. Samuel Myers, M.D., who works as a gastroenterologist and clinician professor of medicine at Mount Sinai School of Medicine of New York University in New York City states that, "smoking slows down the healing of ulcers, increases the risk of relapses, and makes the body mor susceptible to infection-causing bacteria." Dr. Myers also stated that, "both regular and decaffeinated coffee increase levels of stomach acids." They may not cause ulcers by themselves, but they can increase discomfort when an ulcer is trying to heal.

No Alcohol

Alcohol is not only unhealthy for you, but it can erode the stomach's protection lining which creases excess inflammation and can even lead to bleeding in the gut.

Fiber:

Increasing your fiber intake will help digestion become easier and work to reduce any additional workload on the digestive system. It is recommended for women to aim towards 21-25 grams of fiber a day, while men aim between 30-38 grams of fiber a day.

Common sources of Fiber: garbanzo beans, lentils, brussels sprouts, sweet potatoes, avocado, pears, sunflower seeds, flax seeds, hazelnuts, apples and berries (high pectin fruits) and onions.

Coconut

Anthony involving coconut is good for gut health. Cut and eat a raw coconut, drink coconut water regularly, or even add some coconut milk to your day.

Hawthorn Berry

The flavonoids in hawthorn are helpful for stomach disorders such as stomach spasms, stomach acid deficiency, irritations, and ulcers. You may find hawthorn in many items such as jelly or dried fruit snacks. But when consuming this by itself, adults should take doses between 160-1,200 milligram by mouth daily. Follow instructions on labels you may purchase. Hawthorn better also helps with high blood pressure which can also reduce symptoms of an ulcer.

Prickly Pear Cactus

Cutting and peeling the skin off of this fruit and eating whole is helpful for digestive health. You may juice this fruit or simply drink the water from this fruit. This fruit specifically targets the large intestine where most ulcers begin to grow.

Paw Paw (fruit)

Get an unripe paw paw, cut open and remove the seed. Place int container to soak with spring or distilled water for 5 days. After 5 days, strain out the Paw Paw and drink ½ a cup twice a day for 5 days.

Plantains

Take 4 unripe plantains, peel and cut into small bit-sized pieces. Soak in a 4-litre gallon for 2-3 days in a sealed container in the refrigerator. Drink one glass in the AM and one glass in the evening.

Note: disregard the smell and plan to drink this daily for two weeks and you will notice significant progress in addition to following the other steps listed in this section.

Cleaning The Colon

For Adults:

(for children, cut dosages in half to 1/3 the amount listed)

Colon Cleanse Tea: 1 teaspoon of Cascara Sagrada, ½ teaspoons of Black Walnut, and 1 teaspoon of Rhubarb Root for about 10-12oz of tea. This tea is very bitter. But you want this tea to be bitter so that it can break down what is not needed in the body. If this tea is too difficult for you to adjust to, you can always search for these herbs or colon cleanses available in capsule form. You will want to try this tea prior to fasting to identify which option will be best for you during your liquid fast. Cleaning the Colon is vital for survival. The Colon is a part of the gut which is essentially our 2nd brain. It holds onto leftover waste and materials that create inflammation in the body and directly trigger many symptoms of disease. Without a clean colon, the body cannot function well as a whole.

Duration: 5-6 consecutive days at a time. Do for 5 days then take at least 2 days off.

Ingredients:

Cascara Sagrada (1 teaspoon)

Black Walnut hull (1/2 teaspoon)

Rhubarb Root (1 teaspoon)

Prodijiosa (1 teaspoon) – if applicable/available to you.

Water 8oz (boiling)

*You can do any combination of these herbs or take individually for this cleanse. You do not need every ingredient, but this cleanse works best when including all herbs mentioned above.

This cleanse is probably the most important to our health. The colon is essentially our second brain and is a part of the large intestine which works to remove waste from the body. The colon is responsible for holding a temporary storage of feces, but also reabsorbing water and minerals necessary to our health.

Urinary Tract Infection (UTI)

UTI's occur when bacteria from somewhere outside of the body enter the *urethra* (the tube that carries urine from the bladder to be expelled from the body). The body responds by repeatedly sending out any and all materials (urine) through the urethra to help push out the bacteria. Anyone who has had a UTI will experience consistent trips to the bathroom to urinate.

Sex is the most common way to contract a UTI as intercourse can help open up areas making them more susceptible to allowing in external bacteria. UTI's are also very common during menopause due to the body having less estrogen which makes the tissues within the vagina and urethra drier and vulnerable to bacteria. However, sex is not the only ways someone can contract a UTI. Loose-fitting clothing can interact with bacteria outside of the body, as well as not wearing protective coverings to surround any exposed openings of the body near our reproductive organs. But some other common ways of contracting a UTI is, by holding in your urine for too long, consuming too much artificial sugars, not drinking enough water, and even when going through childbirth. Keep in mind that all waste materials and fluids need to be filtered out and leave the body in some way through the urine. Waste materials and bacteria can build up during this process as mentioned above and can create an infection within the urinary tract.

Note: Women are more likely to develop a UTI in their urethra, bladder, or kidneys. Men can get UTI's also, but the male reproductive anatomy makes it harder to get inside of the body.

Remedies:

Hydration

Consuming an adequate amount of water is necessary at all times to help flush out and transport waste materials out of the body. Not only drinking about half of your body weight in ounces (ex. if you weigh 100lbs, drink 50oz) but consuming foods that provide water is necessary. Melons, berries, tomatoes, and cucumbers are only a few items that should regularly be in your die. Consuming items that provide hydration can help wash away and also neutralize the erosive acids that remain in the body from eating things detrimental to our health. For UTI's, an increased water intake will help to dilute bacteria and concentrated salts in the urine which create much of the discomfort those with UTI's experience.

Baking Soda

Once you notice symptoms occurring, mix ¼ teaspoon of baking soda with about 8 ounces of water. Mix together and consume this once a day to help dilute and dissolve some of the harmful bacteria in the urinary tract.

Evian Water

Although distilled water or natural spring water is best, the name brand water *Evian*, contains the same bicarbonate as baking soda but with much less sodium. This helps neutralize acids in the bladder and kidneys to help reduce pain.

Be Cautious With Fruit Juices

Orange juice, apple juice, or any common fruit juices have a higher acid content than many other liquids we consume and can irritate the body when there's an infection present. Typically, these fruit juices provide many benefits, but should be avoided during this time until symptoms completely dissolve.

Avoid Coffee And Alcohol

Not that these substances provide many benefits, but these substances can make it more difficult to urinate according to Dr. Larrian Gillespie, M.D., retired assistant clinical professor of urology and urogynecology and president of Healthy Life Publications. These substances stimulate the muscular walls of the bladder, which trigger "urges" to urinate and cause additional discomfort and pain.

Check Your Vitamin-C

What we refer to as Vitamin-C is a water-soluble nutrient and powerful antioxidant that helps form and maintain connective tissues, including the bones, blood vessels, and the skin. This nutrient can help reduce symptoms of allergic reactions and inflammation which will help to avoid any prolonging issues. However, Vitamin-C is also responsible for manufacturing the adrenal hormones which are needed to combat the stress the body goes through, especially when an area like the urinary tract is under additional pressure as it attempts to remove unhealthy bacteria. Loading up on Vitamin-C will significantly decrease the symptoms of a UTI such as any irritableness or dry/itchy areas.

Common Sources of Vitamin-C: black currants, bell peppers (red), papaya, spring onion, strawberries, cantaloupe, mango, oranges, watercress, raspberries, and tomatoes.

Wash Before Sex

Being preventative is your best by clearing your area(s) before sex. Washing with water (not products with many chemicals) the entire area as well as the anus before sex can help prevent unwanted bacteria from being pushed up into the vaginal area and the urethra.

Urinate After Sex

If you don't feel stimulated to urinate, drink some water that is around room-temperature to help you push out any bacteria that may be sitting around within the urethra after sex.

Use Lubricant

Most bacteria will come to the surface or stick around due to friction. The more friction, the more potential bacteria can be available for infection. If you're experiencing vaginal dryness, discuss with your partner ways to use a water-based lubricant to help decrease friction and help to reduce the chances of bacteria from settling in.

Change Birth Control

Women often get more infections around the time they have a period. The warmth and moisture of the blood that leaves the body can create a breeding ground for bacteria. Larger tampons can obstruct the bladder and prevent it from emptying (urination) in which it is much easier for bacteria to multiply when urine stays in the bladder for a longer period of time.

Use Regular Tampons

Studies have shown that women who use diaphragms and spermicides for birth control have a higher risk of UTI's because they irritate the urethra lining and surrounding tissues.

Wipe Front To Back

After using the bathroom, make sure to wipe front to back away from the anus to ensure no bacteria is pushed forward towards the urethra.

Dandelion Leaf (herb)

Any part of the dandelion plant is very beneficial for the body. the leaf of the Dandelion plant, however, is considered "nature's best natural diuretic" according to Dr. Mark Stengler, N.D., a naturopathic physician from San Diego, California. Unlike pharmaceutical diuretics, you do not flush out many essential minerals. You want to take about 250 milligrams of dandelion root extract three times a day. You may also take 30-60 drops from a dandelion leaf tincture in ½ a cup of water three times a day. This remedy is safe for women while pregnant, but the moment progress appears to be consistent, cut your dosage in half to avoid creating any mineral deficiencies. If you enjoy drinking tea, you can use the dried form of this herb and drink 2-3 cups a day when using 1-2 teaspoons of this herb.

Juniper

This diuretic can also serve as a laxative that helps reduce water retention as well as sodium retention.

Dosage(s):

Generally, 2 to 10 g/day of the whole, crushed, or powdered fruit (corresponding to 20 to 100 mg of essential oil)

Essential oil: 0.02 to 0.1 mL 3 times daily.

Fluid extract: 1:1 (g/mL); 2 to 3 mL 3 times daily.

Infusion: 2 to 3 g steeped in 150 mL of boiled water for 20 minutes 3 times daily.

Vaginitis (and Yeast) Infection

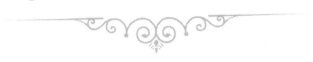

The vagina is essentially its own ecosystem. There are bacteria that is good for protecting this area, and there's harmful bacteria that can invade this area. When there's a bacterial invasion, symptoms such as, soreness, inflammation, pain, irritation, swelling, and discomfort, begin to display itself more often. Doctors will mostly prescribe medications designed to kill this harmful bacterium (which it should), but leftover waste materials and additional bacteria can make its way to this area from consuming these prescriptions and can contribute to these symptoms. What is recommended is improving the vaginal system so it can function well enough so that these harmful bacteria cannot live there.

Note: Proper treatment does depend on knowing which bacteria organism is causing issues. Either (1) Candida albicans, or (2) Protozoa Trichomonas Vaginalis. A standard diagnostic test will tell you which one you are experiencing.

Remedies:

Avoid Sugar (glucose)

Amy Rothenburg, N.D., a naturopathic physician in Enfield, Connecticut states that, "When you want to feed bacteria in a scientific experiment, you coat the petri dish with glucose, or sugar". First step is to not add to the issue that is present by consuming sugar. It is recommended to also avoid refined carbohydrates and alcohol which both turn into glucose when being metabolized and digested.

Completely Avoid: white breads, bagels, waffles, pancakes, white rice, pizza dough, white flours, donuts, white flour pastas, pastries, chips, and cereals, among other items.

Boric Acid

This substance can be a toxic substance you do not want to interact with. However, trace amount of boric acid can be found in many foods you should incorporate more into your diet if you are having any vaginal issues. Items such as apples, bananas, leafy green vegetables, and various nuts. Many fertilizers contain borax but can be tested for being a cause for cancer. In natural soil, it is common to find "sodium borate salt" among other minerals and nutrients which is the scientism name for what we refer to as *boric acid*. Getting foods directly grown in the soil locally will provide additional trace amounts of boric acid to help breakdown infections. Dr. Tori Hudson, naturopathic physician and medical director of A Woman's Time clinic in Portland, Oregon states, "Nothing impresses me more than the success rate of boric acid suppositories for the treatment of candida infections." Dr. Hudson is directly referring to the chemical substances you can find in powder form or in a capsule, so move with caution if you choose any artificial substances to consume when there are many natural options as well.

Dr. Hudson often cites a research study that involved 100 women who all reported having yeast infections and were given boric acid in which 98% had a full recovery within 2-4 weeks. Dr. Hudson recommends 600-milligram capsules that be inserted into the vagina twice a day for 3-7 days for an acute yeast infection and continuing this for 2-4 weeks for a chronic yeast infection.

Triphala (herb)

This herb can work to remove toxins and promote the restoration process of fluids in the body which are both very needed when treating a yeast infection. Soak ½ teaspoon of this dried herb in 1 cup of water for 5 minutes. Let steep, strain out the herb and drink this tea before bed. Once a month you want this herb to be in direct contact with the vagina as well. For this, put 1 tablespoon of this herb in 1 pint of water and bring to a boil. Let cool and then strain. Get a douche bag ready so you can douche your tea. Place the bag directly onto the vaginal area for a few minutes prior to washing the area with water immediately after. Do this at least once a month to help kill harmful bacteria and as a preventative measure later on.

Caution: douching can dry the vaginal area and can upset its natural balance so you will want to talk with your health care practitioner to make sure you are properly douching correctly.

Wear Loose Clothing

All yeast and bacterial infections thrive in warm environments. You can avoid this by wearing loose-fitting clothes so that air can keep this area cool. If you exercise or swim, make an effort to change into dry clothes immediately after. It can also be helpful to sleep in the nude also during this time to prevent this area from getting warmer than needed.

Oil of Oregano

This oil can be applied directly to the skin to reduce inflammation and overgrowths. Consuming this oil orally can benefit the breakdown of yeast infections as well. Pay close attention to instructions on label and check with your physician if your infection is safe enough to apply directly onto infection.

Wear Cotton

Wearing nylon and other synthetic fabrics don't provide the same ability as Cotton does for allowing the skin and area to *breathe*. Cotton panties can help allow air to get in and help prevent any moisture and reduce your symptoms and risk of infection.

Avoid Scented Bathroom Products

Soaps, bath oils, bodywash, and other scented items contain chemicals to produce certain fragrances which can irritate your infection. Avoiding these items can help you become less vulnerable to irritants and help speed up your recovery by keeping your area clean.

Wipe Front To Back

After using the bathroom, make sure to wipe front to back away from the anus to ensure no bacteria is pushed forward towards the urethra and vaginal area.

Varicose Veins

Having varicose veins is mostly seen and treated as a cosmetic issue. We tend to only receive treatments that cover up this issue. However, varicose veins are a disease and a serious one as we cannot replace our veins, and one vein getting clogged can lead to innumerable consequences. Each vein in our legs have specific valves that open to allow blood to flow to the heart and then close so that gravity cannot pull blood right back into the legs. When any of these valves break, blood pools in the vein and create *varicosity* (varicose vein).

Remedies:

Grape Seed or Pine Bark (extract)

Mark Stengler, N.D., naturopathic physician from San Diego, California reports that Grape Seed extract and Pine Bark extract both contain a rich source of anthocyanidins and proanthocyanidins which are bioflavonoids that work well to strengthen the walls of the veins. A daily dose of 150-300 milligrams of either of these extracts can help improve this condition and prevent this condition from getting worse. Berries such as blueberries, blackberries, and cherries are also high in these same flavonoids which can and should be eaten regularly when working to improve upon this condition.

Horse Chestnut (herb)

A *venotonic* is a chemical that helps strengthens the elastic fibers in the vein. There are many prescriptions that are labeled as a "venotonic" but a natural venotonic is an herb called Horse Chestnut. Take 300-milligrams in capsule form or 30 drops of horse chestnut tincture twice a day.

Butcher's Broom (herb)

Varicose veins often involve inflammation and begin to feel painful. When this pain is very persistent it can lead to the development of another condition known as *phlebitis*. To help reduce inflammation, it is recommended to consume a more plant-based diet. In addition to this, an herb known as Butcher's Broom can help directly assist with inflammation in the veins. Take 100 milligrams three times a day.

Bilberry Bark

When you first begin to notice varicose veins, take about 80 milligrams of bilberry bark extract three times a day. This extract helps to shrink the capillaries (blood vessels that become inflamed) so that proper blood flow can be achieved. As you begin to notice improvement start cutting your dosage in half as you wean yourself off of this remedy.

Exercise – "Walk On Water"

Any exercises that work your legs will remain helpful when dealing with varicose veins. You do not want to put much pressure on your legs as you can irritate this condition. A great exercise to do is move around in water. Being in a pool, or water waist-deep water as you simply walk around or work your way up to a complete workout will be best to apply movement and stimulation in the legs, but with low impact and pressure on the muscles, bones, tendons, ligaments, and joints. Aim to walk or gently move around for at least 30 minutes a few days a week while in water. Walking, cycling, swimming, and yoga can be the most helpful forms of exercise to do regularly.

Sleep Position

How you sleep can have a great impact on your condition. Certain sleeping positions can cause the veins in the legs to feel constricted. It is best to sleep with your foot slightly elevated to help reduce and promote circulation. It can be helpful to lie down on the floor, flat on your back and keep your legs elevated for several minutes a day.

Non-restrictive Clothing

Wearing tight-fitting clothes can restrict blood flow. A person may find that their circulation is improved by wearing loose-fitting clothes that do not restrict the blood supply to the lower body. Wearing flat shoes instead of high heels may also help with varicose veins in the legs.

Hydrotherapy

To help continue to improve circulation, incorporate a hot-and-cold foot bath. Fill two large basins, one with warm water and one with ice-cold water. Place your feet first in the cold basin for 30 seconds, and then immediately place your feet into the warm water for about 2 minutes. Repeat at least three times a day to keep the blood vessels active and stimulated. Massaging your legs regularly will remain crucial to reducing your chances of severe symptoms.

Warts

Warts are small colonies of viruses (benign skin tumors) that can anywhere on the body. they can itch, burn, or break open where mucus can ooze out. Besides acne, warts are the most common dermatological condition.

Remedies:

Leave Them Alone

Many warts go away on their own if they are not irritated. If your wart is not getting larger, it may go away on its own after a while.

Stay Dry

Warts are often created in moist spaces. Scan your body and identify areas that become moist such as your feet, hands, or other areas. You will want to keep these areas dry at all times.

Freeze It Off

Going to see your doctor, they can apply ways to freeze your wart off. Freezing the wart can reduce stimulation to the area and also help the wart come off of the skin. There are many products that can be purchased at a local pharmacy or drug store but be cautious to not damage the skin around your wart as this can come with complications.

Olive Leaf

The olive tree contains powerful compounds that break down infections. The active ingredient in olive leaves (oleuropin) should be found on the product label for best effects. Olive leaf can come in dried form, tinctures, or capsules. Make sure to follow instructions on label depending on which form of this plant you decide to use.

Clear Nail Polish

Apply clear nail polish around area to completely cover the wart. Covering the wart with nail polish will create an air-tight seal around the wart, suffocating the virus, and allowing there to be a gradual death where the skin cells can start shedding until the wart can be gone.

Directions:

Brush the polish over the entire surface of the affected area. Allow the polish to dry completely. Reapply three times a day for two to three weeks or until wart is gone. To ensure all sources of oxygen have been eliminated, you may also want to cover the treated area with an adhesive tape.

My Personal Remedy:

Thuja Occidentalis – using 30X potency

Antimonium Crudum – 30X potency

(apply directly onto wart)

Take one dose of Thuja Occidentalis upon awakening and one dose of Antimonium Crudum late afternoon or early evening. Do this for 3-4 days. Dosages for each should be listed on packaging label. Continue this remedy for 3-4 days at a time every 2 weeks until wart goes away.

Thuja Occidentalis is from an evergreen coniferous tree which is extracted from its leaves. Most often used to treat many respiratory and skin infections.

Antimonium Crudum is a product developed from black sulfide out of India. This substance is used for warts and other skin conditions, calluses, and constipation and other stomach ailments.

Water Retention

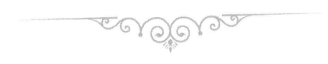

All forms of fluid retention in the body (edema) occur when fluids in the body that usually flow throughout the body, begin to pool together in spaces between the cells. You may feel certain areas of the body appear larger or tighter than usual. Water retention is more common in women since women have additional space in between their cells to support expansion during pregnancy. Doctors will mostly prescribe diuretics (drugs that flush water out of the body) when water retention is present. Although the intention is correct, pharmaceutical drugs that flush water also flush out many essential minerals that are vital to our health such as potassium, magnesium, and iron. Diuretics recommended in this section are natural diuretics which work to flush out water but also provide the body with an abundance of minerals, so they do not contribute to any mineral deficiencies that pharmaceutical drugs create.

Remedies:

Sodium

You cannot absorb water without sodium. You want to avoid excess use of "salt" especially from processed foods and artificial sources. Adding some salt may only help in the short term so you want to rely heavily upon natural sources listed below.

Common sources of sodium: apples, guava, avocado, papaya, mango, carambola, pineapple, banana, melons, beets, pickles, and pears.

Quick Tip: if you boil pieces of hickory, walnuts, and pecan roots, this extracts nutrients such as sodium where you can use this water for meals or to drink after it cools off to boost your sodium intake.

Clean The Kidneys

Water is the best remedy for working to hydrate this detoxifying organ that often holds onto and processes many of the fluids that circulate in the body. It may sound counterproductive to consume more water while your body is retaining water, but a large reason your body has begun retaining water is due to dehydration. When the body is dehydrated it will store water in the kidneys so they can continue to function properly. By consuming more water, you can begin to relieve the kidneys of this additional task and begin working to clean this organ and any accumulated retention of fluids and other waste materials. It is recommended to aim towards half of your bodyweight in ounces a day to remain adequately hydrated.

Dandelion Leaf (herb)

Any part of the dandelion plant is very beneficial for the body. the leaf of the Dandelion plant, however, is considered "nature's best natural diuretic" according to Dr. Mark Stengler, N.D., a naturopathic physician from San Diego, California. Unlike pharmaceutical diuretics, you do not flush out many essential minerals. You want to take about 250 milligrams of dandelion root extract three times a day. You may also take 30-60 drops from a dandelion leaf tincture in ½ a cup of water three times a day. This remedy is safe for women while pregnant, but the moment progress appears to be consistent, cut your dosage in half to avoid creating any mineral deficiencies. If you enjoy drinking tea, you can use the dried form of this herb and drink 2-3 cups a day when using 1-2 teaspoons of this herb.

Burdock

Burdock Root helps purify the blood by cleansing out toxins and increase urine flow. Take up to 3 teaspoons a day in tea form.

Purslane

Purslane inhibits pancreatic *lipase* which reduces work by the pancreas of processing fats and sugars which helps the body avoid retaining water via holding onto collected waste. This herb helps to expel collected waste out through the skin pores and through the urinary tract.

Hawthorn

This herb has long been used in Traditional Chinese Medicine (TCM) for reducing blood pressure. Take 1-2 teaspoons of dried or fresh herb and add to cup. Boil water and pour over herb. Let cool, steep, and drink about 12-ounces a day of this tea for best results.

Juniper

This diuretic can also serve as a laxative that helps reduce water retention as well as sodium retention.

Dosage(s):

Generally, 2 to 10 g/day of the whole, crushed, or powdered fruit (corresponding to 20 to 100 mg of essential oil)

Essential oil: 0.02 to 0.1 mL 3 times daily.

Fluid extract: 1:1 (g/mL); 2 to 3 mL 3 times daily.

Infusion: 2 to 3 g steeped in 150 mL of boiled water for 20 minutes 3 times daily.

Rebounding Exercises

Bouncing up and down by jumping softly on a small trampoline helps to stimulate the lymphatic system which is responsible to managing the fluids in the body. the up and down motions can help to "unlock" much of the water and other fluids that have been held onto or trapped in small pockets within the body over time. Try jumping softly on a small trampoline for about 10-15 minutes a day while fluid retention is present. Remember to bend your knees while jumping to reduce the impact and weight upon your joints.

My Personal Remedy:

The kidneys are one of our main detoxifying organs. When they are backed up, leftover waste materials get pushed into the bloodstream and create stagnation. The blood needs to always flow. We must keep the kidneys clear of toxins and remain hydrated.

Below are 2 examples of something you can do to get started. These should be the only items to consume for 3 days each. Pick one to start with and blend together all ingredients for each meal. Only liquids are to be consumed outside of the items listed below.

Note: neither of these options will completely clean the kidneys but will promote adequate hydration and start the process of naturally cleaning these organs for you to then maintain afterwards.

3 Day Liquid Fast (Option 1)

Morning:

- 2 teaspoons of Key Lime Juice
- 1 tablespoon of Tahini Butter
- 1 Banana
- 1 Cup of Raspberries

- ¼ Cup of Kale
- 1 Tablespoon of Hemp seeds
- 1 Cup of Spring Water

Lunch:

- 1 Cucumber
- 1 Cup of Kale Leaves
- 1 Key Lime (peeled)
- ½ Green Apple
- 1.5 Cups of Walnut Milk
- 1 Cup of Watermelon

Dinner:

- 1 Cup of Blueberries
- ½ Cup of Mango
- 1 Cup of Kale
- ¼ Avocado
- 1 teaspoon of Key Lime Juice
- ¼ teaspoon of Cayenne Pepper
- 1.5 Cups of Coconut Water

3 Day Liquid Fast (Option 2)

Breakfast (AM):

- 1 cup of Spring water
- 1 tablespoon of Hemp Seeds
- 1 Cup of Raspberries
- 1/2 cup of Dandelion Greens
- 1 Burro Banana
- 1 tablespoon of Tahini Butter
- 2 teaspoons of Key Lime Juice

Lunch:
- 1/2 cup of Walnut or Hemp Milk
- 1/2 Cucumber
- 1 cup of Kale
- 1/2 Green Apple
- 1 Squeezed Key Lime
- 1 tablespoon of Coconut Oil
- 1 cup of Mango

Dinner (PM):
- 1.5 cups of Coconut Water
- 1 cup of Blueberries
- 1/2 Cup of Mango
- 1 Cup of Kale
- 1 tablespoon of Key Lime Juice
- 1/2 Avocado
- 1/4 teaspoon of Cayenne Pepper Powder
- 1 tablespoon of Hemp Seeds

Weight Retention

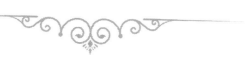

There's nothing particularly healthy about being overweight. However, weight and size can be subjective based upon what you are looking at. A common tool used to measure weight is BMI (body mass index). This involves calculating a formula using a person's height and weight. The formula is BMI = kg/m^2 where kg is a person›s weight in kilograms and m^2 is their height in meters squared. A BMI of 25.0 or more is overweight, while the healthy range is 18.5 to 24.9. BMI applies to most adults 18-65 years. BMI is used to identify when someone may be obese, underweight, or within a "healthy" range. Although a weight does not directly determine one's health, it is more so pointing out the structure of a person. An overweight person may be physically fit, but a BMI can help identify the amount of additional pressure on the joints and ligaments and be used to strengthen certain areas or prepare for any potential injuries over time. An underweight person may have a smaller frame and run the risk of being nutritionally deficient in many areas and want to draw more attention to this. And someone in the "healthy" range may not be very health at all but, having an appropriate BMI, a person can adapt and change without making any drastic changes. The most important piece of BMI is to use what's helpful.

Now, if you do not want to view BMI, you can use a tape measure around each area of your body and identify any areas where there is excess (or lack of) fat, muscle, and size. We are all designed differently, but we want to work without any hindrances that don't involve some outside force. We do not want specific areas of the body to make up for other parts due to them being weaker.

We now live in a world where it is very easy to get larger than what is needed as we have access to many foods high in fat, sugars, refined carbohydrates, and chemicals which promote dependence and an increase consumption of these materials. We often look past or cover up anything we do not want to see or acknowledge. As the population of the world grows heavier, even from a young age, the increase of illness and disease also rise. It's not as if we are not trying to lose any additional weight or hide awareness. We simply live in a world currently where there is much easier access to unhealthy items and sedentary lifestyles are pursued for a variety of reasons. We must work to reduce our overall size (if applicable) as a way to combat the efforts to work further away from obesity and closer towards optimum health and longevity.

Remedies:

Healthier Lifestyle

This is what it all boils down to. the goal is to continue to add more healthy items into your life so that there's less room for any bad habits to contribute to maintaining or gaining weight. Rather than promote specific ways to go about it, take some time and look ahead in your journey towards losing more weight. An important part to remain mindful of is that whatever plan, subscription, or "diet" you initially start out with, they are steps in the correct direction. However, also keep in mind that your first step will not be the same as your next step, nor will it be the same as your last. The most important part is getting started. As this involves a lifestyle change, many other changes will come with this. So also incorporate ways to reduce stress while committing to remaining flexible on your journey. You should encounter a "healing crisis" where the body (and the mind) feel all changes coming at once, which can feel overwhelming, but is a necessary part of this process. Keep in mind that the positive attitude and mindset that you develop over time is yours. Make difficult but necessary changes and enjoy yourself (not indulge) along the way.

General outline for someone wanting to lose weight/waste:

Breakfast (break-fast): a few cups of water to get digestion started. Try to stick with liquids (smoothie, juice, or tea) only but can eat some soft fruit.

Lunch: salad with mostly water-filled veggies, grains and some nuts.

Dinner: something small but filling. Sautee some vegetables and mix together with some leafy green vegetables and your favorite grains.

Note: for specific food recommendations, I encourage variety, whole-food, plant-based items. When you eat better, you can eat in abundance without consequences that you may be used to. Use each item as a necessary step in the right direction towards optimum health and longevity. Set reasonable goals and encourage guidance from others who have achieved success.

Note: the more weight/waste that you remove, the fewer calories overall you will need to consume in order to maintain your new weight. You will thrive off of less and future goals will become simpler and more specific to reach for.

Avoid "Labor-Savers"

Having access to many things that help us "save time" have become unnecessary (although appreciative) at times. Items such as escalators in the mall which only go up one floor, remote controls where we can change the channel from our seat, to remote starting our vehicles to melt the snow/ice off of our cars as we relax and wait. All of these items take a toll off of us but relying on them out of necessity without engaging in regular physical exercise, these items can add to any weight issues one may have. You may not gain more weight from using devices such as the ones named above, but they promote at least a semi-sedentary lifestyle. Avoiding these *labor-savers* can help you not only help you avoid becoming use to maintaining more of a sedentary lifestyle, but help you burn some extra calories, and possible help promote kickstarting your metabolism (which breaks down food in the digestive tract), and lead to you consuming water more often than you typically do.

Try taking the stairs whenever you can. If you feel a need to change channels on your TV, use this as a sign to do another activity rather than continuing to find stations that will leave you sitting in the same place. If it's not too cold, get ready earlier and spend some time brushing off snow and scraping ice off of your car to get moving first thing in the morning.

Keep A Food Journal

In order to change your eating habits and eating behavior, you must start paying attention to what you eat and when you eat; later on, you may discover why you are eating certain items. Note what you consume for a few days and then take a step back so you can review what items you consume that are not helpful in addition to any habits/routines you may notice that you want to adjust.

Get A Full-Length Mirror

These can be purchased for about $20 and can be placed anywhere. If you are only viewing your face in a mirror at home, you will not notice many positive or negative changes your body has on display. Viewing yourself from a full-length mirror will help keep a more accurate view of your entire body as well as serve as a reminder for what you're working on, as well as any noticeable improvements you've been working towards.

Figure Out What You Need

This could include ingredients for meals you want to make, items you plan to incorporate into your lifestyle, or support that you know will be needed. whatever it is, either you "will fail to plan or plan to fail". Plan ahead what you need and create a list of necessary items you want to consume, as well as supports that you want to rely upon. You may have close friends or family you want to check in with regularly, or possibly some comfort item you want close by in times of need as this journey can present its obstacles. Figure out what you need and have everything set ahead of time. If you write it down, you won't waste additional energy thinking about it.

Get Creative

Aside from making newer meals and enjoying this process, get creative in all areas whether you are home or not. Split a meal with a friend, ask your waiter to box up half your meal immediately so you can eat it later and avoid overindulging, take all sides home, or even ask if they could give you a larger portion ("super-size") of a salad as many restaurants do with other dishes.

Movement Is Medicine

Many who are looking to lose weight show signs of depression. Daily exercise should be looked at as a requirement for those who experience any variety of sadness or despair. Not that this is an additional task but viewed as more of being an activity to avoid being stagnant. It's not necessary to develop a body-building schedule or spend all of your free time at the gym. Simply going for a walk for 20-30 minutes a day can be very beneficial to alleviating symptoms of depression. Keith W. Johnsgard, Ph.D., professor emeritus of psychology at San Jose State University in California, USA states that, "the changes in brain chemistry provoked by exercise appear to parallel those of the major antidepressant drugs".

Fiber

Fiber helps promote ease of digestion because it absorbs a lot of water and helps create softer stools, which promote eliminating larger quantities of waste easier. The American Dietetic Association recommends 20-35 grams of fiber daily. This may sound like a lot but, ½ cup of leafy green vegetables can provide about 5g, a small apple is about 3g, and consuming grains like quinoa can provide up to 8g per cup. Just these three items together and you are almost at your daily recommended amount in addition to any other foods you consume that have fiber.

Common sources of Fiber: garbanzo beans, lentils, brussels sprouts, sweet potatoes, avocado, pears, sunflower seeds, flax seeds, hazelnuts, apples and berries (high pectin fruits) and onions.

Note:

If you suspect that you or someone you care about may have an eating disorder, seek out professional help immediately.

National Eating Disorders Association

603 Stewart Street, Suite 803

Seattle, WA, 98101

800-931-2237

www.nationaleatingdisorders.org

National Association of Anorexia Nervosa and Associated Disorders

PO Box 7

Highland Park, IL, 60035

847-831-3438

www.anad.org

Wrinkles

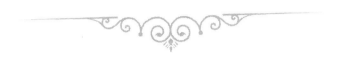

The skin, over time, ages in two different ways: (1) Intrinsic Aging and (2) Extrinsic Aging. Intrinsic aging is genetically programmed into your DNA and will require more attention than it may for other people. Intrinsic aging may prematurely lead to dak spots or other dermatological issues. Extrinsic aging involves how the skin is doing externally such as how it weathers the sun, remaining moist and clear of toxins. Both forms of skin aging will benefit from proper hydration and care; intrinsic aging just involves more attention and specificity. We must reduce the amount of wear and tear, or toll the skin goes through both, internally (intrinsic) and externally (extrinsic).

Remedies:

Sleep On your Back

If your face lays against pillows or sheets for hours while asleep, you are increasing your chances of wrinkles. This can take practice as it's best to try taking naps at first on your back. Many who sleep with their face directly on a pillow often slide around where the face will begin sliding off of the pillow, sheet, or blanket and create temporary wrinkles.

Avoid Squinting

When we squint, we become prone to developing "crow's feet" (wrinkles around the eyes). It is in your best interest to quint whether something is faraway, nearby, or looking too directly into the sun if you are outside during the day. For more on eyesight, review the section in this book under "Eyesight".

Stop Smoking Cigarettes

Dr. D'Anne Kleinsmith, M.D., a cosmetic dermatologist at William Beaumont Hospital in Royal Oak, Michigan, USA states that, "Smokers have more wrinkles than people who don't smoke, especially around the lips". Smoking reduces the body's ability to hold onto oxygen which decreases blood circulation to the areas such as the lips and face. Smoking also involves many facial movements which also add to the amount for wrinkles that can remain present on the face.

Avoid Sunglasses Whenever Possible

Sunglasses are meant to protect the constant glare of the sun from damaging the eyes. However, when you wear sunglasses, the body's natural defense system is turned off in which the sun can penetrate the skin without working through any barriers. This can dehydrate the skin much faster and create wrinkles faster along with many other skin issues.

Refrain from Using Generic Soups

Aside from containing many chemicals, these items will make your skin feel clean even though it robs your skin of many natural oils which will prematurely age your skin and lead to wrinkles.

AHAs (Eat Your Fruit)

Alpha hydroxy acids (AHAs) are natural acids found in fruits and many other plants. These are often used specifically in many lotions, creams, and moisturizers. It is encouraged to not use any products with unnatural chemicals, but making sure products you get contain AHAs to start with. It is best to get your AHAs from the source: nature. Increasing your consumption of fruit and plants will help your skin naturally clear away any blemishes, dark spots, or wrinkles.

Hydration

Not only drinking about half of your body weight in ounces (ex. if you weigh 100lbs, drink 50oz) but consuming foods that provide water is necessary. Melons, berries, tomatoes, and cucumbers are only a few items that should regularly be in your die. Consuming items that provide hydration can help wash away and also neutralize the erosive acids that remain in the body from eating things detrimental to our health.

"Misting"

Aside from drinking enough water and consuming foods that promote hydration, spraying water onto your face will help maintain moisture that is often lost throughout the day.

When dealing with wrinkles, you want to not only eliminate the larger ones, but also the smaller ones that are beginning to form due to reduced moisture.

Massage Oil Recipe

1 ounce of sesame oil, and two drops of sandalwood essential oil. With your fingers, gently massage your forehead horizontally. Do this once a day for a few months.

Apricot Kernal Oil

You can get this oil in tincture form. Massage a light dose onto your face and wash off after about 20-25 minutes. You can also find this oil in tincture form to take orally but make sure to read instructions on label.

My Personal Remedies:

(Taken From my book, *Fasting: A Guide To Health And Wellness*)

Anti-Acne Face Mask

Ingredients:

- 1 Key Lime (juiced)
- 1 teaspoon of Agave Nectar
- 7-10 Fresh Basil Leaves

Instructions:

- Mash fresh Basil leaves. Mix with key lime and agave nectar until smooth.
- Apply this mixture to clean skin. Allow to dry for 30 minutes. Rinse with water and pat dry.
- Repeat three times weekly.

Smoothing Face Mask

Ingredients:

- 1 Cucumber, seeded
- 1 Key lime

Instructions:

- Peel and chop one cucumber. Put the pieces in a blender and mix until smooth.
- Mix 1 teaspoon of fresh Key Lime juice with 1 teaspoon of fresh cucumber juice.

- Use a cotton ball to apply to clean skin. Leave on for 20 minutes. Rinse with cool water and pat dry.
- Repeat daily. You can store cucumber juice in the refrigerator for repeated use.

Remove Dark Spots Mask

Ingredients:

- 1 Papaya
- 1/2 teaspoon of Key Lime Juice

Instructions:

- Blend or mash up a soft ripe Papaya into a puree. Make sure there are no lumps. Add 1/2 teaspoon of Key Lime Juice and mix together.
- Apply the face mask onto your clean face and let it dry for 15-30 minutes.
- Wash away with water. You can do this as needed but no more than three times a week.

Natural Face Mask

Ingredients:

- 1 tablespoon of Agave
- 1 tablespoon of Plum Tomato

Instructions:

- Blend Plum Tomato until you get a smooth puree.
- Stir in with Agave.
- Apply mixture onto your face and let sit for about 15 minutes.
- Wash off with cold water and pat face to dry.
- For more firm skin, mix in 1 tablespoon of Sea Moss Powder and 1 tablespoon of Bladderwrack powder of this mix and leave on your face for 30 minutes before washing off.

Sea Moss Facial Scrub

Ingredients:

- 2 tablespoons of Sea Moss Gel
- Spring Water
- dry brush or exfoliating brush (optional)

Instructions:

- Add 2 tablespoons of Sea Moss Gel to a bowl.

- Add water slowly to bowl (about 1/2 cup). You can add more water if needed but depends on preference.

- Mix together well.

- Apply Gel to face and rub into your skin. you can apply with a dry brush or exfoliating brush if you want a deeper clean.

- Wash off your face with water and pat to dry.

References Section

Acne

Anderson, Gregory J., and Fudi Wang. "Essential but toxic: controlling the flux of iron in the body." *Clinical and Experimental Pharmacology and Physiology* 39.8 (2012): 719-724.

Bowe, Whitney P., and Alan C. Logan. "Acne vulgaris, probiotics and the gut-brain-skin axis-back to the future?." *Gut pathogens* 3 (2011): 1-11.

De Carvalho, Carla CCR, and Maria José Caramujo. "The various roles of fatty acids." *Molecules* 23.10 (2018): 2583.

Fulton Jr, James E., Stephen R. Pay, and James E. Fulton III. "Comedogenicity of current therapeutic products, cosmetics, and ingredients in the rabbit ear." *Journal of the American Academy of Dermatology* 10.1 (1984): 96-105.

Juhl, Christian R., et al. "Dairy intake and acne vulgaris: a systematic review and meta-analysis of 78,529 children, adolescents, and young adults." *nutrients* 10.8 (2018): 1049.

Law, M. P. M., et al. "An investigation of the association between diet and occurrence of acne: a rational approach from a traditional Chinese medicine perspective." *Clinical and experimental dermatology* 35.1 (2010): 31-35.

Ma, Li, Austen Terwilliger, and Anthony W. Maresso. "Iron and zinc exploitation during bacterial pathogenesis." *Metallomics* 7.12 (2015): 1541-1554.

McAskill, Bryan. Fasting: A Guide to Health and Wellness. Balboa Press, 2020.

Pazyar, Nader, et al. "A review of applications of tea tree oil in dermatology." *International journal of dermatology* 52.7 (2013): 784-790.

Pham-Huy, Lien Ai, Hua He, and Chuong Pham-Huy. "Free radicals, antioxidants in disease and health." *International journal*

Samra, George. "The Hypoglycemic Health Association." (2001).

Thompson, Katherine G., et al. "Minocycline and its impact on microbial dysbiosis in the skin and gastro-intestinal tract of acne patients." *Annals of Dermatology* 32.1 (2020): 21.

Addictions

Avena, Nicole M., Pedro Rada, and Bartley G. Hoebel. "Evidence for sugar addiction: behavioral and neurochemical effects of intermittent, excessive sugar intake." *Neuroscience & Biobehavioral Reviews* 32.1 (2008): 20-39.

Fatouros, John G., Allan H. Goldfarb, and Athanasios Z. Jamurtas. "Low carbohydrate diet induces changes in central and peripheral beta-endorphins." *Nutrition Research* 15.11 (1995): 1683-1694.

Gottlieb, Bill. *Alternative Cures: More Than 1,000 of the Most Effective Natural Home Remedies.* Ballantine Books, 2008.

Gomes, Bruno Ramos, and Luis Fernando Tofoli. "A sacred plant of neuronal effect: the use of ibogaine in addiction treatments in Brazil." *Anthropology of consciousness* 33.2 (2022): 333-357.

Wiss, David A., Nicole Avena, and Pedro Rada. "Sugar addiction: from evolution to revolution." *Frontiers in psychiatry* 9 (2018): 385158.

Allergies

Platts-Mills, Thomas AE. "The allergy epidemics: 1870-2010." *Journal of Allergy and Clinical Immunology* 136.1 (2015): 3-13.

Valenta, Rudolf, et al. "Food allergies: the basics." *Gastroenterology* 148.6 (2015): 1120-1131.

Alzheimer's Disease

Bakulski, Kelly M., et al. "Heavy metals exposure and Alzheimer's disease and related dementias." *Journal of Alzheimer's Disease* 76.4 (2020): 1215-1242.

Birks, Jacqueline S., and Richard J. Harvey. "Donepezil for dementia due to Alzheimer's disease." *Cochrane Database of systematic reviews* 6 (2018).

Cisbani, Giulia, and Richard P. Bazinet. "The role of peripheral fatty acids as biomarkers for Alzheimer's disease and brain inflammation." *Prostaglandins, Leukotrienes and Essential Fatty Acids* 164 (2021): 102205.

Fu, Li-Min, and Ju-Tzu Li. "A systematic review of single Chinese herbs for Alzheimer's disease treatment." *Evidence-based Complementary and Alternative Medicine: eCAM* 2011 (2011).

Lee, Hyun Jin, Moo Kyun Park, and Young Rok Seo. "Pathogenic mechanisms of heavy metal induced-Alzheimer's disease." *Toxicology and Environmental Health Sciences* 10 (2018): 1-10.

Megur, Ashwinipriyadarshini, et al. "The microbiota–gut–brain axis and Alzheimer's disease: neuroinflammation is to blame?." *Nutrients* 13.1 (2020): 37.

Anal Itching, Fissures, and Discomfort

Chang, Jason, Elisabeth McLemore, and Talar Tejirian. "Anal health care basics." *The Permanente Journal* 20.4 (2016).

Fargo, Matthew V., and Kelly M. Latimer. "Evaluation and management of common anorectal conditions." *American family physician* 85.6 (2012): 624-630.

Gilani, Artaza, and Gillian Tierney. "Chronic anal fissure in adults." *bmj* 376 (2022).

Anemia

Abramowicz, Beata, et al. "Copper and iron deficiency in dairy cattle." *Journal of Elementology* 26.1 (2021).

Besarab, Anatole, and Stefan Hemmerich. "Iron-deficiency anemia." *Management of Anemia: A Comprehensive Guide for Clinicians* (2018): 11-29.

McNulty, Helene. "The Role of B-Vitamins in Nutritional Anemia." *Nutritional Anemia*. Cham: Springer International Publishing, 2022. 173-185.

Mehta, Sudha W., Mary E. Pritchard, and Charles Stegman. "Contribution of coffee, and tea to anemia among NHANES II participants." *Nutrition Research* 12.2 (1992): 209-222.

Scott, John M. "Nutritional anemia: B-vitamins." *Nutritional Anemia* (2007): 111.

Silva, Carla Sousa, et al. "Trace minerals in human health: Iron, zinc, copper, manganese and fluorine." *International Journal of Science and Research Methodology* 13.3 (2019): 57-80.

Sinha, Nitin, et al. "Effect of iron deficiency anemia on hemoglobin A1c levels." *Annals of laboratory medicine* 32.1 (2012): 17.

Anger

Beck, Richard, and Ephrem Fernandez. "Cognitive-behavioral therapy in the treatment of anger: A meta-analysis." *Cognitive therapy and research* 22.1 (1998): 63-74.

Priyanka, K. *A Study to assess the effectiveness of deep breathing exercise on reduction of anger expression among a*

Rosenwein, Barbara H. *Anger: The conflicted history of an emotion*. Yale University Press, 2020.

Shahrajabian, Mohamad H. "Powerful stress relieving medicinal plants for anger, anxiety, depression, and stress during global pandemic." *Recent patents on biotechnology* 16.4 (2022): 284-310.

Sukhodolsky, Denis G., Howard Kassinove, and Bernard S. Gorman. "Cognitive-behavioral therapy for anger in children and adolescents: A meta-analysis." *Aggression and violent behavior* 9.3 (2004): 247-269.

Angina

Anderson, T. W. "Vitamin E in angina pectoris." *Canadian Medical Association Journal* 110.4 (1974): 401.

Gallacher, J. E. J., et al. "Effect of stress management on angina." *Psychology and Health* 12.4 (1997): 523-532.

Kloner, Robert A., and Bernard Chaitman. "Angina and its management." *Journal of cardiovascular pharmacology and therapeutics* 22.3 (2017): 199-209.

Kinlay, Scott. "Coronary artery spasm as a cause of angina." *Circulation* 129.17 (2014): 1717-1719.

Long, Linda, et al. "Exercise-based cardiac rehabilitation for adults with stable angina." *Cochrane Database of Systematic Reviews* 2 (2018)

Russo, Michele, et al. "Healed plaques in patients with stable angina pectoris." *Arteriosclerosis, Thrombosis, and Vascular Biology* 40.6 (2020): 1587-1597.

Sultan, Sulaiman, et al. "Chelation therapy in cardiovascular disease: an update." *Expert review of clinical pharmacology* 10.8 (2017): 843-854.

Szczurek, Linda, Devin C. Flaherty, and Marc A. Neff. "Colon and Small Bowel." *Passing the General Surgery Oral Board Exa*

Tran, Mongthuong T., et al. "Role of coenzyme Q10 in chronic heart failure, angina, and hypertension." *Pharmacotherapy: The Journal of Human Pharmacology and Drug Therapy* 21.7 (2001): 797-806.

Ankle Sprain

Braund, Rhiannon, et al. "Recommendations of community pharmacists for the treatment of sprains and strains." *International Journal of Pharmacy Practice* 14.4 (2006): 271-276.

Fong, Daniel Tik-Pui, et al. "Sport-related ankle injuries attending an accident and emergency department." *Injury* 39.10 (2008): 1222-1227.

Hing, Wayne A., et al. "Comparison of multimodal physiotherapy and" RICE" self-treatment for early management of ankle sprains." *New zealand journal of physiotherapy* 39.1 (2011): 10-16.

Anxiety

Bull, Barbara Jeanne. *Building chemistry one atom at a time: An investigation of the effects of two curricula in students' understanding of covalent bonding and atomic size.* Diss. Clemson University, 2014.

Choi, Ji Min, et al. "Association between anxiety and depression and nonalcoholic fatty liver disease." *Frontiers in medicine* 7 (2021): 585618.

Coryell, William, et al. "Anxiety responses to CO2 inhalation in subjects at high-risk for panic disorder." *Journal of affective disorders* 92.1 (2006): 63-70.

Daviu, Nuria, et al. "Neurobiological links between stress and anxiety." *Neurobiology of stress* 11 (2019): 100191.

Dogar, I., et al. "Relationship between liver diseases and levels of anxiety and depression." *J Pak Psych Soc* 6.2 (2009): 61-4.

Evans, R. Lee, and Alex A. Cardoni. "Alprazolam (Xanax®, the Upjohn Company)." *Drug Intelligence & Clinical Pharmacy* 15.9 (1981): 633-638.

Jacka, Felice N., et al. "Association between magnesium intake and depression and anxiety in community-dwelling adults: the Hordaland Health Study." *Australian & New Zealand Journal of Psychiatry* 43.1 (2009): 45-52.

Mathew, Roy J., and William H. Wilson. "Cerebral blood flow changes induced by CO2 in anxiety." *Psychiatry research* 23.3 (1988): 285-294.

Nestor, James. *Breath: The new science of a lost art.* Penguin, 2020.

Veleber, David M., and Donald I. Templer. "Effects of caffeine on anxiety and depression." *Journal of Abnormal Psychology* 93.1 (1984): 120.

Weil, Andrew. *Health and healing: The philosophy of integrative medicine.* Houghton Mifflin Harcourt, 2004.

Arrythmia

Alp, Hayrullah, et al. "Protective effects of Hawthorn (Crataegus oxyacantha) extract against digoxin-induced arrhythmias in rats." *The Anatolian Journal of Cardiology* 15.12 (2015): 970.

Gottlieb, Bill. *Alternative Cures: More Than 1,000 of the Most Effective Natural Home Remedies*. Ballantine Books, 2008.

Pippa, Lucio, et al. "Functional capacity after traditional Chinese medicine (qi gong) training in patients with chronic atrial fibrillation: a randomized controlled trial." *Preventive cardiology* 10.1 (2007): 22-25.

Takara, Tsuyoshi, et al. "Passionflower Extract Improves Diurnal Quality of Life in Japanese Subjects with Anxiety: A Randomized, Placebo-controlled, Double-blind Trial." *Functional Foods in Health and Disease* 9.5 (2019): 312-327.

Arthritis

Darlington, L. Gail, and Trevor W. Stone. "Antioxidants and fatty acids in the amelioration of rheumatoid arthritis and related disorders." *British Journal of Nutrition* 85.3 (2001): 251-269.

Hazes, Johanna MW, and Jolanda J. Luime. "The epidemiology of early inflammatory arthritis." *Nature Reviews Rheumatology* 7.7 (2011): 381-390.

Lee, Hea-Young, et al. "Tai Chi exercise and auricular acupressure for people with rheumatoid arthritis: an evaluation study." *Journal of clinical nursing* 21.19pt20 (2012): 2812-2822.

Lin, Chun-Ru, et al. "Willow Bark (Salix spp.) Used for Pain Relief in Arthritis: A Meta-Analysis of Randomized Controlled Trials." *Life* 13.10 (2023): 2058.

Müller, Horst, F. Wilhelmi de Toledo, and K-L. Resch. "Fasting followed by vegetarian diet in patients with rheumatoid arthritis: a systematic review." *Scandinavian journal of rheumatology* 30.1 (2001): 1-10.

Rajendran, A., and R. Sudeshraj. "The therapeutic value of Ayurvedic proprietary medicine Artin oil for chronic musculoskeletal pain relief & Arthritis." (2020).

Rimón, Ranan, and Riikka-Liisa Laakso. "Overt Psychopathology in Rheumatoid Arthritis A Fifteen-year Follow-up Study." *Scandinavian journal of rheumatology* 13.4 (1984): 324-328.

Venetsanopoulou, Aliki I., Paraskevi V. Voulgari, and Alexandros A. Drosos. "Fasting mimicking diets: A literature review of their impact on inflammatory arthritis." *Mediterranean Journal of Rheumatology* 30.4 (2019): 201-206.

Yarnell, Eric. "Herbs for rheumatoid arthritis." *Alternative and Complementary Therapies* 23.4 (2017): 149-156.

Asthma

Escudero, C., et al. "Egg white proteins as inhalant allergens associated with baker's asthma." *Allergy* 58.7 (2003): 616-620.

Frontela-Saseta, Carmen, Carlos A. González-Bermúdez, and Luis García-Marcos. "Diet: a specific part of the Western lifestyle pack in the asthma epidemic." *Journal of clinical medicine* 9.7 (2020): 2063.

Hendrick, D. J., R. J. Davies, and J. Pepys. "Bakers' asthma." *Clinical & Experimental Allergy* 6.3 (1976): 241-250.

Jamalvandi, Mona, et al. "Dairy intake in association with asthma symptoms among a large sample of children and adolescents: a cross-sectional study." *Frontiers in Nutrition* 11 (2024): 1298704.

Kool, Mirjam, et al. "An unexpected role for uric acid as an inducer of T helper 2 cell immunity to inhaled antigens and inflammatory mediator of allergic asthma." *Immunity* 34.4 (2011): 527-540

Lin, Li, Wan Chun, and W. E. N. Fuqiang. "An unexpected role for serum uric acid as a biomarker for severity of asthma exacerbation." *Asian pacific journal of allergy and immunology* 32.1 (2014): 93.

Park, Sohyun, et al. "Association of sugar-sweetened beverage intake frequency and asthma among US adults, 2013." *Preventive medicine* 91 (2016): 58-61.

Song, Feng, et al. "Consumption of milk and dairy products and risk of asthma in children: a systematic review and Meta-analysis." *Archives of Public Health* 81.1 (2023): 147.

Sveiven, Stefanie N., et al. "Milk Consumption and Respiratory Function in Asthma Patients: NHANES Analysis 2007–2012." *Nutrients* 13.4 (2021): 1182

Taylor, Philip E., et al. "Links between pollen, atopy and the asthma epidemic." *International archives of allergy and immunology* 144.2 (2007): 162-17

Woods, Rosalie K., et al. "Do dairy products induce bronchoconstriction in adults with asthma?." *Journal of allergy and clinical immunology* 101.1 (1998): 45-50.

Xie, Luyu, et al. "Association between asthma and sugar-sweetened beverage consumption in the United States pediatric population." *Journal of Asthma* 59.5 (2022): 926-933.

Athlete's Foot

Crawford, Fay. "Athlete's foot." *BMJ clinical evidence* 2009 (2009).

Crawford, Fay, et al. "Athlete's foot and fungally infected toenails." *BMJ* 322.7281 (2001): 288-289.

Zhang, H. W., Z. X. Lin, and Kelvin Chan. "Treatments used in complementary and alternative medicine." *Side Effects of Drugs Annual*. Vol. 37. Elsevier, 2015. 595-601.

Attention Deficit Hyperactivity Disorder (ADHD)

Antshel, Kevin M., et al. "Advances in understanding and treating ADHD." BMC medicine 9 (2011): 1-12.

Arnold, L. Eugene, Nicholas Lofthouse, and Elizabeth Hurt. "Artificial food colors and attention-deficit/hyperactivity symptoms: conclusions to dye for." *Neurotherapeutics* 9.3 (2012): 599-609.

Berner, A., et al. "Higher prevalence of iron deficiency as strong predictor of attention deficit hyperactivity disorder in children." *Annals of medical and health sciences research* 4.3 (2014): 291-297.

Boland, Heidi, et al. "A literature review and meta-analysis on the effects of ADHD medications on functional outcomes." Journal of Psychiatric Research 123 (2020): 21-30.

Campbell-McBride, Natasha. *Gut and psychology syndrome: Natural treatment for autism, dyspraxia, ADD, dyslexia, ADHD, depression, schizophrenia*. Chelsea Green Publishing, 2018.

Chalon, Sylvie. "The role of fatty acids in the treatment of ADHD." *Neuropharmacology* 57.7-8 (2009): 636-639.

Del-Ponte, Bianca, et al. "Sugar consumption and attention-deficit/hyperactivity disorder (ADHD): A birth cohort study." *Journal of affective disorders* 243 (2019): 290-296.

Farsad-Naeimi, Alireza, et al. "Sugar consumption, sugar sweetened beverages and Attention Deficit Hyperactivity Disorder: A systematic review and meta-analysis." *Complementary therapies in medicine* 53 (2020): 102512.

Gillies, Donna, Matthew J. Leach, and Guillermo Perez Algorta. "Polyunsaturated fatty acids (PUFA) for attention deficit hyperactivity disorder (ADHD) in children and adolescents." *Cochrane Database of Systematic Reviews* 4 (2023).

Harms, How Hyperglycemia. "Blood Sugar and the Brain." (2019).

Islam, Kamirul, et al. "A study on association of iron deficiency with attention deficit hyperactivity disorder in a tertiary care center." *Indian journal of psychiatry* 60.1 (2018): 131-134.

Jacobson, Michael F., and David Schardt. "Diet, ADHD & Behavior: A Quarter-Century Review [and] A Parent's Guide to Diet, ADHD & Behavior." (1999).

Kanarek, Robin B. "Artificial food dyes and attention deficit hyperactivity disorder." Nutrition reviews 69.7 (2011): 385-391.

Kleinman, Ronald E., et al. "A research model for investigating the effects of artificial food colorings on children with ADHD." *Pediatrics* 127.6 (2011): e1575-e1584.

Peiper, Howard, and Rachel Bell. *The ADD & ADHD Diet!*. Square One Publishers, Inc., 2012.

Porteous, Sharon Ruth. *HYPOGLYCEMIA AND RELATED EMOTIONAL AND BEHAVIORAL DISORDERS*. Western Michigan University, 1979

Prinz, Ronald J., William A. Roberts, and Elaine Hantman. "Dietary correlates of hyperactive behavior in children." *Journal of consulting and clinical psychology* 48.6 (1980): 760.

Scheffler, Richard M., et al. "The global market for ADHD medications." Health affairs 26.2 (2007): 450-457

Tripp, Gail, and Jeffery R. Wickens. "Neurobiology of ADHD." Neuropha

Back Pain

Cramer, Holger, et al. "A systematic review and meta-analysis of yoga for low back pain." *The Clinical journal of pain* 29.5 (2013): 450-460.

Doshi, A., et al. "Back pain and acute kidney injury." *Clinical medicine* 13.1 (2013): 71.

Gottlieb, Bill. *Alternative Cures: More Than 1,000 of the Most Effective Natural Home Remedies*. Ballantine Books, 2008.

Heffner, Kathi L., et al. "Chronic low back pain, sleep disturbance, and interleukin-6." *The Clinical journal of pain* 27.1 (2011): 35-41.

Kelly, Gráinne A., et al. "The association between chronic low back pain and sleep: a systematic review." *The Clinical journal of pain* 27.2 (2011): 169-181.

Shara, Mohd, and Sidney J. Stohs. "Efficacy and safety of white willow bark (Salix alba) extracts." *Phytotherapy Research* 29.8 (2015): 1112-1116.

Tozzi, P., D. Bongiorno, and C. Vitturini. "Low back pain and kidney mobility: local osteopathic fascial manipulation decreases pain perception and improves renal mobility." *Journal of Bodywork and Movement therapies* 16.3 (2012): 381-391.

Bad Breath (Halitosis)

Charantimath, Shivayogi, and Rakesh Oswal. "Herbal therapy in dentistry: a review." *Innov J Med Health Sci* 1.1 (2011): 1-4.

Gurumurthy, Kaviyaselvi, et al. "Effects of Oil Pulling on Bad Breath and Cavities." *Annals of the Romanian Society for Cell Biology* (2021): 2648-2656.

Messadi, Diana V., and Fariba S. Younai. "Halitosis." *Dermatologic clinics* 21.1 (2003): 147-155.

Pareek, Sunil, et al. "Chlorophylls: Chemistry and biological functions." *Fruit and Vegetable Phytochemicals: Chemistry and Human Health, 2nd Edition* (2017): 269-284.

Pedrazzi, Vinícius, et al. "Tongue-cleaning methods: a comparative clinical trial employing a toothbrush and a tongue scraper." *Journal of periodontology* 75.7 (2004): 1009-1012

Richter, Jon L. "Diagnosis and treatment of halitosis." *Compend Contin Educ Dent* 17.4 (1996): 370-2

Shirakawa, Megumi, et al. "The Effect of Chewing Gum Containing Flavonoid and Chlorophy II on Reducing Bad Breath." *Journal of Psychosomatic Oral Medicine* 10.2 (1995): 142-148

Bed Wetting (Enuresis)

Bogaert, Guy, et al. "Practical recommendations of the EAU-ESPU guidelines committee for monosymptomatic enuresis—Bedwetting." *Neurourology and urodynamics* 39.2 (2020): 489-497.

Bond, Tom. *A controlled examination of the effects of caffeine and liquid consumption on sleep enuresis in children*. Virginia Consortium for Professional Psychology (Old Dominion University, College of William and Mary, Eastern Virginia Medical School, & Norfolk State University), 1994.

Joinson, Carol, et al. "Psychological problems in children with bedwetting and combined (day and night) wetting: A UK population-based study." *Journal of Pediatric Psychology* 32.5 (2007): 605-616.

Thiedke, C. Carolyn. "Nocturnal enuresis." *American family physician* 67.7 (2003): 1499-1506.

Touchette, Évelyne, et al. "Bed-wetting and its association with developmental milestones in early childhood." *Archives of pediatrics & adolescent medicine* 159.12 (2005): 1129-1134.

Belching/Burping (Aerophagia)

Bredenoord, Albert J. "Management of belching, hiccups, and aerophagia." *Clinical Gastroenterology and Hepatology* 11.1 (2013): 6-12

Cigrang, Jeffrey A., Christine M. Hunter, and Alan L. Peterson. "Behavioral treatment of chronic belching due to aerophagia in a normal adult." *Behavior modification* 30.3 (2006): 341-351

Binge-Eating

Chao, Ariana M., Carlos M. Grilo, and Rajita Sinha. "Food cravings, binge eating, and eating disorder psychopathology: Exploring the moderating roles of gender and race." *Eating behaviors* 21 (2016): 41-47.

Dingemans, A. E., M. J. Bruna, and E. F. Van Furth. "Binge eating disorder: a review." *International journal of obesity* 26.3 (2002): 299-307

Fairburn, Christopher G. *Overcoming binge eating: The proven program to learn why you binge and how you can stop*. Guilford Press, 2013.

Katterman, Shawn N., et al. "Mindfulness meditation as an intervention for binge eating, emotional eating, and weight loss: a systematic review." *Eating behaviors* 15.2 (2014): 197-204.

Ng, Longena, and Caroline Davis. "Cravings and food consumption in binge eating disorder." *Eating behaviors* 14.4 (2013): 472-475.

O'Neal, Joanna. "The Light and the Parasite: An Eating Disorders Story." *Yoga and Eating Disorders*. Routledge, 2016. 79-84.

Bites and Stings

Blum, Murray S., et al. "Chemistry of the sting apparatus of the worker honeybee." *Journal of Apicultural Research* 17.4 (1978): 218-221.

Klinghardt, Dietrich K., and Bellevue WA. "Lyme disease: a look beyond antibiotics." *Explor Infect Dis* 14.2 (2005): 6-11.

Klotz, John H., Stephen A. Klotz, and Jacob L. Pinnas. "Animal bites and stings with anaphylactic potential." *The Journal of Emergency Medicine* 36.2 (2009): 148-156.

Overstreet, Maria L. "Tick Bites and Lyme Disease: The Need for Timely Treatment." *Critical Care Nursing Clinics* 25.2 (2013): 165-172.

Schexnayder, Stephen M., and Rebecca E. Schexnayder. "Bites, stings, and other painful things." *Pediatric annals* 29.6 (2000): 354-358.

Stoner, Michael. "Plantain: Its Uses as a Folk Remedy for Insect and Snake Bites." *Kentucky Folklore Record* 20.4 (1974): 96.

Theakston, R. David G., and David G. Lalloo. "Venomous bites and stings." *Principles and practice of travel medicine* (2001): 321-341.

Black Eye

Jackson, Edward. *A Manual of the Diagnosis and Treatment of the Diseases of the Eye*. WB Saunders, 1900.

Schaffer, Susan, Sogol Saghari, and Leslie Baumann. "Prevention and Treatment of Bruising." *Cosmetic Dermatology* (2008): 163.

Würdemann, Henry Vanderbilt. *Injuries of the Eye*. Cleveland Press, 1912.

Bladder Infection

Hudson, Tori. "Treatment and prevention of bladder infections." *Alternative & complementary therapies* 12.6 (2006): 297-302.

Maki, Kevin C., et al. "Consumption of a cranberry juice beverage lowered the number of clinical urinary tract infection episodes in women with a recent history of urinary tract infection."

Mao, Song, and Songming Huang. "Zinc and copper levels in bladder cancer: a systematic review and meta-analysis." *Biological trace element research* 153 (2013): 5-10.

Totsika, Makrina, et al. "A FimH inhibitor prevents acute bladder infection and treats chronic cystitis caused by multidrug-resistant uropathogenic Escherichia coli ST131." *The Journal of infectious diseases* 208.6 (2013): 921-928.

Blisters

Cortese, Thomas A., et al. "Treatment of friction blisters: an experimental study." *Archives of dermatology* 97.6 (1968): 717-721.

Garg, S. C. "Essential oils as therapeutics." (2005).

Knapik, Joseph J., et al. "Friction blisters: pathophysiology, prevention and treatment." *Sports Medicine* 20 (1995): 136-147.

Murphy, Faye, and Jeshni Amblum. "Treatment for burn blisters: debride or leave intact?." *Emergency Nurse* 22.2 (2014).

Sharma, Jyotsana, et al. "Traditional herbal medicines used for the treatment of skin disorders by the Gujjar tribe of Sub-Himalayan tract, Uttarakhand." (2013).

Body Odor

Brocklehurst, John C. "Assessment of Chlorophyll as a Deodorant." *British Medical Journal* 1.4809 (1953): 541.

Hart, Robert. "Human body odor." *NEXUS: The Canadian Student Journal of Anthropology* 1.1 (1980): 1-12

Havlicek, Jan, and Pavlina Lenochova. "The effect of meat consumption on body odor attractiveness." *Chemical senses* 31.8 (2006): 747-752.

Mitchell, Wm. "Chlorophyll as a Deodorant." *British Medical Journal* 1.4810 (1953): 621.

Pause, Bettina M. "Processing of body odor signals by the human brain." *Chemosensory perception* 5 (2012): 55-63.

Boils

Andrews, George Clinton. "The treatment of boils and carbuncles." *The American Journal of Surgery* 6.4 (1929): 458-460.

Hosford, John. "Treatment of Boils and Carbuncles." *British Medical Journal* 1.4024 (1938): 400.

Kuehnert, Matthew J., and William R. Jarvis. "Bacteria and safety of the blood supply." *Annals of internal medicine* 129.2 (1998): 164-165.

Lin, Huang-Shen, et al. "Interventions for bacterial folliculitis and boils (furuncles and carbuncles)." *Cochrane Database of Systematic Reviews* 2 (2021)

Schuetz, Barbara. *Oil of oregano: Nature's antiseptic and antioxidant.* Healthy Living Publications, 2016.

Breast Discomfort

Chan, Cherie YC, Winnie WM Yu, and Edward Newton. "Evaluation and analysis of bra design." *The Design Journal* 4.3 (2001): 33-40.

Chen, Xiaona, et al. "Effect of sports bra type and gait speed on breast discomfort, bra discomfort and perceived breast movement in Chinese women." *Ergonomics* 59.1 (2016): 130-142

Crandall, Carolyn J., et al. "Association of new-onset breast discomfort with an increase in mammographic density during hormone therapy." *Archives of internal medicine* 166.15 (2006): 1578-1584.

Crandall, Carolyn J., et al. "Predictors of breast discomfort among women initiating menopausal hormone therapy." *Menopause* 17.3 (2010): 462-470.

Greendale, Gail A., et al. "Symptom relief and side effects of postmenopausal hormones: results from the Postmenopausal Estrogen/Progestin Interventions Trial." *Obstetrics & Gynecology* 92.6 (1998): 982-988.

Holmes, Helen B., Betty B. Hoskins, and Michael Gross. *Birth control and controlling birth: women-centered perspectives.* Springer Science & Business Media, 1981.

Mason, Bruce R., Kelly-Ann Page, and Keiran Fallon. "An analysis of movement and discomfort of the female breast during exercise and the effects of breast support in three cases." *Journal of Science and Medicine in Sport* 2.2 (1999): 134-144

Mira, Anna. *A biomechanical breast model for the evaluation of the compression and the discomfort perception in mammography.* Diss. Université Grenoble Alpes, 2018.

Bronchitis

Albert, Ross H. "Diagnosis and treatment of acute bronchitis." *American family physician* 82.11 (2010): 1345-1350.

Soilemezi, Dia, et al. "Herbal medicine for acute bronchitis: A qualitative interview study of patients' and health professionals' views." *Complementary Therapies in Medicine* 55 (2020): 102613.

Wopker, P. M., et al. "Complementary and alternative medicine in the treatment of acute bronchitis in children: A systematic review." *Complementary therapies in medicine* 49 (2020): 102217.

Bruises

Jeney, Viktória, et al. "Natural history of the bruise: formation, elimination, and biological effects of oxidized hemoglobin." *Oxidative Medicine and Cellular Longevity* 2013.1 (2013): 703571.

Kouzi, Samir A., and Donald S. Nuzum. "Arnica for bruising and swelling." *American Journal of Health-System Pharmacy* 64.23 (2007): 2434-2443.

Mlambo, Shamiso Shelter, et al. "Treatment of acute wounds and in

Urakov, Aleksandr. "What are bruises? Causes, symptoms, diagnosis, treatment, remedies." *IP Int J Comprehensive Adv Pharmacol* 5.1 (2020): 1-5.

Bunions

Aebischer, Andrea S., and Samuel Duff. "Bunions: A review of management." *Australian Journal of General Practice* 49.11 (2020): 720-723.

Ferrari, Jill. "Bunions." *BMJ clinical evidence* 2009 (2009).

Silfverskiöld, Jan P. "Common foot problems: relieving the pain of bun

Burns

Artz, Curtis P., and Duane L. Larson. "Treatment of burns." *Current Problems in Surgery* 2.3 (1965): 1-40.

Kamolz, Lars-Peter, et al. "The treatment of hand burns." *Burns* 35.3 (2009): 327-337.

Kuroiwa, Kojiro, et al. "Metabolic and immune effect of vitamin E supplementation after burn." *Journal of Parenteral and Enteral Nutrition* 15.1 (1991): 22-26.

Rundus, Christine, et al. "Vitamin E improves cell-mediated immunity in the burned mouse: a preliminary study." *Burns* 11.1 (1984): 11-15

Sheridan, Robert L. "Comprehensive treatment of burns." *Current problems in surgery* 38.9 (2001): 657-756.

Wilson, Ben J., and Jerry A. Stirman. "Initial treatment of burns." *Journal of the American Medical Association* 173.5 (1960): 509-516.

Żwierełło, Wojciech, et al. «Burns: Classification, pathophysiology, and treatment: A review.» *International journal of molecular sciences* 24.4 (2023): 3749.

Bursitis (and Tendonitis)

Aaron, Daniel L., et al. "Four common types of bursitis: diagnosis and management." *JAAOS-Journal of the American Academy of Orthopaedic Surgeons* 19.6 (2011): 359-367

Biundo Jr, Joseph J., Robert W. Irwin, and Enrique Umpierre. "Sports and other soft tissue injuries, tendinitis, bursitis, and occupation-related syndromes." *Current opinion in rheumatology* 13.2 (2001): 146-149

Lanzisera, Rosaria, et al. "A prospective observational study on the beneficial effects and tolerability of a cetylated fatty acids (CFA) complex in a patch formulation for shoulder tendon disorders." *BMC Musculoskeletal Disorders* 23.1 (2022): 352.

Calluses (and Corns)

Mann, Roger A. "Corns and calluses." *Postgraduate Medicine* 90.1 (1991): 268-269.

Nozari, Elnaz, Rasool Asghari Zakaria, and Nasser Zare. "Effect of 17β-estradiol on seedling and callus growth of German chamomile (Matricaria chamomilla L.)." *Journal of Plant Physiology and Breeding* 10.2 (2020): 77-87.

Singh, Dishan, George Bentley, and Saul G. Trevino. "Fortnightly review: callosities, corns, and calluses." *Bmj* 312.7043 (1996): 1403-1406.

Cancer (General)

Ansari, M. S., and N. P. Gupta. "Lycopene: a novel drug therapy in hormone refractory metastatic prostate cancer." *Urologic Oncology: Seminars and Original Investigations*. Vol. 22. No. 5. Elsevier, 2004.

Chandra, Amrish. "Overview of cancer and medicinal herbs used for cancer therapy." *Asian Journal of Pharmaceutics (AJP)* 12.01 (2018)

Ebrahimian, Venus. *Characterization of red diamondback rattlesnake venom proteins on cell death and function.* MS thesis. Wright State University, 2013.

Greay, Sara J., et al. "Inhibition of established subcutaneous murine tumour growth with topical Melaleuca alternifolia (tea tree) oil." *Cancer chemotherapy and pharmacology* 66 (2010): 1095-1102.

Gul, Somia, et al. "Medical Science Turns Deadly Substances into Life Saving Ones: Snake Venom as a Treatment Option." *Open Access Library Journal* 2.3 (2015): 1-9

Korrapati, Supriya, Pallavi Kurra, and Srinivasababu Puttugunta. "Natural and herbal remedies for cancer treatment." *Inventi Impact: Planta Activa* 2016 (2016): 2249-3557.

Maheswari, T. Uma, and S. Sinduja. "Soursop: a promising fruit for cancer mitigation." *Plant Archives* 20.1 (2020): 1653-1656.

Pazyar, Nader, et al. "A review of applications of tea tree oil in dermatology." *International journal of dermatology* 52.7 (2013): 784-790.

Villagran, Marcelo, et al. "The role of vitamin C in cancer prevention and therapy: a literature review." *Antioxidants* 10.12 (2021): 1894.

Vyas, Vivek Kumar, et al. "Therapeutic potential of snake venom in cancer therapy: current perspectives." *Asian Pacific journal of tropical biomedicine* 3.2 (2013): 156-162.

Canker Sores

Chimbo Torres, Cristina Anahis, et al. "A Systematic Review of Cold Sores and Canker Sores." *Journal of Advanced Zoology* 44 (2023).

Sores, What Causes Canker. "Canker Sores." (2008).

Carpel Tunnel Syndrome

De Krom, M. C. T. F. M., et al. "Risk factors for carpal tunnel syndrome." *American journal of epidemiology* 132.6 (1990): 1102-1110.

Genova, Alessia, et al. "Carpal tunnel syndrome: a review of literature." *Cureus* 12.3 (2020).

Jahromi, Behdad, et al. "Herbal medicine for pain management: efficacy and drug interactions." *Pharmaceutics* 13.2 (2021): 251.

Viera, Anthony J. "Management of carpal tunnel syndrome." *American family physician* 68.2 (2003): 265-272

Cataracts

Alvarez-Suarez, José M., et al. "The composition and biological activity of honey: a focus on Manuka honey." *Foods* 3.3 (2014): 420-432.

Garner, Margaret H., and Abraham Spector. "Sulfur oxidation in selected human cortical cataracts and nuclear cataracts." *Experimental Eye Research* 31.3 (1980): 361-369.

Hu, Jindong, et al. "Efficacy and safety of manuka honey for dry eye." *Clinical and Experimental Optometry* 106.5 (2023): 455-465.

Liu, Yu-Chi, et al. "Cataracts." *The Lancet* 390.10094 (2017): 600-612.

Olson, Randall J., et al. "Cataract treatment in the beginning of the 21st century." *American journal of ophthalmology* 136.1 (2003): 146-154.

Philip, Antony Jesu Prabhu, et al. "Dietary zinc, selenium and water temperature during early seawater phase influences the development of vertebral deformities and cataract in adult Atlantic salmon." *Aquaculture* 572 (2023): 739529.

Xu, Baiwei, et al. "Selenium intake help prevent age-related cataract formation: Evidence from NHANES 2001–2008." *Frontiers in Nutrition* 10 (2023): 1042893.

Chapped Lips

Bork, Konrad. "Diseases of the Lips and Mouth." *Braun-Falco's Dermatology.* Springer, Berlin, Heidelberg, 2009. 1081-1107.

Hikima, Rie, et al. "Development of lip treatment on the basis of desquamation mechanism." *International Journal of Cosmetic Science* 26.3 (2004): 165-165.

Hitz Lindenmüller, Irène, Peter H. Itin, and Susanna K. Fistarol. "Dermatology of the lips: Inflammatory diseases." *Quintessence International* 45.10 (2014).

Chronic fatigue syndrome

Afari, Niloofar, and Dedra Buchwald. "Chronic fatigue syndrome: a review." *American Journal of Psychiatry* 160.2 (2003): 221-236.

Bassi, Nicola, et al. "Chronic fatigue syndrome: characteristics and possible causes for its pathogenesis." *The Israel Medical Association Journal* 10.1 (2008): 79.

Chan, Jessie SM, et al. "Qigong exercise alleviates fatigue, anxiety, and depressive symptoms, improves sleep quality, and shortens sleep latency in persons with chronic fatigue syndrome-like illness." *Evidence-Based Complementary and Alternative Medicine* 2014.1 (2014): 106048.

Cleare, Anthony J. "The neuroendocrinology of chronic fatigue syndrome." *Endocrine reviews* 24.2 (2003): 236-252.

Cox, I. M., M. J. Campbell, and D. Dowson. "Red blood cell ma

Earl, Kate E., et al. "Vitamin D status in chronic fatigue syndrome/myalgic encephalomyelitis: a cohort study from the North-West of England." *BMJ open* 7.11 (2017): e015296.

Fukuda, Keiji, et al. "The chronic fatigue syndrome: a comprehensive approach to its definition and study." *Annals of internal medicine* 121.12 (1994): 953-959.

Manuel y Keenoy, Begoña, et al. "Magnesium status and parameters of the oxidant-antioxidant balance in patients with chronic fatigue: effects of supplementation with magnesium." *Journal of the American College of Nutrition* 19.3 (2000): 374-382.

Ockerman, P. A. "Antioxidant treatment of chronic fatigue syndrome." *Clinical Practice of Alternative Medicine* 1 (2000): 88-91.

White, Peter D. "What causes chronic fatigue syndrome?." *Bmj* 329.7472 (2004): 928-929.

Cold Sores

Borazan, Hale, et al. "Oral magnesium lozenge reduces postoperative sore throat: a randomized, prospective, placebo-controlled study." *The Journal of the American Society of Anesthesiologists* 117.3 (2012): 512-518.

Chimbo Torres, Cristina Anahis, et al. "A Systematic Review of Cold Sores and Canker Sores." *Journal of Advanced Zoology* 44 (2023).

Lee, Yi-Chiao, et al. "Management of viral oral ulcers in children using Chinese herbal medicine: a report of two cases." *Complementary Therapies in Medicine* 32 (2017): 61-65.

McIntyre, Anne. *Herbs for common ailments*. Simon and Schuster, 2003.

Slavin, Howard B. "The clinical ramifications of infections caused by the virus of herpes simplex." *Medical Clinics of North America* 35.2 (1951): 563-569.

Tierra, Michael. *The way of herbs*. Simon and Schuster, 1998.

Walsh, David E., Richard S. Griffith, and Ali Behforooz. "Subjective response to lysine in the therapy of herpes simplex." *Journal of Antimicrobial Chemotherapy* 12.5 (1983): 489-496.

Wilson, Michael, et al. "Cold Sores." *Close Encounters of the Microbial Kind: Everything You Need to Know About Common Infections* (2021): 333-343.

Colds and Flu

Bragg, Paul Chappuis. *The miracle of fasting*. Health Science Publications, Inc., 2004.

Carrington, Hereward. *Vitality, fasting and nutrition*. Рипол Классик, 1911.

Eccles, Ronald. "Mechanisms of symptoms of common cold and flu." *Common cold* (2009): 23-45.

Gallacher, Stuart A. "Stuff a cold and starve a fever." *Bulletin of the History of Medicine* 11.5 (1942): 576-581.

Ismail, Halima, and Natalie Schellack. "Colds and flu–an overview of the management." *South African Family Practice* 59.3 (2017): 5-12.

Lee, Wang Jae, and Wang Jae Lee. "Common Cold and Flu." *Vitamin C in Human Health and Disease: Effects, Mechanisms of Action*

Colic

Iacovou, Marina, et al. "Dietary management of infantile colic: a systematic review." *Maternal and child health journal* 16.6 (2012): 1319-1331

Lucassen, Peter. "Colic in infants." *BMJ Clinical Evidence* 2015 (2015).

Roberts, Donna M., Michael Ostapchuk, and JAMES G. O'BRIEN. "Infantile colic." *American family physician* 70.4 (2004): 735-740.

Wheat, J. D. "Causes of colic and types requiring surgical intervention." *Journal of the South African Veterinary Association* 46.1 (1975): 95-98.

Zeevenhooven, Judith, et al. "Infant colic: mechanisms and management." *Nature reviews Gastroenterology & hepatology* 15.8 (2018): 479-496.

Conjunctivitis

Azari, Amir A., and Neal P. Barney. "Conjunctivitis: a systematic review of diagnosis and treatment." *Jama* 310.16 (2013): 1721-1730.

Bayly, Doreen E. *Reflexology today: the stimulation of the body's healing forces through foot massage*. Inner Traditions/Bear & Co, 1984.

Friedlaender, Mitchell H. "A review of the causes and treatment of bacterial and allergic conjunctivitis." *Clinical therapeutics* 17.5 (1995): 800-810.

Hall, Nicola. *Principles of Reflexology: What it is, how it works.* Singing Dragon, 2013.

Lindquist, Thomas D., and T. Peter Lindquist. "Conjunctivitis: an overview and classification." *Cornea, E-Book* 358 (2021).

McLaughlin, Chris, and Nicola Hall. *Secrets of Reflexology.* Ivy Press, 2017.

Wood, Mark. "Conjunctivitis: diagnosis and management." *Community Eye Health* 12.30 (1999): 19.

Constipation

Camilleri, Michael, et al. "Chronic constipation." *Nature reviews Disease primers* 3.1 (2017): 1-19.

Forootan, Mojgan, Nazila Bagheri, and Mohammad Darvishi. "Chronic constipation: A review of literature." *Medicine* 97.20 (2018): e10631

Lembo, Anthony. "Chronic constipation." *Handbook of Gastrointestinal Motility and Disorders of Gut-Brain Interactions* (2023): 263-276.

Piirainen, Laura, et al. "Prune juice has a mild laxative effect in adults with certain gastrointestinal symptoms." *Nutrition Research* 27.8 (2007): 511-513

Schiller, L. R. "The therapy of constipation." *Alimentary pharmacology & therapeutics* 15.6 (2001): 749-763.

Voderholzer, Winfried A., et al. "Clinical response to dietary fiber treatment of chronic constipation." *American Journal of Gastroenterology (Springer Nature)* 92.1 (1997).

Yang, Jing, et al. "Effect of dietary fiber on constipation: a meta analysis." *World journal of gastroenterology: WJG* 18.48 (2012): 7378.

Coughing

Cloutier, Michelle M. "The coughing child: etiology and treatment of a common symptom." *Postgraduate medicine* 73.3 (1983): 169-175.

Fuller, R. W., and D. M. Jackson. "Physiology and treatment of cough." *Thorax* 45.6 (1990): 425.

Irwin, Richard S., and Frederick J. Curley. "The treatment of cough: a comprehensive review." *Chest* 99.6 (1991): 1477-1484

Sultana, Shahnaz, et al. "Cough suppressant herbal drugs: A review." *Int. J. Pharm. Sci. Invent* 5.5 (2016): 15-28.

Wagner, Luise, et al. "Herbal medicine for cough: a systematic review and meta-analysis." *Forschende Komplementärmedizin/Research in Complementary Medicine* 22.6 (2015): 359-368.

Cuts (and Scrapes)

Foster, Steven. "Herbs for Health: Home Remedies for Cuts and Scrapes."

Mlambo, Shamiso Shelter, et al. "Treatment of acute wounds and injuries: Cuts, bites, bruises and sprains." *SA Pharmaceutical Journal* 89.1 (2022): 12-18.

Weigand, Dennis A. "How to treat skin cuts, bruises, burns & blisters." *Diabetes in the News* 12.1 (1993): 36-38.

Dandruff

Borda, Luis J., and Tongyu C. Wikramanayake. "Seborrheic dermatitis and dandruff: a comprehensive review." *Journal of clinical and investigative dermatology* 3.2 (2015).

Hay, R. J., and R. A. Graham-Brown. "Dandruff and seborrhoeic dermatitis: causes and management." *Clinical & Experimental Dermatology* 22.1 (1997).

Meray, Yönter, Duygu Gençalp, and Mümtaz Güran. "Putting it all together to understand the role of Malassezia spp. in dandruff etiology." *Mycopathologia* 183 (2018): 893-903.

Mukti, Ria Andriani, and Agus Ridwan Misbahuddin. "Determination of effectiveness traditional cosmetics of coconut oil and turmeric as anti-dandruff." *2nd International Conference on Social, Applied Science, and Technology in Home Economics (ICONHOMECS 2019)*. Atlantis Press, 2020.

Potluri, Anusha, et al. "A review on herbs used in anti-dandruff shampoo and its evaluation parameters." *Research Journal of Topical and Cosmetic Sciences* 4.1 (2013): 5-13.

Depression

Beck, Aaron T., and Brad A. Alford. *Depression: Causes and treatment.* University of Pennsylvania Press, 2009

Bodnar, Lisa M., and Katherine L. Wisner. "Nutrition and depression: implications for improving mental health among childbearing-aged women." *Biological psychiatry* 58.9 (2005): 679-685.

Emmons, Henry. *The chemistry of joy: A three-step program for overcoming depression through western science and eastern wisdom.* Simon and Schuster, 2006.

Goldman, Larry S., et al. "Awareness, diagnosis, and treatment of depression." *Journal of general internal medicine* 14.9 (1999): 569-580.

Hankin, Benjamin L. "Adolescent depression: Description, causes, and interventions." *Epilepsy & behavior* 8.1 (2006): 102-114.

Lang, Undine E., et al. "Nutritional aspects of depression." *Cellular Physiology and Biochemistry* 37.3 (2015): 1029-1043

Nemeroff, Charles B. "The neurobiology of depression." *Scientific American* 278.6 (1998): 42-49.

Rao, TS Sathyanarayana, et al. "Understanding nutrition, depression and mental illnesses." *Indian journal of psychiatry* 50.2 (2008): 77-82

Zielińska, Magdalena, Edyta Łuszczki, and Katarzyna Dereń. "Dietary Nutrient Deficiencies and Risk of Depression (Review Article 2018–2023)." *Nutrients* 15.11 (2023): 2433

Dermatitis (and Eczema)

Ai, Ping, et al. "Selenium levels and skin diseases: systematic review and meta-analysis." *Journal of Trace Elements in Medicine and Biology* 62 (2020): 126548.

Baral, Priyanka, Vishakha Bagul, and Swati Gajbhiye. "Hemp seed oil for skin care (non-drug cannabis sativa L): A review." *World J. Pharm. Res* 9 (2020): 2534-2556.

Braun-Falco, Otto, et al. "Dermatitis and eczema." *Dermatology* (1991): 316-366.

Hansen, Arild E., et al. "Eczema and essential fatty acids." *American Journal of Diseases of Children* 73.1 (1947): 1-18.

Zohreh, Hajheydari, Saeedi Majid, and Hosseinzadeh Mohammad. "The relationship of serum selenium, zinc, and copper levels with seborrheic dermatitis: a case-control study." *Iranian Journal of Dermatology* 22.1 (2019): 7-12.

Diabetes (Type-1)

Antvorskov, Julie C., et al. "Dietary gluten and the development of type 1 diabetes." *Diabetologia* 57 (2014): 1770-1780.

Atkinson, Mark A., George S. Eisenbarth, and Aaron W. Michels. "Type 1 diabetes." *The lancet* 383.9911 (2014): 69-82.

Diabetes Control and Complications Trial/Epidemiology of Diabetes Interventions and Complications (DCCT/EDIC) Study Research Group. "Intensive diabetes treatment and cardiovascular disease in patients with type 1 diabetes." *New England Journal of Medicine* 353.25 (2005): 2643-2653.

Riddell, Michael C., et al. "Exercise management in type 1 diabetes: a consensus statement." *The lancet Diabetes & endocrinology* 5.5 (2017): 377-390.

Serena, Gloria, et al. "The role of gluten in celiac disease and type 1 diabetes." *Nutrients* 7.9 (2015): 7143-7162.

Shahavandi, Mahshid, et al. "The association between dairy products consumption with risk of type 1 diabetes mellitus in children: a meta-analysis of observational studies." *International Journal of Diabetes in Developing Countries* (2021): 1-8.

Wang, Zhen, et al. "Beyond genetics: what causes type 1 diabetes." *Clinical reviews in allergy & immunology* 52 (2017): 273-286.

Diabetes (Type-2)

Allen, Robert W., et al. "Cinnamon use in type 2 diabetes: an updated systematic review and meta-analysis." *The Annals of Family Medicine* 11.5 (2013): 452-459

Fuangchan, Anjana, et al. "Hypoglycemic effect of bitter melon compared with metformin in newly diagnosed type 2 diabetes patients." *Journal of ethnopharmacology* 134.2 (2011): 422-428.

Gaddam, Arpana, et al. "Role of Fenugreek in the prevention of type

Gainey, Atikarn, et al. "Effects of Buddhist walking meditation on glycemic control and vascular function in patients with type 2 diabetes." *Complementary therapies in medicine* 26 (2016): 92-97.

Jin, Ke-Ke, et al. "Acupressure therapy inhibits the development of diabetic complications in Chinese patients with type 2 diabetes." *The Journal of Alternative and Complementary Medicine* 15.9 (2009): 1027-1032.

Laville, M., and J-A. Nazare. "Diabetes, insulin resistance and sugars." *Obesity reviews* 10 (2009): 24-33.

López-Romero, Patricia, et al. "The effect of nopal (Opuntia ficus indica) on postprandial blood glucose, incretins, and antioxidant activity in Mexican patients with type 2 diabetes after consumption of two different composition breakfasts." *Journal of the Academy of Nutrition and Dietetics* 114.11 (2014): 1811-1818.

Mkhize, Pretty Brightness. *A comparison of the efficacy of Syzygium Jambolanum (Java Plum) 6CH and Syzygium Jamb*

Ryan, Gina J., et al. "Chromium as adjunctive treatment for type 2 diabetes." *Annals of Pharmacotherapy* 37.6 (2003): 876-885.

Taylor, Simeon I. "Deconstructing type 2 diabetes." *Cell* 97.1 (1999): 9-12.

Tsilas, Christine S., et al. "Relation of total sugars, fructose and sucrose with incident type 2 diabetes: a systematic review and meta-analysis of prospective cohort studies." *Cmaj* 189.20 (2017): E711-E720.

Veit, Meike, et al. "The role of dietary sugars, overweight, and obesity in type 2 diabetes mellitus: a narrative review." *European journal of clinical nutrition* 76.11 (2022): 1497-1501.

Wu, Weijing, et al. "Impact of whole cereals and processing on type 2 d

Diaper Rash

Boiko, Susan. "Making rash decisions in the diaper area." *Pediatric Annals* 29.1 (2000): 50-56

Borkowski, Suzanne. "Diaper rash care and management." *Pediatric nursing* 30.6 (2004): 467.

Sharifi-Heris, Zahra, Leila Amiri Farahani, and Seyede Batool Hasanpoor-Azghadi. "A review study of diaper rash dermatitis treatments." *Journal of Client-Centered Nursing Care* 4.1 (2018): 1-12.

Yanti, Dian Anggri. "Differences in The Effects of Coconut Oil and Aloe Vera in Accelerating The Healing of Diaper Rashes in Babies." *JURNAL KESMAS DAN GIZI (JKG)* 6.2 (2024): 381-386.

Diarrhea

Aranda-Michel, Jaime, and Ralph A. Giannella. "Acute diarrhea: a practical review." *The American journal of medicine* 106.6 (1999): 670-676.

Christopher, Nicholas L., and Theodore M. Bayless. "Role of the small bowel and colon in lactose-induced diarrhea." *Gastroenterology* 60.5 (1971): 845-852

Dekate, Parag, M. Jayashree, and Sunit C. Singhi. "Management of acute diarrhea in emergency room." *The Indian Journal of Pediatrics* 80 (2013): 235-246.

Simakachorn, Nipat, et al. "Randomized, double-blind clinical trial of a lactose-free and a lactose-containing formula in dietary management of acute childhood diarrhea." *JOURNAL-MEDICAL ASSOCIATION OF THAILAND* 87.6 (2004): 641-649.

Spapen, Herbert, et al. "Soluble fiber reduces the incidence of diarrhea in septic patients receiving total enteral nutrition: a prospective, double-blind, randomized, and controlled trial." *Clinical Nutrition* 20.4 (2001): 301-305.

Diverticulosis

Burgell, Rebecca E., Jane G. Muir, and Peter R. Gibson. "Pathogenesis of colonic diverticulosis: repainting the picture." *Clinical gastroenterology and hepatology* 11.12 (2013): 1628-1630.

Heaton, K. W., and W. G. Thompson. "Exercise and diverticular disease." *BMJ: British Medical Journal* 310.6990 (1995): 1332.

Martel, Jerry, and Jeffrey B. Raskin. "History, incidence, and epidemiology of diverticulosis." *Journal of clinical gastroenterology* 42.10 (2008): 1125-1127

Ulbricht, Catherine, ed. "Gastrointestinal Disorders: An integrative approach: A natural standard mono-graph." *Alternative and Complimentary Therapies* 16.1 (2010): 34-49

Dizziness

Chang, Chia-Chen, et al. "The relationship between isolated dizziness/vertigo and the risk factors of ischemic stroke: a case control study." *Acta Neurol Taiwan* 20.2 (2011): 101-06.

Furman, Joseph M., and Susan L. Whitney. "Central causes of dizziness." *Physical Therapy* 80.2 (2000): 179-187.

Lee, Eun Jin, and Susan K. Frazier. "The efficacy of acupressure for symptom management: a systematic review." *Journal of pain and symptom management* 42.4 (2011): 589-603

Post, Robert E., and Lori M. Dickerson. "Dizziness: a diagnostic approach." *American family physician* 82.4 (2010): 361-368

Proctor, Conrad A. "Abnormal insulin levels and vertigo." *The Laryngoscope* 91.10 (1981): 1657-1662.

Trinus, Kostiantyn. *Dizziness: etiology, pathogenesis, manifestations.* LITA Corporation, 2010.

Dry Eyes

Baudouin, Christophe. "The pathology of dry eye." *Survey of ophthalmology* 45 (2001): S211-S220.

Clayton, Janine A. "Dry eye." *New England Journal of Medicine* 378.23 (2018): 2212-2223.

Harvey, Daniel, Neil W. Hayes, and Brian Tighe. "Fibre optics sensors in tear electrolyte analysis: Towards a novel point of care potassium sensor." *Contact Lens and Anterior Eye* 35.3 (2012): 137-144.

Dry Mouth

Fox, Philip C. "Management of dry mouth." *Dental Clinics of North America* 41.4 (1997): 863-875.

Joanna, Ngo Di Ying, and William Murray Thomson. "Dry mouth–an overview." *Singapore Dental Journal* 36 (2015): 12-17.

Olsson, Håkan, Carl-Johan Spak, and Tony Axéll. "The effect of a chewing gum on salivary secretion, oral mucosal friction, and the feeling of dry mouth in xerostomic patients." *Acta Odontologica Scandinavica* 49.5 (1991): 273-279.

Peng, Tzu-Rong, et al. "Effectiveness of oil pulling for improving oral health: A meta-analysis." *Healthcare.* Vol. 10. No. 10. MDPI, 2022

Dry Skin

Larmo, Petra, et al. "CO2-extracted blackcurrant seed oil for well-being of the skin."

Pons-Guiraud, A. "Dry skin in dermatology: a complex physiopathology." *Journal of the European Academy of Dermatology and Venereology* 21 (2007): 1-4.

Verdier-Sévrain, Sylvie, and Frédéric Bonté. "Skin hydration: a review on its molecular mechanisms." *Journal of cosmetic dermatology* 6.2 (2007): 75-82.

Earache

Beard, Lillian M. "Earache: beyond chicken soup." *Pediatric News* 38.8 (2004): 19-21.

Mill, W. A. "Earache." *Postgraduate Medical Journal* 12.134 (1936): 464.

Seif, Bernard. "Shingles East and West: a case conference with the doctor as patient." *Townsend Letter for Doctors and Patients* 244 (2003): 85-89.

Smith, Wendy K. "Managing common ear problems: discharge, ache and dizziness." *Pharm. J* (2019).

Young, Robert O., and Shelley Redford Young. *The pH Miracle: Balance your Diet, reclaim your health.* Hachette UK, 2008

Earwax (build-up)

Agrawal, Varun, and P. T. Deshmukh. "Ear Wax and its Impaction: Clinical Findings and Management." *Journal of Pharmaceutical Research International* 33.60A (2021): 176-182.

Rodgers, Rosemary. "Does olive oil prevent earwax build-up? An experimental study." *Practice Nursing* 24.4 (2013): 191-196.

Emphysema (Chronic Obstructive Pulmonary Disease – COPD)

Belman, Michael J. "Exercise in patients with chronic obstructive pulmonary disease." *Thorax* 48.9 (1993): 936-946.

Brashier, Bill B., and Rahul Kodgule. "Risk factors and pathophysiology of chronic obstructive pulmonary disease (COPD)." *J Assoc Physicians India* 60.Suppl (2012): 17-21.

Janssen, Rob. "Magnesium to counteract elastin degradation and vascular calcification in chronic obstructive pulmonary disease." *Medical hypotheses* 107 (2017): 74-77.

Roy, Somdutta Sinha, Shyamali Mukherjee, and Salil K. Das. "Vitamin A, vitamin E, lutein and β-caro-tene in lung tissues from subjects with chronic obstructive pulmonary disease and emphysema." *Open Journal of Respiratory Diseases* 3.02 (2013): 44.

Sethi, Jigme M., and Carolyn L. Rochester. "Smoking and chronic obstructive pulmonary disease." *Clinics in chest medicine* 21.1 (2000): 67-86.

Endometriosis

Bulun, Serdar E., et al. "Endometriosis." *Endocrine reviews* 40.4 (2019): 1048.

Child, Tim J., and Seang Lin Tan. "Endometriosis: aetiology, pathogenesis and treatment." *Drugs* 61 (2001): 1735-1750.

Orr, Andrew, and No Stone Left Unturned. "Category Archives: Refined Carbohydrates."

Parazzini, Fabio, et al. "Diet and endometriosis risk: a literature review." *Reproductive biomedicine online* 26.4 (2013): 323-336.

Eyesight

Cope, Graham. "The effects of smoking on the eye: the role of the ophthalmic nurse." *International Journal of Ophthalmic Practice* 5.5 (2014): 173-177.

Gittleman, Ann Louise. *The Gut Flush Plan: The Breakthrough Cleansing Program to Rid Your Body of the Toxins that Make You Sick, Tired, and Bloated*. Penguin, 2008.

Kaplan, Robert-Michael. *The Power Behind Your Eyes: Improving Your Eyesight with Integrated Vision Therapy*. Simon and Schuster, 1995

Nazrana, Naghma, Tejasvi Jain, and Sanjay Verma. "Role of nutrition in maintaining normal eyesight-a review." *Int J Med Biomed Stud* 4.3 (2020): 194-8.

Scheiner, Gary. *Think like a pancreas: A Practical guide to managing diabetes with insulin*. Hachette Go, 2020.

Sharif, Najam A. "Neuropathology and therapeutics addressing glaucoma, a prevalent retina-optic nerve-brain disease that causes eyesight impairment and blindness." *OBM Neurobiology* 6.1 (2022): 1-51.

Eyestrain

Coles-Brennan, Chantal, Anna Sulley, and Graeme Young. "Management of digital eye strain." *Clinical and experimental Optometry* 102.1 (2019): 18-29.

Kaur, Kirandeep, et al. "Digital eye strain-a comprehensive review." *Ophthalmology and therapy* 11.5 (2022): 1655-1680

Maroof, Saira, et al. "Relationship of screen hours with digital eye strain: a cross sectional survey from teenagers." *Pakistan Armed Forces Medical Journal* 69.1 (2019): 182-86.

Fatigue

Al-Sayegh, Nowall, Saud Al-Obaidi, and Mohammed Nadar. "Smoking impact on grip strength and fatigue resistance: implications for exercise and hand therapy practice." *Journal of Physical Activity and Health* 11.5 (2014): 1025-1031.

Cox, I. M., M. J. Campbell, and D. Dowson. "Red blood cell magnesium and chronic fatigue syndrome." *The Lancet* 337.8744 (1991): 757-760.

Gibson, H., and R. H. T. Edwards. "Muscular exercise and fatigue." *Sports medicine* 2 (1985): 120-132.

Katz, Patricia. "Causes and consequences of fatigue in rheumatoid arthritis." *Current opinion in rheumatology* 29.3 (2017): 269-276.

Lorist, Monicque M., and Mattie Tops. "Caffeine, fatigue, and cognition." *Brain and cognition* 53.1 (2003): 82-94.

Maisel, Peter, Erika Baum, and Norbert Donner-Banzhoff. "Fatigue as the chief complaint: epidemiology, causes, diagnosis, and treatment." *Deutsches Ärzteblatt International* 118.33-34 (2021): 566.

Malaguarnera, Michele, et al. "Acetyl L-carnitine (ALC) treatment in elderly patients with fatigue." *Archives of gerontology and geriatrics* 46.2 (2008): 181-190.

Puri, Basant K. "Long-chain polyunsaturated fatty acids and the pathophysiology of myalgic encephalomyelitis (chronic fatigue syndrome)." *Journal of clinical pathology* 60.2 (2007): 122-124.

Fever

Avner, Jeffrey R. "Acute fever." *Pediatrics in review* 30.1 (2009): 5-13.

Blob, Lawrence F., et al. "Effects of a tyramine-enriched meal on blood pressure response in healthy male volunteers treated with selegiline transdermal system 6 mg/24 hour." *CNS spectrums* 12.1 (2007): 25-34.

Efstathiou, Stamatis P., et al. "Fever of unknown origin: discrimination between infectious and non-infectious causes." *European journal of internal medicine* 21.2 (2010): 137-143

Magnuson, B. A., et al. "Aspartame: a safety evaluation based on current use levels, regulations, and toxicological and epidemiological studies." *Critical reviews in toxicology* 37.8 (2007): 629-727.

Moltz, Howard. "Fever: causes and consequences." *Neuroscience & Biobehavioral Reviews* 17.3 (1993): 237-269.

Fibroids

Giuliani, Emma, Sawsan As-Sanie, and Erica E. Marsh. "Epidemiology and management of uterine fibroids." *International Journal of Gynecology & Obstetrics* 149.1 (2020): 3-9.

Gladish, Samantha. *The 30-day Hormone Solution: The Key to Better Health and Natural Weight Loss.* Page Street Publishing, 2019.

Gupta, Sahana, Jude Jose, and Isaac Manyonda. "Clinical presentation of fibroids." *Best practice & research Clinical obstetrics & gynaecology* 22.4 (2008): 615-626.

Khan, Aamir T., Manjeet Shehmar, and Janesh K. Gupta. "Uterine fibroids: current perspectives." *International journal of women's health* (2014): 95-114.

Lewis, Randine, and L. Ac. "Treatment of endometriosis and fibroids with acupuncture." *Acufinder. com* (2013).

Fibromyalgia

Boulis, Michael, Mary Boulis, and Daniel Clauw. "Magnesium and fibromyalgia: a literature review." *Journal of primary care & community health* 12 (2021): 21501327211038433

Clauw, Daniel J. "Fibromyalgia: an overview." *The American journal of medicine* 122.12 (2009): S3-S13.

Friedman, Michaël. "Fibromyalgia, Thyroid Dysfunction and Treatment Modalities." *Journal of Restorative Medicine* 2.1 (2013): 60.

Michalsen, Andreas, et al. "In-patient treatment of fibromyalgia: A controlled nonrandomized comparison of conventional medicine versus integrative medicine including fasting therapy." *Evidence-Based Complementary and Alternative Medicine* 2013.1 (2013): 908610.

Flatulance

Alvarez, WALTER C. "What causes flatulence?." *Journal of the American Medical Association* 120.1 (1942): 21-24

Kurbel, Sven, Beatrica Kurbel, and Aleksandar Včev. "Intestinal gases and flatulence: Possible causes of occurrence." *Medical Hypotheses* 67.2 (2006): 235-239

Levitt, Michael D., and John H. Bond. "Flatulence." *Annual review of medicine* 31.1 (1980): 127-137.

Saddiqi, Hafiz Abubaker, and Zafar Iqbal. "Usage and significance of fennel (Foeniculum vulgare Mill.) seeds in Eastern medicine." *Nuts and seeds in health and disease prevention*. Academic Press, 2011. 461-467

Sharp, Emily, et al. "Effects of lactose-free and low-lactose dairy on symptoms of gastrointestinal health: A systematic review." *International Dairy Journal* 114 (2021): 104936.

Flu

Eccles, Ron. "Understanding the symptoms of the common cold and influenza." *The Lancet infectious diseases* 5.11 (2005): 718-725.

Earn, David JD, Jonathan Dushoff, and Simon A. Levin. "Ecology and evolution of the flu." *Trends in ecology & evolution* 17.7 (2002): 334-340

Goldschmidt, Vivian. "A Powerful And Natural Way To Prevent The Flu."

Sharma, Raksha, and Girish Palshikar. "Virus causes flu: Identifying causality in the biomedical domain using an ensemble approach with target-specific semantic embeddings." *International Conference on Applications of Natural Language to Information Systems*. Cham: Springer International Publishing, 2021.

Food allergies

Cathcart III, Robert F. "The vitamin C treatment of allergy and the normally unprimed state of antibodies." *Medical Hypotheses* 21.3 (1986): 307-321.

Ortolani, Claudio, and Elide A. Pastorello. "Food allergies and food intolerances." *Best Practice & Research Clinical Gastroenterology* 20.3 (2006): 467-483.

Patel, Bhavisha Y., and Gerald W. Volcheck. "Food allergy: common causes, diagnosis, and treatment." *Mayo Clinic Proceedings*. Vol. 90. No. 10. Elsevier, 2015.

Perrier, C., and B. Corthesy. "Gut permeability and food allergies." *Clinical & Experimental Allergy* 41.1 (2011): 20-28.

Skypala, Isabel J., and Rebecca McKenzie. "Nutritional issues in food allergy." *Clinical reviews in allergy & immunology* 57.2 (2019): 166-178.

Valenta, Rudolf, et al. "Food allergies: the basics." *Gastroenterology* 148.6 (2015): 1120-1131.

Żukiewicz-Sobczak, Wioletta Agnieszka, et al. «Causes, symptoms and prevention of food allergy.» *Advances in Dermatology and Allergology/Postępy Dermatologii i Alergologii* 30.2 (2013): 113-116

Food Poisoning

Aljamali, Nagham Mahmood, M. Najim, and A. Alabbasy. "Review on food poisoning (types, causes, symptoms, diagnosis, treatment)." *Global Academic Journal of Pharmacy and Drug Research* 3.4 (2021): 54-61.

Andargie, Gashaw, et al. "Prevalence of bacteria and intestinal parasites among food-handlers in Gondar town, northwest Ethiopia." *Journal of health, population, and nutrition* 26.4 (2008): 451

Hernández-Cortez, Cecilia, et al. "Food poisoning caused by bacteria (food toxins)." *Poisoning: From specific toxic agents to novel rapid and simplified techniques for analysis* 33 (2017).

Milaciu, Mircea V., et al. "Semiology of food poisoning." *Human and Veterinary Medicine* 8.2 (2016): 108-113.

Foot Aches

Dobrowolski, Christine. *Those Aching Feet: Your Guide to Diagnosis and Treatment of Common Foot Problems.* SKI Publishing, 2005.

Gellman, Richard, and Sandra Burns. "Walking aches and running pains: injuries of the foot and ankle." *Primary Care: Clinics in Office Practice* 23.2 (1996): 263-280.

Milner, Stephen. "Common disorders of the foot and ankle." *Surgery (Oxford)* 28.10 (2010): 514-517.

Foot Odor

Ongsri, Punyawee, et al. "Efficacy of antifungal cream versus powder in the treatment of fungal foot skin infection and unpleasant foot odor at medical department of thai naval rating school." *Southeast Asian Journal of Tropical Medicine and Public Health* 49.2 (2018): 297-303.

Rujitharanawong, Chuda, et al. "Impacts of Foot and Body Odor on Quality of Life." *Journal of the Medical Association of Thailand* 101.10 (2018).

Sharquie, Khalifa E., Adil A. Noaimi, and Saad D. Hameed. "Topical 15% zinc sulfate solution is an effective therapy for feet odor." (2013).

Wulandari, N. F., et al. "Preliminary study on bacterial diversity causing human foot odor." *IOP Conference Series: Earth and Environmental Science.* Vol. 439. No. 1. IOP Publishing, 2020.

Fractures

Cockayne, Sarah, et al. "Vitamin K and the prevention of fractures: systematic review and meta-analysis of randomized controlled trials." *Archives of internal medicine* 166.12 (2006): 1256-1261.

Jackson, Rebecca D., et al. "Calcium plus vitamin D supplementation and the risk of fractures." *New England Journal of Medicine* 354.7 (2006): 669-683.

Olson, Robert A., et al. "Fractures of the mandible: a review of 580 case

Richter, Martinus, et al. "Fractures and fracture dislocations of the midfoot: occurrence, causes and long-term results." *Foot & Ankle International* 22.5 (2001): 392-398.

Frostbite

Hallam, Marc-James, et al. "Managing frostbite." *Bmj* 341 (2010).

Murphy, James V., et al. "Frostbite: pathogenesis and treatment." *Journal of Trauma and Acute Care Surgery* 48.1 (2000): 171

Reamy, Brian V. "Frostbite: review and current concepts." *The Journal of the American Board of Family Practice* 11.1 (1998): 34-40.

Ward, Michael. "Frostbite." *British Medical Journal* 1.5897 (1974): 67.

Zafren, Ken. "Frostbite: prevention and initial management." *High altitude medicine & biology* 14.1 (2013): 9-12.

Gallstones

Carey, Martin C. "Pathogenesis of gallstones." *The American journal of surgery* 165.4 (1993): 410-419.

Lammert, Frank, et al. "Gallstones." *Nature reviews Disease primers* 2.1 (2016): 1-17.

Sanders, Grant, and Andrew N. Kingsnorth. "Gallstones." *Bmj* 335.7614 (2007): 295-299.

Tehrani, Asal Neshatbini, et al. "Dietary fiber intake and risk of gallstone: a case–control study." *BMC gastroenterology* 23.1 (2023): 119.

Gingivitis

Cope, Graham, and Anwen Cope. "Gingivitis: symptoms, causes and treatment." *Dental Nursing* 7.8 (2011): 436-439.

Page, Roy C. "Gingivitis." *Journal of Clinical Periodontology* 13.5 (1986): 345-355.

Singh, Brijendra, and Ritu Singh. "Gingivitis–A silent disease." *J Dent Med Sci* 6 (2013): 30-3.

Varela-López, Alfonso, et al. "A systematic review on the implication of minerals in the onset, severity and treatment of periodontal disease." *Molecules* 21.9 (2016): 1183.

Glaucoma

Bai, Hai-Qing, et al. "Causes and treatments of traumatic secondary glaucoma." *European journal of ophthalmology* 19.2 (2009): 201-206

Belyea, David A., et al. "Marijuana use among patients with glaucoma in a city with legalized medical marijuana use." *JAMA ophthalmology* 134.3 (2016): 259-264.

Green, Keith. "Marijuana smoking vs cannabinoids for glaucoma therapy." *Archives of Ophthalmology* 116.11 (1998): 1433-1437.

Kang, Jae H., et al. "A prospective study of folate, vitamin B6, and vitamin B12 intake in relation to exfoliation glaucoma or suspected exfoliation glaucoma." *JAMA ophthalmology* 132.5 (2014): 549-55

Khaw, P. T., and A. R. Elkington. "Glaucoma—1: diagnosis." *Bmj* 328.7431 (2004): 97-99.

Stone, Edwin M., et al. "Identification of a gene that causes primary open angle glaucoma." *Science* 275.5300 (1997): 668-670.

Sun, Xiaoshen, et al. "Focus: Addiction: Marijuana for Glaucoma: A Recipe for Disaster or Treatment?." *The Yale Journal of Biology and Medicine* 88.3 (2015): 265.

Young, Robert O., and Shelley Redford Young. *The pH Miracle: Balance your Diet, reclaim your health.* Hachette UK, 2008.

Yuki, Kenya, et al. "Reduced-serum vitamin C and increased uric acid levels in normal-tension glaucoma." *Graefe's Archive for Clinical and Experimental Ophthalmology* 248 (2010): 243-248.

Gout

Chang, Hsin-Jen, et al. "Gout with auricular tophi following anti-tuberculosis treatment: a case report." *BMC Research Notes* 6 (2013): 1-3.

Chen, Pei-En, et al. "Effectiveness of cherries in reducing uric acid and gout: a systematic review." *Evidence-Based C*

Choi, Hyon K., et al. "Purine-rich foods, dairy and protein intake, and the risk of gout in men." *New England Journal of Medicine* 350.11 (2004): 1093-1103.

Griffin, Garrett R., et al. "Auricular tophi as the initial presentation of gout." *Otolaryngology-Head and Neck Surgery* 141.1 (2009): 153-154.

Lamb, Kirstie Louise, et al. "Effect of tart cherry juice on risk of gout attacks: protocol for a randomised controlled trial." *BMJ open* 10.3 (2020): e035108.

Grief

Fleming, Stephen, and Paul Robinson. "Grief and cognitive–behavioral therapy: The reconstruction of meaning." (2001).

Grimm, Christie. *Meditations Upon Grief.* Diss. Barnard College, 2014.

Halberstein, Robert, et al. "Healing with Bach® flower essences: testing a complementary therapy." *Complementary health practice review* 12.1 (2007): 3-14.

Hasha, Margot H. "Mindfulness practices for loss and grief." *Bereavem*

Kaminski, Patricia, and Richard Katz. *Flower Essence Repertory.* Flower Essence Society, 1994.

Malkinson, Ruth. "Cognitive-behavioral therapy of grief: A review and application." *Research on Social Work Practice* 11.6 (2001): 671-698.

Stang, Heather. *Mindfulness and grief: With guided med*

Guilt

Do, Y. Nhi, and Georgia Kakaletri. "A Guilt-free Guilty Pleasure: A Qualitative Study of Consumers' Process of Coping with." *Journal of Marketing Research* 49.6 (2023): 900-909.

Gerrard, Cynthia, and Lee Hyer. "Treatment of emotions: The role of guilt." *Trauma Victim.* Routledge, 2013. 445-498.

Kubany, Edward S., and Frederick P. Manke. "Cognitive therapy for trauma-related guilt: Conceptual bases and treatment outlines." *Cognitive and Behavioral Practice* 2.1 (1995): 27-61.

Man, Sonya. "Trauma-informed guilt reduction therapy: overview of the treatment and research." *Current treatment options in psychiatry* 9.3 (2022): 115-125

Yu, Huizi, Edgar Chambers IV, and Kadri Koppel. "Exploration of the food-related guilt concept." *Journal of Sensory Studies* 36.1 (2021): e12622.

Hair Loss

Ali, Alhakim, and N. V. Verma. "Spectroscopic investigation of the hair of diabetic patients." *International Letters of Chemistry, Physics and Astronomy* 3 (2013): 37-45

Frick, David A. "Franklin's Free Will; or, Optimism in Cracow, 1798." *Austrian History Yearbook* 28 (1997): 59-94.

Gasmi, Amin, et al. "Natural Compounds Used for Treating Hair Loss." *Current Pharmaceutical Design* 29.16 (2023): 1231-1244

Inchauspé, Jessie. *Glucose Revolution: The life-changing power of balancing your blood sugar.* Simon and Schuster, 2022.

Jaworsky, Christine. "Alternative Treatments for Hair Loss." *Hair and Scalp Diseases.* CRC Press, 2008. 221-234

Mounsey, Anne L., and Sean W. Reed. "Diagnosing and treating hair loss." *American family physician* 80.4 (2009): 356-362.

Novak, Melinda A., et al. "The role of stress in abnormal behavior and other abnormal conditions such as hair loss." *Handbook of primate behavioral management.* CRC Press, 2017. 75-94.

Phillips, T. Grant, W. Paul Slomiany, and Robert Allison. "Hair loss: common causes and treatment." *American family physician* 96.6 (2017): 371-378

Price, Vera H. "Treatment of hair loss." *New England Journal of Medicine* 341.13 (1999): 964-973.

Rakesh, Kashyap, Dr Mahajan SC Shukla Karunakar, and Mr Sharma. "Formulation and evaluation of hair oil for hair loss disorders." *Seed* 8.11.25 (2016): 12.

Rushton, D. H., et al. "Causes of hair loss and the developments in hair rejuvenation." *International journal of cosmetic science* 24.1 (2002): 17-23

Hangover

Jayawardena, Ranil, et al. "Interventions for treatment and/or prevention of alcohol hangover: Systematic review." *Human Psychopharmacology: Clinical and Experimental* 32.5 (2017): e2600.

Jung, S. J., et al. "Regulation of alcohol and acetaldehyde metabolism by a mixture of lactobacillus and bifidobacterium species in human. Nutrients. 2021; 13: 1875." (2021).

Pittler, Max H., Joris C. Verster, and Edzard Ernst. "Interventions for preventing or treating alcohol hangover: systematic review of randomised controlled trials." *Bmj* 331.7531 (2005): 1515-1518

Swift, Robert, and Dena Davidson. "Alcohol hangover: mechanisms and mediators." *Alcohol health and research world* 22.1 (1998): 54.

Wang, Fang, et al. "Natural products for the prevention and treatment of hangover and alcohol use disorder." *Molecules* 21.1 (2016): 64.

Wiese, Jeffrey G., Michael G. Shlipak, and Warren S. Browner. "The alcohol hangover." *Annals of internal medicine* 132.11 (2000): 897-902.

Headaches

Chen, Ya-Wen, and Hsiu-Hung Wang. "The effectiveness of acupressure on relieving pain: a systematic review." *Pain Management Nursing* 15.2 (2014): 539-550

Cohen, Jay S. *15 Natural Remedies for Migraine Headaches: Proven Effective Treatments for Adults & Children.* Square One Publishers, Inc., 2012.

Day, William Henry. *Headaches: Their nature, causes, and treatment.* Vol. 1877. Lindsay and Blakiston, 1877.

Huang, Hao, and Kaiyin He. "The association between dietary fiber intake and severe headaches or migraine in US adults." *Frontiers in Nutrition* 9 (2023): 1044066.

Lipton, Richard B., et al. "Aspartame as a dietary trigger of headache." *Headache: The Journal of head and face pain* 29.2 (1989): 90-92.

Moffett, Adrienne, Michael Swash, and D. F. Scott. "Effect of tyramine in migraine: a double-blind study." *Journal of Neurology, Neurosurgery & Psychiatry* 35.4 (1972): 496-499

Mullally, William J., Kathryn Hall, and Richard Goldstein. "Efficacy of biofeedback in the treatment of migraine and tension type headaches." *Pain physician* 12.6 (2009): 1005.

Nestoriuc, Yvonne, et al. "Biofeedback treatment for headache disorders: a comprehensive efficacy review." *Applied psychophysiology and biofeedback* 33 (2008): 125-140.

Pareek, Anil, et al. "Feverfew (Tanacetum parthenium L.): A systematic review." *Pharmacognosy reviews* 5.9 (2011): 103.

Schiffman, Susan S., et al. "Aspartame and susceptibility to headache." *New England Journal of Medicine* 317.19 (1987): 1181-1185.

Silberstein, Stephen D. "Evaluation and emergency treatment of headache." *Headache: The Journal of Head and Face Pain* 32.8 (1992): 396-407

Hearing Loss

Eggermont, Jos J. *Hearing loss: Causes, prevention, and treatment.* Academic Press, 2017.

Isaacson, Jon E., and Neil M. Vora. "Differential diagnosis and treatment of hearing loss." *American family physician* 68.6 (2003): 1125-1132.

Le Prell, Colleen G., et al. "Nutrient-enhanced diet reduces noise-induced damage to the inner ear and hearing loss." *Translational Research* 158.1 (2011): 38-53.

Müller, Ulrich, and Peter G. Barr-Gillespie. "New treatment options for hearing loss." *Nature reviews Drug discovery* 14.5 (2015): 346-365

Young, Robert O., and Shelley Redford Young. *The pH Miracle: Balance your Diet, reclaim your health.* Hachette UK, 2008.

Heartburn

Fass, Ronnie, et al. "Treatment of patients with persistent heartburn symptoms: a double-blind, randomized trial." *Clinical Gastroenterology and Hepatology* 4.1 (2006): 50-56.

Hosseinkhani, Ayda, et al. "An evidence-based review of medicinal herbs for the treatment of gastroesophageal reflux disease (GERD)." *Current Drug Discovery Technologies* 15.4 (2018): 305-314

McRorie Jr, Johnson W., Roger D. Gibb, and Philip B. Miner Jr. "Evidence-based treatment of frequent heartburn: the benefits and limitations of over-the-counter medications." *Journal of the American Association of Nurse Practitioners* 26.6 (2014): 330-339

Mulumba, Pie, and One Comment. "Cayenne Pepper: Spicy & Surprising Health Benefits

PeaceHealth, My, and Pay a Bill. "Indigestion, Heartburn, and Low Stomach Acidity (Holistic)."

Robinson, Malcolm, et al. "Heartburn requiring frequent antacid use may indicate significant illness." *Archives of Internal Medicine* 158.21 (1998): 2373-2376.

Heart Disease

Chan, Cecilia Lai-Wan, et al. "A systematic review of the effectiveness of qigong exercise in cardiac rehabilitation." *The American journal of Chinese medicine* 40.02 (2012): 255-267.

Cramer, Holger, et al. "A systematic review of yoga for heart disease." *European journal of preventive cardiology* 22.3 (2015): 284-295.

Emmert, David H., and Jeffrey T. Kirchner. "The role of vitamin E in the prevention of heart disease." *Archives of family medicine* 8.6 (1999): 537.

Heran, Balraj S., et al. "Exercise-based cardiac rehabilitation for coronary heart disease." *Cochrane database of systematic reviews* 7 (2011).

Manchanda, S. C., and Kushal Madan. "Yoga and meditation in cardiovascular disease." *Clinical Research in Cardiology* 103 (2014): 675-680.

Paffenbarger Jr, Ralph S., and Robert T. Hyde. "Exercise in the prevention of coronary heart disease." *Preventive medicine* 13.1 (1984): 3-22.

Pryor, William A. "Vitamin E and heart disease:: Basic science to clinical intervention trials." *Free Radical Biology and Medicine* 28.1 (2000): 141-164.

Turan Kavradim, Selma, Şefika Tuğba Yangöz, and Zeynep Ozer. "Effectiveness of aromatherapy inhalation on anxiety and haemodynamic variables for patients with cardiovascular disease: a systematic review and meta-analysis." *International Journal of Clinical Practice* 75.11 (2021): e14593.

Heat Exhaustion

Armstrong, Lawrence E. "Heat exhaustion." *Exertional Heat Illness: A Clinical and Evidence-Based Guide* (2020): 81-115.

Kenny, Glen P., et al. "Heat exhaustion." *Handbook of clinical neurology* 157 (2018): 505-529

Leithead, C. S., L. A. Leithead, and F. D. Lee. "Salt-deficiency heat exhaustion." *Annals of Tropical Medicine & Parasitology* 52.4 (1958): 456-467.

Ungerer, John T. *Grow, Gather, Heal: Lemon Balm For Everyday Wellness: A Deep Dive Into The Herb's History, Traditional Uses, Medicinal Benefits, Remedies, Recipes and Growing Your own.* John T. Ungerer, 2024

Zhao, Yijie, et al. "Comparison of heat strain recovery in different anti-heat stress clothing ensembles after work to exhaustion." *Journal of Thermal Biology* 69 (2017): 311-318.

Heat Rash

Kamble, Sharad, et al. "A Review on Preparation of Calendula Oil." *Sumer J Med Healthc* 61 (2023)

Opitz-Kreher, Karin, and Johannes Huber. *Twelve Essential Oils of the Bible: Ancient Healing Oils and Their Contemporary Uses.* Simon and Schuster, 2023.

Zondi, Silindelo Minenhle. *The efficacy of a topical application comprising Calendula officinalis Ø and Olea europaea in the management of seborrheic dermatitis of the scalp (dandruff).* Diss. 2017

Heel Pain

Hedaya, Robert. "Five herbs plus thiamine reduce pain and improve functional mobility in patients with pain: a pilot study." *Altern Ther Health Med* 23.1 (2017): 14-9.

Hemorrhoids

Gami, Bharat. "Hemorrhoids-a common ailment among adults, causes & treatment: a review." *Int J Pharm Pharm Sci* 3.Suppl 5 (2011): 5-13.

Lohsiriwat, Varut. "Hemorrhoids: from basic pathophysiology to clinical management." *World journal of gastroenterology: WJG* 18.17 (2012): 2009.

Lohsiriwat, Varut. "Treatment of hemorrhoids: A coloproctologist's view." *World Journal of Gastroenterology: WJG* 21.31 (2015): 9245.

Mott, Timothy, Kelly Latimer, and Chad Edwards. "Hemorrhoids: diagnosis and treatment options." *American family physician* 97.3 (2018): 172-179

Wall, M. "Stoneroot: Collinsonia canadensis. In." *Planting the future: Saving our medicinal herbs* (2000): 215-220.

Herpes Virus

Chakrabarty, Arun, et al. "Emerging therapies for herpes viral infections (types 1–8)." *Expert opinion on emerging drugs* 9.2 (2004): 237-256.

Cole, Shannon. "Herpes simplex virus: epidemiology, diagnosis, and treatment." *Nursing Clinics* 55.3 (2020): 337-345.

Esaki, Shinichi, et al. "Transient fasting enhances replication of oncolytic herpes simplex virus in glioblastoma." *American journal of cancer research* 6.2 (2016): 300.

Ikeda, Keiko, et al. "Arginine inactivates human herpesvirus 2 and inhibits genital herpesvirus infection." *International Journal of Molecular Medicine* 30.6 (2012): 1307-1312.

Mustafa, Murtaza, et al. "Herpes simplex virus infections, Pathophysiology and Management." *IOSR J dent med sci* 15.07 (2016): 85-91.

Rechenchoski, Daniele Zendrini, et al. "Herpesvirus: an underestimated virus." *Folia microbiologica* 62 (2017): 151-156.

Schilling, Ray. "Herpes Medication Successful In Mononucleosis." *Herpes* (2006).

Toulabi, Tahereh, et al. "The efficacy of olive leaf extract on healing herpes simplex virus labialis: a randomized double-blind study." *Explore* 18.3 (2022): 287-292.

Hepatitis C

Coon, Joanna Thompson, and Edzard Ernst. "Complementary and alternative therapies in the treatment of chronic hepatitis C: a systematic review." *Journal of Hepatology* 40.3 (2004): 491-500.

Honda, Akira, and Yasushi Matsuzaki. "Cholesterol and chronic hepatitis C virus infection." *Hepatology Research* 41.8 (2011): 697-710

Liu, Jian Ping, et al. "Medicinal herbs for hepatitis C virus infection." *Cochrane Database of Systematic Reviews* 2010.1 (1996).

Lupberger, Joachim, Daniel J. Felmlee, and Thomas F. Baumert. "Cholesterol uptake and hepatitis C virus entry." *Journal of hepatology* 57.1 (2012): 215-217.

Munir, Saira, et al. "Hepatitis C treatment: current and future perspectives." *Virology journal* 7 (2010): 1-6.

Seeff, Leonard B., et al. "Herbal product use by persons enrolled in the hepatitis C Antiviral Long-Term Treatment Against Cirrhosis (HALT-C) Trial." *Hepatology* 47.2 (2008): 605-612.

Tsai, Fuu-Jen, et al. "Effects of Chinese herbal medicine therapy on survival and hepatic outcomes in patients with hepatitis C virus infection in Taiwan." *Phytomedicine* 57 (2019): 30-38.

Hiccups

Friedman, Nancy L. "Hiccups: a treatment review." *Pharmacotherapy: The Journal of Human Pharmacology and Drug Therapy* 16.6 (1996): 986-995.

Gigot, Albert F., and Paul D. Flynn. "Treatment of hiccups." *Journal of the American Medical Association* 150.8 (1952): 760-764.

Lewis, James H. "Hiccups: causes and cures." *Journal of clinical gastroenterology* 7.6 (1985): 539-552.

High Blood Pressure

Bacon, Simon L., et al. "Effects of exercise, diet and weight loss on high blood pressure." *Sports Medicine* 34 (2004): 307-316.

Calhoun, David A., et al. "Resistant hypertension: diagnosis, evaluation, and treatment: a scientific statement from the American Heart Association Professional Education Committee of the Council for High Blood Pressure Research." *Hypertension* 51.6 (2008): 1403-1419.

Cooper, Richard S., Albert GB Amoah, and George A. Mensah. "High Blood Pressure." *Ethnicity & disease* 13 (2003): 48-52.

Joint National Committee on Prevention, Treatment of High Blood Pressure, and National High Blood Pressure Education Program. *Report of the Joint National Committee on Prevention, Detection, Evaluation, and Treatment of High Blood Pressure*. Vol. 6. Public Health Service, National Institutes of Health, National Heart, Lung, and Blood Institute, 1997.

High Cholesterol

Grundy, Scott M., and Gloria Lena Vega. "Causes of high blood cholesterol." *Circulation* 81.2 (1990): 412-427.

Jayakumari, N., and P. A. Kurup. "Dietary fiber and cholesterol metabolism in rats fed a high cholesterol diet." *Atherosclerosis* 33.1 (1979): 41-47.

Krumholz, Harlan M. "Treatment of Cholesterol in 2017." *JAMA* 318.5 (2017): 417-418.

Lockman, Andrew R., et al. "Treatment of cholesterol abnormalities." *American Family Physician* 71.6 (2005): 1137-1142.

McKenney, James M. "New cholesterol guidelines, new treatment challenges." *Pharmacotherapy: The Journal of Human Pharmacology and Drug Therapy* 22.7 (2002): 853-863.

Ulbricht, Catherine, et al. "Guggul for hyperlipidemia: a review by the Natural Stan

HIV and Aids

Bertozzi, Stefano, et al. "HIV/AIDS prevention and treatment." *Disease control priorities in developing countries* 2 (2006): 331-370.

Deeks, Steven G., and Andrew N. Phillips. "HIV infection, antiretroviral treatment, ageing, and non-AIDS related morbidity." *Bmj* 338 (2009).

Foster, Harold D. "How HIV-1 causes AIDS: implications for prevention and treatment." *Medical hypotheses* 62.4 (2004): 549-553.

Gupta, Praveen Kumar, and Apoorva Saxena. "HIV/AIDS: current updates on the disease, treatment and prevention." *Proceedings of the National Academy of Sciences, India Section B: Biological Sciences* 91.3 (2021): 495-510

Kalichman, Seth C., Lisa Eaton, and Chauncey Cherry. ""There is no proof that HIV causes AIDS": AIDS denialism beliefs among people living with HIV/AIDS." *Journal of behavioral medicine* 33 (2010): 432-440.

Maartens, Gary, Connie Celum, and Sharon R. Lewin. "HIV infection: epidemiology, pathogenesis, treatment, and prevention." *The Lancet* 384.9939 (2014): 258-271.

Oliveira, Julicristie M., and Patrícia HC Rondó. "Omega-3 fatty acids and hypertriglyceridemia in HIV-infected subjects on antiretroviral therapy: systematic review and meta-analysis." *HIV clinical trials* 12.5 (2011): 268-274

Simon, Viviana, David D. Ho, and Quarraisha Abdool Karim. "HIV/AIDS epidemiology, pathogenesis, prevention, and treatment." *The Lancet* 368.9534 (2006): 489-504.

Hives

Greiwe, Justin, and J. A. Bernstein. "Approach to the Patient with Hives." *Allergy and Immunology for the Internist, An Issue of Medical Clinics of North America, E-Book: Allergy and Immunology for the Internist, An Issue of Medical Clinics of North America, E-Book* 104.1 (2019): 15-24.

Guo, Xiaoqing, and Nan Mei. "Aloe vera: A review of toxicity and adverse clinical effects." *Journal of Environmental Science and Health, Part C* 34.2 (2016): 77-96.

Kaplan, Allen P. "Chronic urticaria: possible causes, suggested treatment alternatives." *Postgraduate Medicine* 74.3 (1983): 209-222.

Rosner, David. "Hives of sickness." *Public health and epidemics in New York City. New Brunswick: Rutgers University Press* (1995).

Tierra, Michael. *Chinese traditional herbal medicine*. Lotus Press, 1998.

Zhao, Xiaolan. *Inner Beauty: Looking, Feeling and Being Your Best Through Traditional Chinese Healing*. Random House Canada, 2011.

Hostility

Barefoot, John C., and Redford B. Williams. "Hostility and health." *Handbook of cardiovascular behavioral medicine*. New York, NY: Springer New York, 2022. 503-524.

Von Der Lippe, Anna Louise, et al. "Treatment failure in psychotherapy: The pull of hostility." *Psychotherapy Research* 18.4 (2008): 420-432.

Williams, Redford B., and Virginia P. Williams. "The prevention and treatment of hostility." *Handbook of personality and health* (2006): 159-275.

Hot Flashes

Kronenberg, Fredi. "Hot flashes: phenomenology, quality of life, and search for treatment options." *Experimental gerontology* 29.3-4 (1994): 319-336.

Lieberman, Shari. *Get Off the Menopause Roller Coaster: Natural Solutions for Mood Swings, Hot Flashes, Fatigue, Anxiety, Depression, and Other Symptoms*. Penguin, 1999.

Nelson, Heidi D. "Commonly used types of postmenopausal estrogen for treatment of hot flashes: scientific review." *Jama* 291.13 (2004): 1610-1620.

Philp, Hazel A. "Hot flashes-a review of the literature on alternative and complementary treatment approaches." *Alternative Medicine Review* 8.3 (2003): 284-302

Rattanatantikul, Teerapong. *The Effects of Oral Combined Nutraceuticals on Menopausal Symptoms and Hormonal Changes in Post-menopausal Women*. Diss. Department of Anti-Aging and Regenerative Medicine, College of Integrative Medicine, Dhurakij Pundit University, 2020.

Shanafelt, Tait D., et al. "Pathophysiology and treatment of hot flashes." *Mayo Clinic Proceedings*. Vol. 77. No. 11. Elsevier, 2002.

Hypoglycemia

Conn, Jerome W. "The advantage of a high protein diet in the treatment of spontaneous hypoglycemia: preliminary report." *The Journal of Clinical Investigation* 15.6 (1936): 673-678.

Creery, R. D. G. "Hypoglycaemia in the newborn: diagnosis, treatment and prognosis." *Developmental Medicine & Child Neurology* 8.6 (1966): 746-754.

Shivashankara, A. R., et al. "Antidiabetic and hypoglycemic effects of Syzygium cumini (Black Plum)." *Bioactive food as dietary interventions for diabetes* (2013): 537-554.

Impotence

Brotto, Lori A., Lisa Mehak, and Cassandra Kit. "Yoga and sexual functioning: a review." *Journal of sex & marital therapy* 35.5 (2009): 378-390.

Faleyimu, O., and O. Akinyemi. "Herbal approaches to the problem of erectile dysfunction in Kaduna State, Nigeria." *Egyptian Journal of Biology* 12 (2010): 103-107

Joshi, Anjali Mangesh, Raveendran Arkiath Veettil, and Sanjay Deshpande. "Role of yoga in the management of premature ejaculation." *The world journal of men's health* 38.4 (2020): 495.

Kamatenesi-Mugisha, Maud, and Hannington Oryem-Origa. "Traditional herbal remedies used in the management of sexual impotence and erectile dysfunction in western Uganda." *African Health Sciences* 5.1 (2005): 40-49

Killoren, David. "Causal impotence and veganism." *The Routledge Handbook of Vegan Studies* (2021): 111.

Koolwal, Arpit, et al. "l-arginine and Erectile Dysfunction." *Journal of Psychosexual Health* 1.1 (2019): 37-43.

Kyarimpa, Christine, et al. "Medicinal plants used in the management of sexual dysfunction, infertility and improving virility in the East African Community: a systematic review." *Evidence-Based Complementary and Alternative Medicine* 2023.1 (2023): 6878852

McKay, Alexander. "Sexuality and substance use: The impact of tobacco, alcohol, and selected recreational drugs on sexual function." *The Canadian journal of human sexuality* 14.1/2 (2005): 47.

Morley, John E. "Impotence." *The American journal of medicine* 80.5 (1986): 897-905.

O'Keefe, Mary, and Debra K. Hunt. "Assessment and treatment of impotence." *Medical Clinics of North America* 79.2 (1995): 415-434

Smith, Arthur D. "Causes and classification of impotence." *Urologic Clinics of North America* 8.1 (1981): 79-89.

Incontinence

Kołodyńska, Gabriela, Maciej Zalewski, and Krystyna Rożek-Piechura. "Urinary incontinence in postmenopausal women—causes, symptoms, treatment." *Menopause Review/Przegląd Menopauzalny* 18.1 (2019): 46-50.

Minassian, Vatche A., Harold P. Drutz, and Ahmed Al-Badr. "Urinary incontinence as a worldwide problem." *International Journal of Gynecology & Obstetrics* 82.3 (2003): 327-338.

Nasr, Samer Z., and Joseph G. Ouslander. "Urinary incontinence in the elderly: causes and treatment options." *Drugs & aging* 12 (1998): 349-360.

Park, Seong-Hi, and Chang-Bum Kang. "Effect of Kegel exercises on the management of female stress urinary incontinence: a systematic review of randomized controlled trials." *Advances in Nursing* 2014.1 (2014): 640262.

Patel, Mitul, et al. "Urinary incontinence and diuretic avoidance among adults with chronic kidney disease." *International urology and nephrology* 48 (2016): 1321-1326.

Infertility

Anwar, Shahnaz, and Ayesha Anwar. "Infertility: A review on causes, treatment and management." *Womens Health Gynecol* 5 (2016): 2-5.

Brugo-Olmedo, Santiago, Claudio Chillik, and Susana Kopelman. "Definition and causes of infertility." *Reproductive biomedicine online* 2.1 (2001): 173-185.

Chavarro, Jorge E., et al. "Soy food and isoflavone intake in relation to semen quality parameters among men from an infertility clinic." *Human reproduction* 23.11 (2008): 2584-2590

Hull, M. G., et al. "Population study of causes, treatment, and outcome of infertility." *Br Med J (Clin Res Ed)* 291.6510 (1985): 1693-1697

Ingino, Ashley, and Weiwen Chai. "The Role of Nutrition and Supplements in the Development and Treatment of Female Infertility: A Review of Literature."

Lindsay, Tammy J., and Kirsten R. Vitrikas. "Evaluation and treatment of infertility." *American family physician* 91.5 (2015): 308-314.

Parazzini, F., et al. "Tight underpants and trousers and risk of dyspermia." *International journal of andrology* 18.3 (1995): 137-140

Righarts, Antoinette, et al. "Ovulation monitoring and fertility knowledge: Their relationship to fertility experience in a cross-sectional study." *Australian and New Zealand Journal of Obstetrics and Gynaecology* 57.4 (2017): 412-419

Serder, A. H. "Lifestyle and causes of Male Infertility." *Turkmen Medical* (2010).

Singh, Rajender, and Kiran Singh, eds. *Male infertility: understanding, causes and treatment.* Springer Singapore, 2017.

Wojcik, Malgorzata, et al. "The role of visceral therapy, Kegel's muscle, core stability and diet in pelvic support disorders and urinary incontinence—including sexological aspects and the role of physiotherapy and osteopathy." *Ginekologia Polska* 93.12 (2022): 1018-1027.

Inflammatory Bowel Disease

Baumgart, Daniel C., and Simon R. Carding. "Inflammatory bowel disease: cause and immunobiology." *The Lancet* 369.9573 (2007): 1627-1640.

Ghouri, Yezaz A., Veysel Tahan, and Bo Shen. "Secondary causes of inflammatory bowel diseases." *World journal of gastroenterology* 26.28 (2020): 3998.

Papadakis, Konstantinos A., and Stephan R. Targan. "Current theories on the causes of inflammatory bowel disease." *Gastroenterology Clinics of North America* 28.2 (1999): 283-296.

Sands, Bruce E. "Inflammatory bowel disease: past, present, and future." *Journal of gastroenterology* 42 (2007): 16-25.

Ingrown Hair

DeMaria, Andrea L., et al. "Complications related to pubic hair removal." *American journal of obstetrics and gynecology* 210.6 (2014): 528-e1.

Huang, Jiangxia, et al. "An Interesting Case of Ingrowing Hair." *Clinical, Cosmetic and Investigational Dermatology* (2023): 2329-2331.

Ogunbiyi, Adebola. "Pseudofolliculitis barbae; current treatment options." *Clinical, cosmetic and investigational dermatology* (2019): 241-247.

Inhibited Sexual Desire

Kim, Ha-Na, et al. "Effects of yoga on sexual function in women with metabolic syndrome: a randomized controlled trial." *The journal of sexual medicine* 10.11 (2013): 2741-2751.

Kingsberg, Sheryl A., and James A. Simon. "Female hypoactive sexual desire disorder: a practical guide to causes, clinical diagnosis, and treatment." *Journal of Women's Health* 29.8 (2020): 1101-1112.

Levine, Stephen B. "An essay on the nature of sexual desire." *Journal of Sex & Marital Therapy* 10.2 (1984): 83-96.

McCabe, Marita P. "A program for the treatment of inhibited sexual desire in males." *Psychotherapy: Theory, Research, Practice, Training* 29.2 (1992): 288.

Pfaus, James G. "Pathways of sexual desire." *The journal of sexual medicine* 6.6 (2009): 1506-1533.

Tisserand, Robert. *The art of aromatherapy: The healing and beautifying properties of the essential oils of flowers and herbs.* Inner Traditions/Bear & Co, 1978.

Weeks, Gerald R. "Systematic treatment of inhibited sexual desire." *Integrating sex and marital therapy.* Routledge, 2013. 183-201.

Insomnia

Cunnington, David, Moira F. Junge, and Antonio T. Fernando. "Insomnia: prevalence, consequences and effective treatment." *Medical Journal of Australia* 199 (2013): S36-S40.

Drake, Christopher L., Timothy Roehrs, and Thomas Roth. "Insomnia causes, consequences, and therapeutics: an overview." *Depression and anxiety* 18.4 (2003): 163-176.

Fletcher, David J. "Coping with insomnia: helping patients manage sleeplessness without drugs." *Postgraduate Medicine* 79.2 (1986): 265-274.

Kierlin, Lara. "Sleeping without a pill: nonpharmacologic treatments for insomnia." *Journal of Psychiatric Practice*® 14.6 (2008): 403-407.

Morrison, Jack R., Edward Kujawa Jr, and Brian A. Storey. "Causes and treatment of insomnia among adolescents." *Journal of School Health* 55.4 (1985): 148-150.

Ramakrishnan, Kalyanakrishnan. "Treatment options for insomnia." *South African Family Practice* 49.8 (2007): 34-41.

Singh, Amrinder, and Kaicun Zhao. "Treatment of insomnia with traditional Chinese herbal medicine." *International Review of Neurobiology* 135 (2017): 97-115.

Wing, Y. K. "Herbal treatment of insomnia." *Hong Kong Medical Journal* 7.4 (2001): 392.

Wynchank, Dora, et al. "Adult attention-deficit/hyperactivity disorder (ADHD) and insomnia: an update of the literature." *Current psychiatry reports* 19 (2017): 1-11.

Yeung, Wing-Fai, et al. "Self-administered acupressure for insomnia disorder: a pilot randomized controlled trial." *Journal of sleep research* 27.2 (2018): 220-231.

Irritable Bowel Syndrome (IBS)

Camilleri, Michael. "Management of the irritable bowel syndrome." *Gastroenterology* 120.3 (2001): 652-668.

Canavan, Caroline, Joe West, and Timothy Card. "The epidemiology of irritable bowel syndrome." *Clinical epidemiology* (2014): 71-80.

El-Salhy, Magdy, et al. "Dietary fiber in irritable bowel syndrome." *International journal of molecular medicine* 40.3 (2017): 607-613.

Heitkemper, Margaret, and Monica Jarrett. "Irritable bowel syndrome: causes and treatment." *Gastroenterology Nursing* 23.6 (2000): 256-263.

Horwitz, Brenda J., and Robert S. Fisher. "The irritable bowel syndrome." *New England journal of medicine* 344.24 (2001): 1846-1850.

Naliboff, Bruce D., et al. "Mindfulness-based stress reduction improves irritable bowel syndrome (IBS) symptoms via specific aspects of mindfulness." *Neurogastroenterology & Motility* 32.9 (2020): e13828.

Shaw, G., et al. "Stress management for irritable bowel syndrome: a controlled trial." *Digestion* 50.1 (1991): 36-42

Jet Lag

Arendt, Josephine. "Managing jet lag: Some of the problems and possible new solutions." *Sleep medicine reviews* 13.4 (2009): 249-256.

Herxheimer, Andrew, Keith J. Petrie, and Cochrane Common Mental Disorders Group. "Melatonin for the prevention and treatment of jet lag." *Cochrane Database of Systematic Reviews* 2010.1 (1996).

Sack, Robert L. "The pathophysiology of jet lag." *Travel medicine and infectious disease* 7.2 (2009): 102-110.

Smith, Peter. *Sleep Better with Natural Therapies: A Comprehensive Guide to Overcoming Insomnia, Moving Sleep Cycles and Preventing Jet Lag.* Singing Dragon, 2013.

Kidney Stones

Coe, Fredric L., Joan H. Parks, and John R. Asplin. "The pathogenesis and treatment of kidney stones." *New England Journal of Medicine* 327.16 (1992): 1141-1152

Frassetto, Lynda, and Ingrid Kohlstadt. "Treatment and prevention of kidney stones: an update." *American family physician* 84.11 (2011): 1234-1242.

Khan, Saeed R., et al. "Kidney stones." *Nature reviews Disease primers* 2.1 (2016): 1-23.

Massey, Linda K., Helen Roman-Smith, and Roger AL Sutton. "Effect of dietary oxalate and calcium on urinary oxalate and risk of formation of calcium oxalate kidney stones." *Journal of the American Dietetic Association* 93.8 (1993): 901-906.

Moe, Orson W. "Kidney stones: pathophysiology and medical management." *The lancet* 367.9507 (2006): 333-344.

Knee Pain

Duong, Vicky, et al. "Evaluation and treatment of knee pain: a review." *Jama* 330.16 (2023): 1568-1580.

Jones, Brandon Q., Carlton J. Covey, and Marvin H. Sineath Jr. "Nonsurgical management of knee pain in adults." *American family physician* 92.10 (2015): 875-883.

Post, William R. "Anterior knee pain: diagnosis and treatment." *JAAOS-Journal of the American Academy of Orthopaedic Surgeons* 13.8 (2005): 534-543.

Sanchis-Alfonso, Vicente, et al. "Diagnosis and treatment of anterior knee pain." *Journal of ISAKOS* 1.3 (2016): 161-173.

Schoolmeesters, Laree Jane. *The effect of reflexology on joint pain.* Case Western Reserve University (Health Sciences), 2005.

Yakout, RashaRasha, Narges Seyam, and Hamda Ahmed Mohamed Eldesoky. "Effect of reflexology foot massage on pain intensity and physical functional abilities among patients with knee osteoarthritis." *Egyptian Journal of Nursing and Health Sciences* 3.1 (2022): 17-40

Lactose Intolerance

Catanzaro, Roberto, Morena Sciuto, and Francesco Marotta. "Lactose intolerance: An update on its pathogenesis, diagnosis, and treatment." *Nutrition Research* 89 (2021): 23-34.

Ojetti, Veronica, et al. "High prevalence of celiac disease in patients with lactose intolerance." *Digestion* 71.2 (2005): 106-110.

Scrimshaw, Nevin S., and Edwina B. Murray. "The acceptability of milk and milk products in populations with a high prevalence of lactose intolerance." *The American journal of clinical nutrition* 48.4 (1988): 1142-1159.

Shaw, A. D., and G. J. Davies. "Lactose intolerance: problems in diagnosis and treatment." *Journal of clinical gastroenterology* 28.3 (1999): 208-216.

Laryngitis

Davies, D. Garfield, Anthony F. Jahn, and Anat Keidar. "Medications and the professional voice." *Care of the professional voice*. Routledge, 2004. 78-87.

Dworkin, James Paul. "Laryngitis: types, causes, and treatments." *Otolaryngologic Clinics of North America* 41.2 (2008): 419-436.

Nestor, James. *Breath: The new science of a lost art*. Penguin, 2020

Tulunay, Ozlem E. "Laryngitis—diagnosis and management." *Otolaryngologic Clinics of North America* 41.2 (2008): 437-451.

Wallner, Linden J. "Smoker's larynx." *The Laryngoscope* 64.4 (1954): 259-270.

Wood, John M., Theodore Athanasiadis, and Jacqui Allen. "Laryngitis." *Bmj* 349 (2014).

Macular Degeneration

Holz, Frank G., Steffen Schmitz-Valckenberg, and Monika Fleckenstein. "Recent developments in the treatment of age-related macular degeneration." *The Journal of clinical investigation* 124.4 (2014): 1430-1438.

Mitchell, Paul, et al. "Age-related macular degeneration." *The Lancet* 392.10153 (2018): 1147-1159

Stahl, Andreas. "The diagnosis and treatment of age-related macular degeneration." *Deutsches Ärzteblatt International* 117.29-30 (2020): 513.

Tokarz, Paulina, Kai Kaarniranta, and Janusz Blasiak. "Role of antioxidant enzymes and small molecular weight antioxidants in the pathogenesis of age-related macular degeneration (AMD)." *Biogerontology* 14 (2013): 461-482.

Van Leeuwen, Redmer, et al. "Dietary intake of antioxidants and risk of age-related macular degeneration." *Jama* 294.24 (2005): 3101-3107.

Male Menopause

Channer, K. S., and T. H. Jones. "Cardiovascular effects of testosterone: implications of the "male menopause"?." *Heart* 89.2 (2003): 121-122.

Featherstone, Mike, and Mike Hepworth. "The male menopause: lifestyle and sexuality." *Maturitas* 7.3 (1985): 235-246.

Margolese, Howard C. "The male menopause and mood: testosterone decline and depression in the aging male—is there a link?." *Journal of geriatric psychiatry and neurology* 13.2 (2000): 93-101.

Peate, Ian. "The male menopause: possible causes, symptoms and treatment." *British journal of nursing* 12.2 (2003): 80-84.

Vahter, Marie, Marika Berglund, and Agneta Åkesson. "Toxic metals and the menopause." *British Menopause Society Journal* 10.2 (2004): 60-65.

Marine Bites and Stings

Brown, Graham V., and David A. Warrell. "Venomous bites and stings in the tropical world." *Medical journal of Australia* 159.11-12 (1993): 773-779.

Cegolon, Luca, et al. "Jellyfish stings and their management: a review." *Marine drugs* 11.2 (2013): 523-550.

Theakston, R. David G., and David G. Lalloo. "Venomous bites and stings." *Principles and practice of travel medicine* (2001): 321-341.

White, Julian. "Marine animals: bites and stings." *Current therapeutics* 43.2 (2002): 37-45.

Memory Problems

Hope, Jenny. "Why a whiff of rosemary DOES help you remember: Sniffing the herb can increase memory by 75%." *Daily Mail* 8 (2013).

Uddin, Md, et al. "Medicine that causes memory loss: risk of neurocognitive disorders." *International Neuropsychiatric Disease Journal* 8.1 (2016): 1-18.

Wong, Kah-Hui, et al. "Neuroregenerative potential of lion's mane mushroom, Hericium erinaceus (Bull.: Fr.) Pers.(higher Basidiomycetes), in the treatment of peripheral nerve injury." *International journal of medicinal mushrooms* 14.5 (2012)

Menopause

Al-Azzawi, F. "The menopause and its treatment in perspective." *Postgraduate medical journal* 77.907 (2001): 292-304.

Davis, Susan R., and Rodney J. Baber. "Treating menopause—MHT and beyond." *Nature Reviews Endocrinology* 18.8 (2022): 490-502.

Grindler, Natalia M., and Nanette F. Santoro. "Menopause and exercise." *Menopause* 22.12 (2015): 1351-1358.

Kinney, Ann, Jennie Kline, and Bruce Levin. "Alcohol, caffeine and smoking in relation to age at menopause." *Maturitas* 54.1 (2006): 27-38.

Mishra, Nalini, and V. N. Mishra. "Exercise beyond menopause: Dos and Don'ts." *Journal of mid-life health* 2.2 (2011): 51-56.

Ringa, Virginie. "Menopause and treatments." *Quality of life research* 9 (2000): 695-707.

Rymer, Janice, and Edward P. Morris. "Menopausal symptoms." *Bmj* 321.7275 (2000): 1516-1519.

Santoro, Nanette, et al. "The menopause transition: signs, symptoms, and management options." *The Journal of Clinical Endocrinology & Metabolism* 106.1 (2021): 1-15.

Taneri, Petek Eylul, et al. "Association of alcohol consumption with the onset of natural menopause: a systematic review and meta-analysis." *Human reproduction update* 22.4 (2016): 516-528.

Menstrual Cramps

de Souza, Andrieli Daiane Zdanski, et al. "Menstrual cramps: A new therapeutic alternative care through medicinal plants." (2013).

Eby, George A. "Zinc treatment prevents dysmenorrhea." *Medical Hypotheses* 69.2 (2007): 297-301.

Fugh-Berman, Adriane, and Fredi Kronenberg. "Complementary and alternative medicine (CAM) in reproductive-age women: a review of randomized controlled trials." *Reproductive Toxicology* 17.2 (2003): 137-152.

Hudson, Tori. "Menstrual Cramps,(Dysmenorrhea); An alternative approach.(Women's Health Update)." *Townsend Letter for Doctors and Patients* 225 (2002): 168-172.

Kashani, Ladan, et al. "Herbal medicine in the treatment of primary dysmenorrhea." (2015): 1-5.

Samba Conney, Catherine, et al. "Complementary and alternative medicine use for primary dysmenorrhea among senior high school students in the western region of Ghana." *Obstetrics and Gynecology International* 2019.1 (2019): 8059471.

Morning Sickness

Dugoua, Jean-Jacques. "Vitamins, minerals, trace elements, and dietary supplements." *Clinical Pharmacology During Pregnancy* (2013): 367-382.

Flaxman, Samuel M., and Paul W. Sherman. "Morning sickness: a mechanism for protecting mother and embryo." *The Quarterly review of biology* 75.2 (2000): 113-148.

Hellwig, Jennifer P. "Morning Sickness Treatments: Review Shows Little Evidence." *Nursing for Women's Health* 14.6 (2010): 447-453.

Koren, Gideon. "Treating morning sickness in the United States—changes in prescribing are needed." *American Journal of Obstetrics and Gynecology* 211.6 (2014): 602-606.

PainAssist, Team. "Morning Sickness at Night: Causes, Symptoms, Prevention, Treatment."

Strong Jr, Thomas H. "Alternative therapies of morning sickness." *Clinical obstetrics and gynecology* 44.4 (2001): 653-660.

Motion Sickness

Brainard, Andrew, and Chip Gresham. "Prevention and treatment of motion sickness." *American family physician* 90.1 (2014): 41-46

Glaser, E. M. "Prevention and treatment of motion sickness." (1959): 965-972.

Golding, John F., and Michael A. Gresty. "Motion sickness." *Current opinion in neurology* 18.1 (2005): 29-34.

Huppert, Doreen, et al. "What the ancient Greeks and Romans knew (and did not know) about seasickness." *Neurology* 86.6 (2016): 560-565.

Koch, Andreas, et al. "The neurophysiology and treatment of motion sickness." *Deutsches Ärzteblatt International* 115.41 (2018): 6

Post-White, J., and W. Nichols. "Randomised rrial testing of QueaseEase essential oil for motion sickness." *Int. J. Essent. Oil Ther* 1 (2007): 143-152.

Shupak, Avi, and Carlos R. Gordon. "Motion sickness: advances in pathogenesis, prediction, prevention, and treatment." *Aviation, space, and environmental medicine* 77.12 (2006): 1213-1223.

Muscle Cramps and Spasms

Bergeron, Michael F. "Muscle cramps during exercise-is it fatigue or electrolyte deficit?." *Current Sports Medicine Reports* 7.4 (2008): S50-S55.

Edouard, P. "Exercise associated muscle cramps: Discussion on causes, prevention and treatment." *Science & sports* 29.6 (2014): 299-305.

Maughan, Ronald J., and Susan M. Shirreffs. "Muscle cramping during exercise: causes, solutions, and questions remaining." *Sports Medicine* 49.2 (2019): 115-124.

Miller, Kevin C., et al. "Exercise-associated muscle cramps: causes, treatment, and prevention." *Sports health* 2.4 (2010): 279-283.

Swash, Michael, D. Czesnik, and M. De Carvalho. "Muscular cramp: causes and management." *European Journal of Neurology* 26.2 (2019): 214-221.

Muscle Pain

Cohen, Steven P., et al. "The pharmacologic treatment of muscle pain." *The Journal of the American Society of Anesthesiologists* 101.2 (2004): 495-526.

Mense, Siegfried, and Robert D. Gerwin, eds. *Muscle pain: diagnosis and treatment.* Springer Science & Business Media, 2010.

Noonan, Thomas J., and William E. Garrett Jr. "Muscle strain injury: diagnosis and treatment." *JAAOS-Journal of the American Academy of Orthopaedic Surgeons* 7.4 (1999): 262-269.

Wheeler, Anthony H., and George W. Aaron. "Muscle pain due to injury." *Current Pain and Headache Reports* 5 (2001): 441-446.

Nail Brittleness

Chessa, Marco A., et al. "Pathogenesis, clinical signs and treatment recommendations in brittle nails: a review." *Dermatology and therapy* 10 (2020): 15-27

Dimitris, Rigopoulos, and Daniel Ralph. "Management of simple brittle nails." *Dermatologic therapy* 25.6 (2012): 569-573

Iorizzo, M., et al. "Brittle nails." *Journal of cosmetic dermatology* 3.3 (2004): 138-144.

Shemer, Avner, and C. Ralph Daniel III. "Common nail disorders." *Clinics in Dermatology* 31.5 (2013): 578-586.

Nausea and Vomiting

Cangemi, David J., and Braden Kuo. "Practical perspectives in the treatment of nausea and vomiting." *Journal of clinical gastroenterology* 53.3 (2019): 170-178.

Chepyala, Pavan, and Kevin W. Olden. "Nausea and vomiting." *Current Treatment Options in Gastroenterology* 11.2 (2008): 135-144.

Koch, Kenneth L., and William L. Hasler, eds. *Nausea and vomiting: diagnosis and treatment.* Springer, 2016.

Lacy, Brian E., Henry P. Parkman, and Michael Camilleri. "Chronic nausea and vomiting: evaluation and treatment." *Official journal of the American College of Gastroenterology| ACG* 113.5 (2018): 647-659.

Neck and Shoulder Pain

Cassou, B., et al. "Chronic neck and shoulder pain, age, and working conditions: longitudinal results from a large random sample in France." *Occupational and environmental medicine* 59.8 (2002): 537-544.

Cohen, Steven P. "Epidemiology, diagnosis, and treatment of neck pain." *Mayo Clinic Proceedings.* Vol. 90. No. 2. Elsevier, 2015.

Greenberg, Deborah L. "Evaluation and treatment of shoulder pain." *Med Clin North Am* 98.3 (2014): 487-504.

Krusen, Edward M. "Pain in the neck and shoulder, common causes and response to therapy." *Journal of the American Medical Association* 159.13 (1955): 1282-1285.

Mitchell, Caroline, et al. "Shoulder pain: diagnosis and management in primary care." *Bmj* 331.7525 (2005): 1124-1128.

Nosebleeds

Bishow, Richard M. "Current approaches to the management of epistaxis: treatment of nosebleed varies according to the cause, location, and severity of the hemorrhage. The first step is to thoroughly evaluate the patient." *JAAPA-Journal of the American Academy of Physicians Assistants* 16.5 (2003): 52-61.

Hallberg, Olav E. "Severe nosebleed and its treatment." *Journal of the American Medical Association* 148.5 (1952): 355-360.

Haymes, A. T., and V. Harries. "'How to stop a nosebleed': an assessment of the quality of epistaxis treatment advice on YouTube." *The Journal of Laryngology & Otology* 130.8 (2016): 749-754

Silva, B. Maneesha, et al. "Lifestyle and dietary influences on nosebleed severity in hereditary hemorrhagic telangiectasia." *The Laryngoscope* 123.5 (2013): 1092-1099.

Tunkel, David E., et al. "Clinical practice guideline: nosebleed (epistaxis)." *Otolaryngology–Head and Neck Surgery* 162 (2020): S1-S38.

Oily Hair and Oily Skin

Hazen, H. H., and Florence Biase. "The Care of the Hair." *The American Journal of Nursing* (1933): 123-129.

Hong, Ji Yeon, et al. "Oily sensitive skin: A review of management options." *Journal of Cosmetic Dermatology* 19.5 (2020): 1016-1020.

Kaimal, Sowmya, and Devinder Mohan Thappa. "Diet in dermatology: revisited." *Indian journal of dermatology, venereology and leprology* 76 (2010): 103.

Lanjewar, Ameya, et al. "Review on Hair Problem and its Solution." *Journal of Drug Delivery and Therapeutics* 10.3-s (2020): 322-329.

Shuo, Liu, et al. "Efficacy and possible mechanisms of botulinum toxin treatment of oily skin." *Journal of cosmetic dermatology* 18.2 (2019): 451-457.

Sumit, Kumar, et al. "Herbal cosmetics: used for skin and hair." *Inven. J* 2012 (2012): 1-7.

Osteoporosis

Banu, Jameela. "Causes, consequences, and treatment of osteoporosis in men." *Drug design, development and therapy* (2013): 849-860.

Florence, R., et al. "Diagnosis and treatment of osteoporosis." *Bloomington (MN): Institute for Clinical Systems Improvement (ICSI)* (2013).

Hudec, Susan M. DeLange, and Pauline M. Camacho. "Secondary causes of osteoporosis." *Endocrine practice* 19.1 (2013): 120-128.

Marcus, Robert. "Role of exercise in preventing and treating osteoporosis." *Rheumatic Disease Clinics of North America* 27.1 (2001): 131-141.

Sinaki, Mehrsheed. "Exercise and osteoporosis." *Archives of physical medicine and rehabilitation* 70.3 (1989): 220-229.

Sweet, Mary Gayle, et al. "Diagnosis and treatment of osteoporosis." *American family physician* 79.3 (2009): 193-200.

Overweight

Aronne, Louis J. "Epidemiology, morbidity, and treatment of overweight and obesity." *Journal of Clinical Psychiatry* 62 (2001): 13-22.

Daniels, Stephen R., et al. "Overweight in children and adolescents: pathophysiology, consequences, prevention, and treatment." *Circulation* 111.15 (2005): 1999-2012.

Spear, Bonnie A., et al. "Recommendations for treatment of child and adolescent overweight and obesity." *Pediatrics* 120.Supplement_4 (2007): S254-S288.

Williams, Ellen P., et al. "Overweight and obesity: prevalence, consequences, and causes of a growing public health problem." *Current obesity reports* 4 (2015): 363-370.

Wyatt, Sharon B., Karen P. Winters, and Patricia M. Dubbert. "Overweight and obesity: prevalence, consequences, and causes of a growing public health problem." *The American journal of the medical sciences* 331.4 (2006): 166-174.

Parkinson's Disease

Abou-Raya, Suzan, Madihah Helmii, and Anna Abou-Raya. "Bone and mineral metabolism in older adults with Parkinson's disease." *Age and Ageing* 38.6 (2009): 675-680.

Alizadeh, Mohammad, Sorayya Kheirouri, and Majid Keramati. "What Dietary Vitamins and Minerals Might Be Protective against Parkinson's Disease?." *Brain Sciences* 13.7 (2023): 1119.

Bloem, Bastiaan R., Michael S. Okun, and Christine Klein. "Parkinson's disease." *The Lancet* 397.10291 (2021): 2284-2303.

Calne, Donald B. "Treatment of Parkinson's disease." *New England Journal of Medicine* 329.14 (1993): 1021-1027.

Kalia, Lorraine V., and Anthony E. Lang. "Parkinson's disease." *The Lancet* 386.9996 (2015): 896-912.

Rao, Shobha S., Laura A. Hofmann, and Amer Shakil. "Parkinson's disease: diagnosis and treatment." *American family physician* 74.12 (2006): 2046-2054.

Phlebitis

Goulart, Cristina B., et al. "Effectiveness of topical interventions to prevent or treat intravenous therapy-related phlebitis: A systematic review." *Journal of Clinical Nursing* 29.13-14 (2020): 2138-2149.

Guanche-Sicilia, Aitana, et al. "Prevention and treatment of phlebitis secondary to the insertion of a peripheral venous catheter: a scoping review from a nursing perspective." *Healthcare.* Vol. 9. No. 5. MDPI, 2021

Macklin, Denise. "Phlebitis: A painful complication of peripheral IV catheterization that may be prevented." *AJN The American Journal of Nursing* 103.2 (2003): 55-60.

Matsumoto, Toshiharu, et al. "Zahn Infarct of the Liver Resulting from Occlusive Phlebitis in Portal Vein Radicles." *American Journal of Gastroenterology (Springer Nature)* 87.3 (1992).

Uslusoy, Esin, and Samiye Mete. "Predisposing factors to phlebitis in patients with peripheral intravenous catheters: a descriptive study." *Journal of the American Academy of Nurse Practitioners* 20.4 (2008): 172-180.

Plantar Warts

García-Oreja, Sara, et al. "Topical treatment for plantar warts: A systematic review." *Dermatologic therapy* 34.1 (2021): e14621.

Plasencia, Jorge M. "Cutaneous warts: diagnosis and treatment." *Primary Care: Clinics in Office Practice* 27.2 (2000): 423-434.

Vickers, C. F. H. "Treatment of plantar warts in children." *British medical journal* 2.5254 (1961): 743.

Vlahovic, Tracey C., and M. Tariq Khan. "The human papillomavirus and its role in plantar warts: a comprehensive review of diagnosis and management." *Clinics in Podiatric Medicine and Surgery* 33.3 (2016): 337-353.

Witchey, Dexter Jordan, et al. "Plantar warts: epidemiology, pathophysiology, and clinical management." *Journal of Osteopathic Medicine* 118.2 (2018): 92-105.

Pneumonia

Arancibia, Francisco, et al. "Antimicrobial treatment failures in patients with community-acquired pneumonia: causes and prognostic implications." *American Journal of Respiratory and Critical Care Medicine* 162.1 (2000): 154-160.

Dandachi, Dima, and Maria C. Rodriguez-Barradas. "Viral pneumonia: etiologies and treatment." *Journal of Investigative Medicine* 66.6 (2018): 957-965.

Grief, Samuel N., and Julie K. Loza. "Guidelines for the Evaluation and Treatment of Pneumonia." *Primary Care: Clinics in Office Practice* 45.3 (2018): 485-503.

Mattila, Joshua T., et al. "Pneumonia. Treatment and diagnosis." *Annals of the American Thoracic Society* 11. Supplement 4 (2014): S189-S192.

Pregnancy Discomfort

Greenwood, Connie J., and M. Colleen Stainton. "Back pain/discomfort in pregnancy: invisible and forgotten." *The Journal of perinatal education* 10.1 (2001): 1.

Horan, Mary. "Discomfort and pain during pregnancy." *MCN: The American Journal of Maternal/Child Nursing* 9.4 (1984): 267-269.

Jordan, Robin G., and Anne Z. Cockerham. "Common discomforts of pregnancy." *Prenatal and Postnatal Care: A Person-Centered Approach* 233 (2023).

Zielinski, Ruth, Kimberly Searing, and Megan Deibel. "Gastrointestinal distress in pregnancy: prevalence, assessment, and treatment of 5 common minor discomforts." *The Journal of perinatal & neonatal nursing* 29.1 (2015): 23-31.

Premature Ejaculation

de Carufel, François, and Gilles Trudel. "Effects of a new functional-sexological treatment for premature ejaculation." *Journal of sex & marital therapy* 32.2 (2006): 97-114.

Gillman, Nicholas, and Michael Gillman. "Premature ejaculation: aetiology and treatment strategies." *Medical sciences* 7.11 (2019): 102.

Jannini, Emmanuele A., and Andrea Lenzi. "Epidemiology of premature ejaculation." *Current opinion in urology* 15.6 (2005): 399-403

Jiang, Mingyang, et al. "The efficacy of regular penis-root masturbation, versus Kegel exercise in the treatment of primary premature ejaculation: A quasi-randomised controlled trial." *Andrologia* 52.1 (2020): e13473.

Piediferro, Guido, et al. "Premature ejaculation. 3. Therapy." *Arch Ital Urol Androl* 76.4 (2004): 192-198.

Puppo, Vincenzo, and Giulia Puppo. "Comprehensive review of the anatomy and physiology of male ejaculation: Premature ejaculation is not a disease." *Clinical anatomy* 29.1 (2016): 111-119.

Serefoglu, Ege C., and Theodore R. Saitz. "New insights on premature ejaculation: a review of definition, classification, prevalence and treatment." *Asian journal of andrology* 14.6 (2012): 822.

Waldinger, Marcel D. "Premature ejaculation: different pathophysiologies and etiologies determine its treatment." *Journal of sex & marital therapy* 34.1 (2007): 1-13.

Premenstrual Syndrome (PMS)

Doyle, Caroline, Holly A. Swain Ewald, and Paul W. Ewald. "Premenstrual syndrome: an evolutionary perspective on its causes and treatment." *Perspectives in biology and medicine* 50.2 (2007): 181-202.

Hofmeister, Sabrina, and Seth Bodden. "Premenstrual syndrome and premenstrual dysphoric disorder." *American family physician* 94.3 (2016): 236-240.

Milewicz, Andrzej, and Diana Jedrzejuk. "Premenstrual syndrome: from etiology to treatment." *Maturitas* 55 (2006): S47-S54.

O'Brien, P. M. "Helping women with premenstrual syndrome." *BMJ: British Medical Journal* 307.6917 (1993): 1471.

Roemheld-Hamm, Beatrix. "Chasteberry." *American family physician* 72.5 (2005): 821-824.

Yonkers, Kimberly Ann, PM Shaughn O'Brien, and Elias Eriksson. "Premenstrual syndrome." *The Lancet* 371.9619 (2008): 1200-1210

Prostate Cancer

Chen, Fang-zhi, and Xiao-kun Zhao. "Prostate cancer: current treatment and prevention strategies." *Iranian Red Crescent Medical Journal* 15.4 (2013): 279.

Dunn, Mary Weinstein, and Meredith Wallace Kazer. "Prostate cancer overview." *Seminars in oncology nursing*. Vol. 27. No. 4. WB Saunders, 2011.

Evans, Andrew J. "Treatment effects in prostate cancer." *Modern Pathology* 31 (2018): 110-121.

Litwin, Mark S., and Hung-Jui Tan. "The diagnosis and treatment of prostate cancer: a review." *Jama* 317.24 (2017): 2532-2542

Naitoh, John, Rebecca L. Zeiner, and Jean B. Dekernion. "Diagnosis and treatment of prostate cancer." *American Family Physician* 57.7 (1998): 1531-1539.

Prostate Problems

Ballentine Carter, H., and Donald S. Coffey. "The prostate: an increasing medical problem." *The prostate* 16.1 (1990): 39-48.

Campbell, Joseph D. "Minerals and disease." *Journal of Orthomolecular Medicine* 10 (1995): 177-188.

Rous, Stephen N. *The Prostate Book: Sound advice on symptoms and treatment.* WW Norton & Company, 2002.

Stensvold, Andreas, et al. "Bother problems in prostate cancer patients after curative treatment." *Urologic Oncology: Seminars and Original Investigations*. Vol. 31. No. 7. Elsevier, 2013.

Psoriasis

Duchnik, Ewa, et al. "The impact of diet and physical activity on psoriasis: a narrative review of the current evidence." *Nutrients* 15.4 (2023): 840.

Greaves, Malcolm W., and Gerald D. Weinstein. "Treatment of psoriasis." *New England Journal of Medicine* 332.9 (1995): 581-589.

Peters, Bryan P., Fred G. Weissman, and Mark A. Gill. "Pathophysiology and treatment of psoriasis." *American journal of health-system pharmacy* 57.7 (2000): 645-659

Raharja, Antony, Satveer K. Mahil, and Jonathan N. Barker. "Psoriasis: a brief overview." *Clinical Medicine* 21.3 (2021): 170.

Rendon, Adriana, and Knut Schäkel. "Psoriasis pathogenesis and treatment." *International journal of molecular sciences* 20.6 (2019): 1475.

Rousset, Laurie, and Bruno Halioua. "Stress and psoriasis." *International journal of dermatology* 57.10 (2018): 1165-1172.

Vora, Rita V., et al. "Diet in dermatology: a review." *Egyptian Journal of Dermatology and Venerology* 40.2 (2020): 69-75.

Zangeneh, F. Z., and F. S. Shooshtary. "Psoriasis—types, causes and medication." *Psoriasis-Types, Causes and Medication.* IntechOpen, 2013.

Rashes

Arif, H., et al. "Comparison and predictors of rash associated with 15 antiepileptic drugs." *Neurology* 68.20 (2007): 1701-1709.

Burke, Peter, and Howard I. Maibach. "Jewelry: nickel and metal-based allergic contact dermatitis." *Challenging Cases in Allergic and Immunologic Diseases of the Skin* (2010): 153-168.

Chen, Zhi-Qiang, et al. "Chinese herbal medicine for epidermal growth factor receptor inhibitor-induced skin rash in patients with malignancy: An updated meta-analysis of 23 randomized controlled trials." *Complementary Therapies in Medicine* 47 (2019): 102167.

Ernst, Edzard. "Adverse effects of herbal drugs in dermatology." *British Journal of Dermatology* 143.5 (2000): 923-929.

Hyson, Chris, and Mark Sadler. "Cross sensitivity of skin rashes with antiepileptic drugs." *Canadian journal of neurological sciences* 24.3 (1997): 245-249.

Raynaud's Phenomenon

Coffman, J. D. "Raynaud's phenomenon. An update." *Hypertension* 17.5 (1991): 593-602.

Goundry, Beth, et al. "Diagnosis and management of Raynaud's phenomenon." *Bmj* 344 (2012).

Herrick, Ariane L. "The pathogenesis, diagnosis and treatment of Raynaud phenomenon." *Nature Reviews Rheumatology* 8.8 (2012): 469-479

Hughes, Michael, and Ariane L. Herrick. "Raynaud's phenomenon." *Best Practice & Research Clinical Rheumatology* 30.1 (2016): 112-132

Pope, Janet E. "The diagnosis and treatment of Raynaud's phenomenon: a practical approach." *Drugs* 67 (2007): 517-525.

Repetitive Strain Injury (RSI)

Lau, Roy Yuen Chi, Gabriel Yin Fat Ng, and Chi Keung Yeung. "Healing and Prophylactic Efficacies of Topical Composite Herbal Medication on Overuse-induced Achilles Tendinosis." *Biomedical Journal of Scientific & Technical Research* 42.1 (2022): 33343-33349.

McDermott, Francis T. "Repetition strain injury: a review of current understanding." *Medical journal of Australia* 144.4 (1986): 196-200.

Naiker, Ashok. "Repetitive Strain Injuries (RSI)-an ayurvedic approach." *Journal of Ayurveda and Integrated Medical Sciences* 2.02 (2017): 170-173.

Nainzadeh, Nahid, et al. "Repetitive strain injury (cumulative trauma disorder)." *The Mount Sinai journal of medicine* 66.3 (1999).

O'Neil, Barbara A., Michael E. Forsythe, and William D. Stanish. "Chronic occupational repetitive strain injury." *Canadian Family Physician* 47.2 (2001): 311-316.

Van Tulder, Maurits, Antti Malmivaara, and Bart Koes. "Repetitive strain injury." *The Lancet* 369.9575 (2007): 1815-1822

Restless Legs Syndrome

Allen, Richard P., and Christopher J. Earley. "The role of iron in restless legs syndrome." *Movement disorders: official journal of the Movement Disorder Society* 22.S18 (2007): S440-S448.

Earley, Christopher J., and Michael H. Silber. "Restless legs syndrome: understanding its consequences and the need for better treatment." *Sleep medicine* 11.9 (2010): 807-815.

Ekbom, Karl, and J. Ulfberg. "Restless legs syndrome." *Journal of internal medicine* 266.5 (2009): 419-431.

Gossard, Thomas R., et al. "Restless legs syndrome: contemporary diagnosis and treatment." *Neurotherapeutics* 18.1 (2021): 140-155.

Manconi, Mauro, et al. "Restless legs syndrome." *Nature reviews Disease primers* 7.1 (2021): 80.

Trenkwalder, Claudia, Walter Paulus, and Arthur S. Walters. "The restless legs syndrome." *The lancet neurology* 4.8 (2005): 465-475.

Road Rage

Ayar, Alexander A. "Road Rage: Recognizing a psychological disorder." *The journal of psychiatry & law* 34.2 (2006): 123-150.

Bjureberg, Johan, and James J. Gross. "Regulating road rage." *Social and personality psychology compass* 15.3 (2021): e12586.

Galovski, Tara E., and Edward B. Blanchard. "Road rage: a domain for psychological intervention?." *Aggression and Violent Behavior* 9.2 (2004): 105-127

Wickens, Christine M., et al. "Road rage." *Forensic Psychiatry*. CRC Press, 2017. 297-300.

Rosacea

Cohen, Aaron F., and Jeffrey D. Tiemstra. "Diagnosis and treatment of rosacea." *The Journal of the American Board of Family Practice* 15.3 (2002): 214-217.

Gupta, A. K., and M. M. Chaudhry. "Rosacea and its management: an overview." *Journal of the European Academy of Dermatology and Venereology* 19.3 (2005): 273-285.

Scheinfeld, Noah, and Thomas Berk. "A review of the diagnosis and treatment of rosacea." *Postgraduate Medicine* 122.1 (2010): 139-143

Wilkin, Jonathan K. "Rosacea: pathophysiology and treatment." *Archives of dermatology* 130.3 (1994): 359-362.

Scarring

Baker, Richard, et al. "Cutaneous scarring: a clinical review." *Dermatology Research and Practice* 2009.1 (2009): 625376.

Hameedi, Sophia G., Angela Saulsbery, and Oluyinka O. Olutoye. "The Pathophysiology and Management of Pathologic Scarring—a Contemporary Review." *Advances in Wound Care* (2024).

Potter, Daniel A., David Veitch, and Graham A. Johnston. "Scarring and wound healing." *British Journal of Hospital Medicine* 80.11 (2019): C166-C171

Roseborough, Ingrid E., Mark A. Grevious, and Raphael C. Lee. "Prevention and treatment of excessive dermal scarring." *Journal of the National Medical Association* 96.1 (2004): 108.

Sciatica

Hakelius, Anders. "Prognosis in sciatica: a clinical follow-up of surgical and non-surgical treatment." *Acta Orthopaedica Scandinavica* 41.sup129 (1970): 1-76.

Hurst, Arthur. "The Treatment of Sciatica." *British Medical Journal* 2.4328 (1943): 773.

Kumar, Manish, et al. "Epidemiology, pathophysiology and symptomatic treatment of sciatica: a review." *Int J Pharm Biol Arch* 2.4 (2011): 1050-1061.

Valat, Jean-Pierre, et al. "Sciatica." *Best practice & research Clinical rheumatology* 24.2 (2010): 241-252.

Vroomen, Patrick CAJ, et al. "Conservative treatment of sciatica: a systematic review." *Clinical Spine Surgery* 13.6 (2000): 463-469.

Seasonal Affect Disorder (SAD)

Howland, Robert H. "An overview of seasonal affective disorder and its treatment options." *The Physician and sportsmedicine* 37.4 (2009): 104-115

Magnusson, Andres, and Diane Boivin. "Seasonal affective disorder: an overview." *Chronobiology international* 20.2 (2003): 189-207.

Melrose, Sherri. "Seasonal affective disorder: an overview of assessment and treatment approaches." *Depression research and treatment* 2015.1 (2015): 178564.

Miller, Alan L. "Epidemiology, etiology, and natural treatment of seasonal affective disorder." *Alternative medicine review* 10.1 (2005).

Partonen, Timo, and Jouko Lönnqvist. "Seasonal affective disorder." *The Lancet* 352.9137 (1998): 1369-1374.

Peiser, Benny. "Seasonal affective disorder and exercise treatment: a review." *Biological Rhythm Research* 40.1 (2009): 85-97

Westrin, Åsa, and Raymond W. Lam. "Seasonal affective disorder: a clinical update." *Annals of Clinical Psychiatry* 19.4 (2007): 239-246.

Zauderer, Cheryl, and C. Anne Ganzer. "Seasonal affective disorder: an overview." *Mental Health Practice* 18.9 (2015).

Shingles

Engler, Deirdre, Mncengeli Sibanda, and H. J. Motubatse. "Shingles." *SA Pharmaceutical Journal* 84.6 (2017): 60-64

Johnson, Robert W., and Tessa L. Whitton. "Management of herpes zoster (shingles) and postherpetic neuralgia." *Expert opinion on pharmacotherapy* 5.3 (2004): 551-559

Nazarko, Linda. "Diagnosis, treatment and prevention of shingles: the role of the healthcare assistant." *British Journal of Healthcare Assistants* 13.1 (2019): 20-25.

Peate, Ian. "Preventing shingles: symptoms, treatment and management." *British Journal of Healthcare Assistants* 4.3 (2010): 120-123

Shin Splints

Batt, Mark E. "Shin splints—a review of terminology." *Clinical journal of sport medicine* 5.1 (1995): 53-57.

Kues, Janet. "Literature review: The pathology of shin splints." *Journal of Orthopaedic & Sports Physical Therapy* 12.3 (1990): 115-121.

Moore, Michael P. "Shin splints: diagnosis, management, prevention." *Postgraduate medicine* 83.1 (1988): 199-210.

Ugalde, Viviane, Mark E. Batt, and M. B. B. Chir. "Shin splints: current theories and treatment." *Critical Reviews™ in Physical and Rehabilitation Medicine* 13.2-3 (2001).

Wilder, Robert P., and Shikha Sethi. "Overuse injuries: tendinopathies, stress fractures, compartment syndrome, and shin splints." *Clinics in sports medicine* 23.1 (2004): 55-81.

Sinusitis

Baguley, Campbell J., et al. "Silastic splints reduce middle meatal adhesions after endoscopic sinus surgery." *American Journal of Rhinology & Allergy* 26.5 (2012): 414-417.

Kim, Hyo Young, et al. "The usefulness of nasal packing with vaseline gauze and airway silicone splint after closed reduction of nasal bone fracture." *Archives of plastic surgery* 39.06 (2012): 612-617.

Siqueira Jr, Jose F., et al. "Effects of endodontic infections on the maxillary sinus: a case series of treatment outcome." *Journal of Endodontics* 47.7 (2021): 1166-1176

Snoring

Dzieciolowska-Baran, E., A. Gawlikowska-Sroka, and F. Czerwinski. "Snoring-the role of the laryngologist in diagnosing and treating its causes." *European Journal of Medical Research* 14.Suppl 4 (2009): 67.

Fairbanks, David NF, Samuel A. Mickelson, and B. Tucker Woodson, eds. *Snoring and obstructive sleep apnea.* Lippincott Williams & Wilkins, 2003.

Robin, Ian G. "Snoring." (1948): 151-153.

Vlastos, Ioannis M., and John K. Hajiioannou. "Clinical practice: diagnosis and treatment of childhood snoring." *European journal of pediatrics* 169.3 (2010): 261-267.

Yaremchuk, Kathleen. "Why and when to treat snoring." *Otolaryngologic Clinics of North America* 53.3 (2020): 351-365.

Sore Throat

Angotoeva, I. B., and I. A. Mush'yan. "Sore throat and its causes." *Rossiiskaya otorinolaringologiya* 18.3 (2019): 17-21.

Coutinho, Graça, et al. "Worldwide comparison of treatment guidelines for sore throat." *International Journal of Clinical Practice* 75.5 (2021): e13879.

Krüger, Karen, et al. "Sore Throat." *Deutsches Ärzteblatt International* 118.11 (2021): 188.

McHardy, F. E., and F. Chung. "Postoperative sore throat: cause, prevention and treatment." *Anaesthesia* 54.5 (1999): 444-453.

Tanz, Robert R. "Sore throat." *Nelson pediatric symptom-based diagnosis* (2018): 1.

Sprains and Strains

Altizer, Linda. "Strains and sprains." *Orthopaedic Nursing* 22.6 (2003): 404-409.

Braund, Rhiannon, and J. Haxby Abbott. "Analgesic recommendations when treating musculoskeletal sprains and strains." *New Zealand Journal of Physiotherapy* 35.2 (2007).

Buka, Alfred J. "Strains and sprains." *The American Journal of Surgery* 12.2 (1931): 290-293.

Elmslie, R. C. "The treatment of joint sprains and strains." *British Medical Journal* 1.4026 (1938): 527.

Garrett Jr, William E. "Strains and sprains in athletes." *Postgraduate Medicine* 73.3 (1983): 200-209

Stress

Davis, Douglas A., et al. "Force-induced activation of covalent bonds in mechanoresponsive polymeric materials." *Nature* 459.7243 (2009): 68-72.

Everly Jr, George S., and Robert Rosenfeld. *The nature and treatment of the stress response: A practical guide for clinicians.* Springer Science & Business Media, 2012.

Kaiser, Simon, et al. "Stress relaxation and thermally adaptable properties in vitrimer-like elastomers from HXNBR rubber with covalent bonds." *Soft Matter* 15.30 (2019): 6062-6072.

Konturek, Peter C., Thomas Brzozowski, and Stanisław Jan Konturek. "Stress and the gut: pathophysiology, clinical consequences, diagnostic approach and treatment options." *J Physiol Pharmacol* 62.6 (2011): 591-9.

Surwit, Richard S., and Mark S. Schneider. "Role of stress in the etiology and treatment of diabetes mellitus." *Psychosomatic medicine* 55.4 (1993): 380-393.

Wolkowitz, Owen M., Elissa S. Epel, and Victor I. Reus. "Stress hormone-related psychopathology: pathophysiological and treatment implications." *The World Journal of Biological Psychiatry* 2.3 (2001): 115-143.

Yuen, Eunice Y., et al. "Repeated stress causes cognitive impairment by suppressing glutamate receptor expression and function in prefrontal cortex." *Neuron* 73.5 (2012): 962-977

Stroke

Fugate, Jennifer E., et al. "Infectious causes of stroke." *The Lancet Infectious Diseases* 14.9 (2014): 869-880.

Koroshetz, Walter J., and Michael A. Moskowitz. "Emerging treatments for stroke in humans." *Trends in pharmacological sciences* 17.6 (1996): 227-233.

Markus, Hugh. "Stroke: causes and clinical features." *Medicine* 36.11 (2008): 586-591.

Marsh, James D., and Salah G. Keyrouz. "Stroke prevention and treatment." *Journal of the American College of Cardiology* 56.9 (2010): 683-691.

Matchar, David B., et al. "Medical treatment for stroke prevention." *Annals of internal medicine* 121.1 (1994): 41-53.

Murphy, Stephen JX, and David J. Werring. "Stroke: causes and clinical features." *Medicine* 48.9 (2020): 561-566.

Wajngarten, Mauricio, and Gisele Sampaio Silva. "Hypertension and stroke: update on treatment." *European Cardiology Review* 14.2 (2019): 111.

Sunburn

Danno, Kiichiro, and Takeshi Horio. "Sunburn cell: factors involved in its formation." *Photochemistry and photobiology* 45.5 (1987): 683-690.

Deloughery, Michael N. "Sunburn Prevention and Treatment." *The Nurse Practitioner* 6.3 (1981): 28-30.

Han, Amy, and Howard I. Maibach. "Management of acute sunburn." *American journal of clinical dermatology* 5 (2004): 39-47.

Kaplan, Lee A. "Suntan, sunburn, and sun protection." *Journal of Wilderness Medicine* 3.2 (1992): 173-196.

Land, Victoria, and Leigh Small. "The evidence on how to best treat sunburn in children: A common treatment dilemma." *Pediatric Nursing* 34.4 (2008): 343.

Tachycardia

Amatruda, John M., et al. "Vigorous supplementation of a hypocaloric diet prevents cardiac arrhythmias and mineral depletion." *The American Journal of Medicine* 74.6 (1983): 1016-1022.

Houston, Mark C. "The role of nutrition, nutraceuticals, vitamins, antioxidants, and minerals in the prevention and treatment of hypertension." *Alternative therapies in health and medicine* 19 (2013): 32.

Jeong, Young-Hoon, et al. "Diagnostic approach and treatment strategy in tachycardia-induced cardiomyopathy." *Clinical Cardiology: An International Indexed and Peer-Reviewed Journal for Advances in the Treatment of Cardiovascular Disease* 31.4 (2008): 172-178.

Lerman, Bruce B. "Mechanism, diagnosis, and treatment of outflow tract tachycardia." *Nature Reviews Cardiology* 12.10 (2015): 597-608.

Link, Mark S. "Evaluation and initial treatment of supraventricular tachycardia." *New England Journal of Medicine* 367.15 (2012): 1438-1448.

McSwords, Kayla M. *Registered Dietitian Nutritionists' Knowledge, Education, Impressions, and Utilization of Treatments Regarding Postural Orthostatic Tachycardia Syndrome.* MS thesis. Kent State University, 2023.

Trappe, H-J. "Diagnosis and treatment of tachycardias." *Yearbook of Intensive Care and Emergency Medicine 2000*. Berlin, Heidelberg: Springer Berlin Heidelberg, 2000. 638-648.

Teething

Canto, Fernanda Michel Tavares, et al. "Efficacy of treatments used to relieve signs and symptoms associated with teething: a systematic review." *Brazilian Oral Research* 36 (2022): e066.

Markman, Lisa. "Teething: facts and fiction." *Pediatrics in Review* 30.8 (2009): e59-e64.

McIntyre, G. T., and G. M. McIntyre. "Teething troubles?." *British dental journal* 192.5 (2002): 251-255.

Obiajuru, Ifeanyi OC, et al. "Teething problems and the influence of microbial infections." *of* 6 (2017): 2.

Pereira, Thais Salles, et al. "Parental beliefs in and attitudes toward teething signs and symptoms: A systematic review." *International Journal of Paediatric Dentistry* 33.6 (2023): 577-584

Sood, Sankalp, and Mangla Sood. "Teething: myths and facts." *Journal of Clinical Pediatric Dentistry* 35.1 (2010): 9-13.

Temporomandibular Discomfort

Gauer, Robert L., and Michael J. Semidey. "Diagnosis and treatment of temporomandibular disorders." *American family physician* 91.6 (2015): 378-386.

Karkazi, Frantzeska, and Fulya Özdemir. "Temporomandibular disorders: fundamental questions and answers." *Turkish journal of orthodontics* 33.4 (2020): 246.

Liu, Frederick, and Andrew Steinkeler. "Epidemiology, diagnosis, and treatment of temporomandibular disorders." *Dental Clinics* 57.3 (2013): 465-479.

Michelotti, Ambrosina, and G. Iodice. "The role of orthodontics in temporomandibular disorders." *Journal of oral rehabilitation* 37.6 (2010): 411-429.

Zotelli, Vera LR, et al. "Acupuncture effect on pain, mouth opening limitation and on the energy meridians in patients with temporomandibular dysfunction: a randomized controlled trial." *Journal of acupuncture and meridian studies* 10.5 (2017): 351-359.

Tendonitis

Federer, Andrew E., et al. "Tendonitis and tendinopathy: what are they and how do they evolve?." *Foot and ankle clinics* 22.4 (2017): 665-676.

Hess, Gregory P., et al. "Prevention and treatment of overuse tendon injuries." *Sports medicine* 8 (1989): 371-384.

Kannus, P. "Etiology and pathophysiology of chronic tendon disorders in sports." *Scandinavian journal of medicine & science in sports* 7.2 (1997): 78-85.

Wilson, John J., and Thomas M. Best. "Common overuse tendon problems: a review and recommendations for treatment." *American family physician* 72.5 (2005): 811-818.

Thyroid Issues

Faber, Jens, and Christian Selmer. "Cardiovascular disease and thyroid function." *Cardiovascular Issues in Endocrinology.* Vol. 43. Karger Publishers, 2014. 45-56

Johnson, Cheri A. "Thyroid issues in reproduction." *Clinical techniques in small animal practice* 17.3 (2002): 129-132.

Suter, Paolo M. "The B-vitamins." *Essential and toxic trace elements and vitamins in human health.* Academic Press, 2020. 217-239.

Zhang, Li Rita, et al. "Vitamin and mineral supplements and thyroid cancer: a systematic review." *European journal of cancer prevention* 22.2 (2013): 158-168.

Tinnitus

Dalrymple, Sarah N., Sarah H. Lewis, and Samantha Philman. "Tinnitus: diagnosis and management." *American family physician* 103.11 (2021): 663-671.

Han, Byung In, et al. "Tinnitus: characteristics, causes, mechanisms, and treatments." *Journal of clinical neurology (Seoul, Korea)* 5.1 (2009): 11.

Langguth, Berthold, et al. "Tinnitus: causes and clinical management." *The Lancet Neurology* 12.9 (2013): 920-930.

Levine, Robert Aaron. "Tinnitus: diagnostic approach leading to treatment." *Seminars in neurology.* Vol. 33. No. 03. Thieme Medical Publishers, 2013

Luxon, Linda M. "Tinnitus: its causes, diagnosis, and treatment." *BMJ: British Medical Journal* 306.6891 (1993): 1490

Minen, Mia T., et al. "The neuropsychiatry of tinnitus: a circuit-based approach to the causes and treatments available." *Journal of Neurology, Neurosurgery & Psychiatry* 85.10 (2014): 1138-1144.

Young, Robert O., and Shelley Redford Young. *The pH Miracle: Balance your Diet, reclaim your health.* Hachette UK, 2008.

Toothache

Coleman, Michelle. *Oil Pulling Revolution: The Natural Approach to Dental Care, Whole-Body Detoxification and Disease Prevention.* Ulysses Press, 2015.

De Laat, Antoon. "Differential diagnosis of toothache to prevent erroneous and unnecessary dental treatment." *Journal of Oral Rehabilitation* 47.6 (2020): 775-781.

Fife, Bruce. *Oil pulling therapy: detoxifying and healing the body through oral cleansing.* Piccadilly Books, Ltd., 2017.

Frohn, Birgit. *The Oil Pulling Miracle: Detoxify Simply and Effectively.* Simon and Schuster, 2015.

Spencer, Christopher J., et al. "Toothache or trigeminal neuralgia: treatment dilemmas." *The Journal of Pain* 9.9 (2008): 767-770.

Telgote, Anjali, and Prachi Udapurkar. "An Overview Treatment and Prevention of Toothache." *Journal of Drug Delivery and Biotherapeutics* 1.01 (2024): 120-130.

Yatani, H., et al. "Systematic review and recommendations for nonodontogenic toothache." *Journal of oral rehabilitation* 41.11 (2014): 843-852.

Tooth Decay

Benson, Philip E., et al. "Fluorides for the prevention of early tooth decay (demineralised white lesions) during fixed brace treatment." *Cochrane Database of Systematic Reviews* 12 (2013).

Çolak, Hakan, et al. «Early childhood caries update: A review of causes, diagnoses, and treatments.» *Journal of natural science, biology, and medicine* 4.1 (2013): 29.

Dash, Tapas Ranjan, et al. "Role of medicinal herbs in oral health management." *J. Int. Dent. Med. Res* 1 (2014): 113-119.

Diesendorf, Mark. "The mystery of declining tooth decay." *Nature* 322.6075 (1986): 125-129.

Nagel, Rami. "The cause, prevention, and treatment of early childhood tooth decay." *Townsend Letter: The Examiner of Alternative Medicine* 280 (2006): 99-104.

Wilson, Michael, et al. "Tooth decay." *Close Encounters of the Microbial Kind: Everything You Need to Know About Common Infections* (2021): 273-291.

Tooth Grinding

Bashir, Arwah, et al. "All about bruxism-the teeth grinding." *Journal of Advanced Medical and Dental Sciences Research* 9.5 (2021): 9-23

Saboowala, Hakim, ed. ""Bruxism"(Teeth Grinding or Clenching): Causes, Symptoms, Diagnosis & Management. An Overview." (2020).

Wieckiewicz, Mieszko, Anna Paradowska-Stolarz, and Wlodzimierz Wieckiewicz. "Psychosocial aspects of bruxism: the most paramount factor influencing teeth grinding." *BioMed Research International* 2014.1 (2014): 469187.

Zlatanovska, Katerina, et al. "Bruxism-teeth grinding." *Knowledge-International Journal, Scientific and Applicative Papers* 20.4 (2017): 1719-1723.

Tooth Sensitivity

Clark, Danielle, and Liran Levin. "Non-surgical management of tooth hypersensitivity." *International dental journal* 66.5 (2016): 249-256.

Gillam, D. G., and R. Orchardson. "Advances in the treatment of root dentine sensitivity: mechanisms and treatment principles." *Endodontic Topics* 13.1 (2006): 13-33.

Markowitz, K., and David Henry Pashley. "Discovering new treatments for sensitive teeth: the long path from biology to therapy." *Journal of oral rehabilitation* 35.4 (2008): 300-315.

Panda, Akshyata, et al. "Herbal Agents for Dentinal Hypersensitivity: A Review." *Indian Journal of Public Health Research & Development* 10.11 (2019)

Porto, Isabel CCM, Ana KM Andrade, and Marcos AJR Montes. "Diagnosis and treatment of dentinal hypersensitivity." *Journal of oral science* 51.3 (2009): 323-332.

Tooth Stains

Alazmah, Abdulfatah. "Primary teeth stains and discoloration: a review." *Journal of Child Science* 11.01 (2021): e20-e27.

Hattab, Faiez N., Muawia A. Qudeimat, and HALA S. AL-RIMAWI. "Dental discoloration: an overview." *Journal of Esthetic and Restorative Dentistry* 11.6 (1999): 291-310.

Kapadia, Yash, and Vinay Jain. "Tooth staining: A review of etiology and treatment modalities." *Acta Sci Dent Sci* 2.6 (2018): 67-70.

Noorsaeed, Ashwag Siddik, et al. "Causes and management of tooth discoloration: A Review." *Journal of Pharmaceutical Research International* 33.60B (2021): 969-976.

Rodríguez-Martínez, Jorge, Manuel Valiente, and María-Jesús Sánchez-Martín. "Tooth whitening: From the established treatments to novel approaches to prevent side effects." *Journal of Esthetic and Restorative Dentistry* 31.5 (2019): 431-440.

Volovitz, Benjamin, et al. "Absence of tooth staining with doxycycline treatment in young children." *Clinical pediatrics* 46.2 (2007): 121-126.

Ulcers

Busch, Ch, I. Aschermann, and Ch D. Mnich. "Treatment of chronic ulcers." *Phlebologie* 46.01 (2017): 13-18.

Collins, Lauren, and Samina Seraj. "Diagnosis and treatment of venous ulcers." *American family physician* 81.8 (2010): 989-996.

Mekkes, JR1, et al. "Causes, investigation and treatment of leg ulceration." *British Journal of dermatology* 148.3 (2003): 388-401.

Satoh, Hiroshi. "Role of dietary fiber in formation and prevention of small intestinal ulcers induced by nonsteroidal anti-inflammatory drug." *Current pharmaceutical design* 16.10 (2010): 1209-1213.

Spriggs, Edmund J. "Chronic ulceration of the colon." *QJM: An International Journal of Medicine* 3.4 (1934): 549-550.

Urinary Tract Infection (UTI)

Barnett, Ben J., and David S. Stephens. "Urinary tract infection: an overview." *The American journal of the medical sciences* 314.4 (1997): 245-249.

Flores-Mireles, Ana L., et al. "Urinary tract infections: epidemiology, mechanisms of infection and treatment options." *Nature reviews microbiology* 13.5 (2015): 269-284.

Komala, M., and KP Sampath Kumar. "Urinary tract infection: causes, symptoms, diagnosis and it's management." *Indian Journal of Research in Pharmacy and Biotechnology* 1.2 (2013): 226.

Lee, Jasmine BL, and Guy H. Neild. "Urinary tract infection." *Medicine* 35.8 (2007): 423-428.

Sheerin, Neil S. "Urinary tract infection." *Medicine* 39.7 (2011): 384-389.

Vaginitis (and Yeast) Infection

Hainer, Barry L., and Maria V. Gibson. "Vaginitis: diagnosis and treatment." *American family physician* 83.7 (2011): 807-815.

Hay, Roderick J. "Yeast infections." *Dermatologic clinics* 14.1 (1996): 113-124.

Kükner, S., et al. "Treatment of vaginitis." *International Journal of Gynecology & Obstetrics* 52.1 (1996): 43-47.

Leclair, Catherine, and Amy Stenson. "Common causes of vaginitis." *JAMA* 327.22 (2022): 2238-2239.

Owen, Marion K., and Timothy L. Clenney. "Management of vaginitis." *American family physician* 70.11 (2004): 2125-2132.

Paladine, Heather L., and Urmi A. Desai. "Vaginitis: diagnosis and treatment." *American family physician* 97.5 (2018): 321-329.

Sobel, Jack D. "Vaginitis." *New England Journal of Medicine* 337.26 (1997): 1896-1903.

Varicose Veins

Campbell, Bruce. "Varicose veins and their management." *Bmj* 333.7562 (2006): 287-292

Ernst, E., T. Saradeth, and K. L. Resch. "Hydrotherapy for varicose veins: a randomized, controlled trial." *Phlebology* 7.4 (1992): 154-157.

Jones, Richard H., and Peter J. Carek. "Management of varicose veins." *American family physician* 78.11 (2008): 1289-1294.

London, Nick JM, and Roddy Nash. "Varicose veins." *Bmj* 320.7246 (2000): 1391-1394.

Raetz, Jaqueline, Megan Wilson, and Kimberly Collins. "Varicose veins: diagnosis and treatment." *American family physician* 99.11 (2019): 682-688.

Subramonia, S., and T. A. Lees. "The treatment of varicose veins." *The Annals of The Royal College of Surgeons of England* 89.2 (2007): 96-100.

Warts

Berman, Brian, and Andrew Weinstein. "Treatment of warts." *Dermatologic Therapy* 13.3 (2000): 290-304.

Dall'Oglio, Federica, et al. "Treatment of cutaneous warts: an evidence-based review." *American journal of clinical dermatology* 13 (2012): 73-96.

Hollis, J. M., et al. "Predicting the water retention characteristics of UK mineral soils." *European Journal of Soil Science* 66.1 (2015): 239-252.

Mulhem, Elie, and Susanna Pinelis. "Treatment of nongenital cutaneous warts." *American family physician* 84.3 (2011): 288-293.

Osborne, Earl D., and Edwin D. Putnam. "The treatment of warts." *Radiology* 16.3 (1931): 340-345.

Plasencia, Jorge M. "Cutaneous warts: diagnosis and treatment." *Primary Care: Clinics in Office Practice* 27.2 (2000): 423-434

Rees, Rees B. "The treatment of warts." *Clinics in Dermatology* 3.4 (1985): 179-184.

Water Retention

Cadnapaphornchai, Melissa A., et al. "Pathophysiology of sodium and water retention in heart failure." *Cardiology* 96.3-4 (2001): 122-131.

Martin, Pierre-Yves, and Robert W. Schrier. "Sodium and water retention in heart failure: pathogenesis and treatment." *Kidney International Supplement* 59 (1997).

Moodley, M., et al. "Effects of a water treatment residue, lime, gypsum, and polyacrylamide on the water retention and hydraulic conductivity of two contrasting soils under field conditions in KwaZulu-Natal, South Africa." *Soil Research* 42.3 (2004): 273-282.

Upadhyay, Srishti, et al. "A Review on Water Retention." *Asian Journal of Pharmaceutical Research and Development* (2017): 1-9.

Zeleňáková, Martina, Daniel Constantin Diaconu, and Ketil Haarstad. "Urban water retention measures." *Procedia engineering* 190 (2017): 419-426.

Weight Retention

Bai, Shiping, et al. "Dietary organic trace minerals level influences eggshell quality and minerals retention in hens." *Annals of Animal Science* 17.2 (2017): 503-515.

Lall, Santosh P. "The minerals." *Fish nutrition*. Academic Press, 2022. 469-554.

Truong, Ha H., et al. "Determining the importance of macro and trace dietary minerals on growth and nutrient retention in juvenile Penaeus monodon." *Animals* 10.11 (2020): 2086.

Van der Klis, J. D., M. W. A. Verstegen, and W. De Wit. "Absorption of minerals and retention time of dry matter in the gastrointestinal tract of broilers." *Poultry Science* 69.12 (1990): 2185-2194.

Yeasmin, Sabina, et al. "Influence of mineral characteristics on the retention of low molecular weight organic compounds: A batch sorption–desorption and ATR-FTIR study." *Journal of colloid and interface science* 432 (2014): 246-257.

Wrinkles

Cortiñas, Fabián E., and Abel Chajchir. "Wrinkles, Etiology, Causes, Treatment, and Prevention." *Plastic and Aesthetic Regenerative Surgery and Fat Grafting: Clinical Application and Operative Techniques*. Cham: Springer International Publishing, 2022. 623-639.

Lee, Jin Young, et al. "Loss of elastic fibers causes skin wrinkles in sun-damaged human skin." *Journal of dermatological science* 50.2 (2008): 99-107

Manríquez, Juan Jorge, Daniela Majerson Gringberg, and Claudia Nicklas Diaz. "Wrinkles." *BMJ clinical evidence* 2008 (2008)

Rona, C., F. Vailati, and E. Berardesca. "The cosmetic treatment of wrinkles." *Journal of cosmetic dermatology* 3.1 (2004): 26-34.

Products and Services

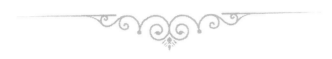

(where to purchase items)

Acupressure

Acupressure Institute

1533 Shattuck Avenue, Berkeley, CA, 94709

www.acupressure.com

This organization can be contacted for audio and video products and body tools used for acupressure.

Jin Shin Do Foundation for Bodymind Acupressure

PO Box 416

Idyllwild, CA, 92549

www.jinshindo.org

This organization provides books, videotapes, audiotapes, acupressure charts, articles, and other materials about Jin Shin Do Bodymind Acupressure.

Affirmations

Brainstickers.com

PO Box 4815

Boise, ID, 83711-4815

www.affirmation.com

Contact this company for information on positive reinforcement stickers for your environment.

Castlegate Publishers

25597 Drake Road, Barrington, IL, 60010

www.midpointtrade.com/castlegate_publishers.htm

This company publishes Spontaneous Optimism: Proven Strategies for Health, Prosperity, and Happiness by Maryann Troiani, Ph.D.

Aromatherapy

Aroma Land

www.buyaromatherapy.com

This website sells oils, blends, and aromatherapy products. They provide a money-back guarantee on all items.

Aroma-Vera

5310 Beethoven Street, Los Angeles, CA, 90066

This company offers essential oils, a large variety of aromatic soaps, candles, bath and massage oils, and hair and skin care products. You can also order a free catalog from the address above.

Dhyana Education and Rejuvenation Centre

6871 Covey Road, Forestville, CA, 95436

www.aromaveda.com

This clinic, educational center and mail-order company offers aromatherapy oils.

Leydet Aromatics

PO Box 2354

Fair Oaks, CA, 95628

This company offers one of the largest selections of essential oils in the USA. Contact the address above for more information in a self-addressed envelope.

Santa Fe Botanical Fragrances

PO Box 282, Santa Fe, NM, 87504

This company carries approximately 75 essential oils. Request a free catalog from the address above.

Breathwork Therapy

Authentic Breathing Resources

PO Box 31376

San Francisco, CA, 94131

www.authentic-breathing.com

This organization offers books, articles, and tapes about therapeutic breathing.

The International Breath Institute

5921 East Miramar Drive, Tucson, AZ, 85715

Write this organization for information on tapes, books, and breathing enhancement products.

Optimal Breathing

PO Box 1551

Waynesville, NC, 28786

www.breathing.com

This organization provides education services, and products for learning breathing techniques that enhance health, performance, and longevity.

Coaching, Guidance, and Consulting

Corey Baker

Business: Kemetic Soul

Address: 7754 Okeechobee Boulevard-932

West Palm Beach, FL 33411

United States

https://www.kemeticsoul.com/

Kemetic Soul, founded by Corey Baker, is a health and wellness business inspired by Sebian Doctrine and the principles of Alternative Naturopathic Health. Located in Palm Beach, Florida, Kemetic Soul offers a range of services and products aimed at holistic well-being, drawing from ancient Kemetic teachings to promote balance and peace within the soul. The business is known for its commitment to helping individuals achieve a harmonious state of health through super-botanical algae known as Irish-moss, natural and spiritual methodologies.

Kemetic Soul provides a unique blend of services that incorporate ancient Kemetic teachings with modern naturopathic practices. One of their standout offerings is the Kemetic Power Station Group Sessions, which are designed to harmonize and recharge the body's energy systems using high-frequency subtle energies. This service, along with others, reflects the company's dedication to fostering spiritual and physical well-being through alternative health methodologies.

Regina Gower

404-615-2315

www.reginaangelina.com

Regina helps people manage their Neurodiversity naturally so they can enjoy a thriving business. This includes, but not limited to: ADHD, autism, high sensitivity, etc.

P. Gibbs LES, MAHS MFT

Business: Better You, Better Us Life Coaching Services

https://betteryoubetterus.com

This business provides individual coaching and free group sessions. They teach skills and concepts to help reduce stress, depression, and anxiety symptoms while strengthening relationships and enhancing effective communication.

Sierra Grana

sierragrana.com

abridgethatmatters.com

@sierragranacoaching

@abridgethat matters

This business provides the following services:

Sierra Grana Coaching – Transformational Life and Business Coaching, and Energy Clearings

A Bridge That Matters – Global Collaborative Networking and resources.

Susan Marco

14 Church Street, Little Silver, NJ, 07739

https://susanmarco.com

https://www.facebook.com/susan.marco.3

This business provides: helping others empower themselves to step into their true selves by releasing old, outdated programming (emotions, beliefs, and thought forms).

Dental Care

Boston Dental

Boston, MA (Seaport District: 22 Boston Wharf Road; Downtown Crossing: 36 Chauncey Street; Government Center: 35 Court Street)

www.bostondental.com

We provide the highest quality, comprehensive dental and aesthetic services – preventative, restorative, and cosmetic dentistry for adults and children alike. You should look forward to visiting the dentist the same way that you look forward to getting a facial or massage – an experience centered around you.

Purely White Teeth

Owner: Markeisha Kelley

999 Broadway St, Saugus, Massachusetts 01906

https://purelywhiteteeth.as.me/schedule.php

This business provides self-care through teeth-whitening services and tooth gems.

Energy Healing

American Polarity Therapy Association

PO Box 19858

Boulder, CO, 80308

www.polaritytherapy.org

This organization offers audiotapes, CDs, videos, and charts about practicing breathwork. You may send a request for product information.

Barbara Brennan School of Healing

500 Spanish River Boulevard, Suite 103, Boca Raton, FL, 33481-4559

www.barbarabrennan.com

This site offers books and audiotapes on energy healing by Barbara Brennan.

Quantum-Touch

PO Box 852

Santa Cruz, CA, 95061

www.quantumtouch.com

This organization offers books and tapes by Richard Gordon, the creator of this technique.

Erotic

Nude Entanglements

Owner: Shataya Pope

50 South Common Street #203 Lynn, MA, 01902

Nudeentanglements.com

Women's online clothing boutique

Exercise/Movement

The Aston Training Center

PO Box 3568

Incline Village, NV, 89450

www.aston-patterning.com

You can visit their website or write a letter to the address above for information on offerings such as articles, videos, and ergonomic products.

Feldenkrais Guild of North America

3611 Southwest Hood Avenue, Suite 100, Portland, OR, 97201

www.feldenkrais.com

This company provides video and audio educational materials for children.

Robin Cotter

Body Rock Fitness By Robin

96 Swampscott Rd, Salem MA. 01970

Cardio Kickboxing & Boxing Classes

Eye Health

Danny Velasquez

Webster Square Vision Center

Address: 120 Stafford St Worcester MA 01602

https://Webstersqvision.com

We are a full-service optical store, providing adjustments, repairs, measurements, frames, lenses, contacts and Vision exams with an on-premises O.D. at all times.

Flower Essences

Flower Essence Services

PO Box 1769

Nevada City, CA, 95959

www.floweressence.com

This organization sells flower essence products, books, audiotapes, and videotapes.

Nelson Bach USA Ltd

100 Research Drive, Wilmington, MA, 91887

www.nelsonbach.com

This company sells flower essences online or through the mail.

Hair Care

Ryan McCauley

Ryan's Fade Factory

Address: Mobile Barber

Facebook: @Ryan'sfadefactory

For booking and portfolio: ryansfadefactory.booksy.com

Herbal and Holistic Medicine

4everevolvn Holistic Health

Owner: Renoda Burns

4everevolvn.com

We specialize in alternative medicine. Herbal remedies. Cold pressed wellness juices. Natural skin/body/oral care. Plant-based E-guides, consultations & more.

A Healthy Crush

Owner: Carl "Crush" Foster (CFO, Executive Chef)

https://ahealthycrush.com/

This business focuses on providing an Alkaline-Electric lifestyle through the use of herbs, cookbooks, workshops, and cooking classes.

African Bio Mineral Cell Food

Owner: Victor Bowman (Dr. Sebi Son)

547 Central Ave (Suite 547), Newark, New Jersey, 07107

www.africanbiomineralcellfood.com

Elevate your health with our premium alkaline foods and herbs.

Alkaline Healing Herbs

Owner: Coralee Montes

4659 North Elston Avenue, Chicago, IL, 60630

www.alkalinehealingherbs.com

This company provides alkaline herbs, capsules, detox packages, personal care products, Seamoss, alkaline juices and teas, and an alkaline mini-mart.

Alkaline Jungle

Owner: Rambo M. Singz

Adept Herbalist, Detox Specialist, Healer, Metaphysician, Nutritionist.

https://alkalinejungle.com/

Provides a variety of packages and products created to heal the body. Detoxes, cleanses, seamoss, diet planning, and health coaching.

Bolingo Balance

Owner: Victor Bowman (Dr. Sebi Son)

https://bolingobalance.com/

Carbonbased Cell Food

5324 Clemons Road, East Rindge, TN, 37412

www.carbonbasedcellfood.com

This business provides detox herbal teas and cleanses, loose herbs, dried sea moss, sea moss gel, herbal capsules, hair oil, and recipe e-books.

Chakra Herbs LLC

Owner: Michael Daily

www.chakraherbs.us

This business provides natural herbs and guidance services to help people transition to a plant-based lifestyle.

Devine Health and Wellness Products LLC

Owners name: Anthony Devine

Address: 1780 Hines Street, Salem, Oregon. Republic 97302

Devine Health and Wellness Products is a company created by Anthony Devine after a friend was diagnosed with stage 4 cervical and ovarian cancer, after the friend drank the juice for 2 years her Cancer went into remission, Anthony then created the Juice, the Alkaline Drops with Trace Minerals, Devine Living Water and " remember good health is true wealth."

Facebook: Metatron's pH Alkaline Drops and Arubah Juice page, Contact : Anthony Devine or Tony @ 971 -283-3741

Evergreen Herbs Inc.

Owner: Marco Mayano Sr.

www.egherbs.com

This business provides bulk herbs that are free from pesticides and herbicides, grown and picked in private fields in Mexico.

262-889-4856

Farmacy For Life

Owner: Adjua Styles and Styles P

"Hip Hop's First Health Store"

https://farmacyforlife.com/

We are dedicated to revolutionizing your health with natural supplements of the highest quality, so that's why our products are non-GMO, organic, vegan, and GMP certified, ensuring that you receive only the best nature has to offer. Our commitment to excellence and purity means you can trust our supplements to support your health journey safely and effectively.

Flourished Lifestyles

Owner: Shanice Martinez

https://www.flourished-lifestyles.com

This business provides all-natural herbal skin care, detox kits, Seamoss and Irish moss.

KBs Creations Inc. (Earthly Treasures Divine)

Owner: Lakisha Buggs

Earthlytreasuresdivine.com

This business provides herbal extracts and capsules. Soon to be offering reiki services, and also have children's books to be released soon.

Monique's Temple

Owner: Trina Esparza

www.moniquestemple.net

This business provides: herbal teas, sea moss, reiki healing, and yoni steaming.

Moore Life and Health

www.moorelifeandhealth.com

Facebook and Instagram: @moorelifeandhealthllc

This business sells homemade vegan soap, herbal tinctures, herbal teas, colon cleanses, sea moss gel, sea moss capsules, etc.

Mothernature.com

This website sells herbal products

Nature's Herbs

47444 Kato Road, Fremont, CA, 94538

This company specializes in medicinal herbs. You can write to this company for a free catalog.

Plants4Medicine

Owner: Samantha Miller

https://plants4medicine.bigcartel.com

Facebook: Plants4Medicine

This business provides holistic herbal remedies, herbal infused shea butters, herbal teas, capsules, sea moss, elderberry syrup, tinctures etc. They also help assist your body in healing naturally.

Rah Healing Inner-G

Seamoss, Herbs, and Sound Healing.

rahhealing.com

A man living in his purpose, a King driven by his vision.

Root'd In Nature by K&C, LLC

Owners: Kekilia Greene and Cilicia Green

https://rootdinnature.com/

Provides wild harvested sea moss, sea moss gel, herbal infused elderberry syrup, hair growth oil, and stress relief tea blends.

Sea Moss Emporium

Owners: Trevor and Shamarian Allen

Mansfield, TX

www.seamossemporium.com

Instagram: www.instagram.com/seamoss.emporium

Facebook: https://www.facebook.com/profile.php?id=100077750073053

Provides wildcrafted sea moss and Irish moss (Chondrus crispus). Items are sold raw, gel, capsule, and in soap form. This business also sells loose leaf healing herbs, cleanses, capsules, syrups.

Sea Moss Tingz

Owner: Danie Paul

Boston, MA

Linktr.ee/SeaMossTingz

This business provides sea moss, herbs, syrups, and body/hair products.

So Ionic Botanicals

Owner: KT The Arch Degree (CEO and Ethnobotanist)

https://www.soionicbotanicals.com/

A proud, family owned and operated business providing preventative herbal solutions.

Tesha Alkaline Watkins

Minneapolis, MN

www.balancemelanin.com

Facebook, Instagram, and Tiktok – Tesha Alkaline Watkins

Her services include: Doula, Herbalist, Plant-based Chef, and Personal Trainer.

The Goddess Collection

Owner: Krystal Alkaline Doula

www.thealkalinegoddess.com

(Celebrating over 1 Million pregnancies and counting!)

2420 Dawson Street, Kenner , LA

Monday - Saturday 9 am - 5 pm CST

Sundays 10am - 3pm

Phone: 504-287-4515

Availability: 10am - 3:30 pm CST

The Goddess Collection provides herbal tea nourishment and divine body collection products serving to helps those with fertility, acne, allergies, eczema, menopause, tooth hygiene and care, congestion, menstrual cramps, fibroids, body butters, organic diapers and pull-ups, crystals, energy healing, beauty products, holistic doula services, and much more!

The Joéful Alchemist

Owner: Arianna Joélle

https://the-joeful-alchemist.square.site/

This business provides Vegan chef, health consultations, alkaline e-cook books, alkaline herbal remedies, seamoss body Butta, etc.

Unbound Abundance / Unbound Wellness

Owner's: Drëka Rochelle F.

www.UnboundAbundance.com

Unbound Wellness offers products and services that merge both ancient ancestral practices with original modern influence.

Our offerings include but are not limited to:

Holistic Skin/Body Care products, herbal remedies, mindfulness tools, and wellness/life coaching.

Vitals by Vida

Owner: Davida Berry

www.vitalsbyvida.com

Facebook.com/vitalsbyvida

Instagram.com/vitalsbyvida

This business makes herbal remedies for chronic and acute illnesses.

Vitanica

PO Box 1285

Sherwood, OR, 97140

www.vitanica.com

This company provides herbal supplements for women that are created by Tori Hudson, N.D., author of The Women's Encyclopedia of Natural Medicine.

Zand Herbal Formulas

1441 West Smith Road, Ferndale, WA, 98248

www.zand.com

This company offers a variety of herbal formulas, herbal extracts, standardized extracts, and sugar-free herbal lozenges.

Homeopathy

Homeopathic Educational Services

2124 Kittredge Street, Berkeley, CA, 94704

Write a letter in a self-addressed envelope to this organization for homeopathy-related products such as software, cassettes, videos, and remedies.

Hydrotherapy

Bodywork Emporium

414 Broadway Santa Monica, CA, 90401

www.bodywork-emporium.com

This company provides books on alternative modalities, including hydrotherapy, on their website. You can request a free catalog through the mail also.

Magnet Therapy

Magnetic Ideas

125 Industrial Park Drive, Sevierville, TN, 37862

www.magneticideas.com

This company offers a variety of therapeutic magnets on their website.

Theramagnets

48 Skyline Drive, Coram, NY, 11727

www.theramagnets.com

This company offers a variety of therapeutic magnets on their website.

Massage Therapy

The International Massage Association

25 South Fourth Street, PO Box 421, Warrenton, VA, 20188

This organization sells a variety of accessories and books related to massage.

SelfCare Catalog

2000 Powell Street, Suite 1350, Emeryville, CA, 94608

This company offers massage and self-massage items. For a catalog, write to the address above.

V.I.E.W. Video

34 East 23rd Street, New York, NY, 10010

For an introduction to Swedish and shiatsu massage techniques, you can order, "Massage Your Mate" a 92-minute, color

Music Therapy and Sound Healing

Inner Peace Music

PO Box 2644

San Anselmo, CA, 94979-2644

www.innerpeacemusic.com

This company provides tapes by Steven Halpern for relaxation and enjoyment. they also provide tapes for better performance, deeper sleep, safer driving, increased creativity, and other self-help areas.

Sound Healers Association

PO Box 2240

Boulder, CO, 80306

www.healingsounds.com

This company provides a variety of information on audiotapes and also sell tuning forks.

Naturopathic Medicine

The American Association of Naturopathic Physicians

8201 Greensboro Drive, Suite 300, McLean, VA, 22102

www.naturopathic.org

This organization maintains a title index of recommended books and software.

Qigong

National Qigong (Chi Kung) Association USA

PO Box 540

Ely, MN, 55731

www.nqa.org

This organization provides a free resource list of recommended books and videos on qigong.

Qi Journal Catalog

Insight Publishing

PO Box 18476

Anaheim Hills, CA, 92817

www.qi-journal.com

This catalog contains a variety of qigong and alternative medicine products.

Wayfarer Publications

PO Box 39938

Los Angeles, CA, 90039

This company sells videos on qigong and martial arts.

Reflexology

American Academy of Reflexology

606 East Magnolia Boulevard, Suite B, Burbank, CA, 91501-2618

This organization offers educational materials and courses on foot, hand, and ear reflexology.

International Academy of Advanced Reflexology and Advanced Reflexology Complementary Health Center

2542 Easton Avenue, PO Box 1489, Bethlehem, PA, 18016

www.reflexology.net

This organization offers videos and charts for sale on their website and by mail.

Reiki

Anna Makoci

The Bridge of Alchemy

Reiki Master & Spiritual Advisor

35 Congress St., Salem MA, 01970

978.907.0664

https://www.facebook.com/profile.
php?id=100095397160599&mibextid=LQQJ4d

Sarah O'Shea

Reki Master

@sosheaa

Email: oshea.sarahe@gmail.com

Spiritual Dictionary

Owner: Sharon Olivier

www.spiritualdictionary.com

KwaZulu-Natal, South Africa

Provides Spiritual healing, reiki, reflexology, access bars, somatic massage, meditation, and luxurious therapeutic bath lavas.

Taina Javier

Reiki Master

@whoelsebuttaina – for Reiki services

@iseeyoucandles – for non-toxic coconut wax, reiki infused candles

Traditional Chinese Medicine

Blue Poppy Press

5441 Western Avenue, #1, Boulder, CO, 80301

www.bluepoppy.com

This company publishes a number of items on Traditional Chinese Medicine. You can visit their website or write to their address. Their website contains free articles to download and has an online book catalog.

Redwing Book Company

44 Linden Street, Brookline, MA, 02445

www.redwingbooks.com

This company publishes books on alternative medicine, including Traditional Chinese Medicine.

Visualization

The Imagery Store at the Academy for Guided Imagery

PO Box 2070

Mill Valley, CA, 94942

This company offers visualization tapes for specific health and behavior problems including, "Mind-Controlled Anesthesia for Systemic Pain", "Restful Sleep", "Chest Pain, Anxiety, and Heartbreak", and "Forgiveness in Healing."

Yoga Therapy

International Association of Yoga Therapists

2400A County Center Drive, Santa Rosa, CA, 95403

www.yrec.org

Send a stamped, self-addressed envelope to this organization for a flyer on product resources.

Yoga Accessories

PO Box 13976

New Bern, NC, 28561

www.yogaaccessories.com

This company offers yoga mats and straps for sale.

Yoga Zone

3342 Melrose Avenue, Roanoke, VA, 24017

www.yogazone.com

This company offers a wide variety of yoga products.

Referrals and Contacts

Practitioners

Alternative Medicine Dictionary

www.altmedicine.net

This web site maintains an international database of practitioners in a variety of areas.

American College for Advancement in Medicine

23121 Verdugo Drive, Suite 204, Laguna Hills, CA, 9263

www.acam.org

For a state-by-state directory of physicians. Additional information is available on their website free of charge.

American Holistic Medical Association

6728 McLean Village Drive, McLean, VA, 22101

www.holisticmedicine.org

This organization represents M.D.'s and D.O.'s who combine mainstream medicine with complimentary therapies. They publish the National Referral of Holistic Practitioners, which is available by mail. Referrals are also listed on their website.

EarthMed.com

2009 Renaissance Boulevard, Suite 100

King of Prussia, PA, 19406

www.earthmed.com

This site maintains a directory of more than 100,000 natural medicine practitioners nationwide. Referrals are also provided by mail.

Health World Online

Professional Referral network

www.healthreferral.com

This site provides a compilation of referral databases from member lists to participating associations. Contains referral information for practitioners of: acupuncture, oriental medicine, flower remedies, guided imagery, homeopathy, naturopathic medicine, and vision training.

Healthy Alternatives

www.health-alt.com

This site provides referral information for practitioners of: aromatherapy, herbal medicine, homeopathy, massage therapy, naturopathy, reflexology, and yoga.

Acupressure

Acupressure Institute

133, Shattuck Avenue, Berkeley, CA, 94709

www.acupressure.com

Referrals are available only for the northern California area. National referrals may be available in the future.

Jin Shin Do Foundation for Bodymind Acupressure

PO Box 416

Idyllwild, CA, 925549

www.jinshindo.org

this organization provides referrals to authorized teachers.

Aromatherapy

National Association for Holistic Aromatherapy

409 Interlake Avenue North, #233, Seattle, WA, 98103

www.naha.org

While there are no standardized certifications or registration of aromatherapy in the USA, you can check with this organization to see if the practitioner is registered with them.

Breath Therapy

The International Breath Institute

921 East Miramar Drive, Tucson, AZ, 85715

www.transformbreathing.com

This organization provides free referrals to breath facilitators who have graduated from their institute.

Energy Healing

American Polarity Therapy Association

PO Box 19858

Boulder, CO, 80308

www.polaritytherapy.org

This organization accepts requests by mail or on their website. Information is sent out by mail.

Barbara Brennan School of Healing

00 Spanish River Boulevard, Suite 103, boca Raton, FL, 33481-459

www.barbarabrennan.com

This school provides referrals to energy healers who have trained there.

International Association for Reiki Professionals

PO Box 104, Harrisville, NH, 03450

www.iarp.org

To locate a free referral to a Reiki practitioner in your area, visit their website or write a letter to the address listed above.

Quantum-Touch

PO Box 82

Santa Cruz, CA, 9061

www.quantumtouch.com

This organization offers nationwide referrals to practitioners of Quantum-Touch.

Flower Essences

Dr. Edward Bach Centre

Mount Vernon, Bakers Lane, Softwell, OX10 0PZ, United Kingdom

www.bachcentre.com

This organization provides an extensive list of international listings of flower remedy therapists.

Flower Essence Society

PO Box 49

Nevada City, CA, 95959

www.flowersociety.org

This organization maintains a registry of practitioners who use flower essences and will provide names of experts in your area.

Herbal Medicine

American Herbalists Guild

1931 Gaddis Road, Canton, GA, 30115

www.americanherbalistsguild.com

This organization provides referral information to certified herbalists.

Homeopathy

The American Board of Homeotherapeutics

801 North Fairfax Street, Suite 306, Alexandria, VA, 22314

For the board directory of the American Board of Homeotherapeutics, send $10.00 to the address above in a self-addressed envelope with letter of inquiry.

The Homeopathic Academy of Naturopathic Physicians

12132 Southeast Foster Place, Portland, OR, 97266

www.healthy.net/pan/pa/homeopathic/hanp

This organization certifies naturopathic homeopaths and makes referrals by mail and on their website.

The National Center for Homeopathy

801 North Fairfax Street, Suite 306, Alexandria, VA, 22314

www.homeopathic.org

This organization provides referrals by mail and on their website.

The North American Society of Homeopaths

1122 East Pike Street, Suite 1122, Seattle, WA, 98122

www.homeopathy.org

This organization provides referrals by mail and on their website.

Hydrotherapy

Note: Naturopathic doctors are the only licensed health care providers who are trained to use hydrotherapy. Review resources listed in "Naturopathic Medicine" later in this section of the book.

Oral Medicine

International Academy of Oral Medicine and Toxicology

PO Box 608531

Orlando, FL, 32860-8531

www.iaomt.org

This organization provides nationwide referrals via mail or on their website to dentists who use alternative methods.

Massage Therapy

American Massage Therapy Association

820 Davis Street, Suite 100, Evanston, IL, 60201-4444

www.americanmassage.org

This association's locator service provides referrals to certified massage therapists nationwide.

Associated Bodywork and Massage Professionals

1271 Sugarbush Drive, Evergreen, CO, 80439-9766

www.abmp.com

This organization provides a complete list of its members by mail and on their website.

The International Massage Association

25 South Fourth Street, PO Box 421, Warrenton, VA, 20188

This organization provides referrals to massage therapists nationwide. You can write them a letter inquiring a complete list.

National Certification Board for Therapeutic Massage and Bodywork

8201 Greensboro Drive, Suite 300, McLean, VA, 22102

www.ncbtmb.com

This organization provides referrals to certified massage therapists nationwide.

Movement Education

Alexander Technique International

1692 Massachusetts Avenue, 3rd Floor, Cambridge, MA, 02138

www.ati-net.com

This organization provides referrals by mail and on their website.

The Aston Training Center

PO Box 3568

Incline Village, NV, 89450

www.aston-patterning.com

This organization provides referrals by mail and on their website.

Feldenkrais Guild of North America

3611 Southwest Hood Avenue, Suite 100, Portland, OR, 97201

www.feldenkrais.com

This organization provides referrals by mail and on their website.

Hellerwork International

3435 M Street, Eureka, CA, 95503

www.hellerwork.com

This organization provides referrals by mail and on their website.

Music Therapy and Sound Healing

American Music Therapy Association

8455 Colesville Road, Suite 1000, Silver Spring, MD, 20910

www.musictherapy.org

This organization can recommend professionals in your area who use this technique.

Naturopathic Medicine

The American Association of Naturopathic Physicians

8201 Greensboro Drive, Suite 300, McLean, VA, 22102

www.naturopathhic.org

This organization has a database on their website locating N.D.'s (Naturopathic Doctors) in your area.

The Canadian Association

1255 Sheppard Avenue East (at Leslie), North York, Ontario, M2K 1E2, Canada

www.naturopathicassoc.ca

This organization makes referrals to N.D.'s in Canada.

The Council on Naturopathic Medical Education

PO Box 11426

Eugene, OR, 97440-3626

www.cnme.org

This is the only accrediting agency that has been recognized by the government's Department of Education.

The Homeopathic Academy of Naturopathic Physicians

12132 Southeast Foster Place, Portland, OR, 97266

www.healthy.net/pan/pa/homeopathic/hanp

This organization certifies naturopaths and makes referrals by mail or on their website.

Qigong

National Qigong (Chi Kung) Association USA

PO Box 540

Ely, MN, 55731

www.nqa.org

This organization provides a free listing of instructors by mail or on their website.

Reflexology

American Academy of Reflexology

606 East Magnolia Boulevard, Suite B, Burbank, CA, 91501-2618

This organization provides referrals to practitioners trained by the academy.

American Reflexology Certification Board

PO Box 740879

Arvada, CO, 80006-0879

Write a brief letter to this organization for a list of certified reflexologists.

International Institute of Reflexology Inc.

5650 First Avenue North

PO Box 12642

St. Petersburg, FL, 33733-2642

This organization provides free referrals by mail.

Reflexology Association of America

4012 Rainbow, Suite K-PMB #585, Las Vegas, NV, 89103-2059

www.reflexology-usa.org

This organization provides nationwide referrals via mail or on their website.

Traditional Chinese Medicine

The American Association of Oriental Medicine

433 Front Street, Catasauqua, PA, 18032

www.aaom.org

This organization provides referrals by mail or on their website.

The National Acupuncture and Oriental Medicine Alliance

14637 Starr Road, SE, Olalla, WA, 9839

www.acuall.org

This organization provides nationwide referrals via mail or on their website.

The National Certification Commission for Acupuncture and Oriental Medicine

11 Canal Center Plaza, Suite 300, Alexandria, VA, 22314

www.nccaom.org

This organization provides nationwide referrals via mail or on their website. There is a small fee for referrals sent by mail.

Visualization

The Academy for Guided Imagery

PO Box 2070

Mill Valley, CA, 94942

www.interactiveimagery.com

This organization provides nationwide referrals via mail or on their website.

The American Society of Clinical Hypnosis

130 East Elm Court, Suite 201, Roselle, IL, 60172-2000

This organization provides nationwide referrals via mail. Send a self-addressed envelope to the address above.

The Society for Clinical and Experimental Hypnosis

PO Box 642114

Pullman, WA, 99164-2114

The organization can refer you to member hypnotherapists around the USA. Send a stamped, self-addressed envelope to the address above.

Yoga Therapy

International Associates of Yoga Therapists

2400A County Center Drive, Santa Rosa, CA, 95403

www.yrec.org

This organization provides nationwide referrals via mail or on their website.

Other Books By Author:

- *Fasting: A Guide To Health And Wellness*
- *An Alkaline Alphabet: Learning The Alphabet With Alkaline Foods*
- *An Alkaline Alphabet: Coloring Your Way Through The Alphabet*
- *Creating Your Own Growing Space: A Step-By-Step Guide Towards Creating A Community Garden and Introduction To Land Ownership*
- *A 21 Day Liquid Fast: A Homemade Alkaline Approach Towards Cleansing The Body and Discovering A New Level Of Health*
- *Healthy Baby Vol. 1: Plant-Based Recipes For Your Growing Baby*
- *Learning To H.E.A.L.: Healthy Eating and Active Lifestyle*
- *Healing Herbs For The Human Body Systems: An Introduction to Human Physiology and Herbal Applications*
- *Guided Meditations and Reflections (Book 1): Finding Stillness*
- *Guided Meditations and Reflections (Book 2): Love Energy*
- *Guided Meditations and Reflections (Book 3): The Zen Mind*

Follow Bryan McAskill On Social Media!

Instagram: **@bryan_mcaskill**

https://instagram.com/bryan_mcaskill?utm

@herbal.healing781

https://instagram.com/herbal.healing781?utm

Facebook:

Herbal Healing by Bryan McAskill

https://www.facebook.com/herbal.healing781/

Website:

www.herbalhealingshop.org

Made in the USA
Middletown, DE
09 September 2024

60045271R00459